W9-CLJ-698

Second Edition

KOZIER - Du GAS'

INTRODUCTION TO PATIENT CARE

a comprehensive approach to nursing

BEVERLY WITTER Du GAS

R.N., B.A. (University of British Columbia)
M.N. (University of Washington)
Ed.D. (University of British Columbia)
LL.D. (Hon.) (University of Windsor)

Nursing Consultant, Department of National Health
and Welfare, Ottawa. Formerly, Nurse Educator,
World Health Organization, University Nursing
Education Project, India (Chandigarh);
Associate Director of Nursing (Education),
The Vancouver General Hospital School of Nursing,
Vancouver, British Columbia.

W. B. SAUNDERS COMPANY/PHILADELPHIA/LONDON/TORONTO

W. B. Saunders Company: West Washington Square
                         Philadelphia, Pa.   19105

                         12 Dyott Street
                         London, WC1A   1DB

                         833 Oxford Street
                         Toronto 18, Ontario

Introduction to Patient Care   ISBN 0-7216-3225-4

Print No.:   9   8   7   6   5   4

PREFACE

This book, which in its first edition was entitled Fundamentals of Patient Care, is intended as an introductory text for nursing students. In preparing the second edition of the text, detailed critiques of the first edition were obtained from several nurse educators in the United States and Canada. In response to their comments, a number of changes have been made in both the content and the organization of material. Particular emphasis has been placed in this edition on helping the student to develop independent judgment in assessing the nursing needs of patients, in selecting and carrying out appropriate nursing measures to meet these needs, and in evaluating the effectiveness of her actions.

The first section of the book (Chapters 1 through 5) has been revised to provide the beginning student with an orientation to the role of nursing in a health care system that is rapidly changing from one which is predominantly hospital- and "cure"-centered to one stressing health maintenance and the prevention of illness. The "health-illness" concept is discussed, and increased emphasis has been placed on the meaning of illness and its effects on the individual and his family.

A new chapter on the nursing process has been included at the beginning of the second section of the book. This section (Chapters 6 through 17) deals with meeting the basic needs of people with health problems. The former chapter on needs of the patient for communication has been deleted because this topic is now covered by most schools in separate courses on communication skills. In its place, a chapter on the needs of the patient for relief from anxiety has been incorporated, because this is such a universal problem of people who are ill.

The third section of the book, commencing with a chapter on the legal implications of nursing practice, introduces the student to her role in diagnostic and therapeutic care. The chapter on legal aspects has been expanded to include a number of topics requested by many nursing students and their teachers, such as the expanding role of the nurse, the nurse's responsibility in regard to wills, and "Good Samaritan" laws.

Common health problems are discussed in the final set of chapters (Chapters 22 through 30). In this section, although the chapter headings remain essentially the same, the content has been reorganized and expanded to assist the student in following through logically the steps of the nursing process in the care of people with such problems as fever, pain, dyspnea and the like.

Each chapter, with the exception of the Introduction, begins with a set of objectives for the student's use in evaluating her own progress in learning. Guides for assessing the nursing needs of patients and for evaluating the effectiveness of nursing action are included at the end of each chapter wherever these are applicable to the content. In addition, a study vocabulary, study situation and bibliography may be found at the end of each chapter.

Beverly Witter Du Gas

ACKNOWLEDGMENTS

The author would like to acknowledge with gratitude the assistance of the many people who contributed to the preparation of this second edition of the textbook. I am especially grateful to the Department of National Health and Welfare for enabling me to make this revision a priority item on my work schedule. The encouragement of Mrs. Verna Splane, Principal Nursing Officer of the Department, and the cooperation and support of Dr. William Hacon and the staff of the Health Manpower Directorate have been deeply appreciated.

I would also like to thank my many colleagues in the Department who contributed time and energy to assisting me with various aspects of the preparation of the text, in particular, Mrs. Marjorie Todd, Dr. Edgar Monagle, Mrs. Elizabeth McCue, Dr. George Evans and Miss Roberta Sametz. Mrs. Louise Segouin and Mrs. Filomena Lucio deserve special thanks for their valuable assistance in the preparation of the manuscript.

I am also very grateful to Miss Barbara Gillies, Senior Instructor and Clinical Coordinator of The Vancouver General Hospital School of Nursing, for reviewing the manuscript and making suggestions for its improvement; to Mrs. Huguette Labelle, Director of the Vanier School of Nursing (Ottawa) and Mrs. Wanda Stratton, Inservice Coordinator, the Riverside Hospital of Ottawa, for making arrangements for and assisting with the taking of pictures for the current edition; and to Miss Jean Leask, Director of Nursing, The Victorian Order of Nurses of Canada, for making available photographs and manuals belonging to the association.

Last, but by no means least, I wish to thank my daughter, Barbara Du Gas, for her assistance, encouragement and critical comments throughout the many months it took to compile this revision.

CONTENTS

26 THE CARE OF PATIENTS WHO HAVE ANOREXIA, NAUSEA
    OR VOMITING 362

27 THE CARE OF PATIENTS WHO HAVE URINARY PROBLEMS 378

KOZIER – Du GAS'

INTRODUCTION TO PATIENT CARE

a comprehensive approach to nursing

1 INTRODUCTION

Nursing is a service profession. The International Code of Nursing Ethics states that "Nurses render health service to the individual, the family and the community. . . . Service to mankind is the primary function of nurses and the reason for the existence of the nursing profession."[1]

In rendering health service, the nurse assists individuals, families and communities in the maintenance of health and the prevention of disease; she ministers to the needs of the sick, helping them to the fullest restoration of health compatible with their illness, or providing comfort and support in the event of incurable disease.[2]

In so doing, the nurse works in close coordination with the members of a growing number of allied health disciplines to provide health services for the people of our country. The provision of these services has become a very large and important part of the nation's business. Today we accept the principle that health is a fundamental right of every citizen, and we believe that access to adequate health services should be guaranteed to all, regardless of race, creed, color or financial status.

One of the major concerns in North America at the present time is to see that the services required to maintain health, to prevent disease and to treat illness, as well as the rehabilitative services needed to restore the sick to an active, functioning role in society, are made available to all persons in our country.

The importance attached to this concern is evidenced by the increasingly large portion of the national budget which is spent annually on health care, and by the rapidly growing numbers of people engaged in providing health care services. In 1960, the amount of money allocated for health services in the Federal Budget of the United States was 3.5 billion dollars; by 1970 this figure had reached 18.8 billion dollars, and the 1971 estimates of Federal spending on health were 20.6 billion dollars, or 10.5 per cent of Federal outlays for all purposes.[3] In the 1971 budget, expenditures on health ranked third on the list of Federal outlays, behind only those allocated for national defense and for income security. In Canada there has been a comparable escalation in the amount of Federal

---

[1]From the *International Code of Nursing Ethics.* Adopted by the International Congress of Nurses, São Paulo, Brazil, 1953.

[2]Ibid. Adapted from the preamble.

[3]Irving J. Lewis: Federal Health Programs – An Inventory. Paper delivered at the Fourth National Congress on the Socio-Economics of Health Care, Chicago, March 20–21, 1970.

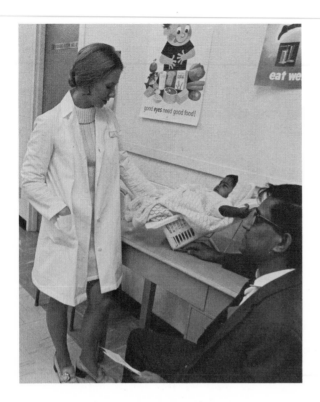

Young children need a considerable amount of health supervision to promote optimum growth and development. Here, Father brings the baby in to the clinic for the nurse to check.

Government monies allocated for health care services.[4]

The increased expenditure on health care has been accompanied by a marked increase in the number of people who provide health care services. Reports indicate that the number of people employed in the health field has been increasing at more than twice the rate of the number of employed persons in the total economy.[5] It has been said that the "health care industry" in the United States now encompasses a combined manpower force larger than that of any other industry. In 1970, it was estimated that over 3 million people in the United States were engaged in occupations directly related to health care, and that by 1975 an additional 1.2 million people will be required.[6] In Canada, in 1970, there were over 350,000 people engaged in health occupations. By 1975 it is expected that this number will have reached 450,000.[7]

---

[4]It is difficult to compare Canadian figures with those of the United States because of the differences in responsibility for health expenditures of the two Federal Governments. The United States budgetary figures for health care expenditures include health resources, medical services and prevention and control of health problems. The Canadian budgetary figures for Federal spending on health include hospital care, general health, public health, medical, dental and allied services. The amount of monies allocated in the Federal Government budget in Canada for health services increased from 3.6 per cent in 1960 to 6.1 per cent in 1970. (*Federal Government Finance, Revenue and Expenditure and Indirect Debt.* Table 2. Dominion Bureau of Statistics Catalogue No. 68211. Ottawa, Canada.)

[5]Eli Ginzberg: Foreword in *Allied Health Manpower: Trends and Prospects* by Harry I. Greenfield. New York, Columbia University Press, 1969. p. vii.

[6]Resolutions. *American Journal of Public Health,* 60:178, January, 1970.

[7]Health Manpower Planning Division, Department of National Health and Welfare, Ottawa, Canada.

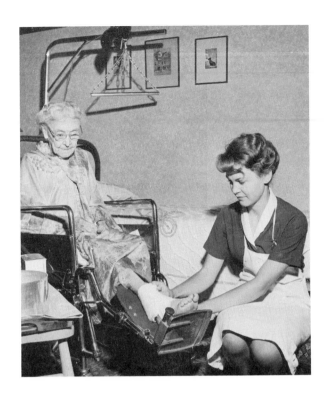

Older people too have increased health needs. The visiting nurse performs a valuable function in helping families to care for older people in their homes.

INCREASED DEMAND FOR HEALTH SERVICES

The fundamental reason for the increased expenditures on health care and the expansion in numbers of health workers has been believed to be an increased demand for health services. The *Manpower Report of the President* in 1970 suggested that several powerful forces have contributed to this increased demand. These forces include: large population growth, increasing public awareness of the value of health care, the expansion of health care insurance and the provision of health care services for low income groups, government subsidies for hospital construction, and enlargement of the scope of medical services through research and technological progress.[8]

One of the most powerful forces contributing to the increased demand for health services has been the rapid rate of growth of our population. Both the

United States and Canada have experienced tremendous population increases, particularly since the end of World War II. The greatest growth has been at both ends of the age spectrum. We have proportionately more older people than we did a generation ago, and also more children and adolescents. Both the older and the younger age groups require more health services than do the remainder of the population. Young children, for example, need a considerable amount of health supervision to promote optimum growth and development and to prevent illness, in addition to the curative and restorative services needed when they are sick. Much of the preventive and health maintenance care is provided by physicians, nurses and other health workers in child care clinics across the nation. In many parts of the country, specially prepared nurses are assuming increasing responsibility for supervising the health care of infants and children.

Older people too have increased health needs. Because of the longer life span, more people in our society today suffer from chronic and degenerative

[8] *Manpower Report of the President.* Prepared by the United States Department of Labor and transmitted to the Congress, March, 1970, p. 174.

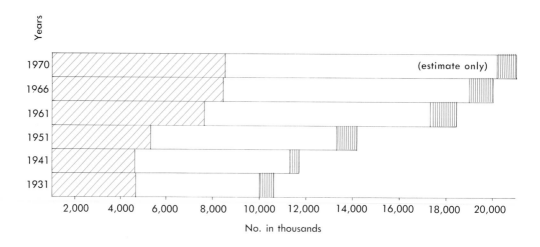

Below 19 yr.

20-69 yr.

70 yr. and over

Years

1970   (estimate only)
1966
1961
1951
1941
1931

2,000 4,000 6,000 8,000 10,000 12,000 14,000 16,000 18,000 20,000

No. in thousands

Number of people in different age groups for selected years in the United States.

diseases than in previous generations. The need for home care and other services for older people has put a strain on existing facilities and added to the demand for health personnel. There has been a major expansion in both the numbers and the capacity of nursing homes to care for the sick among our aged population. This has meant additional requirements for trained workers in general and a heightened demand for professional nurses in particular to carry the major responsibility for supervising care in these homes.

Another major factor contributing to the increased demand for health services has been the growing awareness of the value of health care in our society. Health is no longer considered a privilege but rather a right. People have been made aware, through educational programs in the schools and through radio, television, newspapers and the popular magazines, of the importance of periodic health checkups and the value of seeking medical attention promptly in the event of illness.

The country's growing affluence has meant too that more people can afford to spend a larger portion of their income on looking after their health. There are still segments of our population who cannot afford health care, but increasingly, government-sponsored programs are being established to help look after the health needs of the indigent in our society. The expansion of health care insurance programs has increased the use of health care services and concomitantly the need for more health workers. In Canada all provinces now participate in a system of government-sponsored medical and hospital insurance, which covers an estimated 95 per cent of the population. In the United States, there has been a rapid

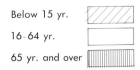

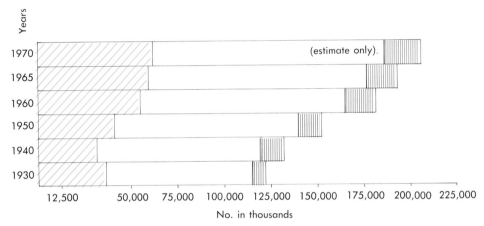

Number of people in different age groups for selected years in Canada.

expansion of private prepaid health insurance plans, and Medicare and Medicaid, two Federal Government programs, have been set up to provide care for persons over 65 and the poor respectively. An increasing number of health services have also been made possible in poverty and ghetto areas by the Economic Opportunity Act in the United States.

Government subsidies for the construction of hospitals, clinics and health centers in both the United States and Canada have also contributed to the rapid growth in demand for health care workers. More doctors, more nurses, more x-ray and laboratory technologists, and a host of other specialized and unspecialized workers are needed to staff the rapidly growing number of hospitals and other health care facilities.

Last, but by no means least, on the list of factors contributing to the increased demand for health services is the explosion of scientific knowledge that has characterized the latter half of the twentieth century. It has been said that the total amount of new information stemming from research in the biomedical sciences in the past 25 years has more than doubled the total amount of knowledge in the field. Rapid advances in medical science have made possible surgery and medical treatment that could not have been contemplated 20 years ago. More complicated surgery, the development of complex machines for the diagnosis and care and treatment of disease, and radical changes in therapy have intensified the need for people with highly specialized skills in the health care field. An ever increasing number of workers are engaged in research to promote still better methods of preventing and treating disease and newer and better ways of delivering health care services.

SHORTAGE OF HEALTH PERSONNEL

As one would expect from the increasing demand for health services, there is everywhere a shortage of highly skilled workers for the health field. In 1970, the Congressional Record indicated that in the United States there was an estimated shortage of 48,000 physicians, 17,800 dentists, 150,000 nurses and 266,000 other allied health personnel. By 1980, it is predicted that the shortage of nurses will have increased to over 200,000.[9]

The increased demand for health services has focused attention on the need to prepare sufficient workers for the field and on the need to utilize health personnel effectively. Methods of health care delivery are being assessed and analyzed to promote the optimum use of the specialized skills of each worker.

Because of the shortage of highly skilled professionals, there has been an increasing delegation of duties and functions to other categories of workers. Nurses are being asked to assume many functions that were previously considered medical practice. In remote and isolated areas, where the shortage of physicians is particularly acute, the nurse may, in many instances, be the only source of medical help in a community. Nurses, in turn, have delegated many routine tasks to licensed practical nurses or to technicians. Nurses are being relieved of many of the non-nursing duties they used to do, such as housekeeping and clerical work. An increasing number of supportive personnel are being utilized to ensure the most effective use of professional workers.

THE ALLIED HEALTH DISCIPLINES

The number of types of worker in the health care field has increased almost as rapidly as has the total number of persons in the field. The shortage of professional workers and the need for people with highly specialized skills have been two major factors contributing to this trend. The term "allied health disciplines" is now used to encompass the large and rapidly growing family of occupational groups who are involved in providing health care services. Over 300 health occupations have been identified in which people have education and training designed specifically to prepare them for work in the health care field.[10] The amount of education and training varies from a few weeks of on-the-job training, as for example, for a nursing orderly, to more than 10 years of post–high school preparation for a specialist physician.

In addition to the traditional health professions of medicine, nursing, dentistry and pharmacy, a cadre of highly specialized workers has developed. Many of these people provide direct care services to patients which are extensions of medical and nursing care, as for example, the physical therapists (physiotherapists) and occupational therapists. Some are technologists whose occupation has evolved because of the need for people with specific skills in handling the complex machinery used in the care of patients, such as the inhalation therapists and the renal dialysis (artificial kidney) technicians. Several of the newer groups have emerged as a result of the delegation of certain functions by the major professionals. These include the "physician's assistant" group, the licensed practical or vocational nurses (or nursing assistants), dental hygienists, dental assistants and pharmacy assistants.

It would be a lengthy task even to list all the occupational groups that are a part of today's health team. The nurse in her day-to-day work will have contact

---

[9]Latest government statistics, furnished to Congress by the National Institutes of Health's Health Manpower Bureau, as reported in *American Medical News*, 13:6, August 3, 1970.

[10]U.S. Department of Health, Education and Welfare: *Health Resources Statistics 1965*. A report prepared by the National Center for Health Statistics. Public Health Service Publication No. 1509. Washington, D.C., U.S. Government Printing Office, 1966, p. 1.

Number of Active Professional Nurses and Nurse Population Ratio
U.S. and Canada Selected Years

	U.S.A.*			CANADA†	
Year	No. of Active Professional Nurses	Nurses/ 100,000 Population	Year	No. of Active Professional Nurses	Nurses/ 100,000 Population
1930	214,292	175	1931	20,474	197
1940	284,159	216	1941	27,142	236
1950	374,584	249	1951	35,204	251
1960	525,374	293	1961	61,699	338
1970	700,000‡	341	1970	110,000‡	515

*Figures from U.S. Departments of Health, Education and Welfare, Public Health Service—National Institutes of Health, Bethesda, Maryland. Public Health Service Publications No. 263 (Revised 1969), p. 9, and No. 1534 (Revised 1970).

†Figures from Health Manpower Planning Division, Department of National Health and Welfare, Ottawa, Canada, 1971.

‡Estimate only.

with many. It is important to remember that each has a special role in the care of the patient. The various members of the health team with whom the nurse comes in frequent contact are discussed in Chapter 5.

THE ROLE OF THE NURSE IN HEALTH CARE

Nurses constitute the largest single group of health care workers in both the United States and Canada. In 1969, there were an estimated 680,000 registered nurses resident and employed in the United States and 100,000 in Canada.[11,12] The number of professional nurses has risen sharply in both countries in the past decade, both in absolute numbers and in proportion to the population. Yet in many areas there is still a shortage of nurses.

With the sometimes bewildering array of other workers in the health field today, the beginning student of nursing may well wonder just what it is

that nurses do. Many of the nurse's traditional duties and functions have been delegated to other workers. The nurse has been relieved of most of the housekeeping duties that formerly occupied much of her time. Ward clerks and unit managers have taken over many of the clerical duties and management functions that nurses used to do. Auxiliary nursing personnel often look after a good deal of the patient's personal care and are now doing a number of treatments that were once carried out only by professional nurses.

The scope of the professional nurse's functions as outlined at the beginning of this chapter implies a much broader area of activity than is represented in the traditional image of the nurse as the "ministering angel" who soothed the patient's fevered brow, changed his linen and dressed his wounds. The nurse still performs many of these activities, but today she is a skilled person who carries out a multiplicity of complex functions. She cares for the patient and about the patient. She assists the physician in carrying out a therapeutic regime for the person who is ill. She is an adviser on health matters. She is expected to coordinate the activities of other members of the nursing team and to

[11]*Facts about Nursing.* 1969 edition. New York, American Nurses' Association, 1969, p. 8.

[12]*Countdown 1970.* Ottawa, Canadian Nurses' Association, 1970, p. 10.

work with a variety of people in allied disciplines as a cooperating member of the health team.

The Care Aspects

From its earliest inception nursing has had a nurturing quality, and this quality is best evidenced in the care aspects of the nurse's role. In caring for the patient, the nurse assists him in carrying out those activities which he would normally do for himself. Caring for the patient involves ministering to his needs and wants, providing comfort and support, protecting him from harm and assisting him to regain his independence as rapidly as possible.[13] Much of nursing action is concerned with the daily living of the patient. Helping him to meet his needs for water, for food, for rest and sleep, and helping him to maintain normal body functioning are primary concerns of the nurse in caring for the patient. In providing comfort and support, the nurse is concerned not only with his physical comfort but also with assisting him to cope with his illness and the stress and anxiety that accompany ill health. The nurse protects the patient and sees that his safety is not endangered. In all these activities the nurse works with the patient, helping him to regain his independence as rapidly as possible and as much as he is able within the limitations imposed by his illness.

In caring for the patient the nurse also cares about him. To many patients these are seen as one and the same; that is, the person who cares for him is perceived as the person who cares about him.[14] Nursing care must be adjusted to suit each individual patient's needs, for no two individuals are alike. Carrying out nursing activities with compassion, with emphathetic understanding and with respect for the patient as an individual of worth and dignity are caring about the patient.

In this regard, a statement from the summary report of the National Commission for the Study of Nursing and Nursing Education seems particularly relevant. In discussing trends in health care delivery and the problem of bringing about change while still retaining good practices from old patterns, the report states that, "It may be that nursing, in particular, holds the key to maintenance of humane, individualistic concern for people and their health problems. And this capacity must be zealously enlarged."[15]

The Cure Aspects

Many of the nurse's activities involve assisting the physician to implement a therapeutic plan of care for the patient. The administration of medications prescribed by the physician and the carrying out of tests and treatments delegated by him are examples of some of the curative aspects of nursing. But the curative role of the nurse is much broader than simply carrying out the doctor's orders. The nurse participates as a member of the therapeutic team. Her observations of the patient's condition and her assessment of the need for medical or nursing intervention are important nursing functions which contribute significantly to the development of a plan of care. The nurse's skill in carrying out therapeutic measures, for example, in giving an intramuscular injection or in operating complicated monitoring equipment, is essential. In innumerable instances the physician relies on the nurse's judgment to initiate action when she feels it is needed. For example, many medication orders are written "to be given as needed" (p.r.n.) and the nurse administers these when, in her judgment, the patient requires them. The nurse also participates in

[13] Frances Reiter Kreuter: What Is Good Nursing Care? *Nursing Outlook,* 5:5:302–304, May, 1957.

[14] Ellen D. Davis: Giving a Bath? *The American Journal of Nursing,* 70:11:2366–2367, November, 1970.

[15] National Commission for the Study of Nursing and Nursing Education: Summary Report and Recommendations. *The American Journal of Nursing,* 70:2:279–294, February, 1970.

evaluating the effectiveness of therapeutic measures. The immediacy of the nurse's presence provides her with a unique opportunity to observe the patient's reactions to medical therapy, and her observations are of invaluable assistance to the physician.

In her curative role the nurse also advises the patient on health matters. Her teaching functions are a very important part of nursing care. They may involve such diverse activities as advising new mothers on the care and feeding of babies, teaching hygiene measures to prevent illness, advising a patient about his diet, teaching deep-breathing exercises to patients before surgery to prevent postoperative complications, or helping a patient to cope with the activities of daily living when he has been handicapped by illness.

The nurse is also frequently involved in helping the patient to carry out activities that have been prescribed or in supervising him while he is doing them. For example, the visiting nurse may go into a patient's home to help him carry out exercises to strengthen his abdominal and leg muscles in preparation for learning to walk again. The nurse also helps the patient and his family to plan for his home care or to work through health problems and develop a plan for overcoming them.

The Coordinating Aspects

The delegation of many routine tasks to auxiliary personnel has freed the nurse for more specialized work, but it has also added to her responsibilities for the administration and coordination of the activities of others. The nurse plans and supervises the care given by such auxiliary nursing personnel as the licensed practical nurse, the nursing orderly and the nurse's aide. In addition, she consults with other professional workers regarding the care given to the patient. She consults with the physician about his plan of therapy. She may need to talk with the dietitian about the foods the patient likes that are permissible on his diet; with the physical therapist

about his exercise program; with the social worker and the community agency about plans for his home care. The nurse sees that appointments for the patient's laboratory tests and x-ray examinations are made and kept. If he is in hospital, she makes sure that the housekeeping staff have cleaned his room and that the aide has brought him drinking water. In most health agencies which have inpatient facilities, nursing is the only service which is provided on a 24 hour a day, seven day a week basis. Other workers come and go, usually during the daytime hours and not on weekends. It is the nurse, then, who establishes a plan for the patient's care and serves as the coordinator for all activities concerned with it. In this, she works cooperatively with the patient and his physician, with the patient's family, and with the other members of the health care team.

The multitude of workers who do things for and to the patient, particularly in a hospital, seems never-ending. Some patients have reported that as many as 50 employees were in and out of their room in one day while they were in hospital. It has been said that what the patient needs is an *ombudsman*, that is, someone who can speak on his behalf and can intercede in his interests. This speaking for the patient and interceding on his behalf is an important part of the nurse's coordinating role.

PREPARATION FOR NURSING

Young nursing and medical students today are much concerned about the need to maintain and strengthen the humanitarian aspects of health care. They usually enter their respective professional schools with a sincere desire to help people. In order to provide skilled and competent help, however, it is necessary for them to learn the scientific foundations on which their profession is based and to acquire the

Fields of employment	United States	Canada
Hospitals, Nursing Homes and Related Institutions	68.7%	79.3%
Public Health and School Health	7.1%	6.6%
Nursing Education	4.2%	3.7%
Occupational Health	3.0%	1.7%
Private Duty, Physicians' Office and other fields	17.0%	8.7%

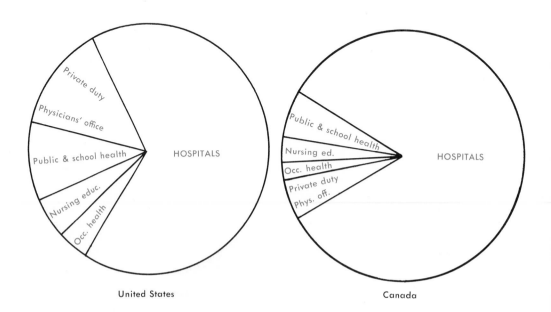

Percentage of registered nurses in various fields of employment in the United States and Canada, 1968. (From Countdown 1969, Canadian Nurses' Association, Research Unit, Ottawa, 1969, p. 15; Facts About Nursing, American Nurses' Association, New York, 1969, p. 11.)

necessary skills to enable them to practice.[16]

The complexity of the nurse's role demands that the nursing student have a firm foundation of knowledge in the biophysical and social sciences. The nurse can no longer depend on traditional or routine nursing techniques. Instead, her skills must be based on a broad background of scientific principles from which she can adjust her nursing care to suit the individual patient's needs and the situation in which these needs must be met. At the present time, the overwhelming majority of nurses are employed in hospitals, and relatively few in the public health field. But there is evidence to indicate that more health care will, in the future, be provided in the community, as for example, in health centers and neighborhood clinics or through hospital-based home care programs. This will mean that considerably more nurses will be required for this field. Indeed, the National Commission for the Study of Nursing and Nursing Education suggested in their report that there may be two distinct career patterns for nurses,

[16]Virginia Henderson: Excellence in Nursing. *The American Journal of Nursing*, 69:9:2133–2137, October, 1969.

with differing preparation for each. In one, the nurse would be primarily concerned with the treatment and rehabilitation of the sick and would work in hospitals or other inpatient facilities; in the other, the nurse's activities would be community-based and she would be concerned more with the prevention of disease and the maintenance of health.[17]

Regardless of where the nurse practices, however, the authors believe that there is a fundamental core of knowledge and skills which are basic to nursing practice. In her introductory course in nursing the student begins to gain some of this fundamental knowledge and to acquire basic skills.

[17]National Commission for the Study of Nursing Education: op. cit., p. 290.

BIBLIOGRAPHY

American Medical News, 13:6, August 3, 1970.

Countdown 1970. Ottawa, Canadian Nurses' Association, 1970.

Davis, Ellen D.: Giving a Bath? *The American Journal of Nursing,* 70:11: 2366–2367, November, 1970.

Facts about Nursing. 1969 edition. New York, American Nurses' Association, 1969.

Federal Government Finance, Revenue and Expenditure and Indirect Debt. Dominion Bureau of Statistics Catalogue No. 68211. Ottawa, Queen's Printer, 1970.

Greenfield, Harry I.: *Allied Health Manpower: Trends and Prospects.* New York, Columbia University Press, 1969.

Health Manpower Source Book. Section 2. Nursing Personnel (Revised 1969). U. S. Department of Health, Education and Welfare. Public Health Service. National Institutes of Health, Bethesda, Md. Available from the Superintendent of Documents, Washington, D.C. 20402.

Health Resources Statistics 1965. A Report Prepared by the National Center for Health Statistics. U.S. Department of Health, Education and Welfare. Public Health Service Publication No. 1509. Washington, D.C., U.S. Government Printing Office, 1966.

Henderson, Virginia: *The Nature of Nursing.* New York, The Macmillan Company, 1964.

Henderson, Virginia: *Basic Principles of Nursing Care.* Basel and New York, published for International Council of Nurses by S. Karger, 1969.

Henderson, Virginia: Excellence in Nursing. *The American Journal of Nursing,* 69:9:2133–2137, October, 1969.

International Code of Nursing Ethics. Adopted by the International Congress of Nurses, São Paulo, Brazil, 1953.

Kreuter, Frances Reiter: What Is Good Nursing Care? *Nursing Outlook,* 5:5:302–304, May, 1957.

Lewis, Irving J.: Federal Health Programs—An Inventory. Paper delivered at the Fourth National Congress on the Socio-Economics of Health Care, Chicago, March 20–21, 1970.

Manpower Report of the President. Prepared by the United States Department of Labor and Transmitted to the Congress, March, 1970.

Mussallem, Helen K.: The Changing Role of the Nurse. *The Canadian Nurse,* 64:11:35–37, November, 1968.

National Commission for the Study of Nursing and Nursing Education: Summary Report and Recommendations. *The American Journal of Nursing,* 70:2:279–294, February, 1970.

Poole, Pamela E.: Nurse, Please show me that you care! *The Canadian Nurse,* 66:2:25–27, February, 1970.

Resolutions. *American Journal of Public Health,* 60:178, January, 1970.

2 HEALTH CARE SERVICES IN THE COMMUNITY

The nurse should be able to:

Describe the spectrum of health care services in a community
Describe the functions of official and voluntary agencies in the
      prevention of illness and the maintenance of health
List the principal providers of primary care services in a
      community
Explain the various functions of a hospital
Describe the functions of various departments within a
      hospital
Describe the nature of home care programs
Describe the nature of rehabilitation services in a community

HEALTH CARE SERVICES 2
IN THE COMMUNITY

INTRODUCTION

People seek the help of health services for a multiplicity of reasons. The new mother may take her infant to the physician's office or to a "well baby" clinic to make sure that he is developing normally, to obtain advice on caring for him to promote his optimum growth and development, and to receive immunizations to protect him from disease. In our health-oriented society a number of people go to their physicians for periodic health checkups, not because they are ill but to be reassured that they are well. A great many people, however, do not seek medical help unless they are worried about their health. The majority of these people receive diagnostic services and are treated in doctors' offices, in clinics or in outpatient departments of hospitals. Many who are ill, however, need to be hospitalized. They may later require rehabilitation services in specialized agencies. People with chronic or prolonged illnesses often need to be cared for in hospitals or nursing homes over a long period of time.

The spectrum of health services in a community ranges from preventive and health maintenance services, through primary care facilities, to inpatient services for the sick and home care and restorative and rehabilitative services for those who require them. A wide variety of agencies provide these services, and many agencies combine a number of them. Hospitals, for example, often have outpatient services for diagnosis and treatment as well as inpatient facilities for the acutely ill and home care

programs for the convalescent. In many instances, two or more agencies combine to provide a more complete range of services for individuals and families. For example, a city health department may work in combination with a visiting nurse service to provide nursing services in the home. Nurses in their practice work in all phases of the health cycle and are therefore concerned with all types of health care agencies.

AGENCIES PROVIDING PREVENTIVE AND HEALTH MAINTENANCE SERVICES

The nurse's role in the prevention of disease and the maintenance of health is an expanding one. At the present time most nurses whose work is primarily concerned with these aspects of health care are employed in official or voluntary agencies. Official agencies are agencies of the government; voluntary agencies are supported by contributions from people within the community. The specific services provided by official and voluntary agencies in any community are largely dependent upon the apparent needs of the people. In an affluent community, most health services may be provided through private physicians; in a community of lower socio-economic status, organized health agencies may offer more extensive programs.

Official Agencies

Official health agencies have been established at the local, state and fed-

15

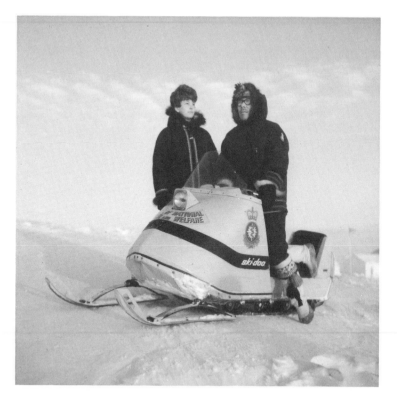

In some rural and remote parts of the country, the public health nurse is the chief source of health care. Here, the nurse and a native community health worker set off from a northern outpost nursing station to make their rounds.

eral levels. At all levels, these agencies are concerned with the prevention of disease and the promotion of health. They often provide services of a curative and rehabilitative nature as well.

The local government agency is usually a city or a county health department, although other branches of a local government may also provide health services as, for example, the welfare department of the school board. The health department of a city or a county usually develops its own health program, based on the needs of the people in the community and the resources available to meet these needs.[1] The general community program usually includes preventive measures such as communicable disease control; the

control of pollution; the safeguarding of water, milk and other food supplies; and the maintenance of cleanliness of public beaches and swimming pools. Health education is also a large part of the program of most local community agencies.

Many official agencies at the local level provide a number of specialized health services in addition to the general community program. These frequently include maternal and child care services; immunization clinics; and often diagnostic, treatment and rehabilitative services, particularly for people in low income groups. The school health program usually consists of health supervision of the students and counselling and consultative services for teachers and parents, as well as the inspection of environmental sanitation. School nurses may also participate in classroom teaching activities that relate to health matters.

[1]Ruth B. Freeman: *Community Health Nursing Practice.* Philadelphia, W. B. Saunders Company, 1970, pp. 89–93.

The local government may also be responsible for the operation of hospitals and related facilities for the care of the sick. These are discussed later in this chapter under inpatient services.

State and provincial public health departments, for the most part, assume leadership and advisory roles to local health agencies, but they may also provide direct services such as the operation of laboratories, the licensure of individuals and agencies, the dissemination of information and the provision of financial assistance. In some states (and provinces) public health agencies serving centers outside the large metropolitan areas may be organized directly by the state department of health. State governments also operate hospitals, particularly tuberculosis hospitals and psychiatric facilities. Community mental health clinics may be directly operated by a state or provincial agency, for example, as are mental hospitals, schools for the mentally retarded and other related psychiatric facilities.

Federal health agencies are concerned with promoting the general health of the nation. In both the United States and Canada, health is primarily the responsibility of the individual states (or provinces). National health policies are therefore initiated at the Federal level, but are implemented by the states. The Federal Government contributes a large share of the monies required to carry out various health programs at the state and community levels, as for example, the Medicare and Medicaid programs in the United States and the Medical and Hospital Insurance programs in Canada. The Federal Government, through its numerous agencies, provides advisory and consultative services for local and state health agencies. Another Federal responsibility is the maintenance of a national information service about health matters. Federal agencies, for example, collect vital statistics and statistics relative to the prevalence of disease, health facilities and health manpower. The Federal Government's role in research in all aspects of health care is also highly significant.

At the direct services level, the Federal Government is concerned with the control of interstate hazards such as pollution, with the control of communicable disease and the setting of standards for food and drug control. The Federal Government is also directly responsible for the provision of health care services to certain segments of the population such as Armed Services personnel and their families, war veterans and the members of the native Indian and Eskimo populations.

Voluntary Agencies

Voluntary agencies are established by the people in a community in response to a particular need that is felt in that community. They are usually supported by donations, and the services they provide serve to supplement or augment the functions performed by official agencies. Voluntary agencies usually provide services of a specific nature. They may be concerned with the preventive, curative and rehabilitative aspects of one disease, as for example, heart disease, tuberculosis, diabetes or arthritis. Some agencies confine their attention to a particular segment of the population such as handicapped children or the mentally retarded. A number of voluntary groups are presently concerned with environmental programs such as pollution control. The visiting nurse agencies which provide care for the sick in the home are organized in many communities by voluntary associations. Voluntary agencies may develop at a strictly local level, at a state level, or they may be national in scope. In the United States, most visiting nurse services are locally organized; in Canada, on the other hand, the major visiting nurse service is the Victorian Order of Nurses, which is a national organization.[2]

---

[2]For additional material on the organization and functions of official and voluntary agencies the nurse is referred to Ruth B. Freeman; op. cit.

PRIMARY CARE FACILITIES

Although many health professionals tend to think of the hospital as the principal place where sick people receive care, in actual fact, it has been estimated that approximately 95 per cent of this care is given outside of hospitals.[3] Most of the health service which people receive is provided in physicians' offices, in clinics or in other community agencies. The term "primary care" is used to designate the initial health care given, that is, the point at which an individual enters the health care system. One of the most pressing concerns in the health field today is the inadequacy of primary care services in many communities. The acute shortage of physicians is given as one of the principal reasons for this inadequacy. Many hospitals are finding their emergency wards overtaxed because people with nonemergency problems are coming there for medical assistance which is not readily available elsewhere. Because of this problem, a number of alternative methods of providing needed health services are being tried. The principal providers of primary care services in the community at the present time are private physicians, clinics operated by community agencies, the outpatient departments of hospitals and newly emerging agencies such as the Neighborhood Health Centers.

Private Physicians' Services

A large number of nurses are employed in physicians' offices. They may work with one physician who is in "solo" practice or with a group of physicians. Although the majority of physicians in the United States and Canada are still in individual practice, group practice is becoming more common. In this type of practice several physicians may work together to provide more comprehensive care for individuals and families. For example, there may be one or two family practitioners in the group, an obstetrician, a pediatrician and a surgeon. Frequently, there is also a psychiatrist, and there may be other specialists as well. Some group practices are small; others are quite extensive. In a large group practice, several nurses may be employed as well as other supportive personnel.

The nurse's role in a physician's office varies. The nurse frequently receives patients in the office, makes appointments and referrals for the patient and assists the physician with physical examinations and treatments. In a number of experimental programs currently being conducted, many nurses are assuming a much expanded role in working with physicians in community practice. Pediatric nurse practitioners in some instances look after much of the well-child care for a pediatrician and do history taking, physical examinations and assessment of a child's condition. They may also make hospital visits to newborn babies and home visits when needed.[4]

Clinic and Outpatient Services

The term "clinic" may be applied to a group practice of private physicians such as that just described or may be used to designate the services provided by a community agency for care and treatment of the sick on an ambulatory basis. In ambulatory care, the patient remains at home but comes into the agency for care and treatment. When community agencies operate clinic services, these usually are provided free of charge to the patient, or a nominal charge may be made. Outpatient services, also of an ambulatory nature, are provided by many hospitals. Again, these may be offered on a charitable basis, or the patient may pay a small fee. In the clinics

---

[3]D. Curiel et al.: *Trends in the Study of Morbidity and Mortality.* (Public Health Paper No. 27.) Geneva, World Health Organization, 1965.

[4]Ethel Gozzi: Pediatric Nurse Practitioner at Work. *The American Journal of Nursing,* 70:11: 2371–2374, November, 1970.

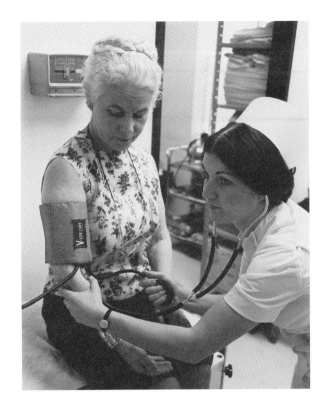

Often, people who are ill receive diagnostic and treatment services in doctors' offices, in clinics or in hospital outpatient departments. This nurse is checking the blood pressure of a patient who is under medical supervision in a Family Practice Unit.

and outpatient departments, diagnostic and treatment services are provided and often rehabilitative services as well. The nurse working in a clinic or outpatient service is frequently responsible for the day-to-day management of the clinic, and she assists the physician with physical examinations and with treatments. She may also perform laboratory tests. The nurse is often involved in health teaching activities in the clinic and in health counselling for individuals and families.

Neighborhood Health Centers

A recent development in the area of primary health services for the people in a community has been the establishment of Neighborhood Health Centers. Originally these centers were set up by the Office of Economic Opportunity in the United States to provide health care services in poverty and ghetto areas. The centers provide comprehensive health services (exclusive of inpatient services) for the residents of a given community in their own neighborhood. They employ a clinic type of approach but are concerned with both health and social problems. They frequently utilize people who live in the community as adjunctive health workers. The concept of the Neighborhood Health Center is rapidly gaining wide acceptance as one possible solution to the problem of providing adequate primary care services in the community to other groups of residents beside the poor.[5]

AGENCIES PROVIDING INPATIENT SERVICES FOR THE CARE OF THE SICK

The majority of registered nurses in both the United States and Canada are

[5]Patterns of Care. *American Journal of Public Health*, 60:9:1723, September, 1970.

employed in hospitals or related institutions which provide inpatient services for the care of the sick. In addition, a large proportion of the clinical experience of nursing students takes place in hospitals. The nurse should therefore be familiar with the functions of hospitals, the kinds of hospitals and related institutions in her community, and the various departments within a hospital.

The Hospital

The hospital is an institution whose chief purpose is the care of sick and injured people. Although not the only agencies concerned with health, hospitals are the centers in which a wide range of specialized functions are brought to bear on health problems. People who are acutely ill generally come to a hospital to avail themselves of the services of the professional people and the facilities necessary for their care.

Hospitals, like public health agencies, perform curative, preventive and rehabilitative functions, but they also are involved in two additional areas of commitment: research and education. The emphasis placed upon any of the three areas varies with the hospital. Generally, the policies of a particular hospital in this regard are determined by the following factors:

1. The cultural, religious and social groups within the community
2. The nature of the diseases of the patients admitted to the hospital
3. The availability of medical and related personnel
4. The specific needs of the particular community and the facilities that are already available
5. The money available to provide these facilities
6. The existence of nearby institutions, for example, a university
7. The size of the community which the hospital serves.

Hospital policies are usually set by the hospital board of directors. Although the membership varies from hospital to hospital, the board usually consists chiefly of people representative of the community served by the hospital. There is usually also one or more representatives of the medical department on the board and, in hospitals operated or financed by government agencies, a member representative of government interests. The hospital administrator almost invariably attends board meetings and frequently serves as secretary to the board. In some hospitals, the director of nursing also attends board meetings, either on a regular or an occasional basis; in others, she does not. Sometimes she is a full-fledged member of the board.

In performing its basic function, the care of the sick and injured, the hospital may render primarily emergency care or it may also render diagnostic, therapeutic and rehabilitative services. Many hospitals also provide facilities for research so that members of the medical profession and allied disciplines avail themselves of the clinical resources of the hospital. Education, the third function of most hospitals, includes the in-service education of institutional personnel and programs for medical students, nursing students, laboratory technicians and dietetic interns.

Kinds of Hospitals. There are many kinds of hospitals; they can be described according to their size, ownership, control, services or the length of stay of the patients. Usually a hospital is described in terms of its available beds. The small community might have a hospital of 10 beds; a large metropolitan area might have one of 2000 beds. Often, smaller hospitals offer limited services, but they may have an arrangement with larger hospitals for the prompt transfer of patients in need of specialized facilities.

Hospitals may be owned or controlled by the government, by private groups or by a single individual. Government ownership of hospitals may be at the federal, state or local level. Often these institutions are governed jointly by representatives of the government and representatives of the community in which the hospital is situated. This arrangement is usually true of the county or municipal hospital. Private groups also own hospitals; for example, it is not unusual for religious organizations to have their own health institutions. An individual or a group of individuals may also operate a hospital or clinic. Physicians in particular often own and operate their own hospitals.

The services offered are another way of describing a hospital. Thus, a hospital may be a general hospital; that is, one that offers a diversity of services, such as surgery, medicine, psychiatry, obstetrics and pediatrics. Or it may be a special hospital, admitting only patients of one sex, people with a particular type of illness or children of a specific age group. In years past psychiatric hospitals were the most obvious special hospitals, and often they were situated in rural areas. Today, however, there is a trend to incorporate a psychiatric nursing unit into the general hospital rather than isolate the mentally ill from the community.

Recently, the length of stay of the patient has become a basis upon which to classify an institution. Generally speaking there are acute care hospitals, chronic care hospitals and day care hospitals. The acute care hospital has restrictions upon the length of stay of patients; some permit patients to stay 30 days at the maximum, after which they are transferred to a chronic care institution. The chronic care hospital, as its name implies, is for long term patients. Often its accent is upon the retraining and rehabilitating of patients over a period of months. Nursing homes also provide long-term care for the sick who require nursing services over an extended period of time.

The day care hospital is a new addition to hospital services. Originally intended for psychiatric patients, it now offers services to patients with various other illnesses. The patient stays at the hospital during the day and returns to his home at night. This arrangement has the obvious advantage of lowering hospital expenses as well as maintaining the home orientation of the patient.

Standards for the quality of service in the hospital have been established by the Joint Commission on Accreditation of Hospitals. Instituted in 1952, the commission is composed of representatives of the American College of Surgeons, the American College of Physicians, the American Hospital Association and the American Medical Association. The commission can accredit a hospital, provisionally accredit it or not accredit it at all.

The Departments Within the Hospital. The many services available within the hospital can be classified as direct or indirect with respect to the patient. Toomay states that the services involved in the operation of a hospital can be divided into three groups: professional services, institutional services and financial services.[6] The services correspond roughly with the departments of the hospital.

Usually, however, the number of separate departments in a hospital is dependent upon its size. The larger the hospital, the greater is the number of departments. The patient is usually aware of the medical department, the x-ray department and the nursing department. He may be less aware of the maintenance department and the purchasing department, yet their services are also important to his comfort and welfare. The following departments are commonly found in the average hospital.

THE MEDICAL DEPARTMENT. The medical department includes the members of the medical staff who are responsible for the care of the patients. Often this department designates a board whose members keep watch on the quality of medical care given by the physicians attending the patients.

THE NURSING DEPARTMENT. The nursing department includes registered nurses, practical nurses, nurse's aides and often orderlies. These people usually give direct care to the patients under the guidance of the head of the department and according to the policies of the hospital administration.

---

[6]Robert E. Toomay: Organization Structure and Hospitals. *Hospital Topics*, 40:55, November, 1962.

The head of the nursing department is usually the director of nursing; she may have an assistant director as well as supervisors and head nurses to carry out administrative duties.

If a hospital has a school of nursing, it is often included within the department of nursing. However, a school of nursing can affiliate with a hospital and yet be a separate entity financially and administratively.

THE DIETARY DEPARTMENT. The dietary department includes dietitians as well as cooks, kitchen maids, tray girls and dishwashers. The chief responsibility of this department is to supply food to the patients, and sometimes to the staff of the hospital. This responsibility usually includes the preparation of therapeutic diets for many patients.

THE LABORATORY DEPARTMENT. The function of the laboratory department is to perform laboratory tests ordered by the physician. These tests include blood serology and chemistry tests, urinalyses, bacteriological tests, and analyses of specimens for pathological diagnosis. The laboratory technician collects some specimens; the nursing staff is responsible for the collection of others.

THE X-RAY DEPARTMENT. One of the obvious functions of the x-ray department is to take x-rays of patients as ordered by the physician. In addition to the x-ray technicians who work in the department, many hospitals employ doctors who are specialists in interpreting x-rays and can aid other physicians in their diagnostic work. The use of x-ray equipment, radium, etc., for therapeutic purposes is also an important function of many x-ray departments.

THE MAINTENANCE DEPARTMENT. The number of services provided by the maintenance department varies from hospital to hospital. The department often performs carpentry, plumbing and electrical services, as well as cleaning, heating and possibly laundry services.

THE PHARMACY DEPARTMENT. The pharmacy department provides pharmaceutical supplies that are ordered by the physician for the patients. The pharmacist prepares some of the medications himself, while others are purchased commercially and are dispensed to the nursing units.

THE BUSINESS DEPARTMENT. This department is responsible for the financial business of the hospital. It prepares the patient's hospital bills, administers the hospital payroll and is involved in budget preparation and general hospital business.

THE CENTRAL SUPPLY DEPARTMENT. The central supply department of the hospital is usually responsible for the cleaning, the sterilizing and often the delivery of equipment used in the institution. It may also be responsible for the purchasing of supplies if the hospital has no purchasing department. In some hospitals the central supply department is included in the nursing department.

THE PERSONNEL DEPARTMENT. This department is responsible for hiring personnel and for job placement within the hospital. Some nursing departments assume the responsibilities for hiring nurses, whereas at other hospitals this task is handled entirely by the personnel department.

THE SOCIAL SERVICE DEPARTMENT. Many hospitals have a separate department to provide welfare services for the patients. Among the concerns of the social worker are family finances and nursing home placement. Usually he maintains liaison between the hospital and other welfare agencies in the community.

OTHER DEPARTMENTS. Large hospitals may have many other departments. There may be separate departments for electrocardiography, physical therapy, public relations, and hairdressing. The services that hospitals supply vary considerably; however, no matter how many departments there may be, they have a common goal: to help meet the needs of the hospital patient and his family.

HOME CARE SERVICES

With the increasing emphasis today on early discharge of patients from hospital and on treating patients within

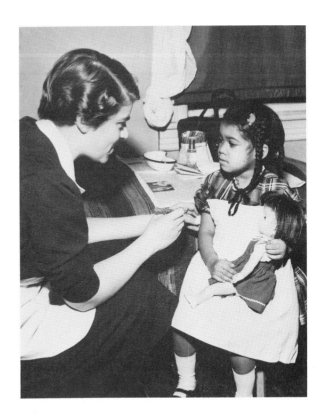

Many nurses are employed in agencies which provide care and treatment to sick people in their homes. This little girl has Dolly ready for her injection when the nurse has finished with hers.

their own home environment as much as possible, many nurses are being employed in home care programs. Home care programs are designed to provide nursing care and other services of a therapeutic nature to people in their own homes.

There are basically two types of home care programs: those that are community-based and those that are hospital-based. Community-based programs are administered by agencies other than a hospital. They may be operated by an official agency, for example, a city health department; by a voluntary agency such as a visiting nurse service; by a combination of agencies; or by a separately incorporated agency. Referrals are made to the agency by the physician who remains in charge of the patient's care. The patient may be admitted to the program either directly from the community or from a hospital where he has been receiving care.

Hospital-based home care programs are usually operated by a hospital in a manner similar to outpatient services.

Nurses and other personnel involved in the home care program may be employed by the hospital, or the services of people attached to another agency may be utilized through a contractual arrangement. A hospital may enter into an agreement with a visiting nurse agency, for example, to provide home care services for its patients. The hospital programs are usually limited to patients who have been discharged from the hospital, or to those who would otherwise be admitted to the hospital as inpatients.

Home care programs frequently offer a wide variety of services, such as direct care nursing services, physical therapy and occupational therapy. Sometimes specialized rehabilitative services or treatment are provided as well. Frequently, a "homemaker service" is a part of the total home care program.[7]

[7]F. Catherine Maddaford: Organized Home Care Programs in Canada. Paper prepared at the School of Hygiene, University of Toronto, 1968.

REHABILITATION SERVICES

One definition of rehabilitation is "the restoration through personal health services of handicapped individuals to the fullest physical, mental, social and economic usefulness of which they are capable, including ordinary treatments and treatments in special rehabilitation centers."[8]

Rehabilitation involves the efforts of members of many disciplines. Doctors, counsellors, therapists, clergymen and social workers, among others, are intimately involved in helping people live happily and productively. Rehabilitation has received increased emphasis in recent years, until today it is a fundamental part of the treatment of most patients.

There are several obvious reasons why rehabilitation has become increasingly important. The first is the enormous socioeconomic problems created by the number of people who are partially disabled. In the United States it has been established that over 20 million people have difficulty or require assistance in moving about.[9] With a longer life span there is an increasing proportion of senior citizens in the population, and certain chronic diseases are most prevalent in this group, for example, cardiovascular disease, mental illness and arthritis. Another reason for the emphasis upon rehabilitation is the increasing number of people who are injured and disabled as a result of accidents.

Medicine has made great advances in saving lives, not only in surgical procedures but in many phases of medical therapy. Many people are living today after accidents which years ago meant certain death. In addition, there have been advances in the control of communicable diseases. Fewer people die today as a result of infectious diseases, although some victims live with residual handicaps.

Chronic disease is a major cause of handicapping people. It has been estimated that 88 per cent of all who could benefit from rehabilitation have chronic diseases. The numbers are enormous and the problem to society — socially, medically and economically — would be overwhelming were it not for rehabilitation services.

Rehabilitation programs in independent centers in the community and as part of the programs of other health agencies and institutions offer comprehensive service to the disabled. A rehabilitation unit coordinates the efforts of many disciplines in order to plan an approach designed to meet individual needs. Generally each patient also follows a plan of therapy during his rehabilitation. The rehabilitation team meets regularly to discuss the patient's progress and revise the plan to meet his changing needs.

In many hospitals a rehabilitation department provides bed services and coordinates its work with that of other hospital departments, such as x-ray and dietetics. It also provides a consultative service to major medical-surgical services such as orthopedics and neurosurgery. Many hospitals have a rehabilitation nursing unit to which a patient can transfer when he is ready. At this time the rehabilitation team assumes the major responsibility for his therapy.

Before a patient in an institution is ready for discharge, he is often visited by a member of a community health agency who assists him and his family in making arrangements for his return home. For example, if a patient cannot climb stairs it may be necessary to change his sleeping arrangements in his home. Some community agencies provide nursing and rehabilitative services within the home. Encouragement and instruction carried on after discharge from a hospital help a person to continue to progress.

Many people require medical rehabilitation in order to restore maximum physical function. Learning to walk and regaining the use of various body muscles are important aspects of therapy. Most rehabilitation centers provide

---

[8]Frank H. Krusen: *Concepts in Rehabilitation of the Handicapped.* Philadelphia, W. B. Saunders Company, 1964, p. 1.

[9]*Ibid.,* p. 3.

gymnasium facilities for corrective and preventive exercises for patients. Such exercises are conducted by a physical therapist both on an individual basis and in classes.

Relearning the activities that are necessary for daily living are most important to patients. To dress oneself, to prepare meals, and so on, represent areas of independence in which the handicapped person can maintain his self-respect. Rehabilitation programs teach the patient to carry out these activities for himself, often providing him with specially constructed tools, such as a fork with an enlarged handle which a person with a partially paralyzed hand can grasp more easily.

Some patients require vocational education before they can obtain employment that is compatible with their limitations. Vocational counsellors can advise patients about fields in which they are likely to succeed and about the employment opportunities in these fields.

The psychologist and the psychiatrist are also important members of the rehabilitation team. Their professional help is often required to help patients cope with the psychological stresses accompanying illness and disability. Moreover, since rehabilitation services can only be fully effective when the patient is motivated to help himself and to cooperate in his plan of therapy, the guidance of the psychologist and the psychiatrist is often necessary to the success of the program.

The Nurse's Role in Rehabilitation

The concept of rehabilitation should permeate all nursing care and be a factor in the nursing care plans of every patient. Planning for his rehabilitation should start with the patient's admission to hospital, and its accomplishment should be a fundamental objective of nursing action throughout his illness. It should be kept in mind that patients require the support of the nurse not just when they are acutely ill but also during the period of convalescence.

Because of her day-to-day contact with patients the nurse has an important role in rehabilitation. She is perhaps the first person to recognize or become aware of many of the patient's needs, since patients often talk easily to a nurse whom they have come to know and who has helped them in the acute phase of their illnesses. Her observations, her understanding and her knowledge, therefore, can be valuable assets to the rehabilitation team.

Another function of the nurse is to encourage and reassure the patient during the period of convalescence. Progress is not always steady; there are sometimes plateaus and during these periods patients feel discouraged. An understanding nurse can help people through these periods of discouragement by reassuring them about their progress. In so doing, the nurse can often reinforce the teaching of other members of the rehabilitation team.

A patient may find it necessary to relearn many skills of living and the nurse can often help him plan his day's activities so that practice and learning sessions are well spaced in order to avoid fatigue.

Above all, the nurse is frequently responsible for coordinating the patient's care. Since she has contact with the various members of the rehabilitation team, the patient's family and the patient, it is often the nurse who is in the best position to schedule the activities of the patient and to help interpret his needs to the various members of the team.

REFERRALS TO HEALTH AGENCIES

When a person comes to a health agency it may be on his own initiative or he may have been referred by his physician or other personnel in allied professions; for example, a teacher might refer a student to the school nurse to have his eyes checked. An acutely injured or ill person may go to the emergency department of a hospital for help, and he may subsequently elect to be admitted to the institution for further care. This is generally an emergency admission, in contrast to an elective admission in which the patient has greater freedom in deciding when and if he will come to a hospital. A person can also transfer from one agency to another. For example, a patient may be transferred to a hospital that has special equipment for treating his particular disease. Patients are frequently referred to public health agencies for continued treatment in the home. Such referrals are becoming much more common today. Many agencies have on their staff a public health nurse who acts as a liaison between hospital and community services.

STUDY VOCABULARY

Hospital	Primary care	Voluntary agency
Official agency	Rehabilitation	

STUDY SITUATION

A group of parents of school children in your district have asked you to talk to them about the health resources in the community. In preparing your talk, you need to answer the following questions:

1. What are the kinds of health agencies? Give specific examples in your community.
2. What factors affect the establishment and utilization of health resources?
3. What are the functions of hospitals generally?
4. Describe the services and the organization of a local hospital.
5. What is rehabilitation?
6. Why is rehabilitation receiving increasing emphasis in care today?

BIBLIOGRAPHY

Curiel D., et al.: *Trends in the Study of Morbidity and Mortality.* (Public Health Paper No. 27.) Geneva, World Health Organization, 1965.
Deaver, George G.: Rehabilitation: A Philosophy. *The American Journal of Nursing, 59:*1278–1279, September, 1959.
Folta, Jeanette R., and Edith S. Deck: *A Sociological Framework for Patient Care.* New York, John Wiley & Sons, Inc., 1966.
Freeman, Ruth B.: *Community Health Nursing Practice.* Philadelphia, W. B. Saunders Company, 1970.
Goldfarb, Alvin I.: Responsibilities to Our Aged. *The American Journal of Nursing, 64:*78–82, November, 1964.
Gozzi, Ethel: Pediatric Nurse Practitioner at Work. *The American Journal of Nursing, 70:*11:2371–2374, November, 1970.
Greene, Georgina, and Lavina Robins: A Rehabilitation Nursing Record. *The American Journal of Nursing, 61:*82–85, March, 1961.
Krusen, Frank H.: *Concepts in Rehabilitation of the Handicapped.* Philadelphia, W. B. Saunders Company, 1964.
Maddaford, F. Catherine: Organized Home Care Programs in Canada. Paper prepared at the School of Hygiene, University of Toronto, 1968.
Morrissey, Alice B.: *Rehabilitation Nursing.* New York, G. P. Putnam's Sons, 1951.
Mussallem, Helen K.: The Changing Role of the Nurse. *The Canadian Nurse, 64:*11:35–37, November, 1968.
Ohlson, Virginia M.: Profile of the Public Health Nurse. *The Journal of the American Medical Association, 198:*3:326–327, October 17, 1966.

Patterns of Care. *The American Journal of Public Health, 60*:9:1723, September, 1970.

Rothberg, June S.: The Challenge for Rehabilitative Nursing. *Nursing Outlook, 69*:37–39, November, 1969.

Rusk, Howard A.: *Rehabilitation Medicine.* Second edition. St. Louis, The C. V. Mosby Company, 1964.

Shannon, Iris R.: Nursing Service at the Mile Square Health Center of Presbyterian St. Luke's Hospital. *The American Journal of Public Health, 60*:9:1726–1732, September, 1970.

Terry, Florence J., et al.: *Principles and Techniques of Rehabilitation Nursing.* Second edition. St. Louis, The C. V. Mosby Company, 1961.

Toomay, Robert E.: Organization Structure and Hospitals. *Hospital Topics, 40*:55, November, 1962.

3   HEALTH AND ILLNESS

The nurse should be able to:

Explain the health-illness concept
Describe differences in the way people view health and
      illness
Explain the role of folk medicine in health care in North
      America today
Explain the role of stress in the causation of illness
List types of stressors
Explain the general adaptation syndrome
Explain the "fight-flight" reaction of the body

INTRODUCTION

Basic to the practice of all the health professions is an understanding of the health-illness concept. Both health and illness are relative states and the words themselves mean different things to different people. As a person gets older, he tends to accept a few aches and pains as a normal part of the aging process, whereas an athlete may feel that he is not in good health unless he can run five miles. Health and illness may be viewed as a continuum which ranges from extreme poor health when death is imminent to peak or "high-level" wellness.[1]

<hr />

[1]Halburt L. Dunn: High-Level Wellness for Man and Society. In *A Sociological Framework for Patient Care* by Jeanette R. Folta and Edith S. Deck (eds.). New York, John Wiley and Sons, Inc., 1966, pp. 213–219.

Neither health nor illness are constant or absolute, but are ever-changing states of being. A person may wake up in the morning with a headache, for example. He may feel so ill, in fact, that he decides he is not well enough to go to work, but he remembers that he has an important appointment. After one or two cups of coffee and breakfast, he may begin to think that perhaps he is not so sick as he thought he was, and, if his appointment goes well, he may feel in excellent health by lunchtime.

What then constitutes health and illness? Extreme states of ill health are usually fairly easy to identify, but a person who is carrying on his normal daily routine may have a serious illness according to his physician and yet appear healthy to other people. Some illnesses which are looked upon as serious deviations from health in our Western society may be considered as normal, or

THE HEALTH CONTINUUM

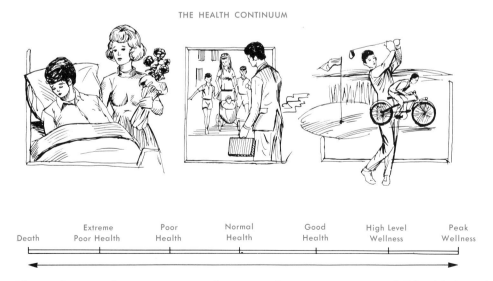

| Death | Extreme Poor Health | Poor Health | Normal Health | Good Health | High Level Wellness | Peak Wellness |

Health may be viewed as a continuum that ranges from extreme states of ill health to peak wellness.

may even be highly desirable in other cultures. For example, in some cultures the person who sees visions or hears imaginary voices talking to him may be highly esteemed, whereas we might consider that this individual has a serious mental disease. Malnutrition in some parts of the world is so common that it is rare to see a child who does not suffer from it.

THE PERCEPTION OF ILLNESS

Illness is not only a biological matter; sociologists tell us that it is also a cultural phenomenon.[2] There is a difference between the scientific definitions of health and illness and the way people view their own health and illness states. In a study to determine differences in the attitudes of people toward illness, Baumann identified three distinct ways in which individuals tend to establish criteria to judge whether they are ill.[3] One was related to the presence or absence of symptoms. Pain is, of course, one of the most common symptoms by which people judge the state of their health. If a person has pain, particularly pain of a severe nature, he usually considers himself ill. As mentioned earlier, however, pain is also relative; a person may live with a backache for years and not consider this an abnormal symptom. The second method by which people judge the state of their health is by the way they feel; they "feel good" or they do not "feel good," they "feel poorly" or they "feel sick."

A third way of establishing the state of one's health is related to the ability to carry out one's daily activities. A person may say he is in good health be-

cause he can work and still have enough energy to play a round of golf in the evening. Another person may decide he is ill on the basis of his inability to walk up a flight of stairs without acute distress in breathing. A woman who cannot carry on her daily household routine of cleaning the house, looking after the children and cooking meals without feeling exhausted may decide that she is not in good health and should perhaps see her physician.

Whether a person determines the state of his health on a symptom basis, a feeling state basis or a performance basis tends to vary with a number of factors. There is no clear-cut delineation of these categories, and it is a mistake to overgeneralize. Socioeconomic status, however, appears to influence to a certain extent whether one uses a symptomatic approach or a feeling-oriented approach; the higher the socioeconomic status, the more symptom-oriented people tend to be, whereas poorer people often determine illness more in terms of how they feel. The level of education also seems to have a bearing on how people judge illness; again, the more education a person has, the more he tends to evaluate health in terms of whether he has the signs and symptoms of disease. This is important to remember in nursing patients. Nurses as well as physicians tend to be highly symptom-oriented, whereas many of the people they care for may view health and illness more in relation to feeling.

Other factors, too, influence an individual's perception of his health. Age, for example, has a great deal to do with it. Older people do not expect to be able to perform gymnastic feats with the ease and vigor they did when they were young. Many adolescents seem particularly concerned with health, and worry over every blemish on their skin. In our stoical American tradition, men are not supposed to complain about pain as much as women are permitted to do, and many men tend to negate the early signs and symptoms of illness. "It is nothing to worry about" is frequently heard from the father in the family.

[2]E. Gartly Jaco (ed.): *Patients, Physicians and Illness.* New York, The Free Press, 1967. Part III —Socio-cultural aspects of Medical Care and Treatment.

[3]Barbara Baumann: Diversities in Conceptions of Health and Physical Fitness. In *Social Interaction and Patient Care* by James K. Skipper, Jr., and Robert C. Leonard (eds.). Philadelphia, J. B. Lippincott Company, 1965, pp. 206–210.

Ethnic background also has an influence, as do the particular values placed upon health in various groups. Again, one should be careful not to generalize because each person is an individual whose personality has been shaped by a multitude of different factors. Many Italian patients and people of Latin origin seem to react more vocally to pain, for example, and to be more feeling-oriented in their attitudes toward health than Anglo-Saxons, but not all patients of Italian background react in the same way. One may find totally different value systems about health in people from the same family. Particularly, differences may be noted between generations. The younger, better educated family members are usually much more informed about nutrition, preventive measures such as immunizations, the signs and symptoms of illness and current methods of treating disease. The young mother does not see herself as restricting her activities or losing her figure just because she has children, although these beliefs may have been accepted by her mother and her grandmother.

SCIENTIFIC MEDICINE AND FOLK MEDICINE

The way a person views health and illness determines to a large extent the type of help he seeks when he is sick. He is also influenced in this regard by the advice of his family and his friends. Studies in communication have shown that people are influenced more by the people around them, their friends, their family and individuals whose opinions they respect, than by any other means of communication. The person who feels in need of medical attention usually receives much advice on where to obtain it. He may elect to go to a physician or a clinic, but he may also choose to seek help from any one of a number of nonmedical practitioners of the healing arts, such as herbalists, naturopaths or spiritual healers.

Although we pride ourselves on our scientific approach to disease in North America, the astounding sales record of numerous long-standing patent medicines attests to the prevalence of many widely held unscientific beliefs about the causes of illness and the methods of curing disease. If an individual is "liverish," has "tired blood," or has kidneys which need "flushing out," he can purchase a medicine in the drug store to cure these conditions. Many women used to rely on (and, indeed, a number still do) a tonic containing iron to cure their "women's ailments." While there may be some value in this, since women are more prone to be anemic than men, it can hardly be considered a cure for everything that ails them. Often people attribute their illnesses to disturbances of the gastrointestinal tract; constipation has frequently been cited as the cause of diabetes, for example. One still sees the copper bracelet used to ward off rheumatism, or a clove of garlic worn around the neck to prevent colds.

The old-wives' tales and guaranteed home remedies are still not far from the surface in scientific North America. One very common belief about the cause of illness is that the individual is being punished for his sins. This belief will, of course, affect a person's reaction to his illness; he may feel guilty about being sick, or feel that he has to atone for his misdeeds through suffering, and sometimes may feel that he does not deserve to get better.

THE CAUSATION OF ILLNESS

Currently, research in the field of medicine has led to acceptance of the belief that many factors may cause disease. The human organism is seen as constantly attempting to maintain a state of equilibrium, or *homeostasis,* both internally and with the external environment. Stresses of any kind upset the delicate balance of the human body and the body reacts by altering certain structures or processes to restore equilibrium. A person may perspire profusely on a very warm day, for example; he then becomes thirsty and increases

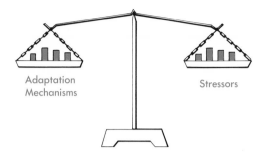

In homeostasis the body attempts to restore a state of equilibrium by counter-balancing the effect of stressors with adaptation mechanisms.

his water intake to restore the fluids he has lost through sweating. The term *stressor* is used to designate any factor which disturbs the body's equilibrium. There are a number of ways of categorizing stressors. They may be classified on the basis of whether they are external or internal; or as biological, psychological and sociological. Freeman has suggested four categories which would seem to be logical and to encompass all types of agents which may act as stressors:

1. Deprivational stress in which there is a lack of some essential factor for the well-being of the individual

2. Stresses of excess, which would be the opposite of deprivation

3. Stresses created by change

4. Stresses of intolerance[4]

Deprivational stressors would include the lack of essential items needed to maintain the chemical balance of the body, as, for example, the lack of water, of oxygen, of vitamins or of food elements. Other types of deprivation might be psychological or sociological in nature. A person who is isolated from contact with other human beings suffers considerable stress. The lack of sufficient parental affection to children in infancy and early childhood is felt to be one of the causes of psychological disorders.

On the other hand, an excess of certain factors may also disturb the body's equilibrium. Exposure to intense heat causes tissue damage in the form of a burn; intense cold may cause frostbite. If a person eats excessively he usually has disturbances of body functioning; he becomes obese and may suffer from gastrointestinal upsets among other things. Excessive interpersonal conflict may also be a source of stress.

Change of any sort may be sufficient to upset the physiological processes in the body. Even the time change experienced by international travelers creates a stress, and an individual may take several days to become adjusted to a different "time clock" for the normal bodily functions of eating, sleeping and elimination. Freeman categorizes the invasion of the body by pathogenic (disease-producing) bacteria under the heading of stress caused by change. This invasion calls forth a strongly protective reaction on the part of the human body.

An intolerance of noxious (or harmful) agents is exemplified in the allergic reactions to certain foods, chemical substances or pollens from which many people suffer. The body's reaction to poisons or toxins would also illustrate this point. If one eats fermented or bad food, the body attempts to remove the substance, frequently through vomiting up the stomach's contents. An intolerance to psychological factors in the environment, such as an unhappy work situation, is also a source of stress. Moving to a different country where customs and social values are different from what one has been accustomed to may cause stress sufficient to result in what is termed "cultural shock." Nurses working with minority groups in our

---

[4]Victor J. Freeman: Human Aspects of Health and Illness: Beyond the Germ Theory. In Folta and Deck, op. cit., pp. 83–89.

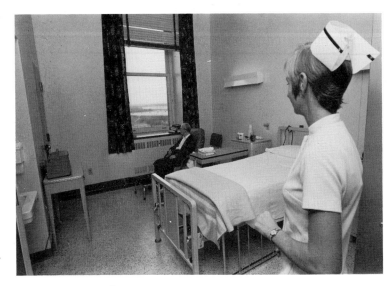

The patient in hospital is often lonely. The lack of social contact can be an added stressor which complicates his illness.

own country or in poverty neighborhoods may experience some of this cultural shock when they encounter customs and ways of life which are different from their own.

THE BODY'S REACTION TO STRESS

The reactions of the body to disturbances in its equilibrium are frequently referred to as *adaptation mechanisms*. Selye pointed out that there is a general nonspecific response which occurs. He described this originally as the phenomenon of "just being sick" and later elaborated on this in his theory of the general adaptation syndrome (G.A.S.). This syndrome, he believed, is the response of the body to any agent that causes physiological stress. The response may be divided into three stages: the alarm reaction in which the body's defenses are mobilized; the "stage of resistance" when the battle for equilibrium is most active; and the stage of exhaustion, which occurs if the stressor is severe enough or is present over a long enough period of time to deplete the body's resources for adaptation.[5]

[5]Hans Selye: *The Stress of Life*. New York, McGraw-Hill Book Company, 1956, p. 31.

The early symptoms of disease are remarkably the same for many illnesses (this was Selye's original "just being sick" response). These symptoms usually include a slight rise in temperature, a loss of energy, a lack of interest in food and a general feeling of malaise. It is in the second stage of the syndrome, the "stage of resistance," that the signs and symptoms characteristic of the body's reaction to specific disorders are seen: the rash erupts on the skin of the child with measles, or the localized pain in the chest and difficulty in breathing occur in pneumonia. If the stress is not relieved, or if it is of sufficient intensity to cause extensive damage to body tissues, the body's adaptive mechanisms may not be able to restore equilibrium, and exhaustion will set in.

Another level of response which represents the body's reaction to immediate danger is the flight-fight reaction. This reaction is called forth when the individual is frightened or feels threatened by harm. There is an emergency mobilization of physiological defense mechanisms as the body prepares for instant action (either fight or flight). This too is an alarm reaction, but of a different sort, in response to psychological stress. The heart beats more forcefully and faster; breathing is increased in rate and depth; blood is withdrawn from surface vessels and the viscera and is shunted to the muscles; blood pressure increases; and the muscles become tense in preparation for action. This is the body's emergency mechanism, designed to protect the individual from real or imagined danger. Anxiety, which is a modified form of fear, usually accompanies illness, and the nurse will often note manifestations of the fight-flight reaction in her patients. She will probably also note them in herself, particularly when she is in new and unfamiliar surroundings or has to do a treatment for the first time. Helping the patient to become familiar with his environment and providing him with an explanation of routines ·and procedures will help to allay many fears. Fear of the unknown is one of the main sources of anxiety for most people. Nurses tend to become so accustomed to the hospital environment that they often forget that everything is strange and frightening for the patient. The subject of anxiety is discussed in Chapter 9.

STUDY VOCABULARY

Adaptation mechanism	Cultural shock	Naturopath
Anemic	Herbalist	Pathogenic
Anxiety	Homeostasis	Stressor

STUDY SITUATION

Mrs. Niccolini is a 64 year old woman of Italian descent who came to New York as a bride in 1927. Her husband, who was a laborer, died one year ago. Mrs. Niccolini now lives with her oldest daughter, who is a school teacher, her daughter's husband and their three teen-age children. Mrs. Niccolini has come to the doctor's office for a physical examination. She tells the doctor that she has not been feeling well for the last few months. Her daughter, who has accompanied her to the doctor's office, adds that Mrs. Niccolini has been having headaches and dizzy spells. Mrs. Niccolini is a very heavy woman, dressed somberly but neatly in black. She does not speak English very well. She states that she has eight children, all of them grown up now, and her health has always been "pretty good."

1. What is the difference between Mrs. Niccolini's point of view and that of her daughter concerning Mrs. Niccoloni's health?

2. What are some of the factors that might cause this difference?

3. What are some of the stresses which may have contributed to Mrs. Niccolini's illness?

BIBLIOGRAPHY

Baumann, Barbara: Diversities in Conceptions of Health and Physical Fitness. In *Social Interaction and Patient Care* by James K. Skipper, Jr., and Robert C. Leonard (eds.). Philadelphia, J. B. Lippincott Company, 1965, pp. 206–210. Reprinted from *The Journal of Health and Human Behavior,* 2:39–46, 1961.

Dunn, Halburt L.: High-Level Wellness for Man and Society. In *A Sociological Framework for Patient Care* by Jeanette R. Folta and Edith S. Deck (eds.). New York, John Wiley and Sons, Inc., 1965, pp. 213–219. Reprinted from the *American Journal of Public Health and Nation's Health,* 49:786–792, 1959.

Freeman, Victor J.: Human Aspects of Health and Illness: Beyond the Germ Theory. In *A Sociological Framework for Patient Care* by Jeanette R.

Folta and Edith S. Deck (eds.). New York, John Wiley and Sons, Inc., 1965, pp. 83–89. Reprinted from the *Journal of Health and Human Behavior, 1:*8–13, 1960.

Gordon, Gerald, Odin W. Anderson, Henry P. Brehm, and Sue Marquis (eds.): *Disease, the Individual, and Society.* New Haven, College and University Press, 1968.

Jaco, E. Gartly (ed.): *Patients, Physicians and Illness.* New York, The Free Press, 1967.

King, Stanley H.: *Perceptions of Illness and Medical Practice.* New York, Russell Sage Foundation, 1962.

Levine, Myra E.: The Pursuit of Wholeness. *The American Journal of Nursing, 69:*1:93–98, January, 1969.

Mechanic, David: *Medical Sociology.* New York, The Free Press, 1968.

Polgar, Steven: Health Action in Cross-Cultural Perspective. In *Handbook of Medical Sociology* by Howard E. Freeman, Sol Levine, and Leo G. Reeder (eds.). Englewood Cliffs, N. J., Prentice-Hall, Inc., 1963.

Selye, Hans: *The Stress of Life.* New York, McGraw-Hill Book Company, Inc., 1956.

Selye, Hans: The Stress Syndrome. In *A Sociological Framework for Patient Care* by Jeanette R. Folta and Edith S. Deck (eds.). New York, John Wiley and Sons, Inc., 1965. pp. 253–257. Reprinted from *The American Journal of Nursing, 65:*97–99, 1965.

Twaddle, Andrew C.: Health Decisions and Sick Role Variations: An Exploration. *Journal of Health and Human Behavior, 10:*105–115, June, 1969.

4 ILLNESS, THE PATIENT AND HIS FAMILY

The nurse should be able to:

Name the three stages of illness
Describe reactions of patients in each of these three stages
Identify some of the needs of patients during each of these
    stages
Describe ways in which the nurse may help to meet these
    needs
Describe the impact of illness on the family

ILLNESS, THE PATIENT   4
AND HIS FAMILY

INTRODUCTION

Some people seek medical advice while believing or hoping that they are not ill, but the majority of people seeking such advice are aware that they are sick and in need of help. Once a person makes the decision to obtain medical help he becomes a patient. As a patient he may or may not be restricted in his activities. Many people continue to carry on with their normal daily work and recreational activities even though they have an illness which requires medical supervision. People with hypertension (high blood pressure) or mild diabetes, for example, may only need to come in to the physician's office or to the clinic for periodic checkups and consultation about their health problems unless complications develop. Other people who are ill may have to give up some of their usual activities but do not require hospitalization. They may instead be cared for in their own homes. Many sick people, however, do require the specialized care and services that are available in hospitals and other institutions on an inpatient basis.

In most cases a person is considered to be sick by his family and friends when there is some restriction in his activities or when his illness necessitates taking precautions which interfere with a normal life-style. The individual may not be able to go to work or to school; he may be confined to bed; or he may not be able to undertake certain activities. There are certain expectations that go along with being sick. There is an implicit assumption on the part of others that the person who is ill requires care and cannot be expected to get better merely by an act of will. The sick person is usually excused from work while he is ill; he is not expected to fulfill all his social obligations, or even to carry out his normal functions within the family. However, the patient also has certain obligations. The state of being ill is considered undesirable in most cultures and the patient therefore has an obligation to want to get well. He is also expected to seek competent help to assist him in doing so, and to cooperate with those who provide this help.[1]

THE STAGES OF ILLNESS

In order to be able to provide the patient with the competent care and support he needs, the nurse should have an understanding of the various stages of illness. The patient, during the early stages of his illness, may require a considerable amount of psychological support to help him to accept his illness. When he is acutely ill, his physical needs and the therapeutic aspects of his care may predominate. As he is

---

[1]T. Parsons: Definitions of Health and Illness in the Light of American Values and Social Structure. In *Patients, Physicians and Illness* by E. G. Jaco. Glencoe, Ill., The Free Press, 1958, pp. 165–187.

getting better he may need the help of various members of the health team to assist him in his return to an active life insofar as he is able within the limitations imposed by his illness. Some patients, of course, do not get better, and they require comfort and supportive measures of a different nature (see Chapter 30).

It has been generally accepted that the experience of illness, insofar as the types of illness in which recovery is expected are concerned, consists of three stages: the initial, or transition, stage, when the individual moves gradually (or sometimes abruptly) from a state of health to a state of illness; the stage of "accepted" illness, when he may be acutely ill; and convalescence.[2]

THE INITIAL STAGE
OF ILLNESS

During the initial stage, the patient frequently remains in his home, although many people are admitted to hospital for investigation and undergo a series of diagnostic examinations as inpatients. During this period the patient may experience many of the discomforts that Selye described as "just being sick" (see Chapter 3). He usually does not feel well; he may have distressing symptoms; and he often finds that he cannot keep up with his normal work load without tiring or, perhaps, cannot enjoy his usual leisure-time activities. He may not feel up to going bowling with his friends or participating in the Saturday night bridge game. People are usually irritable when they do not feel well. In women, this irritability may show itself in easy tears which seem to come at the slightest provocation.

People react to the early signs of illness in a variety of ways. Some attempt

to deny that they are ill and "keep going" despite their fatigue, or they may even try to do more than usual to prove to themselves that they are not really sick. Some people respond to the threat of illness with anger; others become very quiet and withdrawn. A few seem to enjoy their symptoms and the attention they receive from other people. If the individual subscribes to the belief that illness is a punishment, or knows that he has been transgressing some of the laws of health, he may feel guilty. Cigarette smokers, for example, are usually very self-conscious and guilt-ridden if they develop a cough or a chest condition. Often people will try all the preventive measures they have heard of, and many of their family and friends' home remedies as well, before they seek medical advice.

By the time an individual has made a decision to seek medical help, he is usually quite worried. His first appointment in the office or the clinic is fraught with anxiety. He wants to know what is wrong with him, and he doesn't want to know. He would like to begin treatment, yet he may be afraid of what "they" are going to do to him. If he has to undergo diagnostic tests or be referred to a specialist for further examinations, his anxiety mounts and he awaits the final verdict with great trepidation. His fears are usually multiplied if he is told that his condition requires surgery or that he needs to be hospitalized for medical therapy. The hospital for most people is an unknown place; many people think of it as a place to die.

The attitude of the nurse in the physician's office or the clinic, and the initial contacts the patient has with the nurse who receives him in the hospital, can do much to ease the patient through this difficult initial period of illness. Kindness and patience are essential. The patients who are most demanding and critical are usually the most frightened ones. Helping to allay their fears is a large part of the nurse's responsibility. The nurse who takes a personal interest in the patient and shows respect for him as an individual does a great deal to offset the depersonalization the

[2]Henry D. Lederer: How the Sick View Their World. In *Social Interaction and Patient Care* by James K. Skipper, Jr., and Robert C. Leonard. Philadelphia, J. B. Lippincott Company, 1965, pp. 155–167. Reprinted from the *Journal of Social Issues*, 8:4–15, 1952.

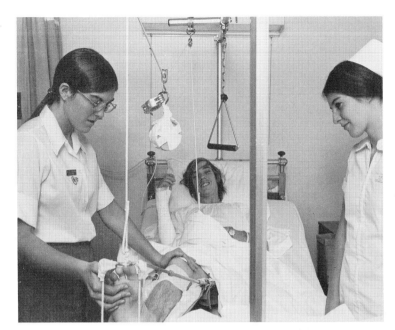

During the acute stage of an illness, the patient may be highly dependent on other people to help him meet his basic needs. This patient, for example, needs help to exercise his leg. The physical therapist is showing the nurse how to move the leg to prevent loss of function of the muscles while the patient is in traction.

patient so often feels in a busy health facility. Explaining treatments and procedures in simple terms, telling him the reason for them and what is going to be done, can take away much of his fear of the unknown. A knowledge of the routines and the physical environment of the nursing unit will help the new patient to feel more comfortable in his new situation (see Chapter 5).

THE STAGE OF ACCEPTED ILLNESS

In the second stage of illness, when a diagnosis (or a tentative one) has been made and therapy has been started, the patient begins to focus his attention and his energies on his illness. He is usually much concerned with his symptoms and wants to know what his temperature is and his blood pressure, and he anxiously awaits the outcome of tests and examinations. The interests of the sick person are usually narrowed; he is much more concerned with himself and with his immediate environment than with anything that goes on outside the sickroom.

The traditional patient-role is essentially a passive-dependent role; for example, the patient accepts prescribed treatments, often with little question. Such acceptance can be particularly difficult for the independent or aggressive person. The patient who has a minor illness may have less need to be dependent and may become critical and demanding.

Three factors contribute to the passive-dependency of the patient. First, a person is usually weakened physically when he is ill; often he simply does not have the strength to carry out his normal activities. Second, the patient is under psychological stress (as well as physical) and so may be less able to cope with situations. The third factor comprises the expectations of the hospital personnel, including nurses. Nurses usually expect the patient to act in a certain way and they communicate their expectations verbally and nonverbally. For example, the patient may be expected to accept a medicine without question.

Today there is much more emphasis on the participation of the patient as a member of the therapeutic team. He is being encouraged to participate in planning his care and in implementing the plan. It is important to create a climate in which this is possible. The patient needs to feel free to express his needs and wants, and to feel that his opinions are respected. When a person participates in planning his care and everything is done, not for him, but rather with him, he assumes more of the responsibility for the outcome. The degree and the type of active participation of a patient vary according to his needs. During the acute stage of an illness the patient may be highly dependent on the nurse. He may need to be bathed, to be changed, he may even need her help in maintaining vital body functions such as breathing, and the nurse is concerned with meeting the patient's dependency needs. It is desirable that each patient become more independent and participate more actively in his own care as he regains his health and as his need for dependence is decreased.

CONVALESCENCE

During the convalescent stage, the patient gradually leaves the sickroom and once again begins to move back into the ordinary everyday world. This is again a transition period and for many a difficult adjustment. The irritability of the convalescent is well known. The attitude of nursing and medical personnel is important in providing the patient with the support and encouragement he requires at this time. Often the patient's family can be of much assistance. Convalescence may be prolonged in some people because they are reluctant to resume the normal responsibilities from which illness excused them. They are often fearful of their ability to resume normal activities. Clear directions on how to care for themselves and simple explanations of what they may expect, combined with the reassurance that help is available if they need it, will often serve to relieve some of the anxiety attendant upon going home from hospital.

THE IMPACT OF ILLNESS ON THE FAMILY

The illness of a family member has an impact on the total family. If the person who is sick is the breadwinner there is a natural concern about loss of his ability to maintain financial responsibility for the family; both he and the other family members may worry about how long he will be unable to work and the using up of sick leave from his place of employment. There may be additional concern over the costs of illness, the payment of medical and hospital bills, and the charges for diagnostic and therapeutic services. The head of the household may not be in a position to make decisions about family matters while he is ill; someone else may have to take over the responsibility for this.

When the mother in the family is sick, household routine is disrupted and other family members must take over the shopping, the planning and cooking of meals, the washing and the ironing. In our small nuclear families, the relatives who might have done this are often thousands of miles away, and the family may have to rely on friends or "homemaker services" to provide help.

If it is an older member of the family who is ill, there is usually much concern. It may be the first member of the household to be seriously ill, and the family is reminded of the mortality of human life. There may be additional worries over who will care for the patient, and again the costs, particularly of prolonged illness, may be a matter to cause considerable concern.

When one of the children is sick, parents are usually very anxious. They may feel guilty of in some way being responsible for the child's illness. Often they feel helpless, and their anxiety and feelings of helplessness may be expressed in hostility and criticism directed toward those who are caring for the child. Many hospitals today permit open visiting on children's wards and encourage parents to share in the care of their children. If the nurse understands some of the reasons behind the parents' behavior and that of

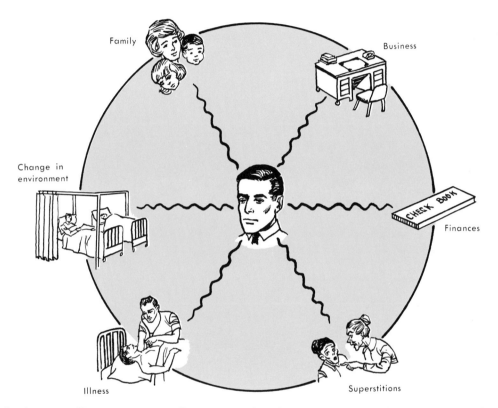

Family

Business

Change in environment

Finances

Illness

Superstitions

Anxiety usually accompanies illness; it is therefore a major consideration in providing nursing care.

family members, and also realizes that her own feelings about this behavior are normal, she is better able to accept hostility and criticism without showing anger and hostility in return.

When a person is hospitalized, his admission has many meanings for him and for his family. While he was ill at home, his care and the responsibility for it probably fell to other family members. After he enters a hospital, the responsibility for his care is transferred from the family to hospital personnel. This transfer of responsibility often produces emotions of mixed relief and guilt on the part of the family: relief because trained people will now provide pro-

fessional care, and perhaps guilt because members of the family feel that the patient would be happier at home or that they have passed on responsibilities that they should be accepting as a family. These feelings are sometimes expressed verbally to hospital personnel or they may be expressed in activities such as bringing food to the patient or by criticizing the personnel and the insitution. If the nurse recognizes the needs of family members and solicits their help in appropriate areas of patient care, such as assisting the patient to eat, the family will feel more comfortable and will be better able to assist in the patient's recovery.

STUDY VOCABULARY

Acute	Hypertension	Patient
Convalescence	Mortality	Transition
Dependency		

STUDY SITUATION

Mr. Lopez is a 34 year old man who works as a truck driver for a large intercontinental van line. He has come to the doctor's office because his back has been bothering him and he finds it difficult to lift the heavy crates he carries in his truck. He also has pain when he drives for long periods. Mr. Lopez is married and has three small children. He asks whether he will have to go to hospital.

1. For what reasons might Mr. Lopez be anxious?

2. What factors might affect how Mr. Lopez reacts to his illness if surgery is needed?

3. What are some of the implications of his illness and how might they affect his family?

4. What can the nurse do to help Mr. Lopez?

BIBLIOGRAPHY

Freeman, Howard E., Sol Levine, and Leo G. Reeder: *Handbook of Medical Sociology.* Englewood Cliffs, N. J., Prentice-Hall, Inc., 1963.

Folta, Jeanette R., and Edith S. Deck: *A Sociological Framework for Patient Care.* New York, John Wiley and Sons, Inc., 1966.

Gordon, Gerald, Odin W. Anderson, Henry P. Brehm and Sue Marquis (eds.): *Disease, the Individual, and Society.* New Haven, College and University Press, 1968.

Jaco, E. Gartly (ed.): *Patients, Physicians and Illness.* New York, The Free Press, 1967. (Also see 1958 edition.)

King, Stanley H.: *Perceptions of Illness and Medical Practice.* New York, Russell Sage Foundation, 1962.

Lederer, Henry D.: How the Sick View Their World. In *Social Interaction and Patient Care* by James K. Skipper, Jr., and Robert C. Leonard (eds.).

Philadelphia, J. B. Lippincott Company, 1965. Reprinted from the *Journal of Social Issues*, 8:4–15, 1952.

Mechanic, David: *Medical Sociology.* New York, The Free Press, 1968.

Tyron, Phyllis, and Robert C. Leonard: Giving the Patient an Active Role. In *Social Interaction and Patient Care* by James K. Skipper, Jr., and Robert C. Leonard. Philadelphia, J. B. Lippincott Company, 1965. pp. 120–127.

5 THE THERAPEUTIC ENVIRONMENT

The nurse should be able to:

Define the term "therapeutic environment"

List the members of the health team in the hospital

Explain some of the main functions of these members

Name factors in the social environment of the hospital which affect the patient

List components of the physical environment of the hospital which contribute to the patient's comfort

Describe the usual procedure for admitting a patient to hospital

Name principles from the social sciences relevant to the care of newly admitted patients

Describe measures which the nurse can take to assist the patient to adjust to the hospital

Describe measures which the nurse can take to assist the patient when he is being discharged from hospital

INTRODUCTION

An environment is the sum total of the external surroundings and influences. It influences people and is in turn influenced by them. It is generally considered that physical, psychological and sociological stimuli of the environment affect the behavior of individuals. The environment therefore affects the way a patient perceives himself and his life situation as well as his role at a given time.

The environment for the care of the sick is made up of two basic components: the physical aspects such as the furniture, the drapes, the lighting, the fixtures and other elements of the furnishings; and the psychosocial aspects that include the people who care for the sick and the customs, cultural values and norms of the agency where this care is provided.

Much attention has been paid in recent years to making the centers and institutions where people receive health care into attractive, warm and friendly places. The cold antiseptic starkness of white and stainless steel that formerly characterized physicians' offices, clinics and hospitals has been replaced in many agencies by color-coordinated decor and comfortable furniture. There is a perceptible change too in the atmosphere of health agencies. Many of the rigid rules and regula-

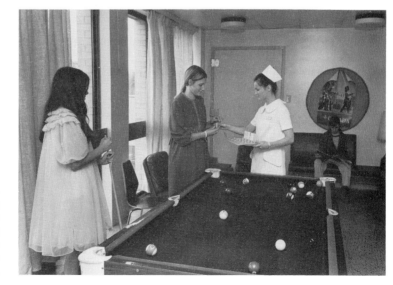

Hospitals today offer many facilities to make the patient's stay more comfortable. A game in the teen-age lounge of a modern hospital is temporarily interrupted for the necessary administration of a medication.

tions that used to govern patient and staff behavior in hospitals are being relaxed. Visiting hours have been extended in most agencies. Families are being encouraged to participate in the care of patients. Patients themselves have greater freedom and are encouraged to do many things for themselves. On many children's wards nurses no longer wear white uniforms but colored smocks or pastel colored uniforms instead. It is not unusual to see the nursing staff in street clothes working with patients on psychiatric units. The nurse should be aware of her role in developing and maintaining an environment which is conducive to health and the recovery from illness.

A THERAPEUTIC ENVIRONMENT

A therapeutic environment is an environment which helps a patient grow, learn and return to health. It is an atmosphere in which the individual is supported in his perceptions of himself as a person of worth. The therapeutic environment is oriented to the needs of the individual, to his importance as an individual capable of solving problems and making decisions.

In such an environment patients are encouraged to participate actively in their care insofar as they are able. Psychological independence is fostered by:

1. Encouraging the patient to participate in his own plan of care

2. Encouraging the patient to assume responsibility and make life decisions for himself within his limitations

3. Helping the patient to develop those patterns of response to stressful stimuli that are compatible with physical and psychological health

4. Helping the patient to function in his sociologically defined roles within his family and the community

5. Helping the patient to gain insight into the limitations within which he must function

6. Helping the patient to make realistic plans for the future

THE HEALTH TEAM

The health team is composed of a variety of personnel representing professional disciplines concerned with the health and welfare of people. The team members, together with the patient and his family, work toward the maintenance or reestablishment of health. The membership varies with the needs of each patient. The physician, the nurse, the dietitian, the social worker often pool information and skills for the benefit of the patient. The clergyman, the public health nurse and the medical specialist are also members of the health team.

Each member of the health team possesses knowledge and skills specific to his discipline. Together, the team is able to make concerted efforts toward a common goal: helping the patient meet his various needs. In many situations the members of the health team meet regularly to confer about the care of patients. In this way, each member augments the services of the other in orienting their functions to goals which will assist the patient and his family.

The patient is often bewildered by the number of different members of the health team beside the physician and the nurse who care for him, particularly in a hospital. It is helpful if the nurse can explain the role and functions of various members of the health care team.

Members of the Nursing Team

The nursing team consists of registered nurses, licensed practical nurses (or nursing assistants), nursing orderlies and nurse's aides. The duties and functions of the different members of the nursing team vary according to the policies of the agency in which they are employed. The registered nurse is responsible for coordinating and supervising the work of other less qualified members of the team. The licensed practical nurse has usually had an educational program of nine months to one year in elementary nursing and may perform many routine nursing procedures and treatments under the direc-

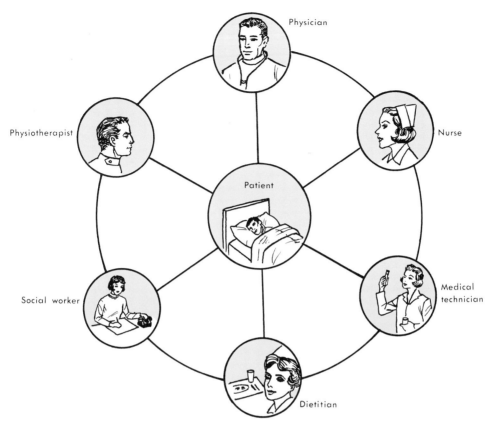

Some members of the health team.

tion of the registered nurse. The nursing orderly usually assists the registered nurse in the personal care of male patients and may do simple nursing tasks. The preparation of the nursing orderly varies from a few weeks of on-the-job training in some places to several months in a program similar to that of the practical nurse. The nurse's aide is frequently trained on the job, or in a course of a few weeks' duration. The nature of the tasks assigned to nurse's aides tends to vary considerably from one agency to another. In some, aides perform tasks that are principally housekeeping in nature, while in others they may assist with the care of patients.

Members of the Medical Team

Patients are admitted to hospital in most instances under the care of their own private physician or a physician on the staff of the hospital to whom they have been assigned. The physician is responsible for directing the therapeutic plan of care for the patient. Most teaching hospitals also have interns and resident physicians. Interns are recent graduates of medical school who have a planned program of clinical experience on the various services of a hospital in order to complete requirements for licensure as practicing physicians. Residents are qualified medical practitioners who are preparing for practice in a medical specialty. In some parts of the country, the internship year is no longer a basic requirement and may instead count toward specialization. If the hospital is affiliated with a medical school there will also be medical students receiving clinical instruction and experience on the hospital wards.

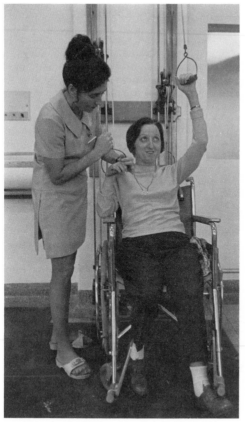

A physical therapist assists a patient with exercises to strengthen her arm muscles.

Other Members of the Health Team

As indicated in Chapter 1, the number of different members of the health team has increased so greatly that it is hard to enumerate them all, let alone describe their roles and functions. Those who work closely with the nurse in the care of the patient include physical therapists and occupational therapists, dietitians, social workers and inhalation therapists.

The *physical therapist* has specialized preparation in physical therapy in a three to four year program of post–high school studies. He assists in assessing the patient's functional ability, strength and mobility; carries out therapeutic treatments, particularly those dealing with the musculoskeletal system; and teaches families and patients exercises and other measures which can contribute to the patient's recovery and rehabilitation.

The *occupational therapist* has a preparation similar to that of the physical therapist; many individuals, in fact, hold a combined degree in physical and occupational therapy. The occupational therapist is primarily concerned, however, with the restoration of bodily function through specific tasks or skills, rather than exercises and treatments. Occupational therapists frequently play a large role in rehabilitation by helping people to develop new skills or to regain skills lessened or lost through illness.

The *dietitian's* special area of expertise is nutrition. The title "nutritionist" is frequently used if the individual is employed in a community agency; "dietitian" if she is employed in a hospital or institutional agency. In a hospital, the dietitian is usually responsible for planning meal service for patients and staff, supervising other workers in the preparation of food and counselling patients about their nutrition problems. The dietitian has usually had a four to five year course of university studies and a year of internship in a hospital.

The *social worker* assists in evaluating the psychosocial situation of the patient and helps patients with their social problems. She (or he) usually has extensive knowledge of community agencies and frequently makes arrangements for home care or for the referral of the patient to other agencies. The majority of social workers hold a baccalaureate or master's degree in social work; however, many community colleges are now offering courses for the preparation of assistant social workers.

The *inhalation therapist* is an expert in diagnostic procedures and therapeutic measures used in the care of patients with respiratory problems. He is skilled in handling oxygen therapy equipment, for example. Programs in inhalation therapy are usually of two to three years' duration and are offered in

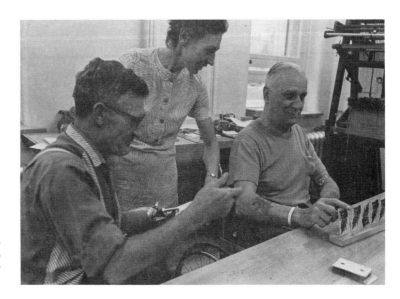

An occupational therapist assists two amputees to learn to play cards, using a specially devised card rack.

community colleges or other types of post–high school educational institutions.

A large variety of medical technicians also assist in patient care. These include the laboratory technicians, the x-ray technicians, and a number of other technicians whose work is highly specialized. As medical technology advances, the number of skilled technicians required to handle the complex equipment used in medical diagnosis and treatment increases correspondingly.

THE SOCIAL ENVIRONMENT OF THE HOSPITAL

The social setting of a hospital includes customs, roles, cultural values and norms. These vary somewhat from community to community, but many characteristics are similar in hospitals throughout this country.

The person outside the hospital sees the hospital as a different world; that is, as a place where life and death are in a delicate balance under the control of those who work there. Actually the personnel of the hospital are part of a highly structured bureaucratic organization, each person having his defined

role and status, which are often indicated by special insignias or uniforms. Lines of authority are well defined, and they become apparent fairly quickly to the new patient. The differences between the student nurse and graduate nurse or between the intern and the resident physician, for example, are made obvious through behavior patterns and verbal communication. This hierarchy of the hospital is justified as being necessary for quick, precise and responsible action in a time of crisis.

The rules and regulations of a hospital, then, govern much of the activity of its personnel. The functions of various groups are often rigidly delimited, a situation which sometimes contributes to the difficulty encountered by the nurse in assuming her primary responsibility of orienting nursing care to patients' needs.

Patients soon become familiar with the rules of the hospital; what is not explained by hospital personnel is explained by the patients already indoctrinated in hospital ways. Indoctrinated patients also initiate the newcomer in the unofficial rules and practices of hospital life, which can be stronger and have a greater influence than the official rules of the institution. Their acceptance by the patient often facilitates his membership in the in-group of his peers.

When patients remain in a hospital for extended periods of time, the social relations among them have considerable influence over their hospital life, although this influence is diminishing in the modern hospital. Today patients stay in the hospital for shorter periods and consequently find that their opportunities to meet other patients have lessened. The changes in hospital design have also affected the social lives of patients. The single room or shared room of today's hospital offers patients more privacy and more comfortable facilities than the large open ward. It also contributes to the safety of the patient by facilitating the prevention and control of infection, but it does provide for fewer contacts than did the open ward with its large groups of people. This restriction is compensated for to some extent in many agencies through the provision of television rooms, patient lounges and dining areas where patients may meet and talk with other patients or with their families. Nevertheless, patients are essentially more isolated than they were in the past, and as a result have less influence upon each other and upon hospital life. This does not mean that one patient does not learn from another, but it does mean that he usually has fewer role models from which to choose.

Although not a part of the bureaucratic organization of the hospital, the patient is the focus of it. He is affected directly and indirectly by most of the rules and policies of the institution. He is affected directly, for example, by a rule which limits smoking to the hours between 6 A.M. and 10 P.M. He is affected indirectly by a policy which allows hospital employees one coffee break a day.

Sometimes the demands of the institution conflict with the professional standards of its personnel, and as a result patients can be affected. For example, the hospital administrators may expect a nurse to care for 10 patients, whereas her professional standards can be met only if she looks after just three patients. Consequently the nurse is confronted with a dilemma.

Different solutions to this problem have been proposed. The nurse often has to set priorities and decide which tasks are essential and which may safely be left. She may have to delegate some of the responsibilities for care to other workers. In this case, she must use her judgment in evaluating the capabilities of other members of the nursing team and deciding on the tasks appropriate for them. Many agencies provide extra nursing personnel who may be called upon and temporarily assigned to a nursing unit if it is particularly busy. Sometimes, the realignment of nursing schedules and routines helps to overcome the problem of too many things for the nurse to do at one time. Not all patients need a bath every day, nor do all baths have to be given in the morning. In a number of hospitals today, many routine nursing procedures are being questioned as to their real value in patient care. The elimination of the early morning taking of temperatures for every patient is an example of one traditional nursing routine which has been dropped by many agencies.

Through media such as television, radio and literature, people have become more sophisticated about hospital life and frequently come to the hospital with definite expectations. The degree to which these expectations correlate with the actual situation has much to do with the person's adjustment to the hospital and to his role as a patient.

THE PHYSICAL ENVIRONMENT OF THE HOSPITAL

The physical environment of the hospital is an important aspect of the patient's care. When a person is ill, his immediate surroundings mean a great deal to him. Frequently he is confined to one room and there he sleeps, eats his meals and entertains his visitors. Factors in the environment which influence his comfort are often not under his control. He may not be able to adjust the lighting or the temperature and humidity of the room himself, nor be able to close the door to lessen noise or open the windows for a breath of fresh air. One of the important aspects of the nurse's responsibility in caring for the patient is adjusting the environment to suit the patient's needs.

Temperature

People differ in the temperatures at which they feel most comfortable; often the elderly person feels the cold more than the younger patient. Generally speaking it has been found that the best room temperature for an adult at sedentary work is 68 to 72° F. for the male and 75° F. for the female. The temperature is higher for the female because she wears lighter clothing. Usually the temperature in the hospital is maintained between 69 and 72° F.

Maintaining a constant temperature usually involves heating during the winter months and air conditioning during the summer months. Traditional steam and hot water heating are still used extensively in institutions throughout the country; however, modern hot air heating is receiving increasing attention. Air conditioning is particularly advantageous in hot humid areas. Some hospitals are entirely air conditioned, whereas others have air conditioned patient units or special areas such as intensive care units and operating room theaters. It is believed that the optimal air movement for air conditioning varies between 10 and 80 cubic feet per minute, depending upon the temperature of the room.

Humidity

Humidity refers to the amount of moisture in the air. The comfort of a person is highly dependent upon humidity, for when the humidity is high there is a decrease in the rate of evaporation of perspiration. A humidity of over 80 per cent is generally unpleasant for most people. A hospital humidity of 40 to 60 per cent is thought to be comfortable. In special situations, high humidity environments are created in order to administer moist air to patients as a therapeutic measure. For this purpose, high humidity rooms are sometimes established, but more often the high humidity is restricted to the air immediately surrounding the patient's head.

Acoustics

Acoustics refers to sound. In hospitals, acoustics are usually concerned with the prevention of noise. People who are ill are frequently highly sensitive to loud noises. Moreover, the hospital patient cannot get away from the noise; it often disturbs his sleep and is particularly bothersome owing to the lack of diversions.

Many of the materials and techniques used in hospitals to dampen noise are based on studies by industry regarding the effect of noise upon efficiency of work. For example, hospitals use special materials on the walls, on the floors and on the ceilings to absorb sound. In addition, architects design nursing units so that work areas are not in the immediate vicinity of the patients' rooms. Movable equipment is fitted with rubber wheels in order that it will move quietly and smoothly. Plastic utensils are used in many agencies now instead of stainless steel, and these also help to lessen noise. All these considerations contribute to a more restful atmosphere.

Lighting

Most hospitals try to make use of natural lighting as much as possible. Not only is sunshine cheerful, but it is also less expensive than electricity. MacEacheren stated that in general artificial lighting should be indirect and that the fixtures should be constructed in such a way that they can be easily cleaned and will not harbor dust.[1] In addition to general lighting most patients require a reading light. Often reading lights are constructed with extendable arms so that they can also be used to provide light during treatments. Hospitals are

---

[1]Malcolm T. MacEacheren: *Hospital Organization and Management.* Third edition. Chicago, Physicians Record Company, 1957, p. 62.

also equipped with night lights in the halls and in the patients' rooms. These are installed in such a way as to provide a subdued light on the floor which is not disturbing to patients in bed.

Decor

The color scheme and the decor of a hospital are extremely important. Years ago hospital walls, ceilings and equipment were entirely white. Recently, however, the importance of the effect of color upon employees and patients has been recognized. Generally, muted pastels are desirable for patients' rooms because they are more restful than strong colors. Psychologists have found that different colors have different meanings. Blue is said to be calming, whereas red often represents anger. Moreover color has an effect upon illumination; lighter colors reflect more light than do darker colors. Today, hospitals are generally attractively decorated. Gone are the white walls and white beds. In their place attractive colors and designs prevail.

Furniture

Furniture should possess certain qualities. It should be easily movable; thus most of the furniture is equipped with rubber castors which turn easily and quietly. The furniture should be easy to clean. This means that corners should be rounded and "dust catchers," such as decorative sculptures, eliminated. In addition, surfaces are hard and durable in order to withstand cleaning and long use.

The patient's room is usually equipped with the following furniture:

The Bed. The hospital bed is 3 feet in width, 6 feet 6 inches in length and 26 inches in height. There are also 7-foot beds available for taller patients. There are adjustable beds that can be lowered to a height which makes it easier for the patient to get out of bed. The adjustable bed is left in the low position unless the nurse is working at the bedside. When the bed is in this position the patient is close to the floor in case he falls or if he wishes to get out of bed.

The hospital bed also has head and knee gatches. These are generally operated by cranks, either at the side or at the foot of the bed. They allow the head of the bed to be raised, and a raised break to be formed about one-third of the distance from the foot of the bed. The bed can also be elevated at the foot by lifting the bed itself and putting locking pins through the inner tubes of the legs at the foot. Some beds can be operated by electricity, and often the buttons to operate these beds are within easy reach of the patient.

The Mattress. The mattresses that are used in hospitals are made of various materials, usually cottons, kapok, or horsehair. Because the hospital patient spends a great deal of time in bed, a firm mattress is of utmost importance for his comfort and for maintaining good body alignment. Some mattresses are covered with a plastic material to protect them and facilitate their cleaning. If the covers are not plastic they should be made of a durable material which cleans easily.

Foam rubber mattresses, water mattresses and sawdust and air mattresses are sometimes used to equalize pressure upon the patient's skin.

Pillows. Each bed normally has at least two pillows, one soft and one firm. The pillows are made of feathers or kapok. The soft pillow is placed on top of the firm pillow. It supports the patient's shoulders and head. Sponge rubber pillows are also used in hospitals, particularly by patients who have allergies.

Pillows are also used to support patients in particular anatomical positions. A pillow at the patient's back while he is on his side offers firm support and comfort.

Linen. Each bed usually has two cotton sheets, a cotton drawsheet, a plastic or rubber drawsheet, two pillow cases, a blanket and a bedspread. The cotton sheets are made of strong, heavy cotton which is long-wearing and can be pulled tightly. The routine use of drawsheets has been discontinued in many hospitals and, increasingly, they are being used only when needed. The purpose of the plastic or rubber drawsheet is to protect the bottom sheet and the mattress from soilage. Unfortunately they often hold body heat and wrinkle uncomfortably under patients. Many agencies are not using blankets on patients' beds any more. The temperature in patient areas of a hospital is often maintained at a sufficiently constant temperature for blankets to be unnecessary. If blankets are used, they are usually made of wool and cotton, although a loose cotton weave is becoming increasingly popular in some areas. The bedspreads are traditionally of white cotton, but colors are being seen more frequently in hospitals today.

The Overbed Table. The overbed table is movable and usually its height is adjustable. Often they have built-in mirrors and book rests. The overbed table is used for a variety of purposes; for example, as a meal tray, as a table for a portable television or as a nursing treatment tray.

The Bedside Table. The bedside table is high enough so that a patient can reach its top surface comfortably. It usually has a small drawer in which the patient can keep his personal belongings and a cupboard in which he may keep his wash basin, mouth care accessories, bath blanket and possibly a bedpan or urinal. Some bedside tables have a rod across the back upon which the patient's towel and wash cloth are hung.

Bedside tables are easily moved and some can be adjusted to different heights. Many patients like to keep their radios on the bedside table, where they may be secured to prevent their falling.

Chairs. There is usually a chair at the patient's bedside which has a straight back and is of simple construction. It can be used by the patient's visitors and by the patient if necessary. Because this chair does not have arms, it does not afford the patient much support if he is sitting for a long period of time.

Usually there is also an armchair in the patient's room. This is more com-fortable and offers good support. The one drawback of many armchairs is that they are so low that it is sometimes difficult for a patient to raise himself out of them. In two- or four-patient bedrooms there is often only one armchair. Armchairs in the hospital are covered by a durable material which is easily cleaned.

The Equipment

The equipment used in hospitals is diverse in design and in purpose. Generally it is portable, quiet, durable, simple to operate, easily cleaned and easily repaired. More and more, facilities are being built into the patient's unit. Facilities for wall suction and piped-in oxygen, for example, are common. The multiplicity of equipment that is used in hospitals precludes a more specific description here.

ADMISSION TO THE HOSPITAL

The admission of the patient to a hospital is a critical period in his hospital stay. The patient is usually apprehensive, and the attitude and behavior of the nurses and other hospital personnel concerned with his admission can do much to make him feel more comfortable. A sincere welcome and genuine interest in the patient help to reassure him that he is a person of worth and dignity. Many hospitals, particularly large ones, have been criticized for their impersonality. Much of the criticism stems from the fact that hospitals are busy places and the personnel are often rushed. But it does not take extra time to be kind or to convey to the patient that he is welcome.

When a patient comes to a hospital he usually goes initially to the admitting office. Here he answers the questions of the admitting clerk or admitting nurse about his financial status, his age, his address, his next of kin and his usual employment. Most hospitals supply an admission sheet for this purpose.

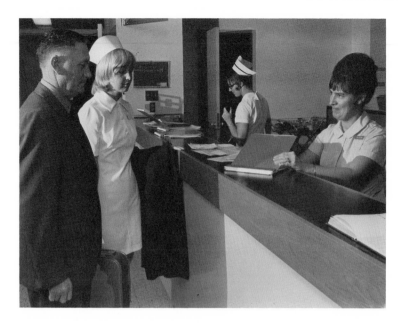

A friendly smile can help to allay some of the anxiety a patient feels on admission to hospital.

Often the patient's initial impression of a hospital is formed in the admitting department. Thus the appearance of the area and the kind of reception provided by the staff is of utmost importance. If a patient is acutely ill, however, he may be admitted to the emergency department of the hospital. In this case it is often a member of the family of the patient who gives the needed information to the admitting clerk. Most hospitals ask patients to sign a consent form during the admitting procedure. This form gives the hospital staff permission to perform any diagnostic and treatment procedures that are considered necessary during the patient's stay.

After the patient has given the requested information to the receptionist in the admitting department, he is usually shown to a nursing unit. In some hospitals, patients who are admitted late at night or will be staying a very short time are often sent to an area called the observation ward. The range of stay in this ward is usually one hour to 48 hours, but this varies according to the hospital policy. In this area the patient is given an orientation to the hospital, his medical history is taken and routine laboratory work is performed.

The patient may also receive a surgical skin preparation and be visited by members of the health team.[2]

When the patient arrives at the nursing unit, a sincere welcome is again important in helping to ease the adjustment to his new environment. The patient should be greeted by name. His family or friends who have accompanied him to hospital should also be made welcome. The patient's room or his bed unit should be ready for him so that he feels expected and welcome. The nurse can help the patient by showing him where showers and bathrooms are located, also telephones and other facilities, and by explaining various routines such as mealtimes and visiting hours. In orienting the patient to his new situation the following points are helpful to keep in mind:

1. The patient needs an introduction to nursing unit personnel and a brief explanation of their duties.
2. He needs an introduction to other patients in the room in which he will be staying.

[2]June Finsterle and Robert S. Vail: An Admitting Suite for the First Critical Hospital Hours. *Hospitals,* 37:45–46, November 1, 1963.

3. He needs an explanation of pertinent hospital routines and policies. These assist the patient to become familiar with what is expected of him and what he may expect. Many hospitals have prepared patient information booklets which are very helpful in this regard.

4. He needs to know how his call light or the intercom system at the patient unit is operated.

The nurse should also find out if the patient has any particular needs or desires which would make his stay in the hospital more comfortable. Some patients, because of their religious or cultural backgrounds, have specific dietary requests, and the dietitian should be informed about these. The nurse should also find out from the patient if he has any allergies and if he has been on any medications at home such as steroids. These observations should be noted on the patient's record and reported to the attending physician.

Once the initial orientation to the hospital has been completed, the patient is usually examined by the hospital physician. This examination includes a medical history, a physical examination and routine screening tests. The Joint Commission on Accreditation of Hospitals requires that all patients admitted to a hospital have a urinalysis and a hemoglobin or hematocrit test.[3] Many hospitals require a chest x-ray and a blood serology test for syphilis as part of the admission routine. Tests for pulmonary function and also tests for blood sugar are performed routinely for all newly admitted patients in some hospitals.

During her contact with the patient, the nurse observes him closely and listens to him carefully. The initial observations of the nurse are of particular importance in assessing the patient's needs. Her observations assist the doctor in his diagnosis and form a basis for the nursing care plan of the patient. In fact, they can assist the entire hospital team in helping the patient meet his physical, sociological and psychological needs.

Basic Principles for the Care of the Patient Admitted to the Hospital

Basic to helping a patient adjust to his illness and to a strange environment are an understanding of certain principles which can serve as guides to action for both the nurse and the patient:

Strange Situations Can Elicit Fear. When people enter a hospital, for example, they encounter a new environment and a new set of behavior norms. Most patients recognize their need to become familiar with the customs and the policies of the hospital. In fact, the patients themselves often provide the new patient with information about the hospital and nursing unit personnel, anticipating his need for information and allaying his fears by explanations.

Illness Can Be a Novel Experience. As a consequence people require an understanding of their illness and of how they view their situation. By assisting the patient to regain or maintain control over his own activities and by helping him to solve the problems he faces, the nurse can support patients in their sick-role.

Patterns of Response Are Learned. A person may fear a situation not because of the situation itself but because of conditioning through previous learning. Thus, a patient may view certain hospital situations as threats to his integrity. By understanding that a person's response is often a result of previous experiences, the nurse can better anticipate her patients' needs and reactions.

Maintaining Personal Identity Is Important. A person's name, clothes and valuables frequently serve as symbols of his identity. They also represent security to many people, since they serve as a link with the understood and the familiar. The nurse can help a patient to maintain his identity by making a point of calling him by name and by encouraging him to use his own clothes

[3]What Tests Are Routine? *The Modern Hospital*, 93:51, September, 1959.

(*Text continued on page 58.*)

AUTHORITY TO DIVULGE INFORMATION:

IF THIS HOSPITAL OR PHYSICIANS ACCOUNT IS TO BE PAID BY ANY FORM OF INSURANCE, OR IN THE CASE OF AN INDIGENT BY A MUNICIPALITY, I HEREBY AUTHORIZE THE RIVERSIDE HOSPITAL TO FURNISH TO SAID PARTIES SUCH INFORMATION AS MAY BE NECESSARY FOR THE SETTLEMENT OF ANY CLAIMS.

CONSENT TO TREATMENT - TRANSFER - OR REMOVAL

I HEREBY AUTHORIZE AND DIRECT THE ATTENDING PHYSICIAN, AND HOSPITAL STAFF TO CARRY OUT SUCH FORMS OF EXAMINATIONS, TESTS, AND TREATMENT AS THEY MAY DEEM NECESSARY FOR THE PHYSICAL IMPROVEMENT OF _James Doe_ . SHOULD IT BE FOUND NECESSARY OR DEEMED ADVISABLE IN THEIR OPINION TO TRANSFER THE PATIENT TO ANOTHER HOSPITAL, I HEREBY CONSENT THERETO. I FURTHER AGREE TO LEAVE THE HOSPITAL OR REMOVE SAID PATIENT WHEN REQUESTED TO DO SO BY THE ADMINISTRATOR OR HIS ASSISTANT.

DATE _October 15 1971_   SIGNED _Mrs. John Doe_

WITNESS _____   RELATIONSHIP _Mother_
                                                    (IF OTHER THAN PATIENT)
RELATIONSHIP _____

OBSTETRICAL CONSENT:

I HEREBY AUTHORIZE AND DIRECT MY ATTENDING OBSTETRICIAN AND/OR HIS ASSOCIATES OR ASSISTANTS TO PROVIDE SUCH SERVICES FOR ME AS THEY MAY DEEM REASONABLE AND NECESSARY, INCLUDING, BUT NOT LIMITED TO, THE ADMINISTRATION OF ANAESTHESIA, AND THE PERFORMANCE OF SERVICES INVOLVING SURGERY, PATHOLOGY AND RADIOLOGY, AND I HEREBY CONSENT THERETO. I FURTHER CONSENT TO THE CIRCUMCISION OF MY BABY SHOULD IT BE DEEMED NECESSARY. THIS CONSENT FURTHER INCLUDES THE AUTHORITY TO DIVULGE INFORMATION AS NOTED TO ABOVE.

DATE _____   SIGNED _____

WITNESS _____   RELATIONSHIP _____
                                                    (IF OTHER THAN PATIENT)
RELATIONSHIP _____

CONSENT TO OPERATION AND ANAESTHESIA:

THE PHYSICAL CONDITION AND THE SURGICAL PROCEDURE CONTEMPLATED TO ALLEVIATE THIS CONDITION HAS BEEN EXPLAINED TO ME BY DR. _D. Smith_ AND I HEREBY AUTHORIZE AND DIRECT HIM AND/OR HIS ASSOCIATES OR ASSISTANTS TO OPERATE UPON _James Doe_ FOR THIS CONDITION, AND/OR TO DO ANY OTHER THERAPEUTIC PROCEDURE HIS/THER JUDGEMENT MAY DICTATE TO BE ADVISABLE FOR THE PATIENTS WELL BEING. AND I FURTHER CONSENT TO SUCH ADDITIONAL SERVICES AS THEY MAY DEEM REASONABLE AND NECESSARY, INCLUDING, BUT NOT LIMITED TO THE ADMINISTRATION AND MAINTENANCE OF ANAESTHESIA AND THE PERFORMANCES OF SERVICES INVOLVING PATHOLOGY AND RADIOLOGY. THIS CONSENT FURTHER INCLUDES CONSENT TO TREATMENT AND AUTHORITY TO DIVULGE INFORMATION AS NOTED AT TOP OF PAGE.

DATE _October 18 1971_   SIGNED _Mrs. John Doe_

WITNESS _Mary Smith_   RELATIONSHIP _Mother_
                                                    (IF OTHER THAN PATIENT)
RELATIONSHIP _____

LEAVING HOSPITAL AGAINST ADVICE:

THIS IS TO CERTIFY THAT _____ AM/IS LEAVING THE RIVERSIDE HOSPITAL AGAINST THE ADVICE OF THE ATTENDING PHYSICIAN AND THE HOSPITAL ADMINISTRATION. I ACKNOWLEDGE THAT I HAVE BEEN INFORMED OF THE RISKS INVOLVED AND HEREBY RELEASE THE ATTENDING PHYSICIAN AND THE HOSPITAL FROM ALL RESPONSIBILITY OF ANY ILL EFFECTS WHICH MAY RESULT FROM THIS ACTION.

DATE _____   SIGNED _____
                                                    (PATIENT/OR PARENT/OR GUARDIAN)
WITNESS _____   RELATIONSHIP _____
                                                    (IF OTHER THAN PATIENT)
RELATIONSHIP _____

Sample of a Patient's Consent Form. (Courtesy of the Riverside Hospital of Ottawa.)

SUMMARY SHEET	NOV 4 71
RIVERSIDE HOSPITAL OF OTTAWA	

DATE OF ADMISSION

DATE OF DISCHARGE (DEATH IN RED INK)

REFERRING PHYSICIAN

ATTENDING PHYSICIAN

DOE   JAMES   SP 1247
123 STATE ST   OTT   234-7566-600
DOE   JOHN   FATHER
SAME
18.10.71   2PM M 12 S SURG   RC
              420   1

STANDARD NOMENCLATURE
CODE NUMBER

FINAL DIAGNOSIS _____

SECONDARY DIAGNOSIS _____

COMPLICATIONS (INFECTIONS, ETC.)

OPERATIONS

CONSULTATIONS   YES ☐   NO ☐

NAME OF CONSULTANT _____

RESULTS: ☐   RECOVERED ☐   IMPROVED ☐   NOT IMPROVED ☐   NOT TREATED ☐   DIAGNOSIS ONLY ☐   DIED ☐

UNDER 48 HRS. ☐   OVER 48 HRS. ☐

CAUSE OF DEATH: _____

_____ AUTOPSY   YES ☐   NO ☐

I HAVE EXAMINED AND APPROVED THIS COMPLETE MEDICAL RECORD ON _____ 19 ___

_____ M.D.
ATTENDING PHYSICIAN

2-8261

(Continued)

RIVERSIDE HOSPITAL OF OTTAWA

RESPONSIBILITY FOR RETAINING PERSONAL POSSESSIONS

I hereby assume all **responsibility for any** items of clothing, toilet articles, jewelry, money, or any other type of personal possessions whatsoever, retained or brought in for the use of

James Doe while a **Patient in the** Riverside Hospital of Ottawa, and I hereby **release** the **Staff and** Hospital Admin- istration from any liability which may **result** from the loss of/or damage to any of the said articles by **any** means whatsoever, while they are in the building. I further agree to comply with any restrictions as to their use which may be requested by either the Medical or Nursing staff for the benefit of any Patient. It is further agreed that this privilege of retention does not extend at any time to any type of previously ordered medication **nor** to alcoholic beverages, neither of which are allowed in the Hospital. Both will be supplied by the Hospital Pharmacy if required on order of the Attending Physician.

DATE: _October 18, 1971_   SIGNED: _Mrs John Doe_

WITNESS: _Mary Smith_   RELATIONSHIP: _Mother_

(if other than Patient signs or if Patient is a minor.)

2-8774

Sample of a Responsibility for Retaining Personal Possessions Form. (Courtesy of the River-side Hospital of Ottawa.)

(when this is hospital policy) and personal possessions when he is admitted to the hospital.

Subgroups Within a Culture Tend to Develop Their Own Norms of Behavior. An understanding of the diversity of habits and modes of behavior and an endeavor to assist each patient to maintain his particular patterns whenever they do not jeopardize his health will help the patient to maintain his identity and will serve to acknowledge respect for him as an individual. Sometimes the behavior of a patient differs from what the nurse expects; nevertheless, acceptance of the patient as a person is basic to the kind of nursing care that enhances his confidence and security.

Articles received for safekeeping

```
SMITH      MARY          SP 1246
2321  MARKET ST  OTT  234-7566-600
JONES     RICHARD    HUS
SAME
11.9.71  2PM  F 23 M    SURG   RC
       420   1
```

Dentures	upper	
	lower	
	partial	
Glasses		
Contact Lenses		✓
Other Prostheses		

Date *September 1, 1971*

Marie Lefebvre
Signature of Nurse

Mary Smith
Signature of Patient

Articles returned

Patient Signature

Signature of Nurse

Sample of an envelope used to receive valuable articles for safekeeping. (Courtesy of the Riverside Hospital of Ottawa.)

Specific Admitting Measures

Two nursing care measures which are concerned specifically with the admission of a patient to a hospital are the care of his clothes and the care of his valuables.

Care of the Patient's Clothes. The manner of caring for a patient's clothes upon his admission to a hospital is dependent upon the policy of the specific hospital. In some hospitals the family is asked to take the patient's clothes home; in others the clothes are stored in a central clothes room after each article of clothing is listed on a hospital form. An increasingly more common procedure is for the patient to keep his clothes in a closet that is provided in his room. In this case a clothing list is usually not made; instead the patient signs a form which states that he assumes responsibility for all the belongings that he brings to the hospital. Occasionally a patient's clothes are infested with vermin; most hospitals provide facilities for sterilizing such clothes before they are returned to the patient.

Because clothes are so often important symbols of identity to a patient, some hospitals suggest that patients wear their own clothes while they are staying there. However, a more common practice is to provide each patient with a hospital gown or pajamas, particularly if he is to have an operation.

Care of the Patient's Valuables. If a patient is unconscious, very ill or otherwise incompetent when he comes to the hospital, his valuables are often sent to the cashier's office for safe-keeping. The valuables of the patient usually include his money, jewelry, personal papers and any other personal effects of value. Valuables which the patient usually wants to keep at his bedside include eyeglasses or contact lenses and dentures. If a patient is lucid and rational upon his admission to the hospital he usually signs a statement in which he assumes responsibility for the valuables which he keeps at his bedside. Patients

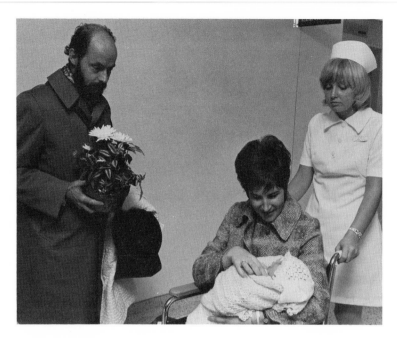

Discharge from a health agency such as a hospital is frequently accompanied by anxiety about the future.

are often encouraged to ask their relatives to take home articles of great value rather than risk their theft or damage. Many hospitals routinely provide facilities for the safe storage of valuables.

DISCHARGE FROM THE HOSPITAL

Hospitals provide a protective environment for their patients, and the world outside often becomes remote, threatening and somewhat awesome to them. Thus, at discharge the joy of being united with one's family and being restored to a state of good health are often mixed with fear and anxiety about the future.

Patients, then, are genuinely concerned about their discharge. They wonder about how they will be able to manage, about being a burden to their families and about their ability to contribute as a functioning member of the family and the community.

Many patients are anxious about the adjustments they must make in their life situations as a result of physical limita-

tions. Changes in occupation and in a way of life are not easily accepted and are often looked upon with fear.

The psychological and physical needs of the patient at discharge can often be met by the patient himself with the support of his family and members of the health team. Some of the common needs of patients are:

1. The need to accept the limitations imposed by illness
2. The need to learn to function effectively within these limitations
3. The need to be accepted as a member of the family and the community
4. The need to learn specific skills and possess specific knowledge pertinent to healthful living

Patients are usually discharged from the hospital, or other health agency, when they no longer require the services it offers. Occasionally, however, a patient leaves a hospital against the advice of the doctor. In such instances, most hospitals require the patient to sign a form that relieves the hospital and the physician of responsibility for any subsequent ill effects. If a person refuses to sign this release the hospital administrator and physician are informed directly.

Should a patient require the services of another agency, the referral is made prior to his discharge. In a hospital the business office must also be notified in order to prepare the patient's financial record so that the patient or his family can make the final business arrangements on the day of discharge.

On the day of discharge the nurse assists the patient with his clothes and personal valuables. She also checks with the patient about any last minute questions he may have about his after-care. New learning material should not be given to the patient just before he leaves the hospital, because patients find it difficult to remember instructions at this time. Moreover, last minute teaching never replaces a teaching plan that has extended over the time of the patient's stay in the hospital. Any final details are written down: for example, the date and time of his appointment with the physician.

When a patient leaves the hospital he is escorted to the door of the hospital. Some hospitals have a policy that all patients are discharged in a wheelchair. In this way a patient does not overtax his strength while leaving the nursing unit.

In summary the nurse has certain responsibilities in a patient's discharge from an agency.

1. Checking that the physician has signed the order for discharge

2. Helping the patient, as he requires, with his transportation, clothing and personal effects

3. Clarifying any questions that the patient might have about after-care

4. Notifying the business office and other related services in advance of the patient's discharge

4. Arranging the necessary referrals with the physician and the patient in cases in which the patient's after-care is to be administered in a hospital department such as the outpatient department

6. Escorting the patient to the door of the hospital upon discharge

An important part of any discharge procedure from a hospital is the entering of dismissal notes on the patient's record. It is general practice to include in the nurse's notes the general condition of the patient, the time of discharge and any particular circumstances relevant to his discharge.

GUIDE TO **ASSESSING** **NURSING NEEDS**	1. What does the patient need to know about his new environment? 2. Does he have any allergies? 3. Has he been taking medications at home? If so, what are they? 4. Does he have any particular food likes and dislikes? 5. Is the social and physical setting in the hospital conducive to health for the individual patient? For example: a. Light b. Noise c. Compatibility of nearby patients

**STUDY
VOCABULARY**

Dietitian	Nurse's aide	Resident
Environment	Nursing orderly	Social worker
Health team	Nutritionist	Therapeutic
Inhalation therapist	Occupational therapist	environment
Intern	Physical therapist	Therapy

**STUDY
SITUATION**

Mr. Austin is a 54 year old businessman. He has a gastric ulcer and he arrives at the hospital to rest for three days before his surgery. Mr. Austin is active and he has a phone put in his room in order that he can continue to take care of his business.

1. What factors would you take into consideration in orienting Mr. Austin?
2. What sociological and psychological principles would guide you and the patient in his orientation?
3. What particular needs might this patient have?
4. Outline an orientation program for this patient.
5. What situations can you anticipate that might be a source of distress to this patient? How should you plan to deal with these?

BIBLIOGRAPHY

Anderson, Barbara J., Hilda Mertz and Robert C. Leonard: Two Experimental Tests of a Patient-Centered Admission Process. *Nursing Research,* 14:151–157, Spring, 1965.

Backmeyer, Arthur C. (ed.): *The Hospital in Modern Society.* New York, The Commonwealth Fund, 1943.

Brown, Esther Lucile: Meeting Patients' Psychological Needs in a General Hospital. In *Social Interaction and Patient Care* by James K. Skipper, Jr., and Robert C. Leonard. Philadelphia, J. B. Lippincott Company, 1965, pp. 6–15. Reprinted from *The Annals of the Academy of Political and Social Science,* 346:117–125, March, 1963.

Burling, Temple, Edith M. Lentz and Robert N. Wilson: *The Give and Take in Hospitals.* New York, G. P. Putnam's Sons, 1956.

Elms, Roslyn R.: Effects of Varied Nursing Approaches During Hospital Admissions: An Exploratory Study. *Nursing Research,* 13:266–268, Summer, 1964.

Finsterle, June and Robert S. Vail: An Admitting Suite for the First Critical Hospital Hours. *Hospitals,* 37:44–46, November 1, 1963.

Friedman, Sigmund L.: The Day Hospital. *Hospital Topics,* 40:47–52, March, 1962.

Ingles, Thelma: Do Patients Feel Lost in a General Hospital? *The American Journal of Nursing,* 60:648–651, May, 1960.

MacEacheren, Malcolm T.: *Hospital Organization and Management.* Third edition. Chicago, Physicians Record Company, 1957.

Malone, Mary F.: The Dilemma of a Professional in a Bureaucracy. *Nursing Forum,* 3:36–60, 1964.

Mauksch, Hans O.: It Defies All Logic but A Hospital Does Function. In *Social Interaction and Patient Care* by James K. Skipper, Jr., and Robert C. Leonard (eds.). Philadelphia, J. B. Lippincott Company, 1965, pp. 245–251.

Siegel, Nathaniel: What Is a Therapeutic Community? *Nursing Outlook,* 12:49–51, May, 1964.

Skipper, James K., Jr., and Robert C. Leonard (eds.): *Social Interaction and Patient Care.* Philadelphia, J. B. Lippincott Company, 1965.

Spencer, Vernon: The Human Side of Admissions. *Hospital Management,* 88:51–100, December, 1959.

Toomay, Robert E.: Organization Structures and Hospital. *Hospital Topics,* 40:55–57, 64–65, November, 1962.

What Tests Are Routine? *The Modern Hospital,* 93:51, September, 1959.

6 THE NURSING PROCESS

The nurse should be able to:

Define "nursing process"

List basic steps in the nursing process

Name sources the nurse uses in gathering information about
    the patient

Describe the nursing history as a tool for gathering informa-
    tion about the patient

Explain Maslow's theory of basic human needs

Describe the formulation of goals for nursing action

Explain the purpose of nursing care plans

Describe methods for evaluating the effectiveness of nursing
    care

THE NURSING PROCESS 6

INTRODUCTION

The term *nursing process* is used to describe the series of steps the nurse takes in planning and giving nursing care. The essential elements of the process are that it is planned, it is patient-centered and it is goal-directed.

The planning and implementation of nursing care are based on scientific principles. The nurse, for example, is aware that strange situations can elicit fear. She therefore plans an orientation program for the patient who is newly admitted to hospital. Her plan is designed to meet the patient's need to overcome his apprehensions about his new environment. Because of the individuality of people, however, the plan must be tailored to suit each patient. Mrs. Jones, for example, who has been a nurse, will need a different type of orientation from Mrs. Smith, who has never been in hospital prior to her present admission. The goal of nursing action will be the same, that is, that the patient becomes familiar with her new environment, but the action taken may be quite different. Mrs. Jones may not need to be instructed in the use of the intercom or other equipment in her room, and she may be quite familiar with the different categories of hospital personnel, but the nurse will probably need to orient her to the particular floor plan of the nursing unit and introduce her to the nursing personnel and the routines on the unit. On the other hand, the nurse may need to give Mrs. Smith detailed instructions on the operation of her bedside equipment and explain the role and functions of different types of workers in addition to orienting her to the physical environment and introducing her to the staff on the unit.

STEPS IN THE NURSING PROCESS

Nursing care may range from the simple act of helping a patient who cannot feed himself to the highly complex measures involved in caring for patients in the intensive care unit of a hospital, or in helping a family with multiple problems to meet their health needs in a community setting. There are, however, certain common steps in the nursing process, whether the care given is a basic comfort measure or a complicated nursing activity. These basic steps are:

1. The collection of information about the patient
2. An assessment of the patient's nursing needs based on an analysis of the data collected
3. The development of goals for nursing action
4. The implementation of nursing action to meet these goals
5. An evaluation of the effectiveness of nursing action

COLLECTION OF INFORMATION

The nurse has many sources of information which she uses to collect information about the patient. Information is obtained from the patient's record, from the nurse's observations of the patient, from talking with the patient and with his family, and through written or oral communication with other members of the health team.

The Patient's Record

The *patient's record* is a valuable source of information, and one which the nurse frequently uses. Before she sees a patient, she can obtain basic information such as the name, age, occupation, religion and other vital statistics of the patient from the admission sheet on the chart. The medical history and progress notes on the record provide the nurse with some insight into the patient's illness. These usually give the tentative diagnosis, past medical history and present signs and symptoms. Often the medical plan of therapy is outlined as well, and this is further clarified on the doctor's order sheet where medications and treatment prescriptions are written. The laboratory sheet furnishes the findings from various tests and examinations performed on the patient. The nurse can also obtain significant data from the notes written by other nurses who are caring for the patient and from those made by other health workers, such as the physical therapist and the social worker.

The Nurse's Observations

Orlando calls any information which the nurse acquires about the patient *observations*.[1] The term is used here, however, to denote the information the nurse obtains about the patient through the use of her senses of sight, hearing, touching and smell. Intelligent observation is important to sound nursing prac-

tice. It is an aid to the physician in his diagnosis of the patient's condition and in his evaluation of medical therapy. It is also essential to the identification of nursing problems and the subsequent evaluation of the effectiveness of nursing measures. A *nursing diagnosis* is the identification of the patient's nursing problems.

Observation should be both systematic and scientific. Although the nurse's observations may intentionally be made to appear casual in order not to arouse anxiety in the patient, in actual fact, her observations are always systematic; the nurse is aware of what to look for and differentiates the normal from the abnormal. It is only through a knowledge of normal behavior that digressions from the normal are recognized. The nurse's observations are scientific in that they are objective and are based on her knowledge of the sciences.

The nurse can consciously develop her skill in observing. It is not possible to note everything that comes within one's range of vision; therefore the nurse must learn to be selective in her observations. She learns what to look for, and her eyes and her ears become trained to observe significant factors in the patient's appearance, in his behavior and in the environment. The nurse should be aware, however, that there is a tendency for people to see and hear what they expect or want to see and hear. Her observations, then, should be as objective as it is possible for her to make them. Observations should be described in terms of a factual record of patient behavior, or of qualitative and quantitative characteristics of the patient's appearance, rather than her interpretations of these.

Observations are made by using the four senses of sight, hearing, smell and touch. These senses are also augmented by tools, such as the clinical thermometer and the stethoscope, which provide more accurate measurements. In addition, an increasing number of technical appliances have been developed to assist in observation and measurement. Closed-circuit television is in use in many hospitals; this equipment pro-

[1]Ida J. Orlando: *The Dynamic Nurse-Patient Relationship.* New York, G. P. Putnam's Sons, 1961, p. 31.

vides for two-way communication between the patient and the nurse and permits nursing personnel to observe the patient without leaving the nursing station. In some centers monitoring systems are in use which automatically and continuously record the patient's vital signs, such as pulse. These systems serve to augment the nurse's field of observation, but they do not substitute for the presence of the nurse at the patient's bedside. Specific skills in observation are discussed in Chapter 7.

Information Obtained From the Patient

Many agencies now use a nursing history to provide a written record of the specific information about a patient which the nurse has obtained through her observations and through interviewing the patient. The nursing history is used as a base for assessing the patient's nursing needs; it provides a means whereby the nurse can plan and modify her care to suit the individual patient's preferences and usual living patterns; it also provides baseline data from which to evaluate the results of nursing action.[2] The format used and the specific information recorded varies in different agencies. Generally the information gathered includes items which nurses in the agency have found helpful for assessing patients' needs and planning nursing care for the majority of patients.[3] Content areas which one agency includes are:

1. Vital statistics about the patient
2. Appearance on first sight
3. The patient's understanding of illness and events leading up to the illness
4. Some indications of the patient's expectations
5. A brief social and cultural history
6. Significant data regarding the patient's usual patterns or habits of living

7. Some indication of that which is important to the patient, statement of what helps him feel secure, comfortable, protected safe and cared for[4]

The nursing history is taken as soon after the patient's admission to the agency as is feasible. It is taken by the nurse who has primary responsibility for planning the patient's care. The technique for obtaining the information is a structured interview; that is, the nurse controls and directs the interview for the purpose of gathering specific data. The data are then used to identify the patient's nursing needs and to individualize his care.

Vital statistics about the patient help to give the nurse some clues as to what the patient is like. The name sometimes helps to identify ethnic origin; age and occupation are important in understanding a patient's reaction to illness. For example, a woman of 40 who is admitted for termination of her first pregnancy may be expected to react quite differently from the 30 year old woman who is in hospital for a therapeutic abortion and already has four children. A singer who is to have even a minor operation on his throat may be extremely anxious about the results of the surgery and its effect on his career. Knowing the patient's marital status assists in the identification of significant family members and also possible sources of conflict. Knowledge of the patient's religion, place of residence and next of kin also help to give the nurse insight into the patient as an individual.

The patient's appearance on first sight is important both to identify present nursing needs and also to provide baseline data for comparison later on. This information is obtained through the observations the nurse makes as already discussed.

The patient's understanding of his illness assists the nurse to recognize potential problems resulting from the patient's condition. The patient may not be aware of his diagnosis and may need help in accepting his illness. He may

---

[2]Dolores E. Little and Doris L. Carnevali: *Nursing Care Planning.* Philadelphia, J. B. Lippincott Company, 1969, p. 66.

[3]Eileen Pearlman: *Manual for the Use of the Nursing History Tool.* Gainesville, Fla., College of Nursing, University of Florida, 1971, p. 15.

[4]Ibid., pp. 24–38.

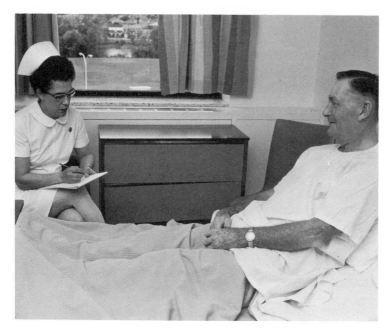

The nursing history is used as a base for assessing the patient's nursing needs.

not understand the implications of his illness. For example, the truck driver with a back injury may not realize that he will possibly have to change his occupation, and he may need considerable help in rehabilitation.

An indication of the patient's expectations regarding his care, what he expects to happen in hospital and the care he anticipates from nursing personnel help the nurse to understand how much explanation the patient will require and may help to clarify some of his reactions to the care he receives. Asking the patient about these matters in itself indicates interest and helps to establish a trusting relationship between nurse and patient.

A brief social and cultural history of the patient includes his level of education, some indication of his work history and a knowledge of significant family members or friends. This type of information helps the nurse to identify some of the strengths and weaknesses of the patient and to assess the potential support of family and friends during his illness.

Significant data regarding the patient's usual patterns or habits of living include such items as sleep patterns,

elimination patterns, usual dietary habits and specific food likes and dislikes as well as activities and patterns of daily living. Problems which the patient has in connection with any of these are noted and reported so that appropriate action can be taken. Information about usual habit patterns also helps the nurse to individualize the patient's care and to modify nursing schedules or environmental factors so that the patient's normal routines are not unnecessarily disrupted. A patient may prefer to have his bath in the evening, for example, and, providing he is capable of taking his bath himself, there seems no reason why he should not do so. If he needs help in bathing and there is sufficient staff on in the evenings, again this hygienic measure can be carried out at the time the patient prefers.

An indication of what is important to the individual helps the nurse to attend to the small details which mean so much to patients. A woman patient may request the nurse to telephone her husband to bring in a clean nightgown and her makeup, for example. This may seem an unimportant detail to the nurse who is busy with medications and treatments, but it is important to the patient in contributing to her sense of well-being. Attention to such requests helps the patient to feel more secure and comfortable in a strange environment; it also helps to maintain the patient's feelings of self-worth.[5]

Information Obtained Through Communication with Other Members of the Health Team

Other members of the health team contribute to the nurse's understanding of the patient and his illness. Observations and interpretations may be communicated by the physician, the social worker, the dietitian and the physical therapist, to name only a few, through written notes on the patient's record, consultations with the nurse or in meetings of various members of the health team.

The physician is responsible for the medical diagnosis of the patient's disease. Through systematic observation and various diagnostic tests, he makes a judgment as to the nature of the patient's condition. The nurse assists the physician in many aspects of diagnosis. Often her observations contribute largely to the data from which the diagnosis is made. She also assists the physician in many diagnostic procedures.

Following the medical diagnosis the patient will have a therapeutic regime prescribed by the physician. His treatment may involve such measures as an operation or exercise. In any case the nursing care plan is dependent upon the specific nursing care problems presented by the patient. These problems involve the disease of the patient, the medical therapy and the individual's own needs and reactions.

The nurse will find it helpful to have a knowledge of medical terminology in order to understand the diagnosis and the objectives of medical therapy.

Pathology refers to the disease process itself; it is generally classified as either organic or functional. *Organic pathology* refers to diseases which can be identified physically, a tumor or a communicable disease for example. *Functional pathology* refers to diseases which have no apparent physical basis; emotional disturbances frequently come under this heading. With the intensive research that is being conducted at the present time, the line between organic pathology and functional pathology has become less distinct and their frequent interrelatedness is recognized. The term *psychosomatic* illness is used to refer to the connectivity between organic illness and emotional factors, for example, between a peptic ulcer and anxiety.

A *medical diagnosis* is the physician's opinion as to the nature of the disease. *Prognosis* means the medical opinion as to the final outcome of the disease process. A prognosis can be described as negative, positive or uncertain; good, poor or fair. Generally the physician is assisted by other members of the health team in establishing the diagnosis and prognosis; for example, he makes use of diagnostic tests performed by technicians.

A *symptom* is evidence that there is a disease process or disturbance in body function. *Subjective symptoms* are those symptoms that can be perceived only by the patient. For example, the patient is the only person who can describe his pain. Perhaps through astute observation of the patient's facial expression or his body position, the nurse might think that a patient has pain, but only the patient himself can actually describe this symptom. An *objective symptom* is one that can be observed and described by others. A flushed face, a swollen ankle, rapid respirations can all be observed and described objectively.

A *sign* is an objective symptom that is detected through special examination. For example, fever is detected by the clinical thermometer, an abnormal heart beat by the stethoscope.

Prefixes and suffixes commonly used in medical terms are listed in the appendix.

---

[5]Ibid. The authors are deeply indebted for much of the material contained here to Dean Dorothy Smith, who made available the *Manual for the Use of the Nursing History Tool* developed at the University of Florida School of Nursing.

ASSESSMENT OF NURSING NEEDS

Nursing care is directed toward those needs of individuals which nursing personnel can help to meet in their professional roles. The nurse determines those areas of need which she can assist the patient to meet by nursing action through an analysis of the information that she has gathered. A helpful basis for categorizing needs and for establishing priorities as guides to nursing action is Maslow's theory of the hierarchy of human needs. This theory is based on the concept that there are certain basic needs which are common to all beings of the human species and that these needs may be arranged in order of priority for satisfaction. Lower-level needs must be satisfied (or at least mostly so) before the individual attempts to satisfy needs of a higher order. The basic human needs identified by Maslow were, in order of priority:

1. Physiological needs
2. Safety needs
3. The need for love and belonging
4. The need for esteem or self-worth
5. The need for self-actualization[6]

Physiological needs take precedence over all others. The maintenance of function of certain bodily processes is so essential that, if there is interference with the process, immediate action must be taken to save the person's life. If there is interference with breathing, for example, prompt measures must be initiated to restore adequate respiration. This may take the form of suctioning of the patient's nasopharynx to remove mucus and secretions, the administration of oxygen, or in some cases, artificial respiration. The relief of pain is another priority item. If pain is severe, the patient cannot think of anything else until he obtains relief from it. The needs of the patient for food, for water, for comfort, for rest and sleep and for activity are basic physiological needs with which the nurse is concerned.

---

[6]A. H. Maslow: A Theory of Human Motivation. *Psychological Review*, 50:370–396, 1943.

Meeting the patient's safety needs is also an important nursing responsibility. When people are healthy they normally take precautions to protect themselves from harm. When they are ill, however, they are dependent on others to do this for them. Safety measures include precautions to prevent accidents, such as siderails to protect the unconscious patient from falling out of bed, and the elimination of fire hazards and other potential dangers in the environment. The prevention of infection is another important aspect of the nurse's role in contributing to the safety of the patient (see Chapters 15 and 16.) The patient's need to feel secure also means that the nurse takes steps to help him to overcome his fears, as for example, by helping him to become familiar with his environment or by explaining tests and procedures which are new to him.

The nurse can also help the patient to meet some of his other needs. Her sincere welcome of the newly admitted patient contributes to his feeling of belonging, and her consideration of his comfort and welfare and that of his family helps to maintain his sense of self-worth and esteem. It is not possible even under the most favorable circumstances for the nurse to meet all the needs of patients, but through her awareness of basic human needs she can direct her actions toward helping the patient to meet those needs which are essential to his well-being and to his recovery.

ESTABLISHING GOALS FOR NURSING ACTION

The identification of patient needs leads to the development of objectives or goals to be attained by the patient with the assistance of nursing action. These goals should be realistic and attainable both in terms of the potentialities of the patient and the ability of the nurse to help him to meet these goals. For example, to set a goal that the patient regain normal musculoskeletal functioning may be completely unrealistic for a patient who has been partially paralyzed by a stroke, but the patient may be able to achieve independence in feeding and dressing himself, and these are goals which the nurse can help him to achieve.

Objectives are stated in terms of patient goals, rather than nursing activities; then nursing action is planned to help the patient to achieve these goals. The goals describe the behavior the patient is expected to attain. For example, "The patient dresses himself each morning without help" might be one objective for the partially paralyzed patient. Behavioral objectives are usually written in sentence form and include: the subject (in this case, the patient), an action verb which describes the desired behavior (dresses himself), the conditions under which the activity is to take place (without help), and a criterion or standard for judging the action (each morning). The conditions need not always be stated.

Long-range general goals, such as "The patient regains optimal musculoskeletal functioning," are important to keep in mind, but for planning specific nursing action for one patient, it is helpful to have goals that are worded more specifically. Another objective for the partially paralyzed patient, for example, might be, "The patient maintains his right arm and leg (if these are the affected ones) in good anatomical position at all times." This type of objective provides scope for the prescription of definitive nursing measures, such as the use of a footboard and pillows to support the arm and leg, and the use of a roll in the patient's hand to maintain normal flexion of the fingers. An objective worded in this manner also helps other personnel by alerting them to the specific needs of this particular patient. Specifically worded objectives also provide the means for evaluating the patient's progress and the effects of nursing action.

For additional help in learning to write objectives in behavioral terms, the nurse is directed to Smith's recent article entitled "The Writing of Objectives as a Nursing Practice Skill" in the *American Journal of Nursing* and Mager's book on *Preparing Instructional Objectives*.[7,8] The book, while originally intended for teachers, is equally useful for nurses.

IMPLEMENTATION OF NURSING ACTION

Once goals have been established, the next step in the nursing process is to determine those nursing measures which will best help the patient to attain these. This involves the exploration of possible courses of action and a decision to try one approach. In assessing the merits of different courses of action, the nurse uses her basic knowledge from the biophysical and social sciences, her understanding of the patient's disease condition and the physician's plan of therapy, and her knowledge about the individual patient as a person.

In implementing nursing action, the nurse may give direct care to a patient or engage in indirect activities which contribute to his care. She may give the patient a bath, administer his medications, change his dressing; or she may supervise others in doing these things for him. She may also teach the patient and his family about his disease process or about measures that he or they can use to assist in his recovery and rehabilitation.

To facilitate the implementation of nursing action, many agencies have developed a system of nursing care plans. The nursing care plan is just what one would expect it to be: the plan of care for the patient. It usually includes a description of the patient's needs, the goals which have been established for nursing care and the specific nursing measures which are to be used in caring for the patient. The care plan is developed as soon after the patient's

---

[7]Dorothy M. Smith: Writing Objectives as a Nursing Practice Skill. *The American Journal of Nursing*, 71:2:319–320, February, 1971.

[8]Robert F. Mager: *Preparing Instructional Objectives*. Palo Alto, Fearon Publishers, 1962.

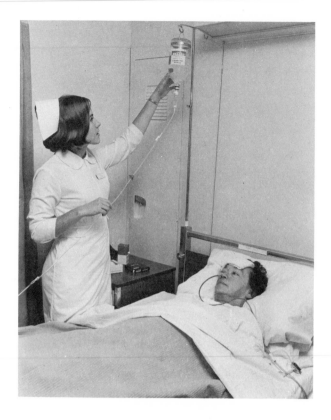

In implementing nursing action, the nurse often gives direct care to the patient, as this nurse is doing in adjusting the intravenous infusion.

admission as sufficient data is available on which to base a plan. It may be developed by the nurse who is in charge of the patient's care or may be jointly determined by the members of the nursing team. Because the patient's nursing needs change from day to day during his illness, the nursing care plan is constantly under revision. Sometimes the nursing care to be given is written in terms of nursing orders, which are prescribed and followed through in much the same manner as doctors' orders. In other agencies, the term "nursing approach" or "nursing action" may be used to identify the specific nursing measures which are to be used in the care of the patient.

The nursing care plan is a means of communicating in writing to other personnel, the nursing needs, objectives of care and specific nursing action to be taken in the care of the patient. In some agencies, care plans are incorporated as part of the Kardex report. Sometimes a separate notebook is used, or the care plan may be placed on the patient's chart or kept at his bedside.

The nursing history, the care plan and the nurse's progress notes not only provide a means of communicating information about the patient to all nursing personnel but they also serve as a basis for evaluating the patient's progress and the effectiveness of nursing care.

Little and Carnevali in their book, *Nursing Care Planning*, discuss the topic of care plans in considerable detail.[9] The nurse is therefore referred to this source for additional material.

EVALUATION OF THE EFFECTIVENESS OF NURSING ACTION

Throughout her care, the nurse constantly evaluates the progress the patient has made toward reaching the pre-

---

[9]Little and Carnevali, op. cit.

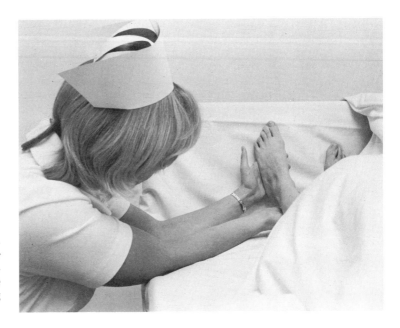

The nurse must constantly evaluate the effectiveness of her actions. This nurse is examining the patient's heel to make sure the skin is not showing signs of pressure.

established goals. Evaluation is the process of determining the extent to which objectives have been attained. It implies measurement against predetermined standards. If the objectives for nursing care have been carefully thought through and the standards have been clearly stated, the nurse can then compare the patient's attainments with these standards. For example, in the case of the partially paralyzed patient described earlier, the criterion for judging the patient's progress is his ability to dress himself each morning. Does he still require help, and if so, how much help does he need? Does he dress himself some mornings and not on others? The answers to these questions enable the nurse to determine whether the goals have been met.

In evaluating the effectiveness of nursing action it is important to have definite criteria in mind. These criteria should be observable and they should be measurable. Then progress can be noted and, if a particular nursing approach does not appear to be effective, an alternative course of action can be tried. The attainment of certain goals may mean that the patient is ready for more far-reaching ones. The patient who has learned to dress himself may be ready to learn other activities of daily living.

Stating criteria in question form helps the nurse to be objective and to look for specific indications that goals have been met. Questions are not always written down, but the beginning nurse may find it easier to develop the habit of asking herself the questions implicit in the nursing goals for the patient if she does put them on to paper.

In some cases the effectiveness of nursing care can be evaluated by the nurse through her observations of the patient. Is his paralyzed arm in good anatomical position, or is the hand in a dependent position? Many times it is necessary to ask the patient if nursing care has been effective. Is he more comfortable? Is he free from pain? While there are some observable signs to indicate that a patient is comfortable or free from pain, these are predominantly subjective feelings which only the patient can tell you.

Other members of the nursing team and of the health team also contribute in evaluating nursing care. The physical therapist and the nurse often work in conjunction to assess the patient's response to therapeutic measures. The patient's family are also frequently involved in evaluating the effect of nursing measures. Evaluation is an ongoing process which reflects the changing needs of the patient and involves a systematic appraisal of nursing activities by all members of the nursing team.

STUDY VOCABULARY

Doctor's order sheet	Nursing care plan	Pathology
Evaluation	Nursing diagnosis	Patient's record
Functional pathology	Nursing history	Prognosis
Medical diagnosis	Nursing process	Psychosomatic
Nursing action	Objective	Sign
Nursing approach	symptom	Subjective symptom
	Organic pathology	Symptom

BIBLIOGRAPHY

Abdellah, Faye G., et al.: *Patient-Centered Approaches to Nursing.* New York, The Macmillan Company, 1960.

Berggren, Helen J., and A. Dawn Zagornik: Teaching Nursing Process to Beginning Students. *Nursing Outlook, 16:*32–35, July, 1968.

Carrieri, Virginia Kohlman, and Judith Sitzman: Components of the Nursing Process. *Nursing Clinics of North America, 6:*1:115–124, March, 1971.

Deutsch, Elizabeth Burki: A Stereotype or an Individual? *Nursing Outlook, 19:*106–108, February, 1971.

Griffith, Elizabeth Welk: Nursing Process: A Patient with Respiratory Dysfunction. *Nursing Clinics of North America, 6:*1:145–154, March, 1971.

Hadley, Betty Jo: Evolution of a Conception of Nursing. *Nursing Research, 18:*5:400–405, September-October, 1969.

Haferkorn, Virginia: Assessing Individual Learning Needs as a Basis for Patient Teaching. *Nursing Clinics of North America, 6:*1:199–209, March, 1971.

Kurihara, Marie: Assessment and Maintenance of Adequate Respiration. *Nursing Clinics of North America, 3:*1:65–76, March, 1968.

Lewis, Lucile: This I Believe . . . About the Nursing Process—Key to Care. *Nursing Outlook, 16:*26–29, May, 1968.

Lewis, Lucile, Virginia Carozza, Maura Carroll, Rita Darragh, Maxine Patrick, Eva Schadt: *Defining Clinical Content, Graduate Nursing Programs, Medical-Surgical Nursing.* Boulder, Colo., Western Interstate Commission for Higher Education, 1967.

Little, Dolores E., and Doris L. Carnevali: *Nursing Care Planning.* Philadelphia, J. B. Lippincott Company, 1969.

Mager, Robert F.: *Preparing Instructional Objectives.* Palo Alto, Fearon Publishers, 1962.

Maslow, A. H.: A Theory of Human Motivation. *Psychological Review, 50:* 370–396, 1943.

McCain, R. Faye: Nursing by Assessment—Not Intuition. *The American Journal of Nursing, 65:*82–84, April, 1965.

Orlando, Ida J.: *The Dynamic Nurse-Patient Relationship.* New York, G. P. Putnam's Sons, 1961.

Pearlman, Eileen: *Manual for the Use of the Nursing History Tool.* Gainesville, Fla., College of Nursing, University of Florida, 1971.

Smith, Dorothy M.: Writing Objectives as a Nursing Practice Skill. *The American Journal of Nursing, 71:*2:319–320, February, 1971.

Wagner, Bernice M.: Care Plans, Right, Reasonable and Reachable. *The American Journal of Nursing,* 69:5:986–990, May, 1969.

Yura, Helen, and Mary B. Walsh: *The Nursing Process.* Washington, D.C., The Catholic University of America Press, 1967.

Zimmerman, Donna Stulgis, and Carol Gohrke: The Goal-Directed Nursing Approach: It Does Work. *The American Journal of Nursing,* 70:2:306–310, February, 1970.

7 SPECIFIC OBSERVATIONAL SKILLS

The nurse should be able to:

Describe ways in which the nurse uses her senses of sight, hearing, touch and smell in making observations about the patient

Describe the technique for taking a person's temperature orally, rectally and by axilla

Outline a basic method for cleaning and disinfecting clinical thermometers

Define pulse

Name sites in the body where an arterial pulse may be felt

Describe the technique for taking the pulse

List qualities of the pulse to be observed

Describe the technique for observing respirations

List qualities of respirations to be observed

Name factors affecting blood pressure

Describe techniques for taking blood pressure

Describe the technique for taking the apical beat

INTRODUCTION

The ability to observe intelligently and scientifically is a basic element of nursing practice. It is essential to the identification of patients' needs and the subsequent planning and evaluating of nursing care. The nurse's skillful observations also aid the physician in his diagnosis of the patient's condition and in his evaluation of medical therapy.

In her observations, the nurse makes use of her physical senses and also utilizes tools such as the clinical thermometer, the sphygmomanometer (the instrument for measuring blood pressure) and the stethoscope, which have been developed to obtain measurements indicative of the functioning of various body processes.

Temperature, pulse and respirations have been traditionally referred to as the cardinal signs of life. Together with blood pressure and the heart beat they indicate basic physiological functions of the human body. Their importance as criteria of physical health should not be ignored in spite of the more intricate methods for measuring body function that have been developed recently.

When a patient first goes to a physician it is customary for his temperature, pulse, respirations and blood pressure to be taken as part of his examination. Most people are familiar with the clinical thermometer and the blood pressure cuff, but the nurse is advised to explain them to those who are not. A simple explanation can often allay unnecessary anxiety.

OBSERVING THROUGH USE OF THE PHYSICAL SENSES

The physical senses of sight, hearing, touch and smell are all used by the nurse in making observations about the patient. The nurse's sense of taste is seldom, if ever, used as an aid to observation. However, a knowledge of how something tastes to the patient can often be of value diagnostically. In addition, the nurse can be guided in her administration of medications by an awareness of how they taste. Unpleasant drugs can often be made more palatable by being given cold, diluted or mixed with food or fluids (see Chapter 21).

Sense of Sight

The sense of sight is basic to the oldest method of examination, that is, *inspection*. Visual acuity is helpful in gaining information about patients; however, the intelligent use of the sense of sight requires more than just good eyesight. It demands skillful observation: the ability to recognize signs and symptoms and to understand their significance in relation to the individual patient.

Through her sense of sight the nurse can identify both covert and overt nursing problems. Symptoms of physical disease as well as symptoms of psychological and sociological dysfunction are evidenced by physical manifestations and patterns of behavior.

General Behavior. Through observation the nurse can often detect both

77

verbal and nonverbal behavior which indicates the general feeling tone and activity of the patient. In describing behavior, the nurse should state exactly what it is that the patient does. For example, "moves slowly," "fidgets with bedclothing," "responds to questions," or "sits quietly in bed" should be used, rather than "patient appears depressed" or "anxious" or "cheerful," which are the nurse's interpretations of the patient's behavior.

Consciousness. The degree of unconsciousness of an individual is frequently important in the determination of nursing and medical diagnoses and the subsequent therapeutic regimes. Consciousness means a normal state of awareness. Unconsciousness may be considered relative, varying in degree and duration. The subject of levels of consciousness is one that requires considerably more elaboration than is possible here. Pertinent observations which the beginning student can make, however, include: the patient's orientation to time and place, that is, does he know what day it is and where he is; does he respond to verbal stimuli, as for example, instructions to raise his arm so that the nurse can give him his injection? The level of consciousness is often tested by the patient's response to questions or reaction to painful stimuli, such as a pinprick. If a patient does not respond to supraorbital (above the orbit of the eye) pressure, he is said to be in deep coma. Coma is a state of unconsciousness from which an individual cannot be aroused. The needs of the unconscious patient are comprehensive.

General Appearance. The general appearance of an individual can give clues to his physical and emotional health. The depressed patient frequently stands with a stooped defeated posture. Some diseases cause patients to adopt a typical gait, for example, the forward angle of the body of the patient with Parkinson's disease (a condition in which there is muscular rigidity). Emaciation or obesity can be an indication of disease and nutritional status. General appearance may be described by such terms as obese, emaciated, thin, pale, flushed, well nourished, stooped, erect, having a normal gait, mobile.

Respiratory System. Many symptoms are significant of disorders of the respiratory tract. A cough may be either productive or nonproductive, spasmodic or constant. Sputum can be described according to its appearance as:
   watery—is thin, colorless, has the appearance of water
   frothy—has the appearance of being light and aerated, contains bubbles
   purulent—may be yellowish or greenish in color, thick in texture, often has a foul odor
   blood-tinged (hemoptysis)—contains red or dark-colored blood
Sputum may also be described in terms of its amount as: copious (large amounts), moderate, or scant (small amounts). As a result of disease processes, a patient can appear *cyanotic* (the skin has a bluish tinge to it), *dyspneic* (the patient has difficulty in breathing), or *orthopneic* (difficulty in breathing is relieved to a certain extent when the patient is in a sitting position). His chest movements may be abnormal and he may exhibit deviations from the normal in the rate and character of his breathing (see the later section of this chapter on respirations).

Gastrointestinal System. A patient's abdomen may appear distended; this is often due to the presence of flatus (gas). His appetite may be good or poor; he may vomit (emesis), and the vomited matter may be described as coffee ground (color and appearance of coffee grounds), sanguineous (pertaining to blood), bilious (containing green and yellow bile), frothy. Fecal elimination can be described according to color, consistency, frequency and amount (see Chapter 24).

Circulatory System. Dysfunction of the circulatory system can give rise to a variety of symptoms which can be detected visually. For example, the skin may appear flushed or pale. Petechiae (pinpoint bleeding in the skin or mucous membrane), ecchymosis (extravasation of blood in tissues), epistaxis (nosebleed) or hemorrhages from a variety of sources may occur. Edema of the tissues or loss of tissue elasticity may arise as a result of fluid or electrolyte disturbances (see Chapter 29).

Integumentary System. The skin and mucous membrane may appear dry, parched, cracked or inflamed. The skin may be coarse, scaly, moist, cyanotic jaundiced; it may show abrasions or other skin lesions. The moistness and texture can also be observed.

Discharges from the body orifices and wounds can be observed for color, consistency and amount. Thus, the discharge may be serous, sanguineous or purulent or any combination of the three; it may be profuse, moderate, small or scant in amount and thick or watery in consistency (see Chapter 22).

Genitourinary System. The visual observations made of the genitourinary system are generally related to secretions, excretions or discharges. Urine may be cloudy, dark, light, smoky or sanguineous (hematuria). A patient may suffer from urinary incontinence, frequency or retention or from anuria (absence of urine) (see Chapter 27).

Nervous System. As part of a physical examination, the physician frequently tests the patient's reflexes. In addition to the physician's observations, the nurse should observe the patient's eye reflexes (e.g., blinking) and the size of his pupils. She should also observe the integrity of the body senses: sight, hearing, smell, taste, touch and cognition.

Sense of Hearing

The sense of hearing is the second most frequently used sense. *Auscultation* is the listening for sounds within the body. For example, during a physical examination the physician usually listens to the heart and lung sounds with a stethoscope. *Percussion* refers to examination by tapping the body. An individual's chest is examined in this manner by placing one hand on the chest and tapping it with the fingers of the other hand.

It is often by listening to the patient that the nurse identifies covert nursing

problems. What a patient says, how he says it, the frequency with which he says it and what he does not say can be significant in the identification of the more obscure needs.

General Behavior. By listening to the patient, the nurse will often find that his words, tone inflections and phraseology reveal emotional tone and general outlook on life. Again the nurse should be careful to report and record what she notes in terms of the patient's observable behavior. Two obvious conditions that can be identified by listening are stammering and stuttering. *Stammering* is hesitant speech; *stuttering* is the spasmodic repetition of the same syllable. The patient may also speak very slowly, or not speak at all; or, conversely, he may speak very rapidly, or in a high-pitched voice. He may not answer certain questions. Observations such as these should be accurately described.

Consciousness. By listening to a patient, the nurse may assess his orientation to his surroundings. To be oriented is to be aware of time, place and circumstances. To be disoriented is to be confused as to time, place and circumstances. Some people do not communicate verbally even though they are conscious. For example, a person who has suffered damage to his organs of speech or who is severely withdrawn may not respond verbally. Some patients speak in a confused or incoherent manner; that is, what they say does not make sense to the listener.

Respiratory System. By listening to a patient's cough the nurse can describe it as dry, loose, harsh, hacking, constant. Breathing can be described as labored, intermittent, moist, gasping, stertorous (noisy) or wheezing.

Gastrointestinal System. The only way that the nurse can know that a patient is nauseated is by having him tell her. Anorexia (loss of appetite) is also frequently verbalized. When an individual's abdomen is tender or painful, he often describes the condition. Pain can be constant, spasmodic or intermittent; crampy, sharp, piercing, acute, burning or tingling; localized or general. Whenever a patient complains of pain the nurse should note its exact character, duration and location (see Chapter 28).

Circulatory System. The patient's apical beat is noted by listening with a stethoscope. His blood pressure can be determined by using a stethoscope, blood pressure cuff and a sphygmomanometer. Blood pressure can be described as fluctuating or constant as well as by the exact level of pressure (see section later in this chapter).

Integumentary System. The nurse can observe a patient scratching himself, but she can only be certain that his skin is itching (pruritus) when he tells her. He may also complain of tingling, numbness, hot, cold and chilling.

Genitourinary System. The patient may describe sensations such as dysuria (difficulty in voiding), burning or painful micturition and urinary frequency.

Sense of Smell

The nurse's sense of smell can also be a means of detecting signs and symptoms.

Respiratory System. The breath of a patient may be described as fruity, fetid, urinous, acetone (sweet), or it may be said that he has halitosis (bad breath).

Integumentary System. The discharge from wounds or body orifices can have a definite odor. For example, the discharge from an infection with *Clostridium welchii* (gas gangrene) has a typically foul odor.

Genitourinary System. The urine of a patient can have a definite odor apart from the normal, faintly aromatic odor; it may be sweet (acetone) or foul, for example.

Sense of Touch

The sense of touch is used as a diagnostic tool by both the physician and the nurse. *Palpation* is the method of examining by using one's fingers. Size, temperature, texture, swelling and hardness are qualities noted by palpation.

Consciousness. The nurse's sense of touch can be used in some respects to help assess the level of consciousness or sensitivity to external stimuli. Testing the patient's response to pressure from one's hand or to pain from a pinprick is frequently done.

Gastrointestinal System. The nurse uses her sense of touch to determine the softness or hardness of the patient's abdomen, which may be indicative of the absence or presence of flatus.

Circulatory System. By using her fingers, the nurse can observe the rate, rhythm, size and tension of the patient's pulse. By pressing an individual's tissues the presence of edema can be ascertained. Edema is the accumulation of intercellular fluid in the tissues; in pitting edema, pressure upon the skin produces an indentation or pit which remains for a few moments.

Integumentary System. The texture of the patient's skin, as well as his tissue turgor, can be significant factors which can be determined by touch. Tissue turgor refers to the normal elasticity of the skin. When the patient is dehydrated, his tissue elasticity is often poor, and if the nurse gently pinches his skin, it stays pinched for a few moments before springing back.

CARDINAL SIGNS

Cardinal or vital signs vary from individual to individual and at different times of the day in one individual, but there is a range that is generally considered to be normal. Thus an oral temperature anywhere between 36.1° and 38°C. (97° and 100.4°F.), a pulse rate between 60 and 80 beats per minute and a respiratory rate between 12 and 18 respirations per minute are normal for most adults. Blood pressure also varies considerably in health. An adult can be expected to have a normal blood pressure anywhere between 90/60 and 140/90 mm. of mercury depending upon his age, amount of activity and so on.

The temperature reflects the balance between the heat produced and the heat lost by the body. It usually varies during the course of a 24 hour period, being

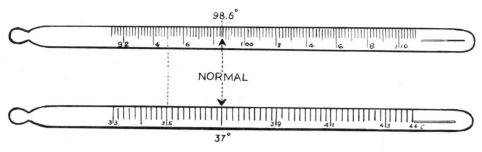

Fahrenheit and centigrade scales are used to measure body temperature. In order to convert Fahrenheit to centigrade, subtract 32 from the Fahrenheit reading and multiply by the fraction ⁵/₉; thus $C = \frac{5}{9}(F - 32)$. To convert centigrade to Fahrenheit, multiply the centigrade reading by ⁹/₅ and add 32; thus $F = \frac{9}{5}C + 32$.

lowest in the early morning hours before a person wakens, and highest in the evening. There are factors other than pathological processes that affect body temperature. The activity of an individual can make some difference, the active person usually having a higher temperature than the sedentary person. Age also affects temperature; the infant and the aged often have body temperatures 0.6°C. (1°F.) higher than that of the young adult. Emotions and anxiety can increase the basal metabolic rate of an individual and thereby elevate the temperature (see Chapter 23).

The heart rate, pulse and blood pressure vary according to age, size, sex and physical and emotional activity. The heart rate and respiratory rate decrease as the child grows, and the pulse decreases in rate until extreme old age. Men generally have a slower heart rate than women, and exercise increases the rate of cardiac contractions.

The rate and depth of respirations is regulated within a range that meets the basic metabolic needs of the body for oxygen. Any activity that necessitates increased oxygen will result in an increased respiratory rate. In addition the respiratory rate is to a limited degree under voluntary control.

Temperature

The source of heat production is cellular activity, particularly that of the muscles and the secreting glands. Heat is lost chiefly through radiation, conduction, convection and evaporation. Radiation is the transfer of heat from one object to another without contact between the two and without a transfer medium. Conduction is the transfer of heat between two objects which are in contact. Convection is the transfer of heat through air or a liquid. Evaporation is the process by which a substance is changed from a liquid to a gas.

Normal body temperature is considered to be 37° C. (98.6° F.) when taken orally. The rectal temperature is expected to be approximately 0.6° C. (1° F.) higher and the axillary temperature 0.6° C. (1° F.) lower. *Pyrexia* and *fever* are two terms used to refer to an elevated temperature. The term *hypothermia* refers to a temperature below normal.

Body temperature is measured with a clinical thermometer, which is an elongated glass tube calibrated in degrees Centigrade or degrees Fahrenheit. Within the tube is a column of mercury which expands in response to the heat of the body. The scale on the thermometer generally starts at about 35° C. (95° F.) and terminates at 43.3° C. (110° F.). Figures beyond this scale are unnecessary, because temperatures above and below these limits rarely occur.

The most common site for obtaining a measure of internal body temperature is the mouth (per ora). The small blood vessels on the under side of the tongue lie close to the surface. When the thermometer is placed under the tongue and the oral cavity is closed, it is possible to obtain a reasonably accurate estimate of the body's internal temperature. The thermometer is wiped off, shaken down and placed sublingually for five to seven minutes. The patient holds the thermometer between his lips and avoids biting it. After the thermometer is removed and the temperature noted, the thermometer is wipped off, shaken down, rinsed under cold running water and dried. If an individual thermometer is used for each patient, the thermometer is then returned to its container, in which it soaks in an antiseptic solution. The method of disinfecting thermometers varies in different agencies. However, the same basic steps are usually followed: that is, wiping off the thermometer to remove mucus and secretions; shaking down the mercury; rinsing in cold water; drying; followed by soaking in a disinfecting agent.

It is frequently necessary to take a patient's temperature via the rectum. This method is indicated when it is either unsafe or inaccurate to take it by mouth, as when a patient is unconscious or irrational; when he is receiving oxygen therapy; when he has a Levin tube in place; or when he has had oral or nasal surgery. The patient lies on his side for this measure. After the thermometer is wiped off and shaken down, it is lubricated with petrolatum or other lubricant. This facilitates the insertion of the thermometer into the rectum and lessens the danger of irritating the mucous membrane. The thermometer is inserted from 1 to 2 inches and held in place for at least two minutes. When it is is removed the temperature is noted, the thermometer is gently shaken down and then washed in cold soapy water before it is returned to its container. It is important to remove all fecal material and to wash in cold or warm water. The use of cold water prevents the coagulation of protein material. Hot water is never used, because it may damage the thermometer.

Rectal and oral thermometers are frequently differentiated by the color of the

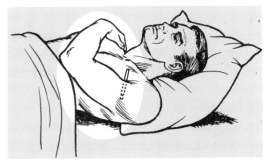

In order to obtain an axillary temperature the thermometer is placed in the patient's axilla, and then his arm is placed across his chest.

bulb; oral bulbs are silver and rectal bulbs are blue. In addition some rectal thermometers are more rounded at the ends, although many thermometers may be used for either rectal or oral temperatures.

Taking an axillary temperature is safer than taking an oral temperature for irrational or mentally disturbed patients. The thermometer is wiped off and shaken down, just as the oral thermometer is. The axilla is dried before the thermometer is inserted, because moisture conducts heat. The thermometer is placed between the inner surface of the patient's arm and his side while his arm is held across his chest. The thermometer is left in place for 10 minutes, then it is removed and the temperature noted. The nurse can expect the axilla temperature to be approximately 0.6° C. (1° F.) lower than the oral temperature. The thermometer should be shaken down and washed in warm soapy water before it is returned to its container.

The clinical thermometer is usually kept in a small vial containing a disinfectant. Various kinds of disinfectants are used to soak the thermometers; the synthetic phenols, isopropyl alcohol (70%) and tincture of Zephiran (1:1000) are all considered suitable. Because thermometers are soaked in a disinfectant when not in use, they need to be washed or wiped off carefully before they are given to patients. Since organic materials can interfere with disinfection, rectal thermometers need to be washed before being returned to the solution; other thermometers should be wiped or washed thoroughly to remove

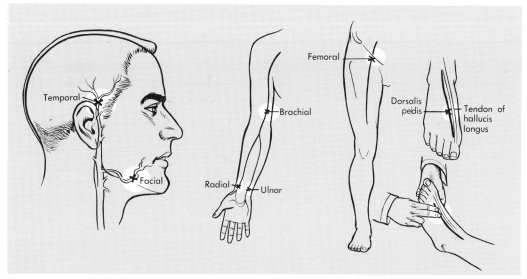

There are many sites on the body where the pulse may be taken; however, the radial pulse is taken most frequently. Other sites which are used, particularly when the radial pulse cannot be obtained, are the brachial, the temporal, the facial, the femoral, and the dorsalis pedis. Pulses are also taken at these points in order to assess arterial circulation to the specific area.

mucus and saliva. In wiping a thermometer, a rotating or twisting motion is used. The thermometer is wiped starting from the tip and working downward to the mercury bulb; that is, from clean to dirty.

Pulse

Pulse is the throbbing of an artery as it is felt over a bony prominence. When the left ventricle of the heart contracts, blood surges through the systemic arteries. This wave of blood is felt as the pulse.

The most common site for obtaining a patient's pulse is the inner aspect of the wrist on the thumb side. This is where the radial artery passes over the radius. With slight pressure the artery is held against the radius so that the pulsations of blood can be felt.

There are other sites in the body where the pulse can be taken if the radial pulse is obscured or if there is a need to test the circulation of blood in a specific area. The temporal pulse is felt anterior to the ear where the temporal artery passes over the temporal bone. The facial pulse is taken at the place where the facial artery passes over the

mandible, that is, on the groove in the mandible approximately one-third of the way forward from the angle of the jaw. The fourth pulse site is that of the femoral pulse. This is taken at the point in the middle of the groin where the femoral artery passes over the pelvic bone. The dorsalis pedis pulse is usually taken to assess circulation in the foot. It can be felt on the dorsum of the foot in a line between the first and second toes, just above the longitudinal arch.

When the nurse takes the patient's pulse, she places her second, third and fourth fingers lightly on the skin at the place where the artery passes over the underlying bone. The reason the thumb is not used to palpate a pulse is that the nurse might feel the pulsations of the radial artery of her own thumb. Usually, counting the rate for one-half minute and then multiplying by 2 gives an accurate record in beats per minute. If the pulse is irregular in any way it is counted for a full minute.

Generally the patient should be quiet so that his pulse rate can be compared with previous observations. Exercise and anxiety accelerate the pulse rate to the extent that it does not reflect the normal rate at rest.

When taking a pulse, the rate, rhythm, size and the tension of the pulse are noted. The *rate* of the pulse is the number of beats per minute. If the pulse rate is greatly accelerated—for example, over 100 beats per minute—the condition is referred to as *tachycardia*. An accelerated rate can be due to disease or stimulation of the cardiac muscle by the sympathetic nerves. A very slow pulse rate, under 60 beats per minute, is called *bradycardia*. It can be a result of parasympathetic stimulation or disease. It is not uncommon to see a slow pulse in a patient who is taking digitalis or any of its derivatives. Not only does digitalis stimulate the heart muscle to stronger systolic contractions, but it also stimulates the vagus nerve, a condition which tends to slow the heart rate.

The *rhythm* of the pulse refers to the pattern of the beats. In health the rhythm is regular; that is, the time between beats is essentially the same—pulsus regularis. The pulse is irregular when the beats follow each other at irregular intervals—pulsus irregularis. An irregular rhythm is called an arrhythmia. There are three basic kinds of irregularities.

1. Sinus irregularities. In this type of arrhythmia the rate is constantly changing, often with respirations, but the beats are of equal strength.

2. Premature contractions. In this type, there is a small beat right after a normal beat, followed by a period of normal rhythm. The finger may not be able to detect the small beat and thus the nurse may perceive long pauses at intervals in the pulse count.

3. Pulsus irregularis perpetuus. This is a pulse that is completely irregular in rhythm and in the strength of the beats.

The *size* of a pulse wave reflects the volume of blood pushed against the wall of the artery in the ventricular contraction. It is actually a measure of pulse pressure. Pulsus magnus refers to a high pulse pressure, pulsus parvus to a low pulse pressure.

The *tension* of the pulse refers to the compressibility of the arterial wall. If under slight pressure the pulse is obliterated, it is a pulse of low tension—

pulsus mollis. A pulse that is obliterated only by relatively great pressure is a pulse of high pressure—pulsus durus. The words "soft" and "hard" are used to describe pulse tension. Pulse tension corresponds to diastolic blood pressure. The hardness of the arterial wall can also be felt by palpation.

An *apical-radial* pulse is ascertained by two nurses. One nurse counts the patient's radial pulse at the same time that the second nurse counts the apical beats of the heart with the same watch. Each is counted for a full minute. In health the apical and radial rates are the same but in illness they sometimes differ, as when some apical beats are not transmitted to the radial artery. The difference between the apical rate and the radial rate is the *pulse deficit*.

Respirations

Respiration is the means by which a person exchanges gases with the atmosphere. External respiration is the exchange of oxygen and carbon dioxide between the alveoli of the lungs and the blood, whereas internal respiration is the exchange of these gases between the blood and the body cells. There are two main types of respirations: thoracic (costal) and abdominal (diaphragmatic). Thoracic respirations are accomplished chiefly by the costal muscles of the chest; abdominal respirations are accomplished by the abdominal muscles. The respirations of women are chiefly thoracic, those of men abdominal.

Respirations are essentially controlled by the respiratory center in the medulla oblongata. This center is sensitive to several factors, such as the carbon dioxide level in the blood and the expansion of the lungs (Hering-Breuer reflex) (see Chapter 25). Respirations controlled in this manner are automatic; however, the rate and depth of respirations are to a certain extent under voluntary control. A person can take deep breaths or shallow breaths, quickly or slowly, within the limitations imposed by the body's need for oxygen.

The nurse observes respirations unobtrusively, often directly after taking the pulse. If a person is aware that his respirations are being counted, he usually finds it difficult to maintain their normal rate. Counting the respirations for one-half minute and then multiplying by 2 gives the number of respirations per minute. Either the inspirations or expirations are counted but not both. Inspiration is the movement of air into the lungs; expiration is the movement of air out of the lungs. Sometimes it is impossible to see a person's chest movements or hear his breathing. By placing a hand on the patient's chest the nurse can often detect these otherwise undetectable respirations. In evaluating respirations the rate, depth, character (digressions from normal breathing), rhythm and symmetry are observed.

The normal respiratory *rate* for an adult is 12 to 18 respirations per minute. An abnormal increase in the respiratory rate is called *tachypnea* (polypnea), and an abnormal decrease is referred to as *bradypnea*. Normal breathing, which is effortless, regular and noiseless, is called *eupnea.*

The *depth* of respirations is determined by observing chest movement. A young adult normally inhales and exhales 500 ml. of air with each breath. This is the *tidal volume.* The inspiratory and expiratory *reserve volumes* are those amounts of air which can be inhaled and exhaled over and above the tidal volume. The *residual volume* is the volume of air remaining in the lungs after a forceful expiration. *Vital capacity* (approximately 5 liters in the adult) is the maximum amount of air which can be expired after a maximal inspiration. The tidal volume and vital capacity (lung capacity) vary from individual to individual. The depth of respirations may be characterized as shallow, normal or deep.

The *character* of respirations refers to digressions from normal effortless breathing. Breathing that is very noisy is called *stertorous. Cheyne-Stokes respirations* are irregular respirations in which, after a period of *apnea* (no breathing), there is a gradual increase in the rate and depth of the respirations, followed by a gradual decline and another period of apnea. *Biot's respirations* are respirations that are irregular in rate and depth, with no emerging pattern. *Kussmaul's respirations,* also called "air hunger," are rapid, intense respirations.

The *rhythm* of respirations refers to the regularity of inspirations and expirations. Normal respirations follow one another evenly, with little variation in the length of the pauses between inspiration and expiration. *Symmetry* refers to the synchronous movements of each side of the chest.

BLOOD PRESSURE

Blood pressure refers to the pressure of the blood within the arteries of the body. When the left ventricle of the heart contracts blood is forced out into the aorta and travels through the large arteries to the smaller arteries, arterioles and capillaries. The pulsations extend from the heart through the arteries and disappear in the arterioles. The *systolic pressure* is the arterial pressure at the height of the pulsation, it is normally 120 mm. of mercury in a young adult. The *diastolic* pressure is the arterial pressure at the lowest level of the pulsation, that is, during ventricular relaxation. It is normally 80 mm. of mercury. The difference between the systolic and diastolic pressures is the *pulse pressure.*

At rest the heart is required to pump only 4 to 6 liters of blood per minute. This volume is increased as much as five times during exercise. Normally each ventricle pumps 70 ml. of blood with each contraction, although wide variations in amount are compatible with life. This volume of output is reflected in the pulsations that can be felt where arteries pass over bones.

A number of variables affect the arterial blood pressure. A decrease in the size of the lumen of the blood vessels, for example, increases the amount of pressure required to pump the blood through the vessels. Any constriction of

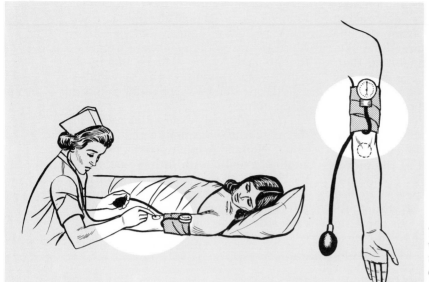

The blood pressure cuff is wrapped evenly around the upper arm so that the lower edge is 1 inch above the antecubital space.

the vessels, or the collection of deposits on the lining of the vessels (for example, fatty deposits) will therefore increase the blood pressure. Changes in the elasticity of the muscular walls of the blood vessels affect the blood pressure. For example, aging decreases the elasticity of muscular tissue, and the older person's blood pressure is usually higher than a younger person's. The viscosity of the blood, which may be altered by fluid balance, affects the blood pressure. The pressure of blood in the arteries is also dependent on the force of the ventricular contractions and on the volume of blood ejected from the heart with each ventricular contraction.[1]

An individual's blood pressure varies from hour to hour and from day to day. It falls during sleep and may be strikingly elevated by strong emotions, such as fear and anger, and by exercise. When a person is lying down, his blood pressure is lower than when he is sitting or standing. Also, the pressure may differ from one arm to the other. Therefore, before taking the blood pressure for a comparison value, the nurse

should check (a) the time of day, (b) the arm and (c) the position of the patient in previous readings.

An abnormal elevation of blood pressure is referred to as *hypertension. Hypotension* refers to abnormally low blood pressure.

There are two practical clinical methods of taking an individual's arterial blood pressure; the auscultatory method and the palpatory method. In the auscultatory method a stethoscope, a blood pressure cuff and a sphygmomanometer are required. Mercury and anaeroid sphygmomanometers are made commercially; the mercury instruments, which are less compact than the anaeroid, are commonly used in physicians' offices.

The cuff is wrapped smoothly and firmly around the patient's upper arm so that the lower border of the cuff is 1 inch above the antecubital space. The bell of the stethoscope is placed over the site of the brachial pulse and the cuff is pumped up until no sounds can be heard through the stethoscope. This means that the artery is collapsed by the pressure of the cuff and no blood is flowing through it. The pressure is then gradually released and, when the blood slips through the artery, sounds are heard in the stethoscope. At the same time the manometer is watched closely. The reading when the first sounds are

[1]Madelyn T. Nordmark, and Anne W. Rohweder: *Scientific Foundations of Nursing.* Second edition. Philadelphia, J. B. Lippincott Company, 1967, pp. 21, 22.

RIVERSIDE HOSPITAL OF OTTAWA

GRAPHIC CHART

SMITH   MARY   SP 1246
2321 MARKET ST OTT 234-7566 600
JONES   RICHARD   HUS
SAME
23.10.71   2PM F 23 M SURG RC

420   1

MONTH & DATE		JULY 1		2		3		4		5		6		7	
POST-OP DAYS						OPERATION 1				2		3		4	
	HOUR	A.M.	P.M.	A.M.	P M	A.M.	P M	A.M.	P.M.	A.M.	P.M.	A.M.	P.M.	A.M.	P.M.
PULSE	TEMP.	4 8 12	4 8 12	4 8 12	4 8 12	4 8 12	4 8 12	4 8 12	4 8 12	4 8 12	4 8 12	4 8 12	4 8 12	4 8 12	4 8 12
200	106°														
190	105°														
180	104°														
170	103°														
160	102°														
150	101°														
140	100°														
130	99 NORMAL														
120	98														
110	97														
100	96														
90	95														
80															
NORMAL 70															
60															
50															
40															

RESPIRATIONS	20	18		18	22 20 20 18 18									
BLOOD PRESSURE	120/80				120/80									

FLUID INTAKE IN C.C.	ORAL		1500					
	I.V.		1800					
	TOTAL-24 HR.		3300					
FLUID OUTPUT IN C.C.	EMESIS AND/OR DRAINAGE		150					
	URINE		800					
	FLUID STOOL							
	TOTAL-24 HR.		950					
STOOL		YES	YES	NO				

DATE	WEIGHT						
JULY 1	124		URINE TO LAB			100% Satu[?] REMOVED	
JULY 7	120						

6562

A sample graphic chart. (Courtesy of the Riverside Hospital of Ottawa.)

heard is the *systolic pressure*. With the continual lowering of the pressure in the cuff, the sounds continue to be heard as the artery alternately collapses and fills. Eventually the sounds diminish in intensity as the artery no longer collapses; weakened beats are usually heard for a few seconds and then disappear altogether. The American Heart Association suggests the onset of muffling (point at which the sounds change) as the best index of *diastolic pressure*. It usually takes practice to learn to distinguish the systolic and diastolic points of pressure with ease and accuracy, and in some patients they are very difficult to discern. Care should be taken, however, to avoid repumping the sphygmomanometer repeatedly within a short space of time.

In the palpatory method of taking arterial blood pressure the blood pressure cuff and sphygmomanometer are used but not the stethoscope; the radial pulse is palpated to ascertain the systolic blood pressure. The cuff is pumped up and then the pressure is slowly released; the reading at the point at which the radial pulse is first felt is the systolic pressure. The diastolic pressure is determined by noting the change in the character of the radial pulsations; however, this reading is not generally considered to be sufficiently accurate.

APICAL BEAT

It is often necessary to determine the rate of the apical beat of the heart. The apical beat is the beat of the heart as felt at its apex. The apex can be considered to be the point of maximal impulse. The apical beat can usually be heard in the fifth intercostal space, 2 to 3 inches to the left of the sternum, just below the left nipple. By reaching with the stethoscope in this area, the point of maximal sound can usually be found.

To determine the apical beat, the bell of the stethoscope is placed over the apex of the heart and the beats are counted for a full minute. A heart beat is heart as "lubb-dubb." The "lubb" represents the closure of the atrioventricular or tricuspid and mitral valves; it occurs at the onset of systole. The "dubb" represents the closure of the semilunar (aortic and pulmonic) valves at the end of systole. The rhythm of the heart beat can also be noted and recorded in the patient's chart.

WEIGHT

It is frequently necessary, as a diagnostic aid or as an aid in the assessment of therapeutic effectiveness, to obtain a patient's weight. For example, a daily weight check is ordered for the obese patient who is on a low calorie diet or for the patient who retains fluid in his tissues. In some health agencies and physicians' offices it is part of the admitting or preliminary procedure to take the weight and height of each patient.

Weight is measured in kilograms or pounds depending upon the policy of the institution. One kilogram is approximately 2.2 pounds. If a patient is to be weighed regularly, the weighing should always be done at the same time of day, since a person's weight may vary as much as several pounds over a 24 hour period. Thus it is not unusual to have the patient weigh himself before breakfast in order to obtain meaningful comparative values.

For the patient who is unable to get out of bed, commercially available bed scales are used. One such model has a hydraulic lift connected to a canvas-like arrangement on which the patient can be lifted off the surface of the bed by turning a handle; his weight is registered on a connected scale.

**STUDY
VOCABULARY**

| Apical beat | Auscultation | Bradypnea |
| Apnea | Bradycardia | Coma |

Conduction	Hypothermia	Residual volume
Consciousness	Inspiration	Stertorous
Convection	Palpation	Systolic
Diastolic	Percussion	Tachycardia
Eupnea	Pulse	Temperature
Expiration	Pulse deficit	Thoracic respiration
Fever	Pulse pressure	Tidal volume
Hypertension	Pyrexia	Vital capacity
Hypotension	Radiation	

STUDY SITUATION

Mr. J. Craig is a patient in a hospital. He is 75 years old. Mr. Craig is unconscious as a result of a cerebral vascular accident. His face is flushed, his respirations are noisy and his respiratory rate is 38 per minute. The patient's pulse rate is 158 beats per minute and his apical rate is 170 beats per minute. His blood pressure at 9 A.M. was 190/140.

1. What factors are significant in your observations of Mr. Craig?
2. Describe how the above data should be recorded.
3. Describe the observations that would be noted about Mr. Craig's pulse and respirations.
4. Define pulse deficit. How should it be taken?
5. What is this patient's pulse pressure?
6. Describe the sites that are possibly suitable for ascertaining his pulse.

BIBLIOGRAPHY

Canetto, Victoria: T.P.R.q.4.h. ad infinitum? *The American Journal of Nursing,* 64:132, November, 1964.

Delp, Mahlon H., and Robert T. Manning: *Major's Physical Diagnosis.* Seventh edition. Philadelphia, W. B. Saunders Company, 1968.

Guyton, Arthur C.: *Textbook of Medical Physiology.* Fourth edition. Philadelphia, W. B. Saunders Company, 1971.

Harmer, Bertha, and Virginia Henderson: *Textbook of the Principles and Practice of Nursing.* Fifth edition. New York, The Macmillan Company, 1955.

Nichols, G. A., and P. J. Verhonick: Time and Temperature. *The American Journal of Nursing,* 67:11:2304–2306, November, 1967.

Nichols, G. A., and P. J. Verhonick: Placement Times for Oral Thermometers: A Nursing Study Replication. *Nursing Research, 17:*159–161, March-April, 1968.

Nichols, G. A., et al.: Oral, Axillary, and Rectal Temperature Determinations. *Nursing Research, 15:*307–310, Fall, 1966.

Nichols, G. A., and B. A. K. Glor: A Replication of Rectal Thermometer Placement Studies. *Nursing Research, 17:*360–361, July-August, 1968.

Nordmark, Madelyn T., and Anne W. Rohweder: *Scientific Foundations of Nursing.* Second edition. Philadelphia, J. B. Lippincott Company, 1967.

Peterson, L. W.: Operant Approach to Observation and Recording. *Nursing Outlook, 15:*28–32, March, 1967.

Poole, Pamela E.: *A Study of the Routine Taking of Temperature, Pulse and Respirations on Hospitalized Patients.* Ottawa, Department of National Health and Welfare, 1968.

Purintun, L. R., and B. E. Bishop: How Accurate Are Clinical Thermometers? *The American Journal of Nursing, 69:*1:99, 100, January, 1969.

Shields, N. E.: Cardiac Anatomy and Physiology. *Nursing Clinics of North America, 4:*563, December, 1969.

Taylor, J. W., et al.: For Effective Thermometer Disinfection. *Nursing Outlook, 14:*56–57, February, 1966.

8 RECORDING

The nurse should be able to:

Explain the purpose of the patient's record
List types of information that are kept on this record
Describe ways in which the record is used
Name four guiding points to keep in mind when recording
Describe the following parts of the patient's record, including
      the type of information contained on it and nursing re-
      sponsibilities in regard to it:
   1. Face sheet
   2. Doctor's order sheet
   3. History sheet
Name five categories of information recorded in the nurse's
      notes
Outline pertinent data that should be included in the nurse's
      notes for each of the five categories of information

INTRODUCTION

The accurate recording and reporting of facts and evaluations of nursing care is considered one of the primary areas of nursing function (see Chapter 18). Recording is the communication in writing of essential facts in order to maintain a continuous history of events over a period of time. Reporting is the communication of information to another individual (or group of individuals) and may be either written or oral.

A number of different records and reports forms are kept by various health agencies, and the nurse will find that these vary from one agency to another. All types of health agencies maintain a patient's record or chart, however. The form of the chart depends on the type of agency. In hospitals, although the exact details of forms may differ from one institution to another, there is a uniformity to the type of information that is kept on the patient's chart.

THE PATIENT'S RECORD

A person's record or chart is a written record of his history, examinations, tests, diagnosis, prognosis, therapy and response to therapy while he is a patient. It is a means by which pertinent data are recorded and communicated to members of the health team. Hospitals are required to keep records by state laws and by regulatory agencies such as the Joint Commission on Accreditation of Hospitals. There are a variety of records kept by health agencies, including personal records, financial records, records of birth, details of communicable diseases and records relevant to narcotic legislation. The nurse is chiefly responsible for the patient's personal record, which contains information regarding his nursing care and his response to medical and nursing therapy.

The chief purpose of the patient's chart is to provide a written record of data about the patient; thus it serves as a means of communication among those whose professional talents are directed toward his care. This concise compilation of data serves as the basis upon which medical therapy is prescribed and nursing care is planned. Other physicians, nurses, social workers and dietitians, for example, contribute information to the chart which aids the physician in his diagnosis and in prescribing the therapeutic regime to be carried out by other members of the health team. The patient's record is also a valuable source of information for the nurse in the development of a plan of care for the patient.

The chart is admissible as evidence in court. Some states, in recognition of the confidentiality of communications between the patient and his physician, have ruled that information gathered in such a setting is inadmissible in court on the objection of the patient. Although the chart is the property of the health agency, it is generally felt that the agency does not have grounds for refusing to provide the information it contains to the patient or his legal representative. The only basis upon which information in a chart could be refused is by showing the court that the patient's medical condition would be adversely affected by disclosure of the information. (The legal implications of nursing practice are discussed in Chapter 18.)

Patients' records also provide material for research. Many disciplines in the health and allied fields avail themselves of this source of information in a diversity of research programs, for example, to show trends in the utilization of the services of a public health agency.

The information in patients' records also serves as an adjunct in the education of many personnel; medical students, interns, nurses and dietitians often use charts as reference sources. The chart also provides learners with a comprehensive picture and enables them to apply theory to a practical situation.

Records are also a source of statistical information. The number of births, deaths, hospital admissions and so on serves as a basis for making plans for the future and for anticipating needs. Some of these statistics are required by law; for example, the record of births must be filed with a government agency.

Another purpose of the patient's chart is to provide a record of the treatment of the patient. In this regard the record enables the medical, nursing and allied professions to fulfill an ethical responsibility, that of providing a check on the quality of the prescribed care. Frequently health agencies have regulations about recording which serve as another governing factor in patient care. For example, a hospital might require that all patients have a physical examination within 24 hours of admission and that this examination be recorded in the patient's chart. The charting then becomes an automatic check on this facet of patient care.

GUIDES TO RECORDING

Policies regarding charting vary with the health agency. Each nurse should be aware of the regulations where she is working. The following guides, however, will help a nurse in her recording

no matter what the particular policy happens to be.

Accuracy

The nurse records all factors accurately and truthfully. The omission of a recording is as inaccurate as an incorrect recording. Time is recorded accurately in the nurses' notes; all treatments and medications are recorded immediately after their administration, never before. Observations are specific and accurate; for example, the pain of a patient is described in detail as to type, exact location, duration and any precipitating factors and concomitant signs and symptoms.

Because the chart is a legal document, most agencies do not permit the use of erasures when an error is made in recording. Each institution has its own method of correcting mistakes. It is not unusual to cross out the error with a single line and initial the error and then to insert the correct information immediately following the error.

Headings on the chart sheets are entered accurately. Many hospitals use Addressograph plates which print data about the patient directly on the sheet. An Addressograph plate usually prints the patient's name, date of admission, nursing unit, hospital unit number (some hospitals have a classification system in which each patient has a number) and the name of the doctor. The Addressograph has the advantage of recording this information quickly and accurately.

Brevity

All recording should be concise and complete. Vagueness is to be avoided. Extra words such as "patient" can usually be eliminated from charting because it is obvious that it is the patient about whom the nurse is recording.

Legibility

Most agencies permit either printing or script on a patient's chart, provided that the script is legible. Ink is used because pencil does not provide a permanent record.

In the nurses' notes, the nurse is required to sign her name following her notations. Her signature includes her first initial and full last name. In some health agencies the nurse is also required to record her status, for example, R.N.

Format

There is usually a standard format used in recording which makes for consistency and facility of communication. For example, all medications and treatments might be recorded in one column of the nurses' notes and all observations in another.

Most agencies use blue or black ink for all charting, but occasionally red ink is used for night charting (12 M.N. to 7 A.M.).

COMMONLY USED TERMS AND ABBREVIATIONS

It is an important part of charting that only correct spelling and acceptable abbreviations be used. Some hospitals provide a list of abbreviations that are acceptable; others accept the commonly used abbreviations (see list in appendix).

THE ADMISSION SHEET

Most agencies have an admission sheet upon which is recorded personal data about the patient. This sheet is generally completed upon admission to an agency and then sent to the nurse or to the nursing unit to become a part of the patient's chart. Admission sheets contain accurate information which the nurse can transcribe to other records when necessary. The material on this sheet, like all the material in the chart, is confidential, to be disclosed only to professional people.

Often admission sheets record a unit number for the patient. This number serves as one means of identification and as a basis for cataloging medical records. The information on the admission sheet generally includes:

1. Patient's full name, including maiden name
2. Address
3. Classification number
4. Nursing unit or agency
5. Date and hour of admission
6. Date of birth
7. Name of physician
8. Details of financial responsibility
9. Sex and marital status
10. Nearest relative
11. Occupation and employer
12. Diagnosis
13. Previous admission or previous call
14. Religion

THE FACE SHEET

The face sheet is the front sheet of a chart, it has a diversity of uses. Frequently it is used to record allergies, but it is also used to record the history at discharge, in which case it is completed by the physician at the end of the patient's care.

The nurse's responsibilities are generlly minimal with respect to the face sheet. Usually the headings and the notation of a patient's allergies are recorded when a patient is admitted to the agency.

THE DOCTORS' ORDER SHEET

The doctors' order sheet is a written record of the orders given by the physician for the patient's treatment. The sheet may be kept in the patient's chart; however, in some hospitals it is kept in a central book on the nursing unit.

Doctors' order sheets are checked regularly by the nursing staff for new orders. Frequently a nursing unit has a method of flagging a patient's chart to indicate that a new order has been

SPEEDISET   MOORE BUSINESS FORMS LTD.

RIVERSIDE HOSPITAL OF OTTAWA	NOV 4 71

PHYSICIAN'S ORDERS

ATTENDING PHYSICIAN _Dr. R S White_

ALLERGIC TO _____

SMITH   MARY   SP 1246
2321 MARKET ST OTT 234-7566 600
JONES   RICHARD   HUS
SAME
23.10.71   2PM F 23 M SURG RC

420 1

DATE	TIME	ORDERS	EXECUTED
Sept 1/71	2 pm	DAT	Noted
		Up as desired	Noted
		APC ⚬ C 30mg tabs ⊤ q4h prn for headache	⊤
	10K	Seconal 100 mg qhs prn	⊤
		Consult ⊼ Dr. Brown regarding headaches	Notified 2:30pm
	WW	Hgb, Hct, WBC, Diff on admission	Done
		AC blood sugar in am.	Req
		Large chest x-ray in am	Req
		Valium 5mg ⊤ id pc ⚬ qhs	⊤ ordered
		Dr White	

NURSE SHALL CLOSE OFF ORDER
SHEET IF NO PHARMACY COPY.

IMPORTANT: NURSE SHALL USE COPY BENEATH AS
PHARMACY REQUISITION.
EACH ORDER MUST BE SIGNED

PHYSICIAN'S ORDER

FORM #2 - 8208

FORM #2 - 8208

PHARMACY COPY A

A sample physician's order sheet. (Courtesy of the Riverside Hospital of Ottawa.)

written. When the nurse has noted and put into effect an order, she indicates this in the prescribed manner on the order sheet.

In some hospitals when the physician orders a medication that is not kept on the nursing unit, he writes his order on a prescription pad as well as on the chart, so that the order can be sent to the pharmacy and a record kept on the nursing unit.

When the physician telephones an order to the nursing staff, the nurse so indicates on the order sheet. She also enters the name of the doctor, the time of the order and her own signature. Frequently doctors are asked to counter-sign their telephone order when they subsequently visit the patient.

THE HISTORY SHEET

The history sheet is a record of the personal and medical history of the patient; it is filled in by the physician. Frequently the doctor also describes the therapeutic regime for the patient and makes notes on the medical progress of the patient after each visit.

The history sheet can be a valuable reference for the nurse in making her nursing care plan for the patient. It provides information about the patient's present medical condition, previous illnesses, family history and current medical therapy.

THE NURSES' NOTES

The nurses' notes in a patient's chart can serve as a record of the medical and related therapies, including nursing, and the responses of the patient to these ministrations. In some agencies only nurses record these notes, whereas in others the auxiliary nursing staff, which includes orderlies and nursing aides, also record their care and observations of patients.

Generally the nurses' notes serve to record and convey five categories of information:

1. Therapeutic measures carried out by various members of the health team

2. Measures ordered by the physician and carried out by nursing personnel

3. Nursing measures which are not ordered by the physician but which the nurse carries out to meet the specific needs of a patient

4. Behavior and other observations of the patient which are considered to be pertinent to his general health

5. Specific responses of the patient to therapy and care

In many situations the nurses' notes serve as a record of the therapeutic measures that are carried out by various members of the health team. For example, when the physician changes a dressing on a patient's wound, it is recorded by the nurse in these notes. She includes not only the name of the doctor performing the procedure but also relevant details such as the appearance of the wound, the amount and nature of any discharge, the application of a medication or dressing and the removal of sutures. In some agencies, the nurse also records visits by the doctor and other members of the health team, such as the physiotherapist and dietitian. This type of charting serves chiefly as a record of care and therapy and therefore as a communication tool for all members of the health team.

Nurses also record measures which are prescribed by the physician and for which the nurse has the primary responsibility. For example, when the physician orders a medication for a patient, and the nurse gives the medication at the prescribed time and assists the patient if he needs help in taking the medicine. This type of charting serves to record either that the physician's orders have been carried out, or, if they are not carried out, the reason why. If a patient refuses to take a medication which has been prescribed, this fact should be noted, together with the patient's stated reason for refusal wherever possible.

The third type of recording comprises the nursing measures which are independent nursing functions. These measures are not ordered by the physician, but rather are measures the nurse judges to be necessary for the patient's care and perhaps supplemental to his medical therapy. The scope that a nurse has in this area depends upon the situation in which she is working. For example, in one situation the nurse shows the patient a position he can assume which she judges might help to relieve his discomfort, whereas in another situation the physician orders the position the patient is to assume.

There are other situations in which the nurse is subject to the physician's order but in which she also uses her judgment about when and if the measure is actually carried out, as when an analgesic is ordered to be given whenever necessary for the relief of pain. The nurse decides when the patient should have the medicine; in making her judgment, she takes into consideration many factors, including the need as perceived by the patient, his safety and comfort and his need for activity and rest. In some agencies the rationale behind nursing decisions is communicated in the nurses' notes or on a nursing care plan in order that other personnel can use the information.

The nurses' notes also serve as a record of that behavior of the patient which is considered pertinent to his general health. Behavior in this sense includes not only body action but emotional tone, verbal communication and autonomic physiological reactions. In this type of recording, objective observations are made and then recorded, the description being as complete and concise as possible. Opinions and interpretations of behavior are omitted. In describing verbal communication which reflects emotional tone, it is better to use direct quotes rather than to paraphrase.

In order that significant behavior can be identified and reported, it is necessary to have a knowledge of the needs of the individual patient and his way of showing physiological, psychological and sociological stress. An understanding of normal behavior and normal body reactions can serve as a guide to the observation of the individual patient. Often, the lack of a bodily reaction can be significant. For example, the lack of shortness of breath in a patient who sits in a chair after spending four weeks in bed can be significant to the physician in determining the need for future exercise.

The fifth area of charting is the specific response of the patient to therapeutic and nursing care measures. This includes the effect of an analgesic on pain, of a sponge bath on a fever and of the application of cold to a swollen joint. In recording such reactions, the nurse may be dependent upon the perception of the patient, as in the case of pain, or she may observe objective criteria such as a reduction in temperature or in the swelling of a joint. When the patient's perceptions are recorded, this fact should be made clear in the record. It is quite possible that a patient could perceive a situation differently from the way the nurse would, and this fact in itself could be important to his care.

When recording in the nurses' notes, the date and time that a patient receives a treatment or a medication are noted accurately. Time is usually denoted by the use of A.M. or P.M., although most agencies use the 24 hour clock to avoid ambiguity. Each entry in the nurses' notes is accompanied by the legal signature of the person who does the recording.

OTHER RECORDS

Various other records are made necessary by the specific needs of the health agency and of the individual patient. Some of the more commonly used records of this kind are discussed in other chapters.

STUDY SITUATION

Mrs. J. Rossten is a patient who has undergone abdominal surgery. She has been on the nursing unit three days postoperatively. Her orders from the physician include dressing changes once a day as necessary and Demerol 100 mg. I. M. p.r.n. for pain.

Her dressing is soaked through with reddish brown fluid and she complains of pain. As her nurse you give her 100 mg. of Demerol and change her dressing.

1. Where should you check for Mrs. Rossten's orders?
2. Give a sample of the charting for the Demerol, including what should be recorded about the patient.
3. What should be included in recording the dressing change? Give an example.
4. Where are these data recorded?
5. How would a change in the physician's orders be indicated to nursing personnel?

BIBLIOGRAPHY

Deschambeau, G. L.: This New Patient Chart Goes the Full Three Rounds. *Modern Hospital, 109*:80, September, 1967.

Dudley, Harry O.: Form for Nurses' Notes Achieves Uniformity in Charting. *The American Journal of Nursing, 41*:72, January 16, 1967.

Hershey, Nathan: Medical Records and the Nurse. *The American Journal of Nursing, 63*:110–112, February, 1963.

Hershey, Nathan: Nurses' Notes—They Can Play a Critical Role in Court. *The American Journal of Nursing, 69*:2403–2405, November, 1969.

Krismer, John R., and J. F. Cordes: Problem-Oriented Record Begins With the Patient. *Modern Hospital, 115*:81–83, November, 1970.

Pfister, Lewis F.: New Forms System. *Hospitals, 44*:53–55, October 16, 1970.

Price, Elizabeth: Medical Records. *Hospitals, 41*:131–134, April 1, 1967.

Smith, Dorothy M.: A Clinical Nursing Tool. *The American Journal of Nursing, 68*:2384–2388, November, 1968.

Sweet, Philothea, and Irmagene Stark: The Circle Care Nursing Plan. *The American Journal of Nursing, 70*:1300–1303, June, 1970.

Walker, Virginia H., and Eugene D. Selmanoff: A Study of the Nature and Uses of Nurses' Notes. *Nursing Research, 13*:113–121, Spring, 1964.

Wright, Harold N.: *Prescription Writing and Medical Jurisprudence.* Sixth edition. Minneapolis, Burgess Publishing Company, 1962.

9 THE NEEDS OF THE PATIENT FOR RELIEF OF ANXIETY

The nurse should be able to:

Differentiate between the expressive and instrumental roles
   of the nurse
Describe the nature and significance of the nurse's expressive
   role in patient care
Distinguish between anxiety and fear
Describe physiological manifestations of anxiety which are
   commonly seen in patients
Describe some behavioral patterns which may be indicative
   of anxiety in patients
List common sources of anxiety for people who are ill
Name guiding principles which are helpful in determining
   nursing action to allay anxiety in patients

THE NEEDS OF THE 9
PATIENT FOR RELIEF OF
ANXIETY

INTRODUCTION

Nursing students have for generations been told that reassuring the patient was an important part of the performance of any nursing activity. It was not uncommon in years past to see "reassure the patient" written as the second step of a nursing procedure, the first step having been to prepare the equipment necessary for carrying out the nursing activity. Whether the reassurance was to take the form of telling the patient that the procedure was not going to hurt or that the nurse really knew how to do the procedure and therefore the patient could safely trust her to do it was usually left to the nurse's imagination.

Gradually, however, there has been a growing realization that reassurance is not a simple matter, nor is it an intuitive process. Today we are much more aware of both the complexities involved in reassuring the patient and the significance of this as a nursing responsibility. The nurse's role in providing psychological comfort and support for the patient is seen as one that is complementary to and quite as important as her role in carrying out specific tasks of a technical nature. The terms "expressive" and "instrumental" are being used to designate these differing aspects of the nurse's role; expressive referring to those activities which contribute to the comfort and well-being of the pa-

tient, as opposed to the instrumental tasks which provide the patient with the technical assistance required to regain his health.[1]

THE EXPRESSIVE ROLE OF THE NURSE

People with health problems are under stress. Their homeostatic balance has been disturbed. They require, in most instances, technical assistance from medical personnel to enable them to overcome their health problems. This technical assistance forms the "curative" aspect of health care. It includes the diagnostic services and therapeutic measures that are carried out by physicians, nurses and allied health workers. The curative aspect is an essential component of health care. But people also need help in maintaining their emotional and psychological equilibrium under the stress of illness. The provision of this psychological support helps the patient to maintain a motivational balance which is conducive to recovery, and this is seen largely as a responsibility of nursing.[2] In her supportive

---

[1]James K. Skipper, Jr.: The Role of the Nurse: Is it Expressive or Instrumental? In *Social Interaction and Patient Care* by James K. Skipper, Jr., and Robert C. Leonard (eds.). Philadelphia, J. B. Lippincott Company, 1965, p. 41.
[2]Ibid.

99

role, the nurse is the person who "cares" for the patient. She maintains an environment that is therapeutic; she looks after the patient's physical comfort; and she helps to allay the fears and anxieties that accompany illness. That these comfort and care aspects of the nurse's role are as important to the patient's recovery as her skilled performance of nursing techniques is being increasingly recognized.

The importance of the patient's mental outlook on his prognosis has long been recognized. Motivation is accepted as essential to recovery; it is difficult to cure the patient who does not want to get well. In the surgical field, the excessively fearful patient is generally considered to be a poor surgical risk; many surgeons refuse to operate on the patient who is convinced that he is going to die under the anesthetic. It is only recently, however, that much attention has been paid to the significance of the alleviation of anxiety as a factor in making the patient's recovery from illness easier and less fraught with complications.

Much of the research to date has been on the effectiveness of preoperative nursing measures in preventing or minimizing postoperative discomfort and complications. There is evidence that nursing action, such as that involved in preoperative teaching, and the time spent in allaying the patient's anxiety can contribute to a smoother postoperative recovery for the patient.[3] Anxiety, however, is such a common concomitant of all illness and its effects on the patient so pervasive that its alleviation is important in every field of nursing.

The nurse should know the signs and symptoms of anxiety and she should be able to identify these in patients. She should be aware of potential sources of anxiety and, whenever possible, take steps to prevent or minimize these. The nurse cannot, of course, anticipate all the fears and anxieties a patient may

experience, but she can help to allay a good many of them.

ANXIETY AND FEAR

Anxiety is considered to be a modified form of fear. Both anxiety and fear are emotional responses of an individual to the threat of real or imagined danger. In fear, the danger is known and identifiable. A person may be afraid of cats, for example, and these pose a very real and recognized threat to him. On the other hand, the uneasiness of anxiety may have no definite basis which the individual can pinpoint; he is afraid, but of what he is afraid he does not know. With people who are ill there are usually elements of both fear and anxiety. The patient may be afraid of pain following surgery, for instance, but he may also be apprehensive about many other things, of the nature of which he is not sure.

Since both anxiety and fear evoke the same physiological reaction in the body and since both are likely to be present in the same individual during illness, the term "anxiety" is used here to encompass both.

SIGNS AND SYMPTOMS OF ANXIETY

The threat of danger causes certain physiological reactions to take place within the body. These vary to a certain extent in different individuals according to their physical makeup, although many are commonly seen in the majority of anxious people. Anxiety also brings about changes in a person's behavior. The nature of these behavioral changes depends on a number of factors, such as the severity of the anxiety, the individual's basic personality structure, and the ways in which he has learned to cope with anxiety in the past. The physical condition of the patient affects his ability to tolerate anxiety. Something which may constitute only a minor worry when one is well may create an overwhelming anxiety when the body's defenses are lowered.

---

[3]Rhetaugh Graves Dumas, Barbara J. Anderson and Robert C. Leonard: The Importance of the Expressive Function in Preoperative Preparation. In Skipper and Leonard, op. cit., pp. 16–29.

Physiological Manifestations

The principal physiological mechanism that is operating in anxiety is the fundamental "alarm reaction" as the body attempts to protect itself from harm (see Chapter 3). It was originally believed that the reaction was due to the outpouring of epinephrine into the bloodstream in response to strong emotion. However, this theory does not account for all the physical signs and symptoms that occur in people with anxiety. It is now believed that these are the result of stimulation of the autonomic nervous system. The sympathetic portion of the system is most usually affected, although, if the stimulus is sufficiently intense, the parasympathetic portion will be affected as well. Thus the anxious individual may show evidence of muscular tension which is a result of sympathetic nervous system stimulation and, at the same time, have diarrhea due to increased gastric motility resulting from overactivity of the parasympathetic system.[4]

Anxiety is such a universal phenomenon that almost everyone has had experience with some of its physical signs and symptoms. There are varying degrees of anxiety, ranging from a mild apprehension to overwhelming panic. In its mild form, anxiety may be beneficial in that it has the effect of putting the body into an alert state and motivating the individual to take some action to alleviate it. Few people would study or get assignments completed on time if there was not a certain amount of anxiety involved. Unresolved anxiety, however, or anxiety in more than mild degree can be harmful.

Among the most easily observable physical signs of anxiety in an individual are the *circulatory changes* which take place. The action of the heart is strengthened and accelerated. The patient's blood pressure may be elevated by 10 mm. of mercury or more above normal. The nurse may find that his pulse rate is considerably above normal. There may be a marked pallor of the skin or sometimes a flushing of the face. Often the skin surfaces are cold.

Muscular tension is almost invariably present. In some people this may be observed in a taut expression of the face or in a clenching of the fists. Some patients assume a very rigid posture. At times muscular tension is revealed by a tremor of the hands; in a facial, arm or shoulder tic; or in a generalized shivering or trembling of the body. The tightening of the abdominal muscles and the "butterflies" in the stomach which one commonly experiences with anxiety are the result of muscular tension. The tension headache is another common symptom of anxiety.

People seek relief from muscular tension in a number of ways: by biting their nails, drumming their fingers on the table, or pacing up and down, for example. Restlessness and overactivity are usually fairly reliable indications that the individual is anxious.

Many people *perspire excessively* when they are in anxiety-provoking situations. It may be the palms of the hands or the soles of the feet that are most affected. This increased perspiration combined with a coldness and pallor of the skin (due to lessened peripheral circulation), results in the typical cold and damp hand of the very anxious individual.

In anxiety, *mental activity is usually increased.* When the anxiety is mild, this may mean that the individual is simply more alert and better able to think clearly than he is usually. When anxiety is increased, however, the heightened mental activity may cause the person to be unable to rest, and insomnia is frequently present.

Changes in the patient's speech should also be noted as possible indications of anxiety. Some people talk very rapidly or constantly when they are anxious and sometimes the voice becomes very loud or high-pitched. In other persons there may be a hesitancy of speech; they may appear to be having difficulty finding the words they want to use. Stammering and stuttering are not uncommon in people with anxiety.

---

[4]For a more detailed explanation of this point, the nurse is referred to the text, *Function of the Human Body,* by Arthur C. Guyton. Third edition. Philadelphia, W. B. Saunders Company, 1969, pp. 352–353.

Often the anxious person has difficulty in concentrating; his attention span may be short and he may be unable to answer even simple questions. The very worried parents who bring a sick child into the emergency unit are sometimes so distraught that they cannot remember their own address.

Psychological Manifestations Of Anxiety

People react to threatening situations in a variety of ways. The psychological manifestations of anxiety in people who are sick usually reflect the ways in which they have learned to cope with life's dangers in the past. While some people can talk easily about their fears, and openly express these to the nurse, others may be saying, "I am frightened" in less easily recognizable form. Some people attempt to *deny* the existence of anxiety. They ask no questions and frequently make a point of keeping conversation off the subject of their illness. In our culture, many men feel that it is unmanly to say that one is afraid, particularly to a woman. Men not infrequently (and sometimes women too) cover up their feelings of anxiety with *loud assurances* that they are not frightened, and they may *joke and laugh* in their attempts to minimize the seriousness of their condition.

Some people react to the threat of danger with *anger and hostility.* They may criticize the care they are receiving and be loud and insistent in their demands for special treatment. People who react in this way often engender hostility on the part of the staff who label them consciously or unconsciously as "difficult" patients. There is an old saying that goes, "When in danger, when in doubt, run in circles, scream and shout." It is perhaps well for the nurse to remember this when she encounters a patient who is being very "difficult." If she can accept this type of behavior as being indicative of the patient's anxiety and not take it as a personal attack on herself she will be in a better position to take positive measures to help the patient.

Crying is another way in which some people react to anxiety. Many nurses are embarrassed to find a patient in tears and find it difficult to know what they should say or do. Attempts to reassure the patient that everything is going to be all right are not usually effective in helping the patient to cope with his feelings. Crying often denotes a feeling of helplessness and inability to handle one's problems. The tears serve to relieve tension, and the nurse can perhaps be most helpful by staying with the patient and being ready to listen when the crying episode is over.

SOURCES OF ANXIETY

Many anxieties which patients experience could be prevented if potential sources of fear were eliminated. Other anxieties, if not preventable, can often be minimized by nursing intervention. The nurse may be able to help the patient either through her own actions or by securing the services of resource people such the chaplain or the social worker, for example, who may be able to provide the assistance the patient needs to work through his problems.

Some of the more common sources of anxiety for patients have been discussed in earlier chapters. The patient is naturally anxious about his condition. Among the most frequently cited sources of anxiety in this regard are: fear of the unknown, fear of pain, fear of death or disfigurement, fear of the loss of love, of strength, or of the ability to return to a normal life.

If the patient is hospitalized, he usually experiences anxiety about the change in his environment. Again, there is a fear of the unknown; he is not sure what is going to happen to him, nor of what is expected of him in his role as a patient. He may fear losing his identity and control over his own destiny. Many people fear loneliness.

The patient may have other anxieties, in regard to his work, for example, or his family. He may wonder how his family are managing without him and what will happen to them if he is ill for a long time. Or, anxieties may result from financial matters such as the cost of illness and hospitalization, or the loss of salary when the patient is unable to work.

Then, there are the superstitions and misconceptions which many people have about illness, and these may be sources of anxiety. In spite of the increasing sophistication of the general public about health matters, many people are still relatively uninformed about modern medical treatment. The word "cancer" immediately draws forth a strong fear reaction in most people, despite assurances that many forms of cancer can be successfully treated if detected early.

MEASURES TO ALLAY ANXIETY

In determining measures which will allay anxiety, the nurse must take into account the fact that her plan of care has to be individualized to suit each patient. No two people are alike in regard to the nature of their anxieties, their reactions to these, or the type of help they need in overcoming them. There is therefore no easy set of rules which the nurse can follow. Instead, she must be guided by her assessment of each patient and an analysis of his particular needs in order to determine the specific action which is most appropriate for him. Some guiding principles may, however, be helpful.

1. *It is easier to allay a known fear than anxiety from an unknown source.* If the nurse can ascertain the cause of the patient's anxiety, she is better able to take specific action to dispel it. Thus, an important first step in helping the patient to overcome anxiety is gathering information about the patient, determining potential sources of anxiety for him and, where possible, identifying the specific source of his anxiety. In doing this the nurse must be tactful; she should not insist if the patient does not want to talk.

2. *People generally feel less anxious when they know what is going to happen to them.* Providing information is important both in preventing and in allaying anxiety. If a patient knows what is going to be done during a laboratory test he is less apprehensive. Similarly, the patient who has been told that a certain procedure may hurt a little is better able to face the pain.

3. *Anxiety is lessened when people feel they have some control over their situation.* Enlisting the patient's cooperation and allowing him to participate in his care whenever possible help to give him this feeling. Permitting the patient to retain a voice in the scheduling of his activities as, for example, his bath, is one way of helping him to feel he still has some control over events.

4. *Loneliness aggravates anxiety.* People need someone to whom they can talk and with whom they can share their feelings. A large part of the nurse's role is learning to listen to patients. Feelings can be shared without words, though, and sometimes words are not necessary. Simply the presence of someone who is sympathetic is helpful to the patient. Some people feel more comfortable in talking over their anxieties with non-medically oriented personnel. The nurse should not overlook the contribution that people such as the chaplain and the social worker can make in helping patients with their anxieties.

5. *A feeling of depersonalization contributes to anxiety.* When the patient feels that he has lost his identity, that he is just a hospital number or an interesting "case," his confidence in the care he is receiving is diminished. It is important to help the patient to retain the feeling that he is a respected person in his own right. Referring to the patient by name, not by bed number, and taking an interest in him as an individual are among the many things a nurse can do to reassure him that he is still an important person.

6. *Anxiety is lessened when the individual feels that he is receiving competent care.* This seems obvious, but the fact that a nurse is careful to attend to the small details of care and shows skill and confidence in carrying out activities does help to reassure the patient that he is in good hands.

7. *Physical activity helps to relieve*

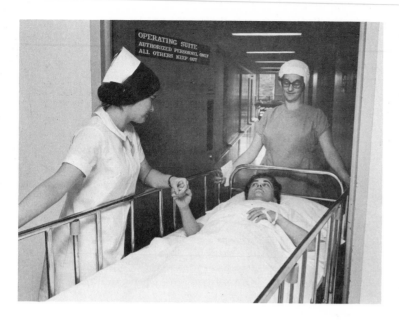

Often the comforting presence of someone who is sympathetic can help to allay some of the anxiety a patient feels in a stressful situation.

muscular tension. Exercise within the patient's limits of tolerance is a good way of relieving the muscular tension accompanying anxiety. If exercise is not feasible or permissible, nursing measures such as a soothing back rub or massage can frequently help to relax tense muscles. The assistance of the physical therapist is often helpful in teaching patients relaxing exercises or suggesting other measures to reduce muscular tension.

8. *Anxiety can often be relieved by diversional activity.* If a person has nothing to occupy his attention, he tends to become introspective and to brood on his troubles. Reading, watching television and playing cards are activities which are usually available in hospitals to help to divert patients from a constant preoccupation with their illness. Women patients often like to knit or to crochet, and these activities should be encouraged. Frequently, the occupational therapist can make suggestions and help to interest patients in activities which divert their attention from themselves.

GUIDE TO ASSESSING THE PATIENT'S NEEDS FOR REASSURANCE

1. Does the patient show physical signs or symptoms of anxiety? For example, is his pulse rate above normal in the absence of a known physical cause for it? Is there evidence of muscular tension?
2. Does the patient appear to treat his illness very lightly, that is, does he laugh and joke a lot about his condition?
3. Is the patient demanding, complaining or hostile toward the staff?
4. Is there evidence that the patient has been crying?
5. Does the patient verbally express any fears?
6. What do you know about this patient as an individual?
7. What are some of the possible sources of anxiety this patient may have?
8. Is the patient lonely?
9. Does the patient have activities to occupy his time?
10. What source people might be able to help this patient?

STUDY
VOCABULARY

Alarm reaction   Expressive activities   Instrumental tasks
Anxiety   Fear   Reassurance
Curative aspects

STUDY
SITUATION

Mrs. Duval is an attractive 38 year old woman who runs a successful hairdressing salon. She has been divorced for a number of years and has one daughter who is now married. The daughter and her husband have a small baby. In a routine physical examination of Mrs. Duval, her physician detected some evidence of tissue changes which could be indicative of early cancer of the uterus. He suggests that Mrs. Duval be admitted to hospital for further diagnostic tests. Mrs. Duval appears to be very upset.

1. For what reasons might Mrs. Duval be anxious?

2. What physical signs and symptoms of anxiety might this patient show? Explain the physiological basis for these symptoms.

3. When Mrs. Duval is admitted to hospital, she is very restless and talks constantly. She tells the nurse that she just cannot sit still. What can the nurse do to help this patient?

BIBLIOGRAPHY

Anxiety—recognition and intervention. *The American Journal of Nursing,* 65:129–152, September, 1965. (Programmed instruction)

Burkhardt, Marti: Response to Anxiety. *The American Journal of Nursing,* 69:2153–2154, October, 1969.

Elms, Roslyn R., and R. C. Leonard: Effects of Nursing Approaches During Admission. *Nursing Research, 15:*39–48, Winter, 1966.

Francis, Gloria M., and Barbara Munjas: *Promotion of Psychological Comfort.* Dubuque, Iowa. William C. Brown Company, Publishers, 1968.

Graham, Lois E., and Elizabeth Myers Conley: Evaluation of Anxiety and Fear in Adult Surgical Patients. *Nursing Research, 20:*2:113–122, March-April, 1971.

Guyton, Arthur C.: *Function of the Human Body.* Third edition. Philadelphia, W. B. Saunders Company, 1969.

Guyton, Arthur C.: *Textbook of Medical Physiology.* Fourth edition. Philadelphia, W. B. Saunders Company, 1971.

Johnson, Jean E.: Psychological Factors in the Welfare of Surgical Patients. *Nursing Research, 19:*1018, January-February, 1970.

Kolb, Lawrence D.: *Noyes' Modern Clinical Psychiatry.* Seventh edition. Philadelphia, W. B. Saunders Company, 1968.

Lewis, Garland K.: *Nurse-Patient Communication.* Dubuque, Iowa. William C. Brown Company, Publishers, 1969.

Little, Dolores E., and Doris L. Carnevali: *Nursing Care Planning.* Philadelphia, J. B. Lippincott Company, 1969.

Mercer, Lianne S., and Patricia O'Connor: *Fundamental Skills in the Nurse-Patient Relationship.* Philadelphia, W. B. Saunders Company, 1969.

Parsons, M. C., H. Faber, N. Hilger, M. J. S. Selg, and S. Stetzer: Difficult Patients Do Exist. *Nursing Clinics of North America, 6:*1:173–187, March, 1971.

Robinson, Lisa: *Psychological Aspects of the Care of Hospitalized Patients.* Philadelphia, F. A. Davis Company, 1968.

Skipper, James K., Jr., and Robert C. Leonard (eds.): *Social Interaction and Patient Care.* Philadelphia, J. B. Lippincott Company, 1965.

Tubbs, A.: Nursing Intervention to Shorten Anxiety-Ridden Transition Periods. *Nursing Outlook, 18:*27, July, 1970.

Walker, Daphne: Reassure the Patient? Yes, but How? *The Canadian Nurse,* 64:27, December, 1968.

10 THE SPIRITUAL NEEDS OF THE PATIENT

The nurse should be able to:

Discuss the relationship of spiritual beliefs and illness

List criteria which are helpful in assessing the spiritual needs of the patient

Identify nursing responsibilities in the spiritual care of patients

Describe the role of the chaplain as a member of the health team

Name specific sacraments and aspects of religious custom of the Jewish, Roman Catholic and major Protestant religions which affect the care of patients with these religious beliefs

Outline nursing responsibilities in regard to these sacraments and religious customs

Establish criteria for evaluating nursing care in relation to the patient's spiritual needs

106

INTRODUCTION

The need of many patients for spiritual counsel is receiving increased recognition from members of the various health and allied professions. In recent years the hospital chaplain has become a valued member of the health team and as such he plays an important role in patient therapy.

Often the nurse is the first person to become aware of a patient's desire or need for spiritual guidance. Frequently it is up to her to inform the patient of the help available to him and to contact the hospital chaplain or the community pastor. The nurse herself may be able to help the patient in spiritual matters, for she has a supportive role as well as the role of maintaining liaison between the patient and his sources of spiritual counsel.

Most people have a religious philosophy. In spite of the highly publicized trend toward secularism in the twentieth century, various studies show that from two-thirds to nine-tenths of the population of the United States profess a belief in a Supreme Being. Moreover, at a time of illness many not included in these figures look for spiritual guidance and consolation.

To provide a person with spiritual counsel is, therefore, in keeping with treating the whole person. Just as people who are ill often require help on a physical level, so they require spiritual aid. In addition, the recent recognition of psychosomatic illness emphasizes the role of emotions in disease. Thus to treat the whole person requires physical, emotional and spiritual help.

The spiritual needs of patients involve answers to such questions as Who am I? What am I like? What kind of world is this? These highly personal questions often become urgent at a time of illness, when the patient finds himself with time to think about himself and the world about him. Shut off from everyday concerns, some patients tend to question their entire system of values.

Some people look for an answer to why they are ill. They may look for moral significance to their illness and hope that religious doctrine will provide the solution. Other patients look for spiritual guidance to assist them in accepting their new role in the family. For example, the husband who normally supports his family but has become dependent upon his wife's earnings while he is ill may face a severe test. The acceptance of such changes in established roles and life patterns can be one of the most difficult adjustments a person must make.

Sometimes a person's values in life change with illness; often his horizons grow smaller, his bed becoming his domain. Spiritual belief can help such a patient to accept his illness and plan for the future. It can help him maintain a realistic perspective of himself and his relationship to the world about him. It can give him that inner strength which is closely interwoven with emotional health and physical well-being.

Religion is a social as well as a spiritual institution within society. Most societies have developed some form of religion, which then serves as an integrative force within the society. Traditionally, the established religions have

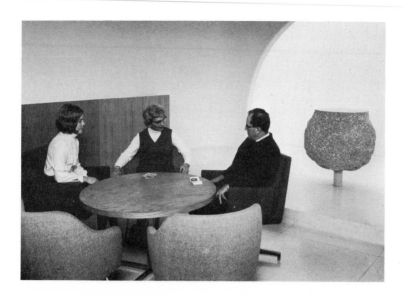

Many hospitals provide a quiet room where the patient and his family can meet with their spiritual counselor.

been concerned with ethics and moral behavior. Many established religions, however, have broadened their activities to include other areas. For example, recreation centers for all age groups have become an accepted part of the facilities of the church. Such centers offer the people of the community opportunities to find new interests and to join groups with which they can identify and in which they feel accepted.

Many churches now have special programs for youth groups designed to help adolescents and young people with their particular problems. "Drop-in centers" and other variously named gathering places are operated by a number of denominations to cater to the needs of young people.

SPIRITUAL BELIEFS AND ILLNESS

Spiritual beliefs, then, often help a patient at a time of stress. Some patients look to religious philosophy to explain illness; others look upon illness as a test of faith. Viewed in this light, illness and injury are usually accepted with forbearance and pose little threat to religious belief.

Still others interpret disease as God's punishment. "What have I done to deserve this?" they may ask. People who believe this interpretation attach a moral significance to disease, and they reason that because they have sinned they are being punished. They often believe that through prayers, promise and penance the cause of the disease will be treated. To them the physician treats only the symptoms. When a patient who believes this gets well, therefore, it is an indication that as a sinner he has been forgiven. On the other hand, should he die, his family either accepts his death as God's punishment or finds it to be unacceptable and unjust.

There are situations in which religious beliefs can be a hindrance to therapy and to health. Some religious groups tend to exalt faith and to disregard science. For example, many practicing Jehovah's Witnesses are by doctrine not permitted to have blood transfusions. The Church of Christ, Scientist, teaches spiritual healing; thus, when a practicing Christian Scientist seeks a physician's help, he may feel guilty because the prayers to relieve his symptoms were inadequate. He rarely blames his beliefs for the lack of cure, even when these beliefs may have caused him to delay his visit to a physician and his condition has worsened considerably during this time.

Generally speaking, religion helps people to accept illness and plan for the future. It can help a person to prepare for death, and it can also strengthen him during life. For example, the Christian belief of eternal life can help a patient face death more serenely. On the other hand, the Christian religion offers an interpretation of life that is based upon love and thus can strengthen a person in his daily life.

A discussion of illness and religious philosophy would not be complete without mentioning faith healing. This is an area that has received considerable publicity and research. There are religious organizations that are active in faith healing, for example, some evangelical groups. The British Medical Association appointed a committee to carry out a program of research on divine healing. The committee was able to categorize all reported instances of divine healing into six areas: mistaken diagnosis, mistaken prognosis, alleviation, remission, spontaneous cure and combined treatment. Although the committee found no evidence to support divine healing as the sole factor in any reported cure, it did not rule out religion as an integral part of patient therapy.[1]

Generally nurses and physicians recognize the importance of spiritual counsel as a part of a patient's therapy, and pastors recognize the close relationship between spiritual, emotional and physical needs.

IDENTIFYING THE SPIRITUAL NEEDS OF THE PATIENT

Spiritual needs, as we have noted, often become particularly apparent during a time of illness. In the hospital, it is usually the nurse who recognizes the patients who would like spiritual guidance, and it is also the nurse's responsibility to make available to the patient the sources of spiritual help.

Some patients bring articles with them which have a religious significance, and from these a nurse often can gain some idea of the importance that religious belief holds for a particular patient. For example, a Roman Catholic patient might have a rosary or a medal; an Episcopalian might have a prayer book.

Nurses should remember that there are patients who are not associated with any particular religious group. To them, spiritual need and spiritual belief are highly personal matters. Others are frankly agnostic, and for them any religious appeal would probably have a negative effect. Still others find the visits of a religious representative to be a source of discomfort rather than comfort; for example, a person might not like the particular hospital chaplain or the religious denomination that he represents. A nurse should cautiously assess the patient's attitude toward religion and his spiritual needs before she proffers suggestions or help.

Westberg has listed nine groups of people who respond best to pastoral care.[2] This list can serve as a guide to the nurse in identifying patients who might like the hospital chaplain to visit. The list should in no way be interpreted to exclude other groups, nor is it intended to replace an assessment of individual needs or to automatically include all patients to whom this classification applies.

1. *The patient who is lonely and has few visitors.* The perceptive nurse will hear a patient express loneliness in obscure ways as well as in obvious terms. The patient who continually has his signal light on to call the nurse may really be saying "I am lonely. Please stay with me." The nurse can also identify the lonely patient by making her rounds of the nursing unit during visiting hours. At this time she has an opportunity to meet patients' families and she can note those who do not have visitors. Patients whose homes are in distant communities may be lonely because their families and friends are far away.

2. *The patient who expresses fear and anxiety.* Some people will state frankly that they are afraid. Others express their fears by their questions, by their silence, by their body tension or facial expression. The taut, pale face and the anxious eyes often express fear as emphatically as words.

[1]Samuel Southard: *Religion and Nursing.* Nashville, Tenn., Broadman Press, 1959, p. 63.

[2]Granger Westberg: *Nurse, Pastor and Patient.* Philadelphia, Fortress Press, 1955, p. 73.

3. *The patient whose illness is directly related to emotions or to religious attitudes.* Because of guilt feelings, occasionally related directly or indirectly to religious doctrine, some people might develop physical symptoms of illness. An example is the single woman who becomes pregnant and, as a result, feels that she faces religious and social condemnation.

4. *The patient who faces surgery.* People who face operations are often afraid, and their fear is not necessarily related to the seriousness of the operation. Many people fear an anesthetic, body disfigurement, pain or even body exposure, but above all they fear death during surgery.

5. *The patient who has to change his pattern of life as a result of illness and injury.* Some people take great pride in their independence, and the prospect of any degree of dependence upon others is frightening. Some people worry about their changing roles within their families or their ability to earn a living. Illness and injury often necessitate abrupt changes in established living patterns that must be met by both the patient and his family.

6. *The patient who is preoccupied about the relationship of his religion and his health.* Such a patient may be seeking the reason for his illness in religious doctrine or may be trying to explain his illness in terms of religious philosophy.

7. *The patient who is unable to have his pastor visit or who would not normally receive pastoral care.* People who come from distant communities may not know a pastor in the immediate area. Other patients may not belong to religious groups in the community, but at a time of illness they may want spiritual counsel.

8. *The patient whose illness has social implications.* For example, the person who has had disfiguring surgery may feel that the hospital chaplain represents social acceptance or social rejection, and acceptance by the community may be important to his future plans.

9. *The patient who is dying.* Facing death, the patient may be filled with uncertainty and worry about his family.

Spiritual guidance can often help him to meet death, and it can help his family accept his death and plan for the future.

THE NURSE AND SPIRITUAL GUIDANCE IN THE HOSPITAL

The nurse can play an important role in providing the patient with spiritual support. One of her most important activities is identifying people's spiritual needs. To do this effectively the nurse must take time to listen to the patient and to ascertain his emotional tone. Usually a patient is not looking for answers from the nurse, he is looking for acceptance and help while he thinks out answers for himself.

Pastors appreciate referrals from nursing personnel and usually welcome the nurse's observations regarding the patient's spiritual needs. Most members of the clergy prefer to look after these needs themselves, however, and nursing responsibilities are usually limited in this regard.

If the nurse feels competent and comfortable in helping to meet the patient's spiritual needs, she can assist him by helping him to read from the Bible, if he so desires. For example, if the patient is unable to read himself the nurse can read to him. If the patient can do his own reading, the nurse can arrange privacy for him. Most hospitals provide Bibles, either at each bedside or at the nursing station or hospital library.

In addition to the Bible and prayer books, there is a great deal of religious literature available. Religious tracts, for instance, are published by many groups. Since tracts are often designed to meet specific needs, particular tracts can be selected to meet particular circumstances.

Prayers are the fourth area in which the nurse can help patients. Prayer takes many forms; to many it is a means of reaching God. However, prayer does not always involve a sense of mutuality; for example, in Buddhism, Gautama is regarded as unconscious and inaccessible.

One patient may prefer to pray silently, and to him prayer is a highly personal activity. Another may like the nurse to say a prayer for him, and this becomes a source of considerable comfort. Prayers need not be long; a simple, sincerely stated prayer can be as comforting as a lengthy one. A simple evening prayer that can be readily learned by the nurse is:

O Lord, support us all the day long of this troublous life, until the shadows lengthen and the evening comes, and the busy world is hushed and the fever of life is over, and our work is done. Then of thy mercy grant us safe lodging, and a holy rest, and peace at last, through Jesus Christ our Lord, Amen.[3]

If the nurse does not feel comfortable praying with the patient or reading to him from the Bible, it is quite acceptable for her to suggest that someone else do this. Most clergymen are happy to assist the patient in these matters, and the nurse may refer the patient to the pastor of his faith.

Finally the sacraments, which constitute a source of strength, are a means of providing spiritual help. Sacraments are usually administered by the designated representative of a religious group, although the nurse can administer the sacrament of baptism to a Roman Catholic patient if a priest is not available. The specific sacraments and the nurse's role in administering them are discussed later in this chapter.

THE HOSPITAL CHAPLAIN

The hospital chaplain may be a minister, priest or rabbi whose chief charges are the patients in a hospital. Large hospitals frequently have full-time chaplains representing several faiths. The Protestant faith is usually represented by ministers of various denominations, for example, Episcopalian, Methodist, Baptist and Congregationalist. The Roman Catholic faith is represented by the priest, the Jewish faith by the rabbi. Small hospitals may not have chaplains but, like their larger counterparts, they extend liberal visiting privileges to the representatives of the established religions in the community.

When the hospital chaplain or pastor comes to see a patient he usually checks with the nurse to make sure his visit is convenient for the patient. At this time the nurse is afforded an opportunity to give him information which may help him in counseling the patient. She can also tell him the names of other patients who want him to visit. Hospital chaplains and community pastors are generally available day or night, and they often leave their telephone numbers with the nurse so that they can be called at any time. It could be imperative, for example, to call a priest quickly for a dying Roman Catholic patient.

Some hospitals have chapels in which religious services are held regularly for the patients and their families. The services are usually conducted by the hospital chaplain or by the pastors from the community. Patients who would like to attend these services should be assisted to do so if it is possible. They may involve rearranging nursing care activities.

The hospital chaplain is an important member of the health team. Kevin describes the Roman Catholic priest as a physician of the soul.[4] McKnight states, "The specific role of the chaplain in a psychiatric hospital is that of helping people come to a healthy relationship with God."[5] The chaplain can contribute much in the care of patients. His knowledge and his spiritual guidance are often important adjuncts to medical care. The hospital chaplain can help people clarify their anxieties and accept illness. The community pastor often maintains liaison between the hospital patient and his family and can lend his support when the patient returns home. He can also assist the physician by interpreting medical instructions for the patient and in planning the patient's future.

Many hospital chaplains are active members of the health team. As such they attend health team conferences and contribute to the plans for the patient's therapy. Their knowledge of the patient's spiritual needs and personal problems can be essential in effectively helping the whole person.

---

[3]Ibid., p. 86.

[4]Barry Kevin: The Catholic Chaplain. *Canadian Nurse,* 57:1142, December, 1961.

[5]Earle T. McKnight: A Chaplain Interprets His Work. *Canadian Nurse,* 57:1139, December, 1961.

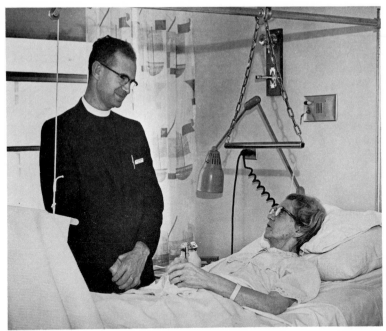

A hospital chaplain can assist many to meet their spiritual needs.

Another service provided by the chaplain is that of serving as a source of information for other members of the health team. For example, his knowledge of religious dietary preferences can be helpful to the dietitian when she plans a patient's menu. The importance of baptism in Roman Catholic doctrine is particularly relevant for nurses in the delivery room. The hospital chaplain can also provide spiritual advice to members of the hospital staff. Counsel at a time of stress can often help a nurse to be more effective in helping patients and their families.

The hospital chaplain also administers the sacraments to patients in the hospital. Through the sacraments, both the patient and his family receive spiritual strength and solace. The specific sacraments of the Roman Catholic, Hebrew, and Protestant faiths are discussed in the following section.

SPECIFIC RELIGIOUS CUSTOMS

The Jewish Faith

Patients who belong to the Jewish faith probably belong to the reform, conservative or orthodox group. Not all Jewish people follow the same practices, so the nurse will need to be sensitive to the patient's individual wishes. Generally the Jewish patient who follows orthodox doctrine will adhere most closely to certain dietary and religious customs. The patient himself, his family or the rabbi will assist the nurse regarding doctrinal customs.

The rabbi is the pastor of the Jewish congregation. Many Jewish patients like to have their own rabbi visit them when they are ill. He provides spiritual counsel to the patient and his family.

To the Hebrew people the act of *circumcision* is a religious rite. It marks the entrance of the male child as a potential citizen to the community. It should take place on the eighth day after birth of a male child; at the conclusion of the ceremony the child is named. Circumcision is called Brith Milah in Hebrew. The elaborateness of the ceremony is dependent upon the preferences of the family. Ten Jewish men must always be present, including all the male members of the infant's family. Following the circumcision there may be a reception for the members of the family and their friends. The nurse will be instructed in advance by the rabbi or the mohel (one who performs the circumcision) as to what equipment will be required for the ceremony.

Upon the death of a Jewish patient, the rabbi should be notified if the family is not present. He will arrange for the patient's burial. There is no need to be concerned about baptism, since the Jewish faith does not practice this rite.

The orthodox Hebrew patient may follow certain dietary regulations. Jewish doctrine forbids the eating of certain foods, including any part of the pig. Also certain other foods may be eaten only when they are specially prepared. The permitted foods are called kosher. They include the meat of animals that are ruminants and have divided hoofs, such as cows and sheep. Kosher fowl are fowl that are not birds of prey, and kosher fish are fish with scales. Examples of kosher fowl are chicken and duck; salmon and sardines can be classed as kosher fish. All shellfish, such as clams, oysters and lobster, are prohibited. Also meat dishes and dishes containing milk or cream may not be eaten at the same meal.

In order for meat to be considered kosher the animals must be slaughtered and the meat prepared in a special manner. No special precautions are required for vegetables. If a hospital is not prepared to provide kosher meat, other protein foods such as vegetable protein products can be substituted. Often a patient's family will arrange to provide kosher food if the patient is anxious about this. The nurse will need to instruct the family regarding any special dietary requirements for the patient.

There are other dietary regulations that apply at the time of the Passover. At this time a Jewish patient may refrain from eating leavened food, for example, bread. The rabbi can arrange to have special Passover matzo (unleavened bread) brought to the patient. Any Hebrew patient can be excused from strict dietary customs when he is ill. If the patient is concerned about this, the nurse can notify the rabbi and he will explain this to the patient.

The Roman Catholic Faith

The Roman Catholic faith recognizes several sacraments which have particular importance for nurses. In the Roman Catholic Church, God is conceived to be a God of mercy and grace, which are mediated through the church. The sacraments are signs and seals of God's expression to his people, and through them a person attains a state of grace, which is necessary for salvation. *Baptism* is the first of the sacraments to be administered to an individual. Because it is necessary for an infant to be baptized in order to receive salvation, it is very important to see to it that an infant in danger of death is baptized. According to Roman Catholic doctrine, an infant has a soul from the minute of conception; therefore a fetus at any stage of development must be baptized if it is born.

A nurse can perform a baptism by sprinkling water on the head of the child and saying, "I baptize thee in the name of the Father and of the Son and of the Holy Ghost." There are forms used in hospitals to record baptism of an infant, one of which is integrated into or attached to the patient's record; the duplicate is sent to the pastor of the family.

Holy Communion is another sacrament of the Roman Catholic Church. Patients are allowed water and medications prior to communion, as well as essential medical procedures up to the time of receiving communion.

When Holy Communion is requested by the patient, the Catholic chaplain of the hospital is called, or a priest from the church which serves the hospital. In either instance, a clean towel is used as a cover on top of the bedside table, on which the nurse places a glass of water and a spoon. Hospitals usually have a communion set on each floor which is taken into the patient's room and left for the use of the chaplain or visiting priest. Privacy is to be observed for the patient and the priest during the communion service.

The *Anointing of the Sick* is a sacrament that is performed for many patients.

Formerly known as Extreme Unction or last rites, it used to be given only to the person who was in danger of dying. Now, however, it is interpreted as an aid to healing and a source of strength. It may therefore be received by a patient one or more times for each illness, and may be received several times in a life-time.

It is felt that this sacrament should be administered when the patient is con-scious. It can be performed any time of the day or night. The priest anoints the eyes, ears, nostrils, lips, hands and feet with oil, for which cotton balls should be provided. Hospitals have a form for the priest to sign after he has adminis-tered this sacrament; the form is then attached to or integrated into the pa-tient's record.

Even if a patient of the Roman Catholic faith dies without receiving the Anointing of the Sick, a priest should be called. He can administer the sacrament immediately following death, thus pro-viding a source of comfort to the pa-tient's family.

With the revisions in dietary practices for Roman Catholics, meat may be eaten on Friday. Hospitals usually have a choice of meat or fish on the Friday menu and, during Lent, on the Wednes-day menu also. The patient is free to select whichever he or she wishes, un-less there is a special diet prescription.

The Protestant Faith

The Protestant faith includes many denominations; Methodists, Baptists, Presbyterians, Episcopalians (Angli-cans) and Congregationalists are but a few of the larger groups. Most Prot-estant patients prefer the chaplain of their own church, but in an emergency the chaplain of another denomination can often help.

The sacrament of *baptism* is a gen-erally universal rite within the Protes-tant faith. Some denominations practice baptism in infancy; others baptize at the age of understanding, often when a child is 12 years old. For a few Protes-tants, baptism is a necessity before death.

Some Protestant denominations hold *Holy Communion* and for many patients this can be a strengthening spiritual food. For this sacrament the clergyman requires a table in the patient's room to be cleared and furnished with a clean white cloth. It is preferable if the patient can assume a sitting position and, of course, privacy should be provided during the service. In communion the patient partakes of wine and bread; the wine represents the blood of Christ and the bread represents the body of Christ. Some Protestants consider this rite to be a cleansing of the soul from sin.

A few Protestant churches, the Epis-copal Church for example, are placing increasing emphasis upon anointing, and for this rite privacy is important.

Some Protestants have dietary cus-toms. Some are vegetarians and some do not drink tea or coffee, for example, members of the Mormon Church. Other people do not smoke or drink alcoholic beverages because of religious doctrine. During Lent, some Protestants practice a variety of dietary restrictions. Gen-erally speaking, however, a Protestant's eating habits are not restricted by reli-gious doctrine.

GUIDE TO ASSESSING NURSING NEEDS	1. Is religion important in the patient's system of values? 2. Does the patient feel spiritual counsel would help his health and well-being? Or does the patient indicate that he does not want assistance with spiritual needs? 3. Is he receiving the spiritual help he wishes? 4. Does the patient have specific spiritual needs with which members of the health team can be of assistance?
GUIDE TO EVALUATING THE EFFECTIVENESS OF NURSING ACTION	1. Is the patient accorded the privacy and facilities required to fulfill his religious needs? 2. Has the chaplain, rabbi or priest been notified if he is needed?

3. Does the patient have access to the Bible or other religious literature in accordance with his wishes?

STUDY VOCABULARY

Annointing of the sick	Communion	Priest
Baptism	Kosher	Rabbi
Chaplain	Pastor	Religion
		Sacrament

STUDY SITUATION

Mrs. J. C. D. is a 43 year old woman who has been in the hospital for 10 days. She states that her religion is Protestant. Mrs. D. was pregnant before she came to the hospital, but she lost her baby as a result of an automobile accident. She was scheduled to go home several days ago; however, she appeared very tired and depressed. The doctor suggested that she stay in the hospital for another week. One afternoon when the nurse walked into Mrs. D.'s room, she found the patient reading the Bible. The patient looked embarrassed and immediately put the Bible away. She said, "I am so unhappy. I lost my baby and I am sure it was a girl."

The nurse answered, "But Mrs. D., you have four wonderful sons at home now. You are really very lucky and you should think about them."

Mrs. D. said nothing more.

1. For what reasons might Mrs. D. be depressed?
2. What kinds of behavior might indicate to the nurse that this patient is worried?
3. What might the nurse have said?
4. What could the nurse do to help Mrs. D.?
5. If Mrs. D. had belonged to the Roman Catholic Church, what should the nurse consider?

BIBLIOGRAPHY

Allport, Gordon W.: *The Individual and His Religion.* New York, The Macmillan Company, 1961.

Blum, Richard H.: *The Management of the Doctor-Patient Relationship.* New York, Blakiston Division, McGraw-Hill Book Company, 1960.

Brown, Ester L.: *Newer Dimensions in Patient Care. Part III. Patients as People.* New York, Russell Sage Foundation, 1964.

Cabot, Richard C., and Russel L. Dicks: *The Art of Ministering to the Sick.* New York, The Macmillan Company, 1936.

Daoust, J. M.: Spiritual Care of the Sick. *L'hôpital d'Aujourd'hui,* 16:7:20, July, 1970.

Kevin, Barry: The Catholic Chaplain. *Canadian Nurse,* 57:1142–1143, December, 1961.

McKnight, Earle T.: A Chaplain Interprets His Work. *Canadian Nurse,* 57: 1139–1141, December, 1961.

Naiman, H. L.: Nursing in Jewish Law. *The American Journal of Nursing,* 70:10:2378–2379, November, 1970.

Nottingham, Elizabeth K.: *Religion and Society.* New York, Random House, 1954.

Pederson, W. Dennis: The Broadening Role of the Hospital Chaplain. *Hospitals,* 42:9:58, May 1, 1968.

Southard, Samuel: *Religion and Nursing.* Nashville, Tenn., Broadman Press, 1959.

Spiro, David: Jewish Patients in Hospital. *Canadian Nurse,* 57:1144, December, 1961.

Westberg, Granger: *Nurse, Pastor and Patient.* Philadelphia, Fortress Press, 1955.

Williams, Daniel D.: *The Minister and the Care of Souls.* New York, Harper & Brothers, 1961.

Young, Richard D.: *The Pastors' Hospital Ministry.* Nashville, Tenn., Broadman Press, 1954.

11 THE MOVEMENT AND EXERCISE NEEDS OF THE PATIENT

The nurse should be able to:

Define posture

Explain the functions of skeletal bones, body muscles and
    spinal nerves in body movement

Explain the principle of leverage

List other principles derived from the biophysical sciences
    which underlie body mechanics

Describe methods of carrying out common nursing measures
    utilizing these principles

Explain the importance of muscular activity for the person
    who is ill

Differentiate between active and passive exercise

Name the kinds of joints found in the body

List types of movements permitted by each kind of joint

Describe full range of motion exercises for different parts of
    the body

Describe methods for helping an individual to relearn to
    walk with and without mechanical aids

116

THE MOVEMENT AND 11
EXERCISE NEEDS OF
THE PATIENT

INTRODUCTION

A knowledge of the principles of body movement and skill in their application are important to both the patient and the nurse. Exercise and body movements are often prescribed as supportive measures to meet the patient's particular health needs. When these are not prescribed specifically, it becomes a nursing responsibility to plan a daily program of activities to meet the patient's needs for movement and exercise.

It is equally important that the nurse use her body in a way which not only avoids muscle strain but uses energy efficiently. But the practice of good body mechanics is not restricted to nursing care; it is integral to healthy living for all people. In health and in illness, good posture and efficient body movement are essential therapeutically and aesthetically. Courses in beauty often stress the importance of posture and facility of movement.

Once a person has a knowledge of the principles underlying body mechanics, he should put them into practice in order to establish good habit patterns of body movement. As these patterns are established, movements become smooth and place a minimum of strain upon the body muscles. The nurse will find that she can help patients to move more easily, and the patient will find that he is more comfortable.

Kinesiology is the science of human motion; its study dates back to Aristotle, who is considered the father of kinesiol-ogy. To understand body motion, the nurse needs a knowledge of anatomy, physiology and physics as well as a knowledge of the principles underlying body movement.

PHYSIOLOGY AND ANATOMY OF BODY MOVEMENT

Posture is "the relationship of the various parts of the body at rest or in any phase of activity."[1] Posture is considered to be good when the proper function of the body systems is favored. It is poor when undue strain is placed upon the muscles, ligaments, and joints in maintaining balance.

Body movements are made principally by means of the skeleton, the muscles and the nervous system. The skeleton is made up of bones, two of the functions of which are to provide an attachment for muscles and ligaments and to act as levers. The proximal end of a skeletal muscle is attached to the less movable bone; this point of attachment is called the origin of the muscle. The distal end of the muscle is attached to a freely movable bone; this point is called the insertion of the muscle.

The muscles, which are composed of fibers, contract to produce motion. Skel-

---

[1]Jessie L. Stevenson: *Posture and Nursing.* Second edition. New York, Joint Orthopedic Nursing Advisory Service of the National Organization for Public Health Nursing and the National League of Nursing Education, 1948, p. 8.

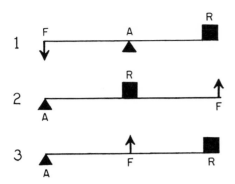

F = Force
A = Axis or fulcrum
R = Resistance or weight

Three types of levers.

etal muscle is continuously in slight contraction, or tonus. General good health, good nutrition, alternate rest and activity help to maintain the extensibility of muscle without stretching and thus affect muscle tone favorably.[2]

The bones of the body also act as levers, and in body mechanics the principle of leverage is frequently used. A lever is "a rigid bar which revolves about a fixed point, the fulcrum."[3] The fulcrum of the lever is a fixed point. The resistance arm is the area between the resistance or weight and the fulcrum. The effort arm is the area between the point at which the energy is applied and the fulcrum. The levers of the body vary in shape and even in rigidity. The principles of leverage are applied in procedures described later in the chapter.

The spinal nerves are directly involved in trunk and limb movements. Each spinal nerve has an anterior and a posterior root. The anterior root conducts impulses to the muscles from the central nervous system; the posterior root conducts impulses from the sensory receptors to the central nervous system.

Body movement is also affected by gravity, the force which pulls all objects toward the center of the earth. Most movement, then, involves pulling to at least some extent against the force of gravity. To describe the movement of the body parts, terms such as abduction, adduction, flexion and extension are used. Abduction refers to movement away from the central axis of the body. Adduction refers to movement toward the axis of the body. Flexion is the act of bending; extension can be described as the act of straightening. Illustrations of abduction, adduction, flexion and extension are given later in this chapter.

Body movements can also be described relative to three planes: the sagittal, frontal and transverse. When the body is in the anatomical position, the sagittal plane divides it into right and left sections, the frontal plane into dorsal and ventral sections and the transverse plane into upper and lower sections.

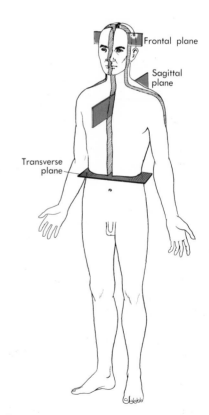

Sagittal, frontal and transverse planes of the body.

[2]Margaret C. Winters: *Protective Body Mechanics in Daily Life and in Nursing.* Philadelphia, W. B. Saunders Company, 1952, p. 9.

[3]John M. Cooper and Ruth B. Glasgow: *Kinesiology.* St. Louis, The C. V. Mosby Company, 1963, p. 37.

PRINCIPLES UNDERLYING BODY MECHANICS

Certain principles underlying body movement can serve as guides for the patient and the nurse.

Muscles tend to act in groups rather than singly. For example, breathing requires the coordinated activity of a number of muscles including the intercostals, the diaphragm and the sternocleidomastoid muscles, the scalenes, the thoracohumeral and the thoracoscapular muscles. To move the thigh alone involves all the gluteus muscles as well as the adductor muscles.

Large muscles fatigue less quickly than small muscles.

Using a group of large muscles places less strain on the body than using a group of smaller muscles or a single muscle. For example, less strain results when a heavy object is raised by flexing the knees rather than by bending from the waist. The former movement utilizes the large gluteal and femoral muscles, whereas the latter utilizes the smaller muscles such as the sacrospinal muscle of the back.

Active movement results in the contraction of muscles. Active and passive exercises are often prescribed for patients. Active movement involves the contraction of the muscles; the energy is supplied by the patient. Passive movement does not require muscle contraction; the energy is essentially supplied by a second person. The nurse can assist a patient with both active and passive movements as a part of nursing care.

Muscles are always in slight contraction. This condition is called muscle tone. If the nurse prepares her muscles for action prior to activity, she will protect her ligaments and muscles from strain and injury. For example, she will be better prepared to lift a heavy object if she first contracts the muscles of her abdomen and pelvis and the gluteal muscles of the buttocks.

The stability of an object is greater when there is a wide base of support and a low center of gravity and when a vertical line from the center of gravity falls within the base of support. In her motions the nurse can assume a broad stance and bend her knees rather than bend at the waist. This practice keeps the vertical line of her center of gravity within her base of support, thus providing her with greater stability. For example, in helping a patient to move, the nurse's position is more stable and she is therefore better able to maintain her balance if she stands with her feet apart and bends her body at the knees rather than at the waist.

The amount of effort required to move a body depends upon the resistance of the body as well as the gravitational pull. By utilizing the pull of gravity rather than working against it, the nurse can reduce the amount of effort required in movement. For example, it is easier to lift a patient up in bed when he is lying flat and his center of gravity has been shifted toward the foot of the bed than it is when he is in a sitting position in which the resistance of the body to movement is much greater.

The force required to maintain body balance is greatest when the line of gravity is farthest from the center of the base of support. Therefore, the person who holds a weight close to his body uses less effort than the person who holds the weight in his extended arms. For example, when moving a patient from a bed to a stretcher, it is easier for the lifters if they hold the patient's body close to their own.

Changes in activity and position help to maintain muscle tone and avoid fatigue. If a person changes his position even slightly while he is carrying out a task, and if he changes his activity from time to time, he will maintain better muscle tone and avoid undue fatigue.

The friction between an object and the surface upon which the object is moved affects the amount of work needed to move the object. Friction is a force that opposes motion. The smoothest surfaces create the least friction; consequently less energy is needed to move objects on smooth surfaces. The nurse can apply this principle when a patient changes his position in bed by providing a smooth foundation upon which the patient can move.

Pulling or sliding an object requires less effort than lifting it, because lifting necessitates moving against the force of gravity. If, for example, the nurse lowers the head of a patient's bed before she helps him to move up in the bed, less effort is required than when the head of the bed is raised.

Mechanical devices can lessen the amount of work required in movement. If, in lifting heavy objects, the nurse uses her arm as a lever whenever possible, she will utilize less energy than she would in direct lifting.

Using one's own weight to counteract a patient's weight requires less energy in movement. If a nurse uses her own weight to pull or push a patient, her weight increases the force applied to the movement.

LIFTING THE PATIENT AND HELPING HIM TO MOVE

Often the nurse is called upon to help a patient to move or to change his position. Gentle, sure motion on the nurse's part, based on her knowledge of body mechanics, not only helps patients to move easily but also gives them a sense of confidence in the nurse. Some patients, unable to move by themselves, are completely dependent upon the nurse for their changes in position and their exercise. The nurse is frequently called on to assist her patients to make the movements described in this section. It should be noted that there are various methods of performing each movement. The techniques and illustrations used here present one way of doing them.

Helping the Patient Move to the Side of the Bed

The nurse may be called upon to help a patient who is lying on his back (dorsal recumbent position) to move to the side of the bed, as when she is planning to change his surgical dressing. To lift the patient would require a great deal of effort upon the nurse's part, possibly putting unnecessary strain on her muscles

as well as upon the patient. The patient can be helped to move more easily, however, if the nurse uses her own weight as a force to counteract the patient's weight and her arms to connect her with the patient so that they move as one.

1. The nurse stands facing the patient at the side of the bed toward which she wishes the patient to move.

2. She assumes a broad stance with one leg forward of the other and with her knees and hips flexed in order to bring her arms to the level of the bed.

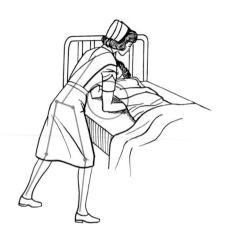

3. The nurse places one arm under the shoulders and neck of the patient and the other arm under the small of patient's back.

4. She shifts her body weight from her front foot to her back foot as she rocks backward to a crouched position, bringing the patient toward her to the side of the bed. The nurse's hips come downward as she rocks backward. The patient should be pulled rather than lifted in this procedure.

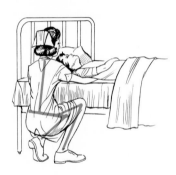

5. The nurse then moves the middle section of the patient in the same manner by placing one arm under the small of the patient's back and one arm under the thighs. Then the patient's feet and the lower legs are moved with the same motion.

Care should be taken not to pull the patient off the side of the bed. If the patient is unable to move her arm that is nearer the nurse, it should be placed across the patient's chest so that it will not hinder movement or be injured. In moving a patient in this manner, the nurse should feel no strain across her shoulders; it is her own weight that supplies the power to move the patient.

Raising the Shoulders of the Helpless Patient

Some patients are unable to raise their shoulders, even for a short time. When the nurse finds it necessary to raise such a patient, as when changing the pillows, she should proceed as follows:

1. The nurse stands at the side of the bed and faces the patient's head. She assumes a wide stance with her foot that is next to the bed behind the other foot.

2. She passes her arm that is farther from the patient over the patient's near shoulder, and rests her hand between the patient's shoulder blades.

3. In order to raise the patient the nurse rocks backward, shifting her weight from her forward foot to her rear foot, her hips coming straight down in this motion.

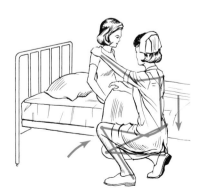

The nurse can either guide the patient with her free arm or use it for balance. Again it is the nurse's weight which counteracts the patient's weight.

Raising the Shoulders of the Semihelpless Patient

The semihelpless patient can move to some extent; however, he needs considerable support in most of his movements. In order to help the semihelpless patient raise his shoulders, the nurse uses her own arm as a lever and her elbow as the fulcrum.

1. The nurse stands at one side, facing the head of the patient's bed. Her foot next to the bed is to the rear and the other foot is forward. This position provides a wide base of support.

2. She bends her knees to bring her arm that is next to the bed down to a level with the surface of the bed.

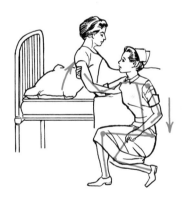

3. With her elbow on the patient's bed the nurse grasps the posterior aspect of the patient's arm above the elbow, and the patient grasps the nurse's arm in the same manner.

4. The nurse then rocks backward, shifting her weight from her forward foot to her rear foot and bringing her hips downward. Her elbow remains on the bed and acts as the fulcrum of the level.

Moving the Helpless Patient Up in Bed

Helpless patients are best assisted to move up in bed by two persons rather than one; however, one nurse can help a patient to move up in bed by moving him diagonally toward the side of the bed. By moving the patient in sections and by using her own weight to counteract the patient's weight, the nurse can safely move the helpless patient up in bed. This is most easily done if the head of the bed is lowered; then the nurse is not working directly against the force of gravity.

1. The nurse stands at the side of the patient's bed and faces the far corner of the foot of the bed. She places one foot behind the other, assuming a broad stance.

2. She flexes her knees so that her arms are level with the bed and puts her arms under the patient. One arm is placed under the patient's head and shoulders, one arm under the small of his back.

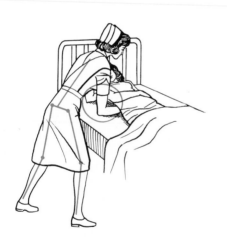

3. The nurse rocks forward, then shifts her weight from her forward foot to her rear foot, her hips coming downward. The patient will slide diagonally across the bed toward the head and side of the bed.

4. This is repeated for the trunk and legs of the patient. (See the procedure for moving the patient to the side of the bed.)

5. The nurse then goes to the other side of the bed and repeats steps 1 to 3. She continues this process until the patient is satisfactorily positioned.

Moving the Semihelpless Patient Up in Bed

This movement is facilitated if the patient can assist by flexing his knees and pushing with his legs. In assisting the patient to make this movement, the nurse should take precautions that his head does not hit the top of the bed. Thus the nurse can lower the head of the bed and put the patient's pillow at the head of the bed, where it can act as a pad. Helping the patient move up in bed can be done by one or two nurses; in the latter instance one nurse stands at each side of the patient's bed. The procedure for one nurse is described here.

1. The patient flexes his knees, bringing his heels up toward his buttocks.

2. The nurse stands at the side of the bed, turned slightly toward the patient's head. One foot is a step in front of the other, the foot that is closer to the bed being to the rear; her feet are directed toward the head of the bed.

3. The nurse places one arm under the patient's shoulders and one arm under his thighs. Her knees are flexed to bring her arms to the level of the surface of the bed.

4. The patient places his chin on his chest and pushes with his feet as the nurse shifts her weight from her rear foot to her forward foot. By grasping the head of the bed with his hands, the patient can help pull his own weight.

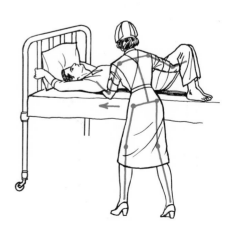

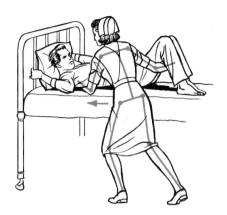

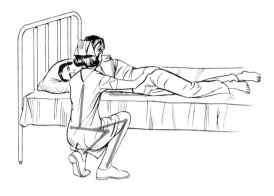

Helping the Patient Turn on His Side

When a patient needs help in order to turn on his side, the nurse must take particular care that the patient does not fall off the bed. She can control his turning by placing her elbows on the bed as a brace to stop his roll.

1. The nurse stands on the side of the bed toward which the patient is to be turned. The patient places his far arm across his chest and his far leg over his near leg. The nurse checks that the patient's near arm is lateral to, and away from, his body so that he does not roll upon it.

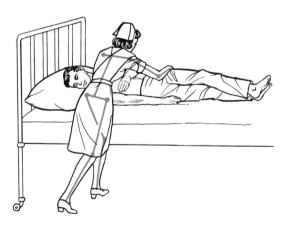

2. The nurse stands opposite the patient's waist and faces the side of the bed with one foot a step in front of the other.

3. She places one hand on the patient's far shoulder and one hand on his far hip.

4. As the nurse shifts her weight from her forward leg to her rear leg, the patient is turned toward her. The nurse's hips come downward during this motion.

5. The patient is stopped by the nurse's elbows, which come to rest on the mattress at the edge of the bed.

Helping the Semihelpless Patient Raise Her Buttocks

In this motion the nurse's arm acts as the lever, her elbow as the fulcrum.

1. The patient flexes her knees and brings her heels toward her buttocks.

2. The nurse faces the side of the bed and stands opposite the patient's buttocks. She assumes a broad stance.

3. With her knees flexed to bring her arms to the level of the bed, the nurse places one hand under the sacral area of the patient, her elbow resting firmly on the foundation of the bed.

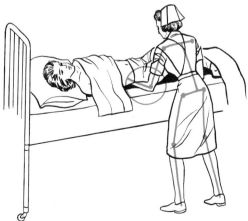

4. As the patient raises her hips, the nurse comes to a crouching position by bending her knees, while her arm acts as a lever to help support the patient's buttocks. The nurse's hips come straight down in this action. While the nurse supports the patient in this position she can use her free hand to place a bedpan under the patient or to massage the sacral area.

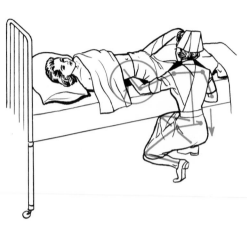

Assisting the Patient to a Sitting Position on the Side of the Bed

1. The patient turns on her side toward the edge of the bed upon which she wishes to sit. (See the procedure for helping the patient turn on her side.)

2. After ensuring that the patient will not fall off the bed, the nurse raises the head of the bed.

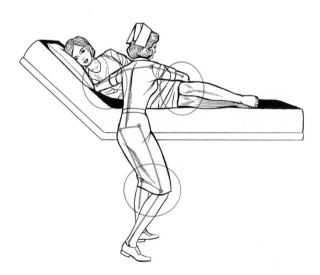

3. Facing the far bottom corner of the bed, the nurse supports the shoulders of the patient with one arm, while with the other she helps the patient to extend her lower legs over the side of the bed. She assumes a broad stance, with her foot that is toward the bottom of the bed being to the rear of the other foot.

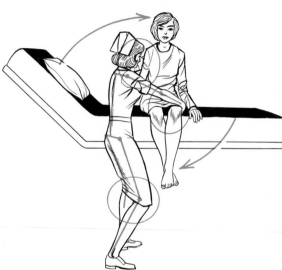

4. The patient is brought to a natural sitting position on the edge of the bed when the nurse, still supporting the patient's shoulders and legs, pivots her body in such a manner that the patient's lower legs are swung downward. The nurse's weight is shifted from her front leg to her rear leg.

Assisting the Patient to Get Out of Bed and Into a Chair

In this procedure the bed should be at a height from which the patient can step naturally to the floor. If the bed cannot be lowered sufficiently, the nurse should obtain a footstool for the patient. The footstool must be stable and have a surface upon which the patient is unlikely to slip. Also, it is advisable for the patient to wear low-heeled shoes rather than loose slippers. The former enable the patient to walk comfortably, yet provide support and are not as likely to slip.

1. The patient assumes a sitting position on the edge of the bed and puts on shoes and dressing gown.

2. A chair is placed at the side of the bed with its back toward the foot of the bed.

3. The nurse stands facing the patient, her foot that is closer to the chair is a step in front of the other, to give her a wide base of support.

4. The patient places her hands upon the nurse's shoulders, and the nurse grasps the patient's waist.

5. The patient steps to the floor, and the nurse flexes her knees so that her forward knee is against the patient's knee. This prevents the patient's knee from bending involuntarily.

6. The nurse turns with the patient while maintaining her wide base of support. She bends her knees as the patient sits in the chair.

Lifting the Patient From a Bed to a Stretcher (Three Man Carry)

To move a patient who must remain in the horizontal position from one place to another, for example, from a bed to a stretcher, three persons are usually needed. The tallest person should take the top third of the patient, because he probably has the longest reach and can most easily support the patient's head and shoulders. The second person supports the middle third of the patient, usually the heaviest part. He will be helped if the first and third persons put their arms beside his. The shortest person supports the patient's legs.

Before the patient is moved, a stretcher is placed at right angles to the bed, with the head of the stretcher almost touching the foot of the bed. The stretcher wheels should be locked. To coordinate their movements, the three persons must work by the numbers; the person who takes the head of the patient calls the numbers.

1. The three who are to move the patient face the side of the patient's bed. Each assumes a broad stance, with his foot that is toward the stretcher being forward.

2. At the call of "one," the three bend their knees and place their arms under the patient. The first person places one arm under the neck and shoulders and the other arm under the small of the patient's back. The middle person places one arm under the small of the patient's back and the other arm under his hips. The person at the foot of the bed places one arm under the patient's hips and the other arm under the patient's legs.

3. At the call of "two" the patient is turned toward those who are lifting him. This is accomplished by rolling the patient toward the lifters. The patient's arms should not be allowed to dangle freely. The lifters hold him close to their bodies in order to avoid backstrain.

4. At the call of "three," they rise, step back (with the forward foot), and walk in unison to the stretcher.

5. At the call of "four," they bend their knees and rest their elbows on the stretcher.

6. At the call of "five," each lifter extends his arms so that the patient rolls to his back at the middle of the stretcher. Protection is needed at the far side of the stretcher to prevent the patient from rolling off.

7. At the call of "six," each lifter withdraws his arms.

In lifting the patient, the lifters should hold the patient close to their bodies. It is also important to lift and lower the patient with an easy smooth motion in order not to jar or frighten him.

SOME DEVICES FOR ASSISTING THE PATIENT TO MOVE

The Drawsheet

A drawsheet placed under a helpless patient as an aid in moving him has proved useful in many situations. The drawsheet should extend from the patient's arm level to the inferior aspect of the buttocks.

At least two nurses are needed to move a patient by this means. One nurse stands at each side of the patient, grasps the drawsheet firmly near the patient, and moves the patient and drawsheet to the desired position—up in the bed or toward the side, for example.

To turn a patient on his side, his arms and legs are first positioned safely (see p. 123). The nurse then reaches over the patient, grasps the drawsheet on the far side, and pulls it toward her in such a way that the patient rolls on his side toward the nurse. Again the nurse should take precautions to ensure that the patient does not roll off the side of the bed.

Mechanical Devices

There are several mechanical devices available for moving a patient. One is the hydraulic lift, which can elevate a person and move him—from his bed to a stretcher for example. Some models have heavy canvas supports which fit under the patient's buttocks and behind his back to provide support. These lifts can be used to assist a patient in and out of the bathtub and in and out of bed.

EXERCISE

Most patients require some type of exercise; there are very few for whom all exercise is contraindicated. The physician generally orders the degree of activity for patients in the hospital, that is, whether he is to be confined to bed, have bathroom privileges and so on; however, the patient who has a specific need for remedial exercises, for example, the patient with a paralyzed arm, is often guided in his exercise by the physical therapist (physiotherapist) and the nurse. For many patients, exercise is part of their nursing care and most of the guidance they receive is provided by the nurse. It is an important independent nursing function to assess the patient's needs and provide for suitable exercise for patients within existing limitations and contraindications.

Patients who remain in bed for a prolonged period are prone to complications as a result of their inactivity. Loss of mobility and muscle strength are often evident in bed patients, particularly the elderly. Exercise helps maintain and create good muscle tone and prevent atrophy. For the person in bed this means that the strength of his muscles is maintained or developed in readiness for greater activity. Exercise also helps in the elimination of waste products from the muscles. The contraction of muscles increases circulation and the removal of wastes from the body. Increased circulation, particularly an increase in venous return from the extremities, is particularly important for the person who remains in bed. Stasis of blood is a predisposing factor in the formation of clots, which can lead to serious complications.

The increased basal metabolic rate which results from exercise increases the body's need for oxygen. This in turn results in an increase in both the rate and depth of respirations, thus improving lung aeration and helping to prevent infectious processes in the lungs which occur as a result of inactive lung areas and stagnant secretions. Improved blood circulation also increases the delivery of oxygen and nutrients to tissues, thus maintaining their health and preventing deterioration and ulcer formation.

Contracture of the muscles and stiffening of the joints are other unfortunate side effects of prolonged inactivity. By putting joints through their full range of motion, these can often be avoided.

Kinds of Exercise

Exercise can be described as isotonic or isometric. In isotonic exercise, the muscle shortens, causing the limb to move. Isotonic exercises increase muscle strength and help joint mobility. Isometric exercises are also of value in strengthening muscles, but they do not improve joint movement. In this type of exercise the patient consciously increases the tension of his muscles, but there is neither joint movement nor is the length of the muscle changed.

Exercise can be either active or passive. In active exercise the patient supplies the energy to move the various parts of his body. In passive exercise the body part is moved by someone else, and the muscles do not actively contract. Regardless of the kind of exercise the physician suggests, the nurse can assist the patient. She should help him plan his exercises in order that he may avoid fatigue. If passive exercises are prescribed, she can exercise the various parts of the patient's body. During the bed bath, for example, the nurse has an excellent opportunity to move the patient's limbs through their full range of motion. Very often a patient can learn to carry out his exercises independently.

Types of Joints

In order to understand the types of movement that are included in a full range of motion, it is necessary to keep in mind the various kinds of joints in the body. These include six.

Hinge. This is a uniaxial joint which permits flexion and extension. An example of a hinge joint is the knee.

Pivot. This is also a uniaxial joint. It permits rotation. An example is the atlantoaxial (the joint between the first cervical vertebra and the base of the skull).

Condyloid. This is a biaxial joint. It permits flexion, extension, abduction and adduction. A combination of these four movements is called circumduction. The wrist is a condyloid joint.

Saddle. This is another biaxial joint. It permits flexion, extension, abduction, adduction, circumduction. An example is the thumb.

Ball and socket. This type of joint is polyaxial. Movements permitted include flexion, extension, abduction, adduction, circumduction and rotation. The hip joint is a ball and socket joint.

Gliding. This is a *plane* joint and permits gliding movements. An example is the acromioclavicular joint of the shoulder.

Range of Motion

When a patient is exercising, his joints should go through their full range of

motion. For example, the normal shoulder and upper arm movements are flexion, extension, hyperextension, abduction, adduction, and circumduction; inward rotation and outward rotation. The chief muscles involved in these movements are the deltoid (abducts upper arm), pectoralis major (flexes and adducts the upper arm), trapezius (raises and lowers the shoulders), latissimus dorsi (extends and adducts the upper arm) and serratus anterior (pulls the shoulder forward).

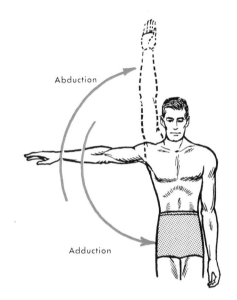

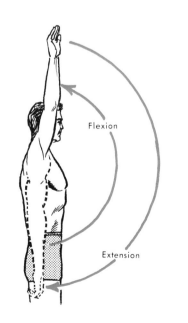

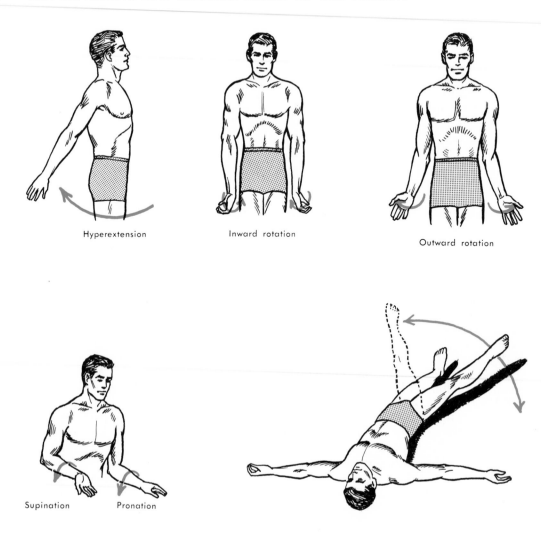

Hyperextension   Inward rotation   Outward rotation

Supination   Pronation

Hand and finger exercises are often a part of a patient's therapy. Flexing, abducting, extending and adducting the hand, as well as flexing and extending the joints of the fingers, are exercises commonly carried out by patients who have some functional impairment as a result of a stroke. It is particularly important to exercise the thumb. The ability of man to bring the thumb in opposition to the tip and base of the fingers is a key factor in using the hands. It permits the individual to hold a pencil and write, for example, to hold a fork and eat, or to do any number of ordinary activities.

The knees and the elbows can be flexed and extended. The biceps, quadriceps and hamstring muscles are active in these movements. The forearm can be supinated and pronated. The four principal muscles that move the forearm are the biceps brachii (flexes and supinates), brachialis (flexes and pronates), triceps brachii (extends) and pronator quadratus (pronates).

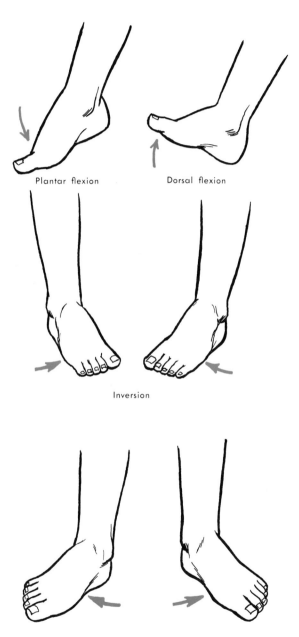

Plantar flexion   Dorsal flexion

Inversion

Eversion

Thigh movement involves the gluteus muscles and the adductor muscles. The gluteus muscle (maximus, medius and minimus) extend, rotate and abduct the thigh. The adductor muscles adduct the thigh and adduct and flex the leg. Flexion, extension, abduction, adduction, and inward and outward rotation from the hip are usually possible. Circumduction of the hip involves all the movements of the hip. Most hip movements involve movement of the pelvis as well.

Movements of the feet and toes are also important. The ankle is a hinged joint that permits plantar flexion and dorsal flexion. Inversion and eversion of the feet take place in the gliding joints. The joints of the toes permit flexion, extension, abduction and adduction.

Normally the vertebral joints permit flexion, extension, lateral flexion and rotation of the cervical spine and trunk. The rectus abdominus, the external and internal oblique muscles and the sacrospinal muscle are involved in these movements.

The degree to which people can tolerate exercise varies considerably. A patient should avoid fatigue and pain while exercising. Joints need to be exercised to their full range of motion, but the nurse should not force movement when it is painful to the patient or when she meets resistance.

AMBULATION

It is sometimes necessary for patients to relearn to walk, often with the aid of crutches, braces or canes. This is usually the responsibility of the physical therapy department, but there are some situations in which it is necessary for the nurse to assist the patient.

It is sometimes necessary for the nurse to help the patient to walk again following an extended period of bed rest. Preparing the patient for this task involves both psychological and physical measures. The nurse can help the patient to gain confidence in his ability to walk again. Often her encouragement and her faith in his ability can bolster his. If an appropriate exercise program has been maintained throughout his illness, the task is easier. Before attempting to stand, it is important for the patient to learn to maintain good trunk balance in a sitting position; then in a standing position before he attempts to walk. When he can maintain a standing position and feels confident in his balance, a few steps should be tried. Since good balance is essential and the patient must feel steady on his feet, it is important that he wear shoes with good support rather than slippers when he is standing or walking. The patient should not be allowed to become fatigued and should attempt only short distances at first. The nurse can help to promote the patient's feelings of self-confidence by helping him to set small goals for each day's activity and acknowledging his accomplishment of these goals.[4]

Most patients who are learning to walk again following a lengthy period of bed rest require physical support when they are first starting. In these efforts, the patient can be well supported by being held at his waist from the rear. This can easily be accomplished with a towel folded lengthwise and encircling the patient's waist. Such support helps the patient to maintain his balance and keep his center of gravity within his base of support.

If the patient has weakness on one side of his body, the nurse supports the patient on his unaffected side. This may be done by having the patient put his good arm around the nurse's shoulder and clasp her hand. The nurse puts her other arm around the patient's waist. Together, they step forward, the patient using his weak foot first and the nurse her opposite foot to provide as wide a base of support as possible.

Another method of assisting the patient who has a one-sided weakness is for the nurse to place her arm under the patient's good arm, at the axilla; she then clasps the patient's hand with her other hand, thus providing a secure hand hold for the patient on which he can lean or support himself.[5]

---

[4]*Rehabilitation Nursing Supplement.* Ottawa, Victorian Order of Nurses for Canada, 1966.
[5]Ibid.

Braces give support to a particularly weak leg. There are also a variety of walkers available which provide support for a person while he is walking. When a patient uses a walker, much of his weight is borne by his hands and arms as he pushes the walker forward.

Some patients find it necessary to use crutches for a period of time. There are many kinds available: underarm, elbow extension and Lofstrand crutches for example. Often the nurse measures a patient for crutches and helps him learn to walk with them. Several methods are used to measure a person for an underarm crutch. One method is to measure the distance from the patient's axilla to the heel of his foot while he is in bed. To this distance, 2 inches is added. A second method is to measure from the anterior fold of the axilla to a point 6 inches lateral to the heel. When crutches are of appropriate length the hand bar permits slight flexion of the elbow, and the weight is borne by the hands and arms rather than at the axilla. The nerves in the axilla are not protected against pressure except by a layer of fat, which is compressible. If weight is borne on the axilla, then, the pressure may result in nerve damage and possibly paralysis. For this reason the top of the crutch should be 2 inches below the axilla and should not be padded initially.

Gaits

There are seven basic crutch gaits:

Two Point Crutch Gait. This gait has the following sequence: right crutch and left foot simultaneously; left crutch and right foot simultaneously.

Three Point Crutch Gait. This gait has the following sequence: both crutches and the weaker limb; then the stronger limb.

Four Point Crutch Gait. This gait has the following sequence: right crutch, left foot, left crutch, right foot. This is a particularly safe gait because there are always three points of support on the floor at one time.

Tripod Gaits. There are two tripod gaits: in one, the patient puts the crutches forward simultaneously and then drags his body forward; in the other, he puts his crutches forward one at a time, and then drags his body forward.

Swing Gaits. There are two swing gaits: in one, the patient puts his crutches forward and then swings his body up to his crutches; in the other, he swings his body beyond them.

The advantage of possessing skill in more than one gait is twofold: the patient can use a slow or fast gait as he wishes and, since each gait requires a different combination of muscles, he can change gaits when he becomes fatigued.

Before a person uses crutches he would be wise to strengthen the muscles he will need, particularly the shoulder depressors (trapezius), triceps and the latissimus dorsi muscles. These can be strengthened by simple exercises that the patient can carry out in bed, for example, rising himself with the help of a trapeze and doing push-ups in which his buttocks are raised off the bed from a sitting position.

GUIDE TO ASSESSING NURSING NEEDS

1. Does the patient understand his need for rest and exercise?
2. Is the patient changing his position as necessary? Does he require help?
3. How often should the patient's position be changed?
4. Has a specific exercise program been prescribed for the patient?
5. If not, what should be included in a daily exercise program for the patient? How much help will the patient need with this?

6. Can the patient learn to do exercises himself?
7. Can the family learn to help the patient with exercises or changes in position?
8. Is the patient in need of specific skills, for example, crutch walking?

GUIDE TO EVALUATING THE EFFECTIVENESS OF NURSING ACTION

1. Do the patient's body positions enable him to be comfortable and maintain good body alignment?
2. Are the patient's exercises compatible with preventing complications such as muscle contractures or atrophy?
3. Are the objectives of the exercises being met? For example, are increased strength and mobility noticeable?
4. Does the nursing care plan outline appropriate nursing measures to meet the patient's needs for rest, exercise and change in position so that all nursing personnel are alerted to these?

STUDY VOCABULARY

Abduction	Gravity	Posture
Active (exercise)	Insertion (muscle)	Pronation
Adduction	Isometric	Sagittal (plane)
Extension	Isotonic	Supination
Flexion	Kinesiology	Transverse
Friction	Origin (muscle)	(plane)
Frontal (plane)	Passive (exercise)	

STUDY SITUATION

Mr. C. R. Lee is admitted to your nursing unit and you assigned to look after him. Mr. Lee is a 54 year old businessman who had a stroke at home and is now paralyzed on his right side. He is conscious, speaks coherently and is anxious to regain the use of his right arm and leg. The physician has ordered that Mr. Lee be given passive exercises for his paralyzed limbs three times a day.

1. What factors should you consider when planning Mr. Lee's exercises?
2. What exercises should Mr. Lee carry out?
3. What are the objectives of his exercises?
4. Explain the difference between passive and active exercise.
5. When should these exercises be done?
6. What are some of the advantages of having Mr. Lee learn to do his own passive exercises?
7. What observations would indicate that exercises should be terminated?
8. How is the effectiveness of the exercises evaluated?

BIBLIOGRAPHY

Cooper, John M., and Ruth B. Slassow: *Kinesiology.* St. Louis, The C. V. Mosby Company, 1963.
Day, M. A. C.: Postural Reflex Patterns. *Nursing Research,* 13:139–147, Spring, 1964.

Fash, Bernice: *Body Mechanics in Nursing Arts.* New York, McGraw-Hill Book Company, Inc., 1946.

Kelly, Mary M.: Exercises for Bedfast Patients. *The American Journal of Nursing,* 66:10:2209–2213, October, 1966.

Kottke, Frederic J., and Russell S. Blanchard: Bedrest Begets Bedrest. *Nursing Forum,* 3:57–72, 1964.

Larson, Carroll B., and Marjorie Gould: *Calderwood's Orthopedic Nursing.* Sixth edition. St. Louis, The C. V. Mosby Company, 1965.

Nordmark, Madelyn, and Anne Rohweder: *Scientific Foundations of Nursing.* Second edition. Philadelphia, J. B. Lippincott Company, 1967.

Olsen, Edith V.: The Hazards of Immobility. *The American Journal of Nursing,* 67:4:780–797, April, 1967.

Rehabilitation Nursing Supplement. Ottawa, Victorian Order of Nurses for Canada, 1966.

Rehabilitative Aspects of Nursing. A Programmed Instruction Series. New York, National League for Nursing, 1966.

Rusk, Howard A.: *Rehabilitation Medicine.* Second edition. St. Louis, The C. V. Mosby Company, 1964.

Stevenson, Jessie L.: *Posture and Nursing.* Second edition. New York, Joint Orthopedic Nursing Advisory Service of the National Organization for Public Health Nursing and the National League of Nursing Education, 1948.

Sutton, Audrey L.: *Bedside Nursing Techniques in Medicine and Surgery.* Second edition. Philadelphia, W. B. Saunders Company, 1969.

Terry, Florence J., et al.: *Principles and Technics of Rehabilitation Nursing.* Second edition. St. Louis, The C. V. Mosby Company, 1961.

Winters, Margaret C.: *Protective Body Mechanics in Daily Life and in Nursing.* Philadelphia, W. B. Saunders Company, 1952.

12 THE HYGIENIC NEEDS OF THE PATIENT

The nurse should be able to:

Describe changes that take place in the skin during the
life cycle

List principles from the biophysical and social sciences relevant to personal hygiene

Explain the significance of the bath as a part of the patient's
total care

Describe one method of giving a bed bath

List precautions to be taken when patients have a tub bath

Describe how to give a back rub

Define the term "decubitus ulcer"

List factors contributing to the development of decubitus
ulcers

Describe nursing measures which can be taken to prevent the
development of decubitus ulcers

Outline a regime for mouth care for the patient who requires
assistance

Describe measures for assisting patients in the care of:
1. The hair
2. The nails
3. The eyes

Outline measures to be taken in the care of patients with
pediculosis

134

THE HYGIENIC NEEDS OF   12
THE PATIENT

INTRODUCTION

Hygiene is the science of health and its preservation; it also refers to practices that are conducive to good health. Good personal hygiene is important to a person's general health. It is usually important to his comfort also, although habits of personal cleanliness vary from individual to individual and from culture to culture. The extent to which cleanliness is esteemed as a virtue depends to a large extent on the cultural background of the individual and the social values he and his peer group hold.

The person who is ill usually has a lowered resistance to infection; consequently the presence of pathogenic bacteria in his environment poses a constant threat of infection. Helping the patient to keep clean, by removing dirt, excretory products and secretions, eliminates many substances in which these bacteria flourish. In addition, hygienic measures help the patients to be comfortable and relaxed. Most people feel better when they are fresh and clean, and many who have been unable to rest will sleep soundly after a relaxing bath.

People who are ill are frequently concerned about unpleasant odors. Excessive perspiration and the presence of bacteria in the mouth and on the skin are common causes of such odors. Bad breath (halitosis) is most frequently caused by bacteria and old food particles in the mouth. Good oral hygiene usually eliminates this source of unpleasantness.

Another reason that good personal hygiene is desirable for the sick person is that a clean, refreshed feeling helps his morale. Generally, a well-groomed appearance is indicative of good mental health. Thus the nurse often observes that a patient who is very ill does not care about grooming; however, once the patient begins to feel better, he often suggests to the nurse that he shave or, in the case of a female patient, asks for her cosmetics. In fact, such requests are usually signs that a person is feeling better, and that he is more aware of his immediate environment.

Hygienic practices vary widely among individuals. These differences are accounted for by cultural patterns and home education, as well as by individual idiosyncracies. For example, some people are accustomed to bathing daily, others once a week. Not every patient needs a bath every day, and indeed for some patients a complete bath daily may be harmful. This is particularly true of the elderly, whose skin tends to be thinner, drier, and less elastic than the young person's.

The nurse should be aware of differences in individual needs and habit patterns when she plans patient care. The patient who is accustomed to a tub bath before retiring may feel more comfortable and sleep better if he can continue this pattern. The fewer changes in habits that a person has to make, the easier is his adjustment to new situations. As a person gets older his habit patterns tend to become more deeply ingrained, and older people usually find it more disturbing than young people do to have their day-to-day routines altered. In spite of individual patterns the nurse can help the patient to adopt healthful practices and she should utilize every opportunity to teach the patient sound hygienic measures.

ANATOMY AND PHYSIOLOGY WITH RESPECT TO HYGIENE

The skin is composed of two main layers, the outer, thinner layer or epidermis, and the inner, thicker layer or dermis. Underlying these layers is subcutaneous tissue and adipose tissue. The epidermis itself has four layers on most areas of the body except the palms of the hands and the soles of the feet, where there are five. The outermost, horny layer of epidermis continually flakes off. This horny layer is particularly thick on elderly people.

The nails of the fingers and toes are composed of epidermal cells that have been converted to keratin. Epithelial cells lie under the crescent of each nail, and it is from these cells that the epidermal cells of the nails grow. The mucous membrane, which is also composed of epithelial tissue, lines the body cavities and passageways. For example, mucous membrane lines the digestive tract, the respiratory passages and the genitourinary tract.

There are three kinds of skin glands in the body. The sebaceous glands secrete oil and are present wherever there is hair. The oil (sebum) keeps the hair supple and pliable. A second type of gland is the sweat gland. These are most numerous in the axilla, on the palms of the hands and the soles of the feet and on the forehead. Their function is to help maintain body temperature and to excrete waste products. Sweat from these glands has a distinctive odor which is distasteful to some people of Western culture. The ceruminous glands, located in the external ear canal, secrete cerumen (wax). Some people accumulate a large amount of cerumen

in their ears and this can impair hearing. In such cases, a physician can syringe the ears to remove excessive wax.

The skin changes throughout life. An infant's skin is less resistant to injury and infection than the adult's skin; therefore, his skin should be handled particularly carefully in order to prevent injury. Often infants need special soaps and lotions which are mild and non-irritating.

The adolescent's skin is often a source of embarrassment to him. Excessive secretions from the oil glands, together with excessive perspiration, predispose the adolescent to acne. To treat acne, physicians often order special low-fat diets and prescribe astringent lotions. An astringent is a substance which, when applied to the skin, has a drying and contracting effect. Cleanliness is of utmost importance during this period in order to prevent secondary infections.

As the adult advances in age two kinds of skin change take place. First, there is wrinkling, sagging and increased pigmentation due to exposure to sunlight. Secondly, there is a general thinning of the skin accompanied by increased dryness and inelasticity. This aging takes place in the epidermis and dermis and in the subcutaneous fat. The epidermis is generally thinned and flattened and sometimes there is an increased growth of the outer layer of the epidermis. A decrease in oil secretions leads to increased dryness and scaliness, and as a result, older people tolerate soap less well than younger adults. If the elderly person bathes too frequently his skin will become very dry. An oily liquid or a skin cream is often used by the elderly patient in place of soap and alcohol rubs.[1]

The skin is nourished by nutrients that are delivered by the blood. Since the skin itself has limited absorbent ability, the nutrient creams that are so widely advertised on television and in magazines have only a limited value in

[1]Robert G. Carney: The Aging Skin. *The American Journal of Nursing*, 63:112, June, 1963.

promoting skin health. If food and fluid intake is interfered with, the skin will very likely show some ill effects. If fluid intake is insufficient, the patient becomes dehydrated and his skin appears dry and loose, a condition called poor tissue turgor. The skin of a patient who has suffered prolonged nutrient insufficiency heals very slowly after injury.

PRINCIPLES OF PATIENT HYGIENE

The skin and mucous membranes act as the first line of defense against trauma to the body. It is important to a patient's care that his skin and mucous membranes be kept healthy and intact. Any break in the continuity of these tissues can result in infection.

The health of the skin and mucous membranes is highly dependent upon adequate nourishment and an adequate fluid intake. Any situation which interferes with the intake of nourishment and water or with the supply of oxygen, fluid and nutrients to a part of the body is often reflected in the health of the skin. Nurses are frequently challenged to help a patient maintain healthy skin and mucous membranes in spite of a depleted supply of food, water and oxygen.

Skin and mucous membranes vary in their resistance to injury. Factors which affect a person's resistance include his general health and the amount of subcutaneous tissue. Good general health increases resistance to injury; a very small amount or a large amount of subcutaneous tissue lowers resistance.

Hygienic practices are learned. People learn most of their hygienic practices at home during their childhood. For example, children are taught by their parents how to brush their teeth and how often to bathe. The wide diversity of hygienic practices within our society reflects the cultural norms of the various groups that make up the society.

Hygienic practices vary according to socioeconomic class. Patients of lower socioeconomic class often live under poor sanitary conditions, and it is difficult for them to follow many hygienic measures. For example, a person who has to carry his water up three flights of stairs may not make a practice of bathing regularly.

THE PATIENT'S BATH

Bathing has several purposes: It cleanses and it promotes comfort. Bathing also stimulates blood circulation and affords an opportunity to exercise. When a nurse assists a patient to bathe she has an opportunity to teach him desirable hygienic measures and incorporate other health teaching. In addition, she has an opportunity to assess many of his needs. For example, during the bath is a good time to observe the condition of the patient's skin, nails and hair and to note such factors as the presence of edema, the quality of respirations, and any difficulty or pain the patient has on moving.

It is also a good time to assess the patient's mental state. Many patients find it much easier to talk to the nurse when she is assisting them with their bath than at other times. Davis suggests that the reason for this is that the act of giving physical care is perceived by many patients as caring about them.[2] Thus the bath provides an excellent opportunity for the nurse to establish rapport with the patient and facilitate communication between patient and nurse.[3]

The hospital patient may have a bed bath, a tub bath or a shower. The physician usually orders the type of bath that a person can safely have. He will consider not only the amount of activity

---

[2]Ellen D. Davis: Giving a Bath? *The American Journal of Nursing*, 70:11:2366–2367, November, 1970.

[3]Ibid. See also Virginia Henderson: *Basic Principles of Nursing Care.* Basel and New York, published for the International Council of Nursing by S. Karger, Revised, 1969, pp. 33–35.

involved but also the specific needs of the individual. For example, a patient who has had a recent abdominal operation will probably not have a tub bath or shower until his incision is healed, because of the danger of getting it wet and contaminated. (To contaminate is to soil or make unclean.) Both the tub bath and the shower require more activity on the part of the patient than a bath in bed.

In the bed bath, the nurse may give the entire bath to the patient, or the patient may participate within the limits of his physical condition. Very often patients are encouraged to help themselves as much as possible. This provides an opportunity to exercise muscles and stimulate blood circulation, and gives the patient a feeling of accomplishment and increasing independence.

It is believed by many, however, that the nurse should be careful to retain some aspects of assisting the patient with personal hygiene. If she does not, she loses a valuable time for free and spontaneous talk with the patient for which other opportunities must be found.[4]

Not all patients require a bath every day while they are in hospital; nor is it necessary for all patients to receive a bath in the morning. Many people prefer to take theirs in the evening. For the patient who tires very easily or who is very ill, the bath may be contraindicated. The geriatric patient's skin will often become overly dry if he bathes often. For these people as well as for other patients who do not require complete bed baths, abbreviated personal hygiene is indicated. Abbreviated hygiene includes washing the patient's hands and back, axilla and perineal area, as well as providing for oral hygiene and massaging bony prominences. The nurse makes these judgments based upon the needs of the patient and the orders of the physician.

The Bed Bath

The equipment required for the bed bath includes bath towels, wash cloths,

a water basin and soap. A bath blanket is also required to cover the patient so as to avoid embarrassing exposure and to keep him warm. The kind of soap used will depend largely on the individual needs of the patient and on the policy of the health agency. Some institutions permit patients to use their own soap; others supply a special bacteriostatic soap or preparations such as pHisoderm or one that has a pH similar to that of the skin. It is thought that preparations such as pHisoderm do not destroy the normal protective acid coating of the skin.

Before a patient bathes he may wish to use a bedpan or the toilet. This is a desirable practice for hygienic reasons as well as for the comfort of the patient.

Principles Relevant to the Bed Bath General. When bathing the patient, the nurse folds the wash cloth in such a way that the corners are folded on the palm of the hand to form a pad. It is suggested that the patient be bathed in the following manner:

a. eyes — inner to outer canthus (no soap)
b. face
c. arms, hands and axilla
d. chest and breasts
e. abdomen
f. legs
g. back and buttocks
h. perineal area

Only the area being washed should be exposed. This lessens the patient's embarrassment and helps him keep warm. Each area of the skin is dried immediately after it has been washed and rinsed and before the next area of the body is exposed.

If the patient soaks his hands and feet in the basin of water he will feel more refreshed. This practice also serves to soften the patient's nails so that they can be easily cut and cleaned. The pan of water should not be too full or the water may spill when the hands or feet are immersed. Washing the patient's back is best done with the patient lying on his abdomen. If this is impossible the patient can turn to one side while the nurse

---

[4]Ibid.

washes the other side of his back and then can reverse his position.

The nurse should take special care to wash, rinse and dry well the creases in the patient's skin and to massage bony prominences. These areas are particularly prone to irritation. The body skin creases become excoriated if they remain moist; the bony prominences are irritated by constant friction and pressure against the bed clothes. Excoriation is the superficial loss of skin substance. Also, the areas that bear the weight of the patient while he is in bed are prone to irritation.

The patient's skin is then dried well. Skin that remains wet over a long period is uncomfortable and becomes irritated.

Heat is conveyed from the body by the convection of air currents. Care should be taken not to expose the body surface unduly. Drafts are to be avoided and the patient should be kept warm during his bath. The nurse can close the windows of the patient's room if it is cool outside or if there is any danger of a draft. The bed unit is screened for privacy, the patient's spread and blanket are removed and a bath blanket is placed over the patient. The top sheet is then slipped out from under the bath blanket to prevent exposing the patient unnecessarily. The patient then removes his gown. Dirty linen should be placed in a container (dirty linen hamper) as soon after it is removed from the bed as possible. Agency procedures vary in this regard, but it is generally accepted that bed linen is a potential source of infection and suitable precautions are taken in handling it.

People differ in their tolerance of heat. Most patients require bath water between 43.3° C. to 46.1° C. (110° F. and 115° F.). Water at this temperature is comfortable to most patients and it does not injure skin or mucous membranes. Water at 50° C. (120° F.) in the basin will cool to the safe temperature range by the time it comes in contact with the patient's skin. The nurse collects the equipment and takes it to the patient's bedside before she gets the water so that the water does not cool too much before it is used. It may be necessary to add additional hot water during the procedure, or to change the water. Patients who are particularly sensitive to heat may require cooler water.

The skin is sometimes irritated by the chemical composition of certain soaps. Soap can be irritating to a patient's skin and particularly to his eyes. Therefore patients are often advised not to use soap on their faces.

Long smooth strokes on the arms and legs that are directed from the distal to the proximal increase the rate of venous flow. Distal means farther from the point of attachment; proximal means closer to the point of attachment. For example, the hand is distal to the elbow.

Moving the body joints through their full range of motion helps to prevent loss of muscle tone and improves circulation.[5] The nurse can use the bed bath as an opportunity to help the patient to put his joints through their full range of motion. A nurse should know the individual patient's needs and limitations for exercise. The advisability of exercise is discussed in Chapter 11.

The Tub Bath

Tub baths are taken for hygienic and therapeutic reasons. The physician may order a therapeutic bath for some patients as, for example, hip baths for the patient who has had rectal surgery. Patients with skin diseases often have oatmeal or medicated baths. Various types of therapeutic baths are discussed in Chapter 20. Aside from these therapeutic measures, a tub bath is most often a hygienic measure enjoyed by most people.

Bathtubs in hospitals frequently have rails, or the adjacent wall is equipped with handles to help the patient climb in and out of the tub. Most tubs also now have safety strips on the bottom which help to prevent the patient

---

[5]Edith V. Olson et al.: The Hazards of Immobility. *The American Journal of Nursing,* 67:4: 780–797, April, 1967.

from slipping. No sick person should lock himself in the bathroom unattended; he may require help. The nurse or attendant should know when a patient is bathing, and often it is wise to check that he is all right. If a patient is out of bed for the first time after even a few days of bed rest, it is generally unwise to leave him alone in the bath; an attendant can stay just outside the curtains if the patient prefers privacy.

The bathtub is filled one-third full of water. Unless the physician orders otherwise, the water is drawn at 40 to 41° C. (105° F.), a comfortable and safe temperature for most people. The length of time that a person bathes depends upon his endurance and strength. If the bath is too lengthy it may fatigue him unnecessarily. A very hot bath will cause the blood to be diverted away from the vital centers of the brain to the surface areas of the body; as a result he may feel faint and lose consciousness.

Getting in and out of the bathtub is often a difficult maneuver, and the patient may need assistance from the nurse. Usually it is easier if the patient first sits on the edge of the tub with his feet inside the tub, then reaches over to grasp the rail on the other side and gradually eases himself down. In helping the patient out of the tub, it is a good practice to let the water out before the patient attempts to stand up. There are many mechanical devices available today for assisting with the tub bath procedures. A mechanical lift (or hoist),

for example, can be used in either hospital or home situations. The use of a shower stool, so that the patient can sit while having a shower, is another solution to the bath problem.

THE BACK RUB

After the bath, the patient's back is often rubbed with an emollient lotion or cream. Although alcohol has been the traditional solution for rubbing the backs of patients in hospital, it should be used with caution. Alcohol dries and hardens the skin, leaving it more susceptible to cracking.[6] This is a particular hazard in the elderly, whose skin tends to be dry and thin, and in patients whose nutritional status or hydration is poor. Emollient creams and lotions are considered preferable. Most agencies have their own preference as to the type of cream or lotion used for back care.

When the nurse gives the patient a back rub, the best position for the patient is the prone position. The side-lying position is the next most preferable. These positions permit the nurse to use long, firm strokes, which are both soothing to the patient and stimulating to the blood circulation. A circular motion over the bony prominences of the shoulder blades and at the base of

---

[6]Ibid., p. 790.

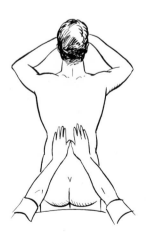

Long, smooth and circular motions increase the blood circulation to the skin.

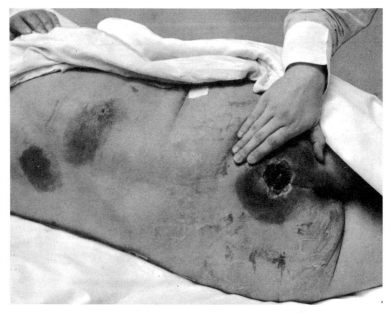

A decubitus ulcer. Note the dark necrotic tissue in the center of the ulcer and the reddened areas on upper back. (From Brunner, L. S., Emerson, C. P., Jr., Ferguson, L. K., and Suddarth, D. S.: Textbook of Medical-Surgical Nursing. J. B. Lippincott Company, Philadelphia, 1964.)

the spine helps to keep the skin in good condition.

When giving a back rub, the nurse should warn the patient that the solution may feel cold. It is more comfortable for the patient if the nurse warms the solution in her hands before she applies it to the patient's back. The nurse starts at the sacrum and moves up to the center of his back. Here circular motions are made to increase circulation to these bony prominences. The pressure of the nurse's motions should be sufficiently firm to stimulate the muscle tissue. However, if the patient is very thin or the skin is in poor condition, the nurse should be careful not to use undue pressure in rubbing or massaging. After the circular motions over the shoulders, the nurse brings her hands down to the lower edge of the patient's buttocks and to the patient's sacrum, where the circular motion is repeated. This process is continued until the circulation to the skin has been stimulated and all lotion is rubbed in well. The nurse also rubs the patient's knees, elbows, heels and any other reddened areas on bony prominences. Care should be taken however not to massage reddened areas on the patient's thighs or lower legs.

Sometimes when circulation is poor, a person may develop a clot in one of the blood vessels supplying the limbs. Surface areas in the vicinity of the clot often become reddened, warm to the touch and tender. Massage may loosen the clot and cause it to circulate in the blood stream. This can be dangerous because the clot may subsequently block another vessel, for example, in the heart, where it can cause much damage. The nurse should always report the presence of reddened areas on the patient's skin and particularly those which may be indicative of clot formation in the blood vessels below the surface.

DECUBITUS ULCERS

Decubitus ulcers (bedsores, pressure sores) are areas from which the skin has sloughed. These sores may develop in persons who are ill in bed for a long period of time, especially if the patient is unable to move about freely, or they may occur in people who sit in wheelchairs for several hours at a time, as, for example, patients who are paralyzed or who, for other reasons, are confined to a wheelchair. They occur as a result of prolonged pressure on one part of the body with resultant loss of circulation to the area and subsequent tissue destruction. Although decubitus ulcers may occur in any patient, if there is sufficient pressure on one area to cause ischemia, they are seen most frequently in individuals with poor nutritional status, especially if there is a negative nitrogen balance.[6] They are most often seen on the bony prominences of the body. If decubitus ulcers are not treated, they quickly increase in size and become very painful. Secondary infection often complicates the picture.

The conditions that predispose to decubitus ulcers include continuous pressure on one area, dampness, a break in the skin surface, poor nutrition, dehydration, poor blood circulation, thinness (bony prominences unprotected by adipose tissue) and the presence of pathogenic bacterial. Early signs of a decubitus ulcer include redness and tenderness of an area. The patient usually complains of a burning sensation. Other early warning signs include coldness of an area and the presence of edema. Unless special measures are taken at this time to relieve pressure and increase local tissue nourishment, a break in the patient's skin usually follows. Then the sore increases in depth and the tissue gradually sloughs off. Decubitus ulcers are difficult to cure; consequently preventive measures are always indicated.

There are many nursing care measures that can be employed in order to prevent decubitus ulcers. Frequent changes in position to rotate the weight-bearing areas relieve pressure on any single group of bony prominences. The normal healthy individual shifts his body position every few minutes. For the patient who is unable to do this himself, it is the nurse's responsibility to see that his position is changed. A regular schedule should be set up for turning the patient as often as necessary to keep the skin in good condition.

Massage and exercise stimulate circulation and thus improve the nourishment to the cells of the skin. Keeping the skin dry and clean inhibits the growth of disease-producing bacteria and prevents skin from becoming excoriated; body sections and excreta are particularly irritating to a patient's skin. The nurse should take particular care that a patient's linen and dressings are dry and clean. In areas where secretions cannot be prevented, protective ointments, such as zinc oxide or petrolatum, can be used to prevent excessive irritation.

Another preventive measure for decubitus ulcers is the use of devices to relieve pressure on specific areas of the patient's body. An overbed cradle will keep bedclothes off the patient, and other aids such as alternating pressure mattresses, oscillating beds and fluidized air or water mattresses may also be used. Many hospitals use a special frame, such as a Stryker frame or Foster bed, which permits the patient to be turned easily. Another measure which has been found helpful in the prevention of decubitus ulcers is the use of sheepskin under pressure areas. It is considered preferable to use the whole skin, but small pads have been found effective in protecting areas such as the heels or elbows of the patient.[7] The woolskins are being used extensively in many hospitals and nursing homes. They are particularly helpful in home situations where expensive mechanical devices may not be available.

Attention to the patient's nutritional status is essential. Since decubitus ulcers occur most frequently in patients with a negative nitrogen balance, the protein intake should be increased. Foods which contain complete proteins, such as eggs, milk and meat, are recommended. The proteins are needed for the regeneration of body tissue. Usually, supplementary amounts of vitamin

---

[6]Ibid., p. 789.

[7]Miriam A. Brownlowe, Florence R. Cohen, William E. Happich: New Washable Woolskins. *The American Journal of Nursing*, 70:11:2368–2370, November, 1970.

C are prescribed also because of the role of this vitamin in the healing process. Care must be taken also that an adequate fluid intake is maintained. Dehydration results in poor tissue turgor, which is another predisposing factor in the development of decubitus ulcers.

When a decubitus ulcer develops, the nurse faces a challenge in curative nursing care. The outside area of the decubitus ulcer is often less extensive than the inside area. The preventive measures just mentioned can be employed therapeutically and, in addition, the application of dry heat, such as that from an infrared lamp, increases circulation to the area and dries secretions. The latter measure is generally ordered by the physician. Decubitus ulcers are prone to infection by bacteria; the moist, poorly nourished tissue provides a good medium for the growth of pathogenic bacteria. The use of aseptic technique in the care of an infected ulcer prevents secondary infection and the transfer of bacteria to other areas of the body and to other patients.

The physician usually orders a therapeutic regimen for the care of the patient who has a decubitus ulcer. Antiseptic solutions, soap and water and antibiotic creams are all advocated at one time or another. Sometimes it is necessary to graft skin over a decubitus ulcer. Ulcers are very difficult to cure; the best nursing care is prevention.

MOUTH CARE

Good oral hygiene is essential to health and to comfort. Infections of the mouth and the parotid glands can frequently be avoided through regular care.

Oral care includes regular care by a dentist as well as adequate cleansing of the teeth. Brushing the teeth removes food particles that provide a likely medium for bacterial growth. Brushing also massages the gums and thus stimulates circulation and subsequent nutrition.

Most people brush their teeth at least twice a day, in the morning and before going to bed. Many dentists advocate brushing the teeth after every meal or at least rising the mouth after food is taken. These measures help to prevent the accumulation on and between the teeth of food particles which predispose to dental caries. Patients usually bring their own toothbrushes with them to hospital and their own dentifrice. If they do not, they should be provided with a brush and toothpaste or other substance to use. Salt, baking soda and precipitated chalk make effective dentifrices. Many agencies now are using disposable toothbrushes for patient use.

If a patient cannot brush his teeth himself the nurse should assist him. When brushing teeth, the brush should be moved from the gum to the crown of the tooth. This motion is carried out on both the inner and outer aspects of the teeth.

A patient's nutritional status can affect the condition of his mouth, and the condition of the mouth can affect a person's nutritional status. Adequate fluid and a balanced diet help maintain a healthy mouth and healthy gums. Sometimes, because of disease processes, a patient's intake of fluid is inadequate. This often results in a furry tongue and a bad taste and the development of sordes. Sordes is the collection of microorganisms, food and epithelial tissue which accumulate in the mouth. The unpleasant taste may have a negative effect upon a person's appetite.

Mouth care is also essential for patients with artificial dentures. Usually the patient with dentures prefers to take them out and clean them himself with a dentifrice and water, then to rinse his mouth before reinserting the dentures. A mouthwash is often refreshing to these patients. If a person cannot remove his own dentures, the nurse can remove and clean them for him. Care should be taken in removing dentures, in handling them while cleaning, and in storing them. Dentures are expensive articles; their replacement takes time;

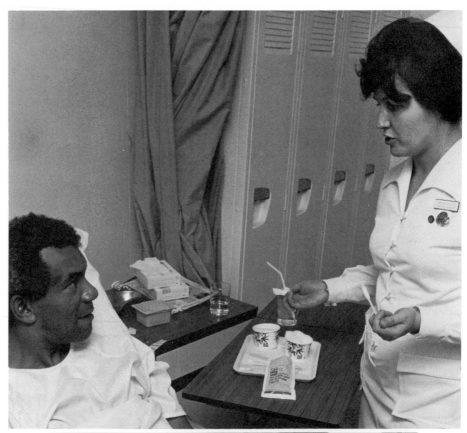

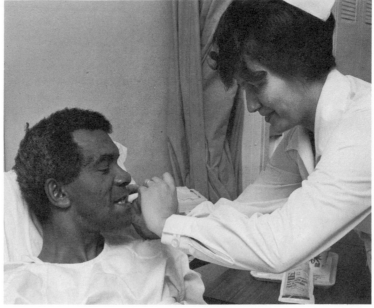

Many agencies use disposable trays for special mouth care. The nurse is explaining the procedure to the patient.

and the person who wears them is uncomfortable without them. He cannot eat anything that has to be chewed, and he finds speech difficult.

In removing dentures, it is usually easier to remove the upper plate first, place it in a container and then remove the lower plate. For washing, it is safer to put the plates in a basin full of water than to wash them under the tap. The plates are often slippery and hard to hold. The teeth should be brushed with a dentrifrice and rinsed with cold water. Care should be taken not to use water that is too hot on dentures; they may crack or become misshapen. Since many people remove them at night, a container should be provided for the safe storage of dentures when they are not in use. Agencies often have a special container for this purpose; it should be labeled with the patient's name, hospital and bed number. Dentures are one of the most frequently lost articles in a hospital, and precautions should be taken for safeguarding them.

Patients are usually provided with antiseptic mouthwashes while they are in the hospital. If a patient is very weak or unconscious, special preparations are indicated to cleanse his mouth. Oral hygiene includes cleaning the teeth and gums, also the palate, the tongue and inner cheeks. With the unconscious patient, care must be taken that the fluid used for cleansing is not aspirated. Lemon juice, glycerin in water, lemon juice and water, and hydrogen peroxide solutions have all been used for cleansing. These agents, however, tend to be drying, and other substances such as Lubrafax and milk of magnesia, which do not have astringent qualities, appear to be equally effective. With a cotton tipped applicator or gauze sponges wrapped around a tongue depressor, the nurse cleanses the patient's mouth every four hours or as it becomes necessary. This is particularly important for patients who are not taking fluids by mouth. Care should be taken while cleansing the patient's mouth not to injure the mucous membrane. Petrolatum can be used to lubricate dry lips.

HAIR CARE

Care of the patient's hair is important to both his grooming and his sense of well-being. As part of the daily toilet each patient's hair needs to be brushed and combed. Thorough brushing stimulates circulation to the scalp and improves the nourishment of the epithelium. Most patients can tend to this themselves, but the nurse may have to assume the responsibility for the aged or very ill patient.

The nurse, by seeing to daily care of the hair, can ensure that the patient's hair does not become matted. Often, long hair is braided so that it will stay neatly in place and make the patient feel more comfortable. Patients who are in the hospital for some length of time may want a shampoo, which is usually ordered by the physician. For the patient who is out of bed a shampoo is no problem. The sink in his room or the shower bath affords facilities for hair washing.

If a patient must remain in a supine position, however, the shampoo is given while he is in bed or on a stretcher. If a stretcher is used, it is best to move the patient to a sink and support his head on the edge of the sink. If it is necessary for the patient to remain in bed, then the nurse can use a folded plastic sheet or a specially constructed waterproof pad to direct the water from the patient's hair into a pail. The nurse uses pitchers of water, taking precautions to keep the patient's bed dry. The patient's hair needs to be dried quickly after the shampoo in order to avoid chilling. Most hospitals have hair dryers for this purpose. Many brands of dry shampoo are now available, and these may be used for patients whose condition contraindicates a regular shampoo.

Today many large hospitals have hair dressing and barber services for patients. Often the patient will request the services of the barber and the nurse then arranges for this. The nurse is usually responsible for telling the patient what services are available and what charges are made for them.

SHAVING THE MALE PATIENT

Male patients usually feel better when they are shaved. If the male patient cannot shave himself the nurse may be asked to do this for him. If the patient has an electric razor this is no problem, but a safety razor requires more skill. Very warm water is needed to give an adequate shave. After the skin has been lathered with shaving soap, the skin is held tautly and the razor is drawn over the skin in short strokes. The nurse will find that the safest way to shave the patient is to stretch the skin over the bone in a particular area and then to shave in the direction in which the hair is growing. Areas around the mouth and nose are particularly sensitive; in these areas the nurse's motions need to be firm but gentle. After the patient has been shaved he will likely prefer a shaving lotion for his skin. Most shaving lotions are refreshing and have a slightly antiseptic effect.

After a shave, the male patient will not only look better but he will in all probability feel better. Relatives are often reassured when the male patient is well groomed, chiefly because this is the way they are accustomed to seeing him.

Many women are accustomed to shaving the hair in the axilla and to removing superfluous hair from their faces and legs. Opportunity should be provided for them to maintain these practices while they are ill if they so desire. Women are usually particularly sensitive about unwanted hairs on the chin and upper lip. A number of good depilatory creams are available. These preparations should be used with caution, however, because they are irritating to the skin and many people cannot tolerate them. Tweezers may be used instead to remove facial hairs.

NAIL CARE

Care of the nails is another area of grooming that most patients can attend to themselves. For the very ill patient or the patient who has difficulty in moving, however, nail care may be the nurse's responsibility. Often nail polish is not advised for a patient because the physician or the nurse may want to check the color of the tissue underneath the nails. This is particularly true for patients who are to undergo surgery. Most hospitals prohibit the use of colored nail polish for these patients.

The responsibility for cleaning and trimming the nails of patients who are unable to do this themselves usually falls to the nurse. For patients who are particularly prone to infection, for example, patients with diabetes mellitus or circulatory problems, it is advisable not to cut the nails for fear of injuring the skin or cuticle around the nail. Toenails are cut straight across, fingernails in an oval shape. Many people prefer that their fingernails be filed rather than cut so that they can be shaped attractively.

To prevent hangnails, it is best to keep the cuticle of the nail pushed well back and lubricated with oil. Some patients have very hard fingernails and horny toenails. If the patient soaks his feet for 10 to 15 minutes in warm water, the nails will soften sufficiently so that they can be cut with nail cutters. Special nail clippers are available which are particularly helpful in cutting thick toenails. If the nails are too thick and difficult to cut, the services of a podiatrist (foot specialist) should be obtained.

EYE CARE

Nursing care involves the care of the eyes. On occasion the nurse will be called on to help a patient to care for his eyes when they have become irritated or infected. The physician usually orders a special solution to cleanse the eyes. Tap water or normal saline are also used. With absorbent cotton dipped in the solution, the eye is wiped from the inner canthus to the outer canthus. The nurse uses a clean piece of cotton each time she wipes the eye. Water or normal saline will soften crusts so they are easily removed. The motion from the inner to the outer canthus washes the discharge away from the nasal lacrimal duct, which is located on the inner aspect of the orbit of the eye.

Unconscious patients require special attention to protect their eyes from damage. The upper and lower lids should be kept clean and free from discharge. The lids should be closed when the patient is being turned to prevent scratching of the cornea.

Patients' glasses, contact lenses and other prostheses should be looked after carefully and the patient assisted with their care if he is unable to care for them.

CARE OF PATIENTS WITH PEDICULOSIS

Occasionally a patient will be found to have pediculosis (infestation with lice). His care involves killing and removing all the pediculi (lice) and their eggs (nits) that have infected the skin, hair and clothing. There are three main types of pediculosis: pediculosis capitis or infestation of the scalp with lice, pediculosis corporis or infestation with body lice and pediculosis pubis or infestation of the pubic hair with lice. There are several methods for ridding patients of pediculi. Initially the patient's clothing is sterilized. Then a combination of baths and the application of dusting with insecticide powder is commonly used. Infested patients are separated from other patients for 24 hours after treatment has been initiated to avoid spreading the pediculi. The treatment is repeated until pediculi cannot be found on the patient. Precautions are normally taken for one week after treatment is commenced.

Pediculi are spread by direct contact and through vehicles such as clothing, eating utensils and combs. Pediculi are usually found in environments where poor hygienic measures are practiced.

GUIDE TO ASSESSING NURSING NEEDS

1. Is the patient receiving adequate personal care, for example, oral and eye care?
2. Does the patient require assistance with hygienic measures?
3. Does the patient require measures to prevent complications such as bed sores? For example, does he require assistance in changing his position?
4. Is his body position compatible with good health?
5. Does the patient's fluid intake record indicate adequate fluid consumption?
6. Is he taking an adequate diet?
7. Are devices such as overbed cradles needed to take pressure off?
8. Do the patient and his family require knowledge or skills in hygienic care?
9. Is there a need for information about nutrition, such as the importance of diet and fluid consumption?

GUIDE TO EVALUATING THE EFFECTIVENESS OF NURSING ACTION

1. Is the patient clean and dry?
2. Is his skin in good condition?
3. Are microorganisms in the environment and on the patient

kept at a minimum through adequate cleanliness, ventilation and other hygienic measures?

4. Is the bath safe, comfortable and therapeutically effective?

STUDY
VOCABULARY

Astringent	Epidermis	Pediculosis
Cerumen	Excoriation	Perspiration
Ceruminous	Halitosis	Sebaceous
Contaminate	Hygiene	Sebum
Dermis	Keratin	Sordes
Distal	Mucous membrane	

STUDY
SITUATION

Your patient, Mr. J. C. Jones, was admitted to the nursing unit yesterday. He is a 53 year old bachelor who is unemployed and lives in a rooming house in a low socioeconomic area of the city. He stopped school in the third grade. When he was admitted to the hospital, Mr. Jones appeared to be very dirty and his clothes were sent to the laundry. Your patient is thin and malnourished, and he is in the hospital for investigative procedures.

1. What principal factor would you take into consideration in planning and teaching Mr. Jones hygienic measures?
2. What factors would affect his learning of desirable hygienic practices?
3. Why is good skin care particularly important for him?
4. What factors could contribute to the sloughing of Mr. Jones's skin?
5. Outline the preventive nursing care measures for decubitus ulcers.
6. Explain how you should teach Mr. Jones good oral hygiene.
7. How could you evaluate the effectiveness of your teaching?

BIBLIOGRAPHY

Brownlowe, Miriam A., Florence R. Cohen and William F. Happich: New Washable Woolskins. *The American Journal of Nursing,* 70:11:2368–2369, November, 1970.

Carney, Robert G.: The Aging Skin. *The American Journal of Nursing, 63:* 110–112, June, 1963.

Davis, Ellen D.: Giving a Bath? *The American Journal of Nursing,* 70:11: 2366–2367, November, 1970.

Dorland's Illustrated Medical Dictionary. Twenty-fourth edition. Philadelphia, W. B. Saunders Company, 1965.

Ginsberg, Miriam K.: A Study of Oral Hygiene Nursing Care. *The American Journal of Nursing,* 61:67–69, October, 1961.

Guyton, Arthur C.: *Functions of the Human Body,* Philadelphia, W. B. Saunders Company, 1969.

Harmer, Bertha, and Virginia Henderson: *Textbook of the Principles and Practice of Nursing.* Fifth edition. New York, The Macmillan Company, 1955.

Harvin, J. Shand, and Thomas S. Hargest: The Air-Fluidized Bed: A New Concept in the Treatment of Decubitus Ulcers. *Nursing Clinics of North America,* 5:1:181–187, March, 1970.

Henderson, Virginia: *Basic Principles of Nursing Care.* International Council of Nurses. Basel and New York, S. Karger, Revised, 1969.

Olson, Edith V. et al.: The Hazards of Immobility. *The American Journal of Nursing, 67:4:*780–797, April, 1967.

Schreiber, Frederic C.: Dental Care for Long-term Patients. *The American Journal of Nursing, 64:*84–86, February, 1964.

Tassman, Gustav C., Gilbert M. Zayon, and Jack N. Zafran: When Patients Cannot Brush their Teeth. *The American Journal of Nursing, 63:*76, February, 1963.

13 THE COMFORT NEEDS OF THE PATIENT

The nurse should be able to:

Describe the basic anatomical position

List guiding principles to follow when helping bed patients to maintain a position of good body alignment

Describe methods which utilize these principles to assist bed patients to maintain good body alignment in different positions

Name principles from the biophysical sciences relevant to bed-making that contribute to the patient's comfort and safety and to the nurse's safety in carrying out this procedure

Describe methods of bed-making which utilize these principles

Describe various types of mattresses, mechanical and other supportive devices that may be used for therapeutic or comfort reasons on the sick person's bed

150

THE COMFORT NEEDS OF 13
THE PATIENT

INTRODUCTION

Comfort has been defined as "support; contented well-being; . . . consolation in trouble or worry."[1] Comfort then is a state of mind in which the individual is generally at peace with himself and with his environment.

Discomfort can result from stimuli from both psychological and physical sources. Thus, a person who is afraid or worried is uncomfortable; as is one who is cold or in pain.

There are many causes of emotional discomfort, some of which have been mentioned earlier in the text. For example, the newly admitted hospital patient is subjected to the stresses concomitant with entering any strange environment. The ill person often fears pain, death and disability, and he worries about his ability to cope with forthcoming stresses. Neglect by the nursing staff or care by an unyielding, unconcerned nurse also contributes to a patient's discomfort. The patient looks to the nurse for understanding and support in order to attain some degree of psychological comfort.

Many people are aware of the sources of their discomfort and when given the opportunity, they make them known. The nurse who communicates her understanding of the patient's needs and who takes the time to listen to him can do a great deal to relieve his worry and discomfort.

There are avenues of expression other than the verbal. The patient who is uncomfortable may appear restless, pale or tense, or he may perspire profusely or lie rigidly in bed. He may also be irritable. All in all there are a multitude of ways of expressing discomfort, and the nurse needs to be aware of them and be alert to their possible meanings.

Physical discomforts can contribute to a patient's anxiety and interfere with his health. Pain, nausea, heat and even an untidy environment are stimuli which the patient finds uncomfortable or even unbearable. By the selection of appropriate nursing care measures, the nurse can prevent the development of many situations which could be a source of discomfort. In addition, many discomforts can be alleviated once they occur; therefore, the nurse should be alert to the earliest signs of discomfort in a patient and aware of the measures that will prevent their extension.

The nurse has many resources at her disposal to relieve a patient's discomfort, but it is only through a systematic approach to the problem that the effective measure or measures can be defined. It is important that the nurse record her observations of the results of her nursing care measures in order that other members of the health team may be made aware of her findings and can avail themselves of this knowledge for the patient's benefit. For example, pain can often be relieved by a change in position, exercise, physical support,

---

[1]*Webster's Seventh New Collegiate Dictionary.* Springfield, Mass., G. & C. Merriam Company, 1963.

heat, or analgesics. Sometimes the relief of anxiety contributes to the lessening of pain. These measures vary in their effect from one person to another, and consequently the nurse should find the measure or combination of measures which is most effective for a specific patient.

The various nursing measures which the nurse can employ to treat physical discomfort are discussed separately in this chapter; however, the nurse can use them singly or in combination as her judgment indicates. It should be noted that comfort measures are often therapeutic measures and as such may be ordered by the physician. For example, food may be a comfort and a pleasure at the same time that it is specific in the treatment of the patient's illness. It is equally true that a therapeutic measure can serve as a comfort to the patient. The hot water bottle, the clean dressing and the supportive binder can be comforting and reassuring to the patient while serving their therapeutic purposes.

POSITIONS FOR THE PATIENT

Generally patients assume the positions which are most comfortable for them. For the patient who can move easily and freely in bed without therapeutic considerations, the nurse's chief responsibility in regard to his position is his comfort. The astute use of pillows and the provision of a firm foundation will help him remain comfortable.

Patients assume positions for therapeutic reasons as well as for comfort. The possible reasons for positioning a patient therapeutically are many: to maintain good body alignment, to prevent contractures, to promote drainage, to facilitate breathing and to prevent decubitus ulcers are but a few.

The physician usually orders the appropriate therapeutic position for a patient. There are also situations, however, in which it is left to the nurse's judgment as to which position is best. Intelligent assessment of a patient's needs and a knowledge of anatomy and physiology are important bases for such judgments. Also, the nurse needs to be aware of the variety of positions that it is possible for the patient to assume and the supportive measures which promote his comfort in these positions.

The following are guides with which the nurse should be familiar in assisting patients to assume different positions:

1. Joints should be maintained in a slightly flexed position. Prolonged extension creates undue muscle tension and strain.

2. Positions as close as possible to the basic anatomical position provide good body alignment, which is, of course, desirable.

3. Positions should be changed frequently, at least every two hours. Prolonged pressure on one area of the skin may cause decubitus ulcers. The tolerance of the skin of individual patients is not generally known.

4. All patients require daily exercise unless it is medically contraindicated.

5. When a patient changes his position, his joints should go through the full range of motion unless this too is medically contraindicated.

Anatomical Position

In the anatomical position, the patient stands with his hands at his sides, thumbs adducted and hands pronated. The head is erect and the feet are directed forward. The knees and fingers are slightly flexed.

This position is used as the basis upon which to refer to the three planes of the body: the sagittal, the frontal, and the transverse (see Chapter 11, page 118).

Dorsal Recumbent Position

In the dorsal recumbent position the patient lies on his back with his head and shoulders slightly elevated. Usually one pillow suffices for this purpose. The lumbar curvature of the back is best supported by a small pillow or a folded towel if necessary.

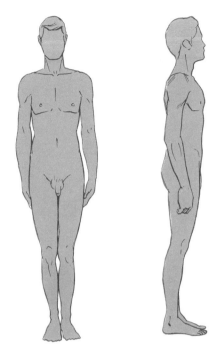

The anatomical position.

In the dorsal recumbent position, the patient's feet will normally assume a plantar flexion position. Prolonged positioning in plantar flexion, however, can result in foot drop, a condition in which the gastrocnemius and the soleus muscles remain involuntarily contracted. Preventive measures for this complication include the use of the footboard, which helps the patient to maintain his feet in dorsal flexion and removes the weight of the bedclothes from his toes. Flexion, extension and circumduction of the patient's ankles help maintain muscle tone and ankle joint mobility.

When the patient is lying in the dorsal recumbent position (and in all positions described subsequently), care should be taken to maintain the fingers in a functioning position, that is, fingers flexed and thumb in opposition. A small hand roll may be placed in the palm of the hand and the fingers curved around it. This is particularly important for unconscious patients and for those who have difficulty of movement in one or both hands. Wrist drop must also be prevented. The hand should never be left in a dependent position.

In some cases, the patient's head and shoulders are not elevated by pillows and rolls. The patient lies on his back with his head and shoulders on the flat surface. Supports similar to those just described are used when indicated.

This position is frequently prescribed for patients who have had spinal anesthetics.

Prone Position

The prone position is a position in which the patient lies on the abdomen with the head turned to one side. Many people are relaxed and sleep well in

If the patient does not have support for his thighs, they will tend to rotate outward. Two rolled towels or a rolled bath blanket tucked in at the lateral aspects of the thighs under the trochanter of the femur will maintain the patient's legs in alignment. His legs should be slightly flexed for maximal comfort. This is attained by placing a small pad under his thighs just superior to the popliteal space. Direct pressure should be avoided upon the popliteal area because of possible interference with circulation to the extremities and injury to the popliteal nerve.

Dorsal recumbent position with padding for support and to prevent pressure on bony prominences.

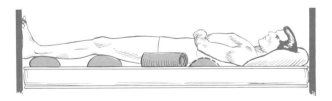

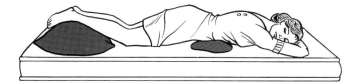

Prone position with padding for support and to prevent pressure on bony prominences. Note that the head is turned to the side and no pillow is provided.

this position; and some find it most comfortable to flex their arms over their heads.

Supportive measures for the patient in this position include a small pillow or pad, as needed, under the abdomen at the level of the diaphragm in order to give support to the lumbar curvature and, in the case of the female patient, to take weight off the breasts. A small pillow or towel roll under each shoulder helps to maintain the anatomical position. In addition, a pillow under the lower legs elevates the patient's toes off the bed and permits slight flexion of the knees. Alternatively, the patient can extend the toes over the end of the mattress to take the weight off the tips. Plantar flexion is minimized if the patients's lower legs are also supported. When the patient is in a prone position, there is pressure on the knees. A small pad under the thighs can be used to relieve this pressure. Sheepskin or sponge rubber pads may also be used under the knees.

The patient may prefer a pillow for her head. Unless the physician wishes the patient's head on a flat surface, in order to promote drainage of mucus for example, a small pillow is often more comfortable; however, it should not be so thick as to hyperextend the patient's head.

Lateral (Side-Lying) Position

In the lateral position the patient lies on his side with both arms forward and his knees and hips flexed. The upper leg is flexed more than the lower leg. Weight is borne by the lateral aspects of the patient's ilium and by his scapula.

The upper knee and hip should be at the same level; the upper elbow and wrist should be at the same level as the upper shoulder to prevent the limbs from being in a dependent position. The patient's heels and ankles may be protected by using small pads (for example, of sheepskin or sponge rubber) to keep them from rubbing on the bedclothes.

If the patient's upper arm falls across his chest, his lung capacity may be restricted; a pillow to support the patient's arm permits greater chest expansion and enables the nurse to readily observe the character and rate of his respirations.

The person who lies laterally will probably prefer a pillow for his head. A pillow of proper depth should prevent lateral flexion of the head. Frequently the patient will also require the support of a pillow placed lengthwise behind his back.

The lateral position is prescribed in order to take weight off the sacrum of the patient; and in addition, the patient

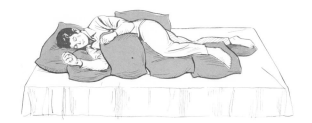

Lateral position. Notice the pillow supporting the patient's upper arm in order to allow for chest expansion.

can eat more easily in this position than in the supine position. It also facilitates some kinds of drainage. Finally many people find it a relaxing position.

Fowler's Position[2]

Fowler's position is probably one of the most frequently assumed positions. It is a sitting position in which the head gatch of the patient's bed is raised to at least a 45 degree angle.

In Fowler's position the patient is usually comfortable with at least two pillows for the back and head. The first pillow is best placed far enough down the patient's back to provide support for the lumbar curvature. A second pillow supports the head and shoulders. An emaciated patient will probably need three pillows. For patients who are very weak, pillows placed laterally will support the arms and help to maintain good body alignment.

Small pillows or a pad under the patient's thighs permit slight flexion of the knees, and a footboard permits dorsal flexion and prevents the patient from sliding toward the foot of the bed. Sometimes the knee gatch of the bed is used to support flexion of the knee. If the knee gatch is used, it should not be flexed too much because of the danger

of putting pressure on the popliteal nerve and major blood vessels which are close to the skin surface in the popliteal area. Prolonged pressure can cause serious interference with both nerve supply and circulation to the lower limbs.

In Fowler's position the main weight-bearing areas of the patient are the heels, sacrum, and posterior aspects of the ilium. The nurse should pay particular attention to these areas when she gives skin care.

Fowler's position is indicated for patients who suffer either cardiac or respiratory distress, since it permits maximal chest expansion.

Two variations of Fowler's position are the *semi-Fowler* and *high Fowler* positions. The semi-Fowler position refers to an elevation of the head of approximately 30 degrees. This is a comfortable position for the patient who must remain with his head and chest slightly elevated. The high Fowler position refers to the full sitting position, that is, with the head of the bed elevated to a 90 degree angle. The head gatches of most hospital beds can be elevated to this height. A position somewhat similar to the high Fowler is the sitting position in which the patient leans over an overbed table upon which several pillows have been placed for comfort. Some patients with respiratory problems find this position makes breathing easier for them. Patients who have difficulty exhaling tend to lean forward to compress the chest for additional expiratory force.[3] The pillows on the overbed table provide support for the arms and help to maintain the individual in as erect a position as possible to increase his total lung capacity.

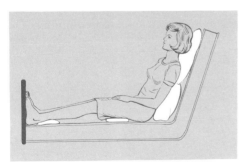

Fowler's position. Pillows can be provided for the patient's arms if such support is required.

Sims's Position (Semiprone Position)

The Sims position is similar to the lateral position except that the patient's

[2]In some hospitals, Fowler's position refers to the elevation of the upper part of the body without flexion at the hips; any elevation with hip flexion is referred to as the semi-Fowler position.

[3]Jane Secor: *Patient Care in Respiratory Programs.* Saunders Monographs in Clinical Nursing, Vol. 1. Philadelphia, W. B. Saunders Company, 1969, p. 75.

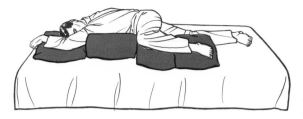

Sim's position (semiprone position). A small pillow may or may not be placed under the patient's head.

weight is on the anterior aspects of the patient's shoulder girdle and hip. The patient's lower arm is behind him and his upper arm is flexed at the shoulder and elbow. The upper leg is acutely flexed at the hip and knee, and the lower leg is slightly flexed at the hip and knee.

A rolled pillow placed laterally and in front of the patient's abdomen will support the patient in this position. Pillows for the patient's upper arm and upper leg will prevent adduction of these limbs, and a small pillow for the patient's head will prevent lateral flexion. If, however, the patient is unconscious and the nurse wants to promote mucus drainage from the mouth, a pillow under his head is contraindicated.

In the Sims position the patient's feet naturally assume the plantar flexion position. If the patient is to maintain the Sims position for some time, supports should be provided in order that his feet assume the dorsal flexion position. A footboard or sandbag can be used for this purpose.

The Sims position can be established on both the left side and the right side. The patient's position should be changed frequently; if he is unable to move himself, the nurse can help him turn every two hours, or oftener as needed. When turning the patient who is unconscious, the nurse should be sure that the patient's eyelids are closed to prevent the possibility of the cornea being scratched by the bedclothes. Good skin care, particularly to the anterior aspects of the patient's ilium and shoulder girdle, is also indicated.

This position is prescribed for patients who are either unconscious or unable to swallow. It permits the free drainage of

mucus. The Sims position also allows maximal relaxation and is therefore a comfortable sleeping position for many people.

Knee-Chest Position

The knee-chest position is used chiefly in examinations of the rectum and colon. In this position the patient kneels, with the buttocks upward. The patient's chest and head rest upon the bed surface.

It is important that the patient who assumes this position be adequately draped in order to prevent embarrassment and to provide warmth. Many hospitals have special rectal drapes which completely cover the buttocks of the patient except for a circular cutout over the anus. The patient will generally need additional covering for his shoulders and a pillow for his head.

If the health agency does not have special drapes, the nurse can improvise with a cotton drawsheet. The drawsheet is placed across the patient so that the lower edge just covers the buttocks. The corners are tucked around the medial aspect of the patient's thighs. By raising

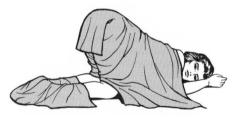

Knee-chest position. The drape is arranged so that the patient is suitably covered and the center fold can be raised to expose the anal area.

the fold of the sheet, the anal area is exposed.

Lithotomy Position

The lithotomy position is used chiefly for examinations and operations involving the reproductive and urinary tracts. In this position the patient lies on her back with a small pillow for her head. Her hips are flexed and slightly abducted and her knees are also flexed. The patient needs support for her feet if she is to maintain this position for more than a few minutes.

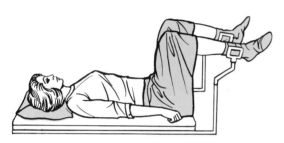

The lithotomy position is often used for urinary and vaginal examinations and operations.

A variation of the lithotomy position is the position assumed by the female patient who is having a urinary catheterization. In this position both the hips and knees are flexed and the legs are abducted, with the feet being brought together on the surface of the bed. This affords the nurse a field that exposes the perineum and permits the insertion of the catheter into the urethra.

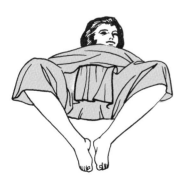

The lithotomy position is modified for treatments such as a urinary catheterization.

Because the lithotomy position is an embarrassing one for most patients, it is important that adequate drapes be provided. One way of draping the patient is to place a drawsheet across the patient so that the lower border is 4 inches below the symphysis pubis. Then each of the lower corners of the drawsheet are brought to the medial aspect of the patient's thighs and tucked around the patient's legs. When the upper fold of the drawsheet is lifted the patient's perineum is exposed. The nurse should also provide the patient with a covering for the upper part of the body. Another method is to place a bath blanket diagonally over the patient. The opposite corners (at each side of the patient) are wrapped around the legs and anchored at the feet. The lower corner can be drawn back and tucked under the top layer of the bath blanket to expose the perineum.

Trendelenburg Position

This position is used for some kinds of surgery and occasionally in situations involving shock and hemorrhage. In the modified Trendelenburg position shown (page 158), the patient lies on her back. The foot of the bed is elevated at a 45 degree angle so that the patient's hips and legs are higher than her shoulders.

This adaptation of the Trendelenburg position is sometimes used for a patient who requires vaginal irrigation. In this procedure it is important that the patient's hips are higher than her chest in order that the irrigating fluid will reach the posterior fornix of the vagina. Draping for this position is similar to that used in the lithotomy position.

In a regular Trendelenburg position the foot of the bed is elevated but the patient is not flexed at the waist. This position is also used in some situations when the patient is in shock.

There are other positions for patients, and the nurse will see them used in the nursing unit and in the operating room. But regardless of the position of the patient, certain principles apply: In positioning the patient in bed, it is most im-

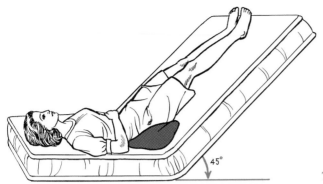

The modified Trendelenburg position.

portant that the nurse drape the patient adequately. In many situations it is equally important that she change the patient's position frequently. Adequate exercise, good skin care and supportive measures for maintaining good body alignment should also be carried out.

THE BED OF THE ILL PERSON

The bed is especially important to most people who are ill. To the patient in the hospital, the bed may be the one thing that he feels is entirely his. Moreover, much of a patient's comfort is dependent upon the condition of his bed, particularly if he is in it for long periods of time. When a patient appears to be unduly particular about his bed, the nurse should remember that he may spend 24 hours of his day in bed. To him a neat, clean and wrinkle-free bed is necessary for comfort. Other patients who are exacting in regard to their beds and bed units may be clinging to a position from which they can control some aspect of their environment at a time when they believe that many decisions and activities are beyond their control. The ill patient's horizons often narrow, and matters about which he normally

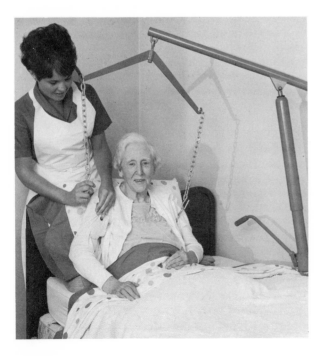

The bed of the patient at home can often be equipped with mechanical devices which add to the comfort of the patient. The nurse is adjusting a mechanical lift which will help her to move this patient.

would have no concern become important.

Traditionally, the hospital bed is made in the morning after the patient's bath. When the bed is made, soiled linen is changed and the entire bed is aired and remade. It is equally important that linen be changed whenever it becomes damp or soiled. As was pointed out in Chapter 11, soiled or wet linen predisposes a patient to decubitus ulcers and to infections.

Types of Beds According to Purpose

There are several ways of making a bed and each has its purpose. The *closed bed,* which is defined as an empty bed, is made after its occupant is discharged from the hospital. In a closed bed the spread extends over the bedclothes to the top of the mattress and the pillows are placed on top of the spread. In some hospitals the spread covers the pillows as well as the entire mattress.

The *open bed* refers to a bed that has been assigned to a patient. The spread is folded back with the blankets, and the top sheet is turned back on the spread. One side of the top bedclothes is sometimes turned back so that the patient can get into the bed easily.

The *occupied bed* refers to a bed which is occupied. Generally in this situation the person must remain in bed continuously, even while the nurse is making the bed. It is important for the nurse to learn to change linen and make a bed smoothly and quickly while the patient remains in it. Often the patient in an *occupied bed* is seriously ill and a great deal of activity is contraindicated.

The *anesthetic bed* or *recovery bed,* a variation of the basic hospital bed, is provided for the patient immediately after surgery. Its purpose is to provide a clean area into which a patient can be easily moved. It is also important that the bed linen can be easily changed, with a minimum of disturbance to the patient. Frequently this type of bed is made in such a way that a part of it can be changed without remaking the entire bed; for example, a separate short sheet might be placed under the patient's head in such a manner that it can be removed when it is soiled without disturbing the rest of the bedclothes.

The *diagonal toe bed* is designed to expose the leg or foot of the patient and at the same time to provide warmth and adequate covering. A variation of the open bed, it is often used to air wet casts and for the patient whose leg is in traction. In the latter situation, ropes and pulleys extend from the patient's leg over the end of the bed, thus making it impossible to completely tuck the covers under the mattress at the foot of the bed.

Linen for the Hospital Bed

The linen required for the basic hospital bed comprises two sheets, two pillow cases, one plastic or rubber drawsheet (optional), one cotton drawsheet (optional), one or two blankets and one spread. (Blankets are also optional.)

Cotton and rubber drawsheets have been traditionally used on the sick person's bed for two reasons: They are easier to change than the bottom sheet, and they protect the mattress. With the availability of plastic-covered mattresses, however, and increasing use of cotton mattress pads, (similar to the ones that are commonly used in the home), the routine use of drawsheets, both rubber (or plastic) and cotton, is disappearing. In many agencies the use of drawsheets is now reserved for the beds of patients who need them; they are no longer put on every bed.

When a plastic or rubber drawsheet is used, it is placed under a cotton drawsheet since the rubber (or plastic) retains heat and is uncomfortable. The drawsheet usually extends from above the patient's waist to his midthigh. Thus it can serve to absorb secretions in cases of urinary or fecal incontinence.

The cotton that is used for sheets, pillow cases and drawsheets must be of a heavy weight that wears well in spite of strong pulling and frequent washing. Moreover, because linen is often washed in disinfectant solutions in order to kill microorganisms, a heavy weight is necessary to withstand the laundering.

The blankets that are used in hospitals and most other health agencies are frequently made of a loose cotton weave or a mixture of flannel and cotton. The blankets should be able to withstand frequent washings without damage or shrinkage. In many hospitals, the temperature of patients' rooms is such that no blankets are needed. However, blankets are sometimes necessary for warmth. Usually one or two blankets suffice. An extra blanket is sometimes used as a throw blanket over the spread but there is a danger that it will be taken to another bed, thus transferring microorganisms from one patient to another. For this reason it is best to put both blankets under the spread or to put the extra blanket in the patient's closet until he wishes to use it. Elderly patients are often more sensitive to the cold than younger patients and therefore require more covers for warmth.

Changing the Hospital Bed

Generally there are two basic procedures in changing a hospital bed: stripping the bed and making the bed. When the nurse is changing a bed, she should be cognizant of the microorganisms that are present in the environment and the methods by which they are spread. The following principles should be kept in mind.

1. Microorganisms are present on the skin and in the general environment.

2. Some microorganisms are opportunists; that is, they can cause infections when conditions are favorable. For example, a break in the skin or mucous membrane of the patient may become a site of infection.

3. Patients are often less resistant to infections than healthy people because of the stress resulting from an existent disease process.

4. Microorganisms can be transferred from one person to another or from one place to another by air, by fomites or by direct contact among people. A fomite is an inanimate object other than food which can harbor microorganisms. Therefore the nurse should avoid holding soiled linen against her uniform, should never shake linen and should wash her hands before going to another patient.

The use of good body mechanics is also important in making a bed. The principles that underlie body movements in helping the patient to move are equally applicable in bedmaking (see Chapter 11). Some of these principles are reviewed here.

1. Maintain good body alignment. For example, the nurse stands facing the direction in which she is working and works in such a way that she does not twist her body.

2. Use the large muscles of the body rather than the small muscles. For example, flexing the knees in order to bring the body to a comfortable working level is preferable to bending at the waist. The former uses the large abdominal and gluteus muscles, whereas the latter puts strain upon the back muscles and shifts the center of gravity outside the base of support.

3. Working smoothly and rhythmically is less fatiguing because the muscles are alternately contracted and relaxed.

4. Pushing or pulling requires less effort than lifting.

5. Using one's own weight to counteract the weight of an object decreases the effort and strain. For example, if the nurse shifts her weight when she is pulling a mattress, it requires less effort than if she pulls the mattress with her arms. In addition, she places little strain upon her back and arm muscles.

The method of stripping and making a bed differs from place to place. Basically, however, every health agency wants the end product to be neat, clean, comfortable and durable, and the bed changing process to be economical in time, equipment and the patient's and nurse's energies. The following methods are suggested as guides to the student.

Stripping the Bed. Stripping a bed necessitates removing the linen and detachable equipment from the bed.

1. *Obtain the necessary equipment.* Generally all that is needed to strip a bed is a receptacle for soiled linen. Some hospitals provide a small hamper cart which the nurse takes to the door of the patient's room and into which she places the soiled linen. Care must be taken that microorganisms are not transferred by means of the hamper cart from one patient to another. Ideally, a linen hamper is provided for each patient.

If hampers are not provided, the nurse can tie the bedspread by its corners to the post at the foot of the bed to serve as a receptacle for soiled linen. Soiled linen on the floor is not only unclean, it also facilitates the spread of microorganisms.

The nurse can avoid extra trips by taking several bundles of linen out to the linen hamper at one time. The nurse would also be wise to bring all her clean linen and clean equipment in order to save time and effort. (See the procedures for making the open bed).

2. *Remove the equipment from the bed.* First the nurse places the patient's bedside chair beside his bed. The back of the chair is in line with the foot of the bed and the front faces the head of the bed. Sufficient room is left between the chair and the bed for the nurse to pass in order to save her steps when she goes around the foot of the bed. If a chair is not available, a movable table may be used. The patient's call light, refuse bag and so on are detached from the bed and placed on the bedside table. The patient's pillows are placed on the seat of the bedside chair; soiled pillow cases are put in the linen hamper.

3. *Remove the linen from the bed.* Starting at the head of the bed, the nurse loosens the top and bottom bedding from the mattress as she walks around the bed. When she returns to the first side of the bed, she grasps the spread at the center and near side and folds it to the bottom of the bed. She then picks up the spread at the center and lays it

folded in quarters across the back of the bedside chair. This step is repeated for the blankets and the sheets, if they are to be reused. None of the linen should touch the floor.

If drawsheets are used they are folded with as little contact as possible and then picked up in the center and placed over the back of the chair. The reason for folding linen in such a manner is that it is ready to be placed back on the bed with a minimum of movement. Conservation of energy and movement is important to a nurse's efficiency and to the quality of her care.

4. *Turning the mattress.* After the linen has been removed from the bed, the mattress may be turned from side to side, if the nurse feels this is needed, and pulled to the head of the bed. By grasping the lugs at the side of the mattress and by using good body mechanics, the nurse can turn a mattress with little effort. The following guides should be kept in mind:

a. Flex your knees to bring your arms to the work level.

b. Use your own weight to counteract the object's weight.

c. Pushing or pulling requires less effort than lifting.

d. Use the large muscles of the body.

e. Attain a wide base of support.

f. Maintain good body alignment.

Making the Open Bed. Frequently patients who are in bed much of the day are able to get up while the nurse makes the bed. However, the decision regarding the patient's activity is the physician's, and the nurse should not help a patient out of bed without the physician's approval. Because a patient states that he feels well enough to get up is not sufficient reason for him to do so. On the other hand, even though the patient has permission to get up, his condition may change and the nurse may suggest that he stay in bed until further instructions are received from the physician. In order to meet the needs of her patient, the nurse must continually use her judgment and her knowledge.

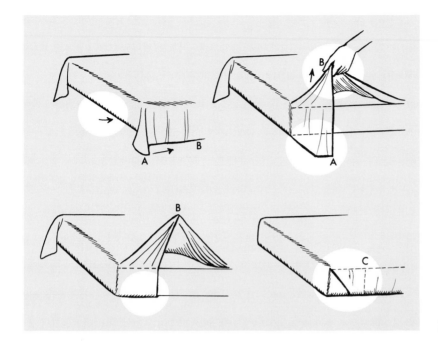

Mitering a corner.

1. *Obtain the necessary equipment.* The nurse brings all the linen and equipment that she needs for making the bed in as few trips as possible. A few minutes' thought beforehand can often save time later. Clean linen for the bed and equipment for patient hygiene can often be collected at the same time. The linen is placed on the bedside chair in the order in which it is to be used.

2. *Make the bed.* The bottom sheet is placed on the bottom half of the mattress in such a way that the open edge is away from the center and the sheet just hangs over the bottom edge of the mattress. The sheet is then opened to the head of the bed and centered over the mattress. The sheet is tucked under the mattress at the head of the bed and the corner is mitered or squared on one side. The sheet is then tucked in smoothly along the sides. To miter the corner of a sheet the following steps are performed.

   a. Tuck the sheet in securely under the mattress at the head of the bed.

   b. Lift the sheet at *A* (see illustration above), and bring it along the side of the mattress.

   c. Grasp the sheet at *B* and bring this point directly up, releasing the sheet at *A*.

   d. Tuck in the part of the sheet that hangs below the mattress.

   e. Bring *B* down firmly and tuck under the mattress. The underfold of the corner (*C*) should be even with the edge of the mattress.

To square a corner means to tuck in the end of the sheet and then to fold the side under so that the fold runs parallel to the corner and gives a boxed appearance to the corner.

After the bottom sheet has been tucked in on one side of the bed, the drawsheets are placed on the bed if they are indicated. They are tucked in on the near side.

The top sheet is then placed across the foundation near the foot and opened so that the bottom half of the bed is covered. It is then carried to the head of the bed until the edge of the sheet is even with the edge of the mattress. The blankets and bedspread are applied in the same manner but are brought to within approximately 9 inches of the edge of the mattress.

When the bed has been made completely on one side, the other side is made up in the same manner. The foundation is pulled tightly so that it is free of wrinkles. Wrinkles are uncomfortable and can be irritating to the skin.

Many agencies now use contour sheets which make it easier to provide a firm wrinkle-free foundation for the bed.

The head of the bed is completed by folding back the top covers. The pillows are replaced on the bed.

3. *Replace the equipment.* Before the nurse leaves the bedside she replaces any equipment that the patient requires. This includes attaching the signal light to the bed, placing the bedside chair beside the bed and arranging the bedside table within the patient's reach. All unnecessary equipment is removed, and small articles that the patient is not using are placed safely in his bedside table. The nurse should ask the patient's permission before discarding any of his belongings, including flowers.

Making the Closed Bed. To make a closed bed the nurse follows the same method as for an open bed except that the spread is brought to the head of the bed so that it is even with the top sheet, and the top sheet and blanket are not folded back. There are many variations of this pattern in hospitals.

Making the Occupied Bed. Making an occupied bed is similar to making an open bed except that the nurse is concerned with maintaining the patient's body alignment, safety and comfort. It is preferable to make the bed while the bed is level; however, some patients are unable to assume the dorsal recumbent position because of their condition—for example, because of difficulty in breathing. In such cases the nurse is challenged to make a comfortable, neat bed while the head of the bed is elevated. Although the physician usually orders the position in which the patient is to be maintained, it is often the nurse's decision whether the patient's position can be changed while the bed is made.

When a bed is stripped while the patient remains in it, a pillow is left for the patient's comfort. After the spread and blankets have been removed, a bath blanket is placed over the top sheet, which is then removed by drawing it down from under the bath blanket. If the patient is to be washed, it is done at this time, before the foundation of the bed is changed, to prevent the clean sheet from becoming damp or soiled during the bath.

It is easier to change the foundation of the bed if the patient is moved to the far side of the bed. The foundation on the near side is loosened and if the linen is to be removed, it is folded to the center of the bed. Clean linen is placed on the near side of the bed and tucked in. The patient then rolls over the folded linen to the near side of the bed. The soiled linen is removed, and the clean linen is pulled tightly across the bed and tucked in.

The patient is assisted to the center of the bed and the second pillow is replaced. The top covers are replaced as for an open bed. The nurse must remember to withdraw the bath blanket after she has put on the top sheet. For some patients, as for example, orthopedic patients in traction, the bed may be made from top to bottom rather than from side to side.

When the nurse replaces the top covers, she should allow sufficient room for the patient to move his feet. Toe pleats in the top covers will provide this

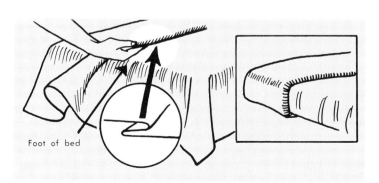

A vertical toe pleat is made while the nurse is standing at the foot of the bed.

Foot of bed

extra space for the patient. To make a vertical toe pleat, the upper sheet and the blankets are raised and a 2 inch fold is made in the sheet and blankets perpendicular to the foot of the bed. The linen is then tucked in. As an alternative, the nurse can loosen the top covers at the foot of the bed, or the patient can cross his feet before the corners are mitered in order to ensure sufficient foot room.

After the nurse completes the bed she tidies the unit. This involves putting away personal utensils that the patient is not using and placing articles such as his water glass and radio within easy reach. The hospital patient's signal cord is attached to the bed so that it is always within easy reach. It gives the patient a feeling of security to know that the nurse may be easily and quickly summoned.

Today, hospitals often employ a housekeeping staff which is responsible for cleaning the patient's unit. It is the staff's responsibility to clean the bed-unit tables, change the patient's drinking water and look after his flowers. Floor washers are assigned to clean the hospital floors regularly. In a hospital where a specialized staff is not employed for these purposes, these duties may very likely become the nurse's responsibility. In any case, the nurse is often responsible for checking that the patient's environment is clean and comfortable.

Making the Anesthetic Bed (recovery bed). The anesthetic bed is an adaptation of the basic hospital bed. It is customarily made directly after the patient goes to surgery. If the patient is to go to the recovery room (postanesthetic room or P.A.R.) after surgery, the bed is usually taken there so that the patient is transferred to his own bed immediately after the operation is over.

The purpose of the anesthetic bed is to provide a safe, comfortable and convenient bed for the postsurgical patient. Usually the foundation for an open bed is completed, and then one or two rubber (plastic) and cotton drawsheets are placed over it to protect the bottom sheet. This is done because a short

drawsheet is more easily changed than an entire bottom sheet; therefore the patient will be disturbed less if it is necessary to change any part of the foundation of the bed.

The top covers on the anesthetic bed are generally folded back in order to make it easier for the patient to be transferred into the bed. One method of arranging the top covers is to fold the bedclothes up on both sides and both ends. Then all the covers can be quickly folded to one side or the other when the patient is transferred to the bed.

The anesthetic bed is always made with clean linen, as free from microorganisms as possible. A clean bed lessens the danger of infection and is generally more comfortable. If a pillow is needed for the postoperative patient, it should have a plastic covering to protect it from vomitus and drainage. In many agencies today, all pillows are plastic covered for easy cleaning.

The bed unit for the postoperative patient is arranged for efficiency of care. The patient's personal belongings are put safely away and the bedside table is left clear. Tissues should be immediately available and a kidney basin should be nearby so that it can be quickly obtained if it is needed. Siderails should be attached to the bed. An intravenous standard should be either attached to the bed or available in the patient's room. Blood pressure equipment is needed also. Since oxygen or suction equipment is often required at the bedside the nurse must check that a space is set aside for this equipment and that the equipment is ready for the patient when he returns from the operating room.

THE MATTRESS

There are many different kinds of mattresses available for both therapeutic and comfort purposes. The regular mattress for the hospital bed is firm and often covered with a plasticized material. Patients who are allergic to these mattresses require mattresses made of foam rubber. This type offers the patient support but molds somewhat to his body. The foam rubber mattress also has an advantage in that it places less pressure upon the patient's bony prominences. Because of this it is often used in the prevention and treatment of decubitus ulcers in patients who must remain in bed for long periods of time.

Also available are split foam rubber mattresses. These mattresses are divided horizontally into three sections. The sections at the head and foot of the bed are approximately 2½ feet in length and the middle section 1½ feet in length. The middle section is in turn divided lengthwise into two parts, one of which can be pulled out in order to insert a bedpan without moving the patient. The split foam rubber mattress is generally used for debilitated patients and for those who are unable to move.

A third type of mattress is the alternating pressure mattress, which is run by a small motor. This mattress can be filled with either air or water. Areas of the mattress are alternately deflated and inflated with the result that there is a continual change in the pressure upon the various parts of the patient's body. These alternations of pressure stimulate circulation to the skin, thus facilitating the nourishment of tissues and the removal of waste products. Before a patient is placed on an alternating pressure mattress he requires an explanation of the use of the mattress and reassurance about his safety. Some patients feel nauseated initially because of the motion, but this usually disappears within several hours. The nurse must also warn the patient and staff not to prick the mattress with safety pins or sharp instruments. This bed is more effective with only a single layer of linen between the mattress and the patient. Care must be taken not to pinch or shut off the tubing to the motor when the bed is being made.

Another type of bed, the air-fluidized bed, uses the flotation principle to provide uniform support to all parts of the body. The mattress portion of the bed is made of very fine medical-grade optical glass spheres. Air is blown through these spheres to keep them constantly moving, and the patient experiences a comfortable sensation of floating without feeling unstable.[4]

Sawdust mattresses are also used by some agencies for patients whose movement is limited, to provide more equal distribution of pressure. Gel flotation and Silastic flotation pads are frequently used when the patient is transferred to a normal bed. These pads are often used in home care.

THE OVERBED CRADLE

The overbed cradle is a device that attaches to the mattress of the bed and extends over the top of the bed. It is used to keep the top bed covers off the patient. Some overbed cradles are hoop arrangements which extend from one side of the bed to the other; others extend only to the midline of the bed. Overbed cradles are usually made of metal or plastic.

The primary purpose of the overbed cradle is to keep the weight of the top bedclothes off the patient. Patients who have burns, uncovered wounds or wet casts often need to keep the top bedclothes away from the injured area. When the nurse is applying a cradle to the patient's bed, she should ensure that it is securely fastened to, or under, the mattress. The cradle is carefully positioned so that the area of the patient's body that is to be free from the weight of the top bed covers is directly under the cradle. The top bedclothes must be pulled up higher than normally so that they cover the shoulders of the patient.

THE FOOTBOARD

The footboard is a device that is placed toward the foot of the patient's bed to serve as a support for his feet.

---

[4] J. Shand Harvin and Thomas S. Hargest: The Air-Fluidized Bed: A New Concept in the Treatment of Decubitus Ulcers. *Nursing Clinics of North America*, 5:1:181–186, March, 1970.

Some footboards fit onto the bed frame across the foot of the bed; others attach to the sides of the bed frame and thus may rest on the mattress at any point along the bed. Footboards are usually made of wood, plastic or heavy canvas.

Footboards are also used to keep the weight of the top bedding off the patient's feet as well as to support the patient in maintaining his feet in a neutral position. Normally the feet of the patient who is lying in the dorsal position assume plantar flexion. In time if his feet are not exercised or supported they may become fixed in plantar flexion. This condition, known as foot drop, is the result of contractures of the gastrocnemius and soleus muscles. With this complication, the patient is unable to stand with his heels on the floor. Foot drop is usually treated by physiotherapy, but sometimes it can be modified only by surgery.

When the nurse applies a footboard to the bed, it is placed so that the patient can rest the soles of his feet against it while the rest of his body is in good alignment. The top bedclothes need to be brought higher up on the bed so that they cover the patient's shoulders. The footboard is securely fastened to the frame of the bed; it usually has to be removed when the foundation of the bed is stripped.

A *footblock* is a block of wood or a box that is placed at the foot of the bed. Its purpose is the same as that of the footboard. The footblock has a disadvantage: it is not adjustable to the height of a patient. On the other hand it is easily obtainable for the patient who is confined in bed at home.

THE FRACTURE BOARD

The fracture board (bed board) is a support that is placed under the patient's mattress to give added rigidity to the mattress. It is usually made of wood or of wood and canvas and is constructed to fit the standard hospital bed. One type of fracture board has hinges so that the head and knee gatches of the bed can be used with the

board in position. Another type is made of slats, which provide for flexibility so that the head and knee gatches of the bed can be raised or lowered if desired.

The fracture board is used in situations in which the patient needs additional support for his back. Patients who have spinal injuries often have fracture boards ordered by the physician.

The fracture board is easily applied to an unoccupied bed. Usually an orderly can slide the fracture board from a stretcher to the bed, making sure that the hinged joints of the board correspond to the gatches of the bed. The nurse should explain to the patient that the purpose of the board is to provide firmness and thus should not be modified by the extensive use of pillows.

THE BALKAN FRAME

The Balkan frame is a frame made of wood or metal which extends lengthwise above the bed and is supported at either end by a pole. A trapeze may be attached to the frame just above the patient's head as an aid to the patient in lifting himself up in bed. Often the Balkan frame serves as an attachment for the pulleys and weights of traction equipment, which is used for patients who have fractures of the lower limbs, particularly the femur.

Often the sole purpose of the Balkan frame is to provide a trapeze. Some of the new frames use only one pole when

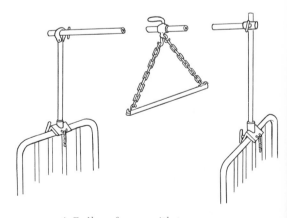

A Balkan frame with trapeze.

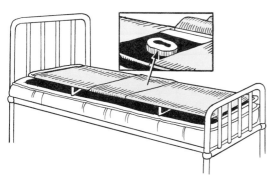

The Bradford frame. Note the removable canvas strip in the center to enable the insertion of a bedpan.

the frame is used solely to support a trapeze. The nurse can show the patient how to use this as an exercise device or as an aid in moving.

THE BRADFORD FRAME

The Bradford frame is a canvas, stretcher-like device that is supported by blocks on the foundation of the bed. It is used to immobilize patients who have injured spines. The canvas is divided into three parts so that the small center portion can be removed to insert a bedpan. In the newer type of fracture beds the canvas covering of the frame is in strips to facilitate care to the patient.

One of the nurse's responsibilities is to reassure the patient that he is not likely to fall off the frame and that it is preferable that he lie quietly. Bradford frames have been replaced in many instances by CircOlectric beds, Stryker frames and Foster beds.[5]

OTHER SUPPORTIVE DEVICES

There are several kinds of supportive rolls available to patients. These rolls have been referred to earlier in this chapter. The *trochanter roll* is often made from a bath towel. The towel is folded lengthwise once and then rolled to within 6 inches of one end. The roll is secured by two safety pins that are fastened between the body of the roll and the tail of the roll. To support the thigh of the patient so as to prevent external rotation, the tail of the roll is placed under the patient's thigh, with the safety pins away from the patient. The roll is then firmly secured along the patient's leg. Trochanter rolls are also used to raise a patient's heels off the foundation of the bed.

Sponge rubber pads, sheepskin pads and *small pillows* also serve as supportive devices. Placed under bony prominences they relieve pressure; placed in the lumbar curve or under a limb they support or elevate an injured part. A small sponge rubber pad placed in the patient's hand can be used as an exercise implement. It can also be used to

---

[5] For a more detailed discussion of beds and frames used in the care of orthopedic patients, the nurse is directed to *Bedside Nursing Techniques in Medicine and Surgery* by Audrey L. Sutton. Second edition. Philadelphia, W. B. Saunders Company, 1969, pp. 197–200.

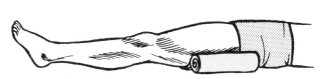

A trochanter roll can be used to prevent external rotation of the hip. The safety pins used to secure the roll initially are placed so that they face away from the patient.

prevent severe flexion of the hand and to separate skin surfaces in conditions of spastic contraction. The size of the pad allows slight flexion of the hand and fingers, with the thumb comfortably placed in normal anatomical position.

Sandbags also serve as a means of providing support to the patient. They are firmer than trochanter rolls and, because of their weight, are less easily moved. For this reason sandbags are desirable when body alignment must be maintained, for example, in fractures. Sandbags should be pliable so that they can be shaped to the contours of the body.

GUIDE TO ASSESSING NURSING NEEDS

1. Does the patient require assistance to maintain a position of good body alignment?
2. What position is best for this patient?
3. Is the patient able to change his position as he needs to?
4. Does he require supportive devices or a different type of mattress or bed for therapeutic reasons?
5. What nursing measures are needed to prevent physical discomfort for this patient?

GUIDE TO EVALUATING THE EFFECTIVENESS OF NURSING ACTION

1. Is the patient comfortable? For example, is he warm and free from pain?
2. Is his body alignment anatomically sound?
3. Are the measures used to promote comfort recorded so that other members of the health team are aware of them?
4. When the patient is in bed, is the bed comfortable?

STUDY VOCABULARY

Anatomical position	Emaciated	Lithotomy position
Anesthetic bed	Fomite	Miter
Balkan frame	Footboard	Open bed
Bradford frame	Fowler's position	Popliteal
Closed bed	Fracture board	Sims's position
Comfort	Knee-chest	Supine
Cradle	position	Trendelenburg
Dorsal recumbent position	Lateral	position

STUDY SITUATION

Mrs. R. Rogers is a 56 year old woman who was admitted to the hospital with acute rheumatoid arthritis involving her back, her knees and her feet. Mrs. Rogers is an obese woman and she finds it difficult to breathe when the head of her bed is flat. She complains of pain in her joints continually. Mrs. Rogers has a limited income and lives by herself in a small apartment. Her husband died four years ago, and her one daughter rarely comes to see her.

The physician has ordered that Mrs. Rogers be maintained in good body alignment at all times. Her position is to be changed every four hours. She is on a low calorie diet.

1. What particular needs of this patient can you discern from the foregoing data?

2. Which other members of the health team could assist with Mrs. Rogers' care?
3. What might be some of the reasons for her discomfort?
4. What positions would Mrs. Rogers best assume? Describe them.
5. Which supportive devices might make Mrs. Rogers more comfortable? How should you use them?
6. How can the nurse ascertain the patient's comfort?

BIBLIOGRAPHY

Dorland's Illustrated Medical Dictionary. Twenty-fourth edition. Philadelphia, W. B. Saunders Company, 1965.

DuGas, Beverly: An Analysis of Certain Factors in the Diffusion of Innovations in Nursing Practice in the Public General Hospitals in British Columbia. Unpublished doctoral dissertation. Vancouver, The University of British Columbia, 1969.

Harmer, Bertha, and Virginia Henderson: *Textbook of the Principles and Practice of Nursing.* Fifth edition. New York, The Macmillan Company, 1955.

Harvin, J. Shand, and Thomas S. Hargest: The Air-Fluidized Bed: A New Concept in the Treatment of Decubitus Ulcers. *Nursing Clinics of North America,* 5:1:181–186, March, 1970.

Kaufman, Margaret A.: Autonomic Responses as Related to Nursing Comfort Measures. *Nursing Research, 13:*45–55, Winter, 1964.

Secor, Jane: *Patient Care in Respiratory Problems.* Saunders Monographs in Clinical Nursing, Vol. 1. Philadelphia, W. B. Saunders Company, 1969.

Sutton, Audrey L.: *Bedside Nursing Techniques in Medicine and Surgery.* Philadelphia, W. B. Saunders Company, 1969.

Webster's Seventh New Collegiate Dictionary. Springfield, Mass., G. & C. Merriam Company, 1963.

14 THE NUTRITIONAL NEEDS OF THE PATIENT

The nurse should be able to:

Explain how food helps to satisfy basic human needs
Give examples of the role of food in the traditions, customs,
    superstitions and religions of different cultures
Explain differences between the nutritional needs of the sick
    and those of the well
Describe the four basic types of diet commonly used in
    hospitals
List some of the factors to be considered in the acceptance of
    food by patients
Describe the nurse's responsibility in providing nourishment
    for the patient
Outline essential factors in tray service to patients
List guiding principles to follow when feeding a patient
Outline factors to be considered in attempting to change a
    person's food habits

THE SIGNIFICANCE OF FOOD

Food and the partaking of meals have a significance in human society that goes far beyond the provision of nourishment for the body.[1] In addition to fulfilling a basic physiological need, food may also help to satisfy one or more of an individual's many other needs. It has long been recognized, for example, that food is closely related to feelings of security. This is not merely the presence or absence of food in sufficient quantity to appease hunger, but the availability of specific foods. For many people, milk is a basic security food; for others, it may be meat, potatoes, rice, or some other familiar food which helps to foster feelings of security most.[2] When a person is ill, it is sometimes necessary to deprive him of certain foods. If any of these foods hold strong security meanings for him, it is understandable that the individual may feel threatened by its absence from his diet.

Food is often used to promote a feeling of social acceptance. Sitting down to eat with another person, even if the food that is taken is simply a cup of coffee, conveys to the other person that you consider him your equal. Offering someone a cup of tea or coffee, our "ritual of hospitality," can do much to foster an atmosphere of warmth and friendliness that is often difficult to attain in other ways. In some hospitals, obstetrical nurses use a "coffee-get-together" with the patients to provide a relaxed and informal setting in which to teach new mothers about the care of their infants.

Then, too, some foods are used for their prestige value, to enhance feelings of self-esteem. In many cultures, bread is a prestige food. In our North American society, steak and roast beef are generally considered prestige or "status" foods, and these are usually the most expensive items on a restaurant menu. Food may also be used to express creativity. Many women, and a good many men also, enjoy using their creative talents to prepare gourmet meals or exotic dishes to please their families and friends.

The partaking of food in one form or another plays an important role in many religious ceremonies. One has only to think of the Christian ceremony of Communion to be aware of the significance of food in this regard. At Communion, one partakes of bread, which symbolizes the flesh of Christ, and of wine, which symbolizes His blood. In some religions, as for example, in Judaism, the preparation of food is in itself a ritual, and some hospitals maintain a kosher kitchen to cater to the needs of their orthodox Jewish patients. There are also many food taboos associated with religious doctrines. The Orthodox Muslim will not eat pork, for example, nor the Hindu, beef.

---

[1]Miriam E. Lowenberg, E. Neige Tidhunter, Eva D. Wilson, Moira C. Feeney, and Jane R. Savage: *Food and Man*, New York, John Wiley & Sons, 1968, p. 109.

[2]Ibid.

Food is, in fact, intertwined with the traditions, superstitions, and prejudices of virtually every culture. The Easter ham in our country and the Devali[3] gift of sweets in India are but two examples of the incorporation of food into traditional customs. To spill salt is considered by many people to be bad luck, and this is a common example of a superstition involving food. Most of us have prejudices against certain foods; yet these foods may be eaten with great enjoyment by others. Until fairly recently, few North Americans would have eaten snails, for example, although these are considered a delicacy by most people in France.

Mealtime, in most parts of the world, is a significant aspect of family life. In many cultures, eating is considered a private affair, to be shared and enjoyed only with one's family or intimate friends. Meals often play an important role in reaffirming solidarity within the family group. In most North American homes, the mother usually likes to have all members of the family present for the evening meal. The traditional gathering of the family for Thanksgiving or Christmas dinner serves to strengthen family ties within the extended family unit. Meals, too, may provide a time when family roles are defined and clarified; Father sits at the head of the table, a tangible symbol of his role as head of the family.[4]

In our culture, we usually like to think of mealtime as a pleasant time — a period of relaxation, when we can enjoy the company of others and engage in social conversation. Hospitals today are doing much to make mealtimes more pleasurable for patients. Trays are attractively served; there is usually a choice of menu from which the patient may select the foods that he likes; and many hospitals now have small dining areas adjacent to the nursing units, where patients who are able may gather to eat their meals.

FOOD AND THE SICK PERSON

Food as a source of nourishment is particularly important for those who are ill. It has been reported that almost all sick persons have some disturbance in gastrointestinal functioning.[5] They may lose their appetite or be unable to tolerate food and fluids; there may be a problem in the digestion of food or in the absorption of nutrients from the gastrointestinal tract. Whatever the problem, the sick person's nutritional needs are usually different from those of the well. Lack of exercise because of illness may decrease the body's need for energy-giving foods but, at the same time, there is a greater need for tissue-building nutrients.

The nutrients that are taken into the body, normally via the gastrointestinal tract, are digested and then absorbed into the blood stream and taken to the cells of the body. In the cells, metabolic activity takes place. Metabolism has two phases: catabolism and anabolism. In catabolism the glucose derived from carbohydrates, and the ketones and glycerol derived from fat, are broken down into carbon dioxide, water and energy. Proteins are broken down into carbon dioxide, water, urea and energy. In anabolism this energy is used in the synthesis of enzymes and proteins needed by the body cells. The restructuring of amino acids to form protein elements of the body is a particularly important part of anabolism.

In the well person, the processes of anabolism and catabolism are normally equal. In the sick, particularly those who are incapacitated, the catabolic activities are increased, which leads to a breakdown of cellular materials and a subsequent deficiency of protein.[6]

---

[3]Devali, the "Festival of Lights," is a major religious festival in India.

[4]Anne Burgess and R. F. A. Dean (eds.): *Malnutrition and Food Habits.* New York, The Free Press, 1963, pp. 63–64.

[5]Edith V. Olson et al.: The Hazards of Immobility. *The American Journal of Nursing,* 67:780–797, April, 1967, pp. 785–787.

[6]Ibid.

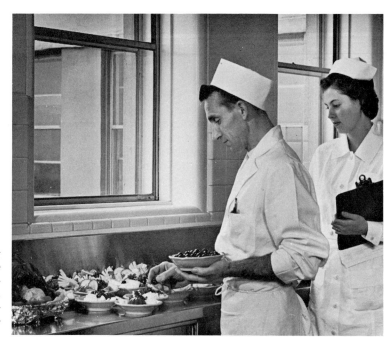

People who are ill frequently require special diets which are designed to meet their particular needs. In health agencies, such as hospitals, food is usually prepared under the direction of a dietitian.

Thus, there may be a decreased need for food for energy requirements but an increased need for specific nutrients in the person who is ill. Additional protein foods are important for almost all sick people. There are, of course, some conditions in which a high-protein diet is contraindicated, but the foregoing statement is a good general rule.

There are certain conditions, too, in which metabolic activity, both anabolic and catabolic, is increased, as in patients with a fever, and in these cases there is a need for additional energy-giving foods as well as proteins.

In a good many disease conditions, the patient may be unable to tolerate food or fluids, or may lose these through vomiting, diarrhea or other means. In these cases, the replacement of lost fluids and nutrients is an important part of the patient's therapeutic care. In some disease conditions, there is interference with the absorption of food. These cases require special adaptation of the diet.

Because foods vary in the amount and kinds of nutrients they contain, physicians often order special diets for pa-

tients—diets designed to meet the patients' particular needs. Nurses should know the main constituents of the common foods in order to be able to explain diets to patients and also teach patients and their families how to meet their nutritional needs.

KINDS OF DIET

Food for the sick person may then be thought of as a therapeutic agent as well as a source of pleasure and nourishment. As a part of the patient's therapeutic regime, food is usually prescribed in the form of a diet. There are many kinds of diet. For example, the average patient is on a regular or full (normal) diet. This means that he eats any or all of the foods that he normally eats in health. Generally fried and highly seasoned foods are not served to patients because of the difficulty many people normally have in digesting them. A modification of the full, or regular, diet is the light diet. The foods on this diet are cooked simply, with an avoidance of fried foods, rich desserts and other fat-rich foods. Coarse gas-forming foods such as corn, turnips, radishes, onions, cabbage, cauliflower and cucumbers are also usually avoided.

A third type of diet is the soft diet. This diet consists of food that requires little chewing and contains no harsh fiber or highly seasoned foods. Because soft-diet foods are easily digested, they are often indicated for people who have gastrointestinal disorders or difficulty in masticating food.

A fourth kind of diet is the liquid diet. There are usually two types of liquid diet: full liquid and clear liquid. A full liquid diet is free of irritating condiments and cellulose. Often gelatin, jelly and junket are included in a full liquid diet, and also soft drinks and ice cream. A clear liquid diet permits water, tea with lemon, or coffee. Often a patient on a clear liquid diet is restricted in the amount of fluid he may take at one time.

Therapeutic diets are special diets which vary greatly in their composition and purpose. Many special diets are designed to eliminate substances that are irritating to the gastrointestinal tract. The amount and kind of nutrients may be varied or certain nonnutritive compounds eliminated. For example, restrictions may be placed on the flavoring or seasoning used or on the amount of cellulose to be consumed. There are also diets that restrict the amount of sodium, sugar or protein. There are high calorie diets and low calorie diets, high protein diets and low protein diets. There are also diets which control the quantity and type of fat. Each therapeutic diet is ordered by the physician to meet the patient's specific needs. The quantity of each kind of food is calculated by the dietitian and each meal is served carefully in the prescribed amounts of specific foods.

Regardless of the kind of diet it is important that the patient understand why he is served certain foods. The physician and the dietitian can help gain the patient's cooperation and thereby his acceptance of the prescribed food as part of his prescribed therapy.

FACTORS THAT AFFECT FOOD ACCEPTANCE

Many factors have a bearing upon the acceptance of food. Some of these factors can be modified by the nurse; others she can use as guides to the provision of satisfactory nourishment. For example, the sedentary patient is less likely to have a good appetite than the patient who exercises regularly. If a patient is able to perform some activity he should be encouraged to do so, for it will stimulate his appetite. It is important, however, that this activity be carried out well before meals, not directly afterward, and that the amount of exercise is not exhausting.

Attractively served food is more conducive to a good appetite than food served in a disorganized setting. Moreover, food should always be served either hot or cold, never lukewarm. If the nurse serves the patient, she should check that the liquids are not spilled and that the food is served at its most desirable temperature. The patient who needs assistance should, of course, be helped immediately after his food is served.

Another factor which affects appetite is the environment in which a person eats. If a patient is served in his room, the air should be fresh and free from unpleasant odors. Those nursing measures which are uncomfortable or unpleasant should not be carried out just prior to the meal.

As noted in the section on the meaning of food at the beginning of this chapter, cultural, moral and religious values play a considerable role in food acceptance. Most Europeans are accustomed to a small "continental" breakfast of coffee and rolls, and may reject the hearty meal which so many North Americans enjoy in the morning. A large number of people from Eastern cultures are vegetarians and find it difficult to obtain a sufficient variety of nutrients from our predominantly meat-dominated menus. Beans and rice form an important part of the diet for many

Spanish-Americans, but the rice may be unacceptable if mixed with raisins and sweetened in a pudding. With the highly diversified ethnic origins of the people of our country, it is important that all these factors be taken into consideration in the preparation of hospital diets.

There is also the matter of individual differences in taste and preference for food, as any one from a large family knows. From the moment of birth various factors such as good or poor digestion, allergies and differences in taste, the extent of one's imagination, his education and the food habits in the home will influence an individual to develop his own particular set of eating habits.[7]

Illness has a very great bearing upon a person's acceptance of food. Those who are nauseated, dyspeptic, in pain or febrile are less desirous of food than healthy people. The nurse has a responsibility to modify these factors as much as possible in order that the patient will accept nourishment. Small, frequent meals are often more acceptable to the sick person than large servings at regular meal hours. It is necessary to cater to the particular tastes of the individual, to find out what he does and does not like in the way of food, in order to encourage him to take a sufficient amount of nourishment. Every effort should be made to see that the patient is free of pain and is comfortable when food is offered. A frequent concomitant of illness is anxiety, which may well affect a patient's desire for food as well as his ability to digest it. Sometimes anxiety is manifested in complaints about the food. The coffee is cold, the meat may be too well done. Often these complaints are a vocalization of a deeper anxiety. Understanding and acceptance on the part of the nurse can do much to help the patient to accept his illness and his diet.

THE NURSE'S ROLE IN THE PROVISION OF NOURISHMENT

Rarely is the nurse of today responsible for the cooking and preparation of food. Usually other personnel are employed to prepare and, often, to serve food to the patient. The nurse, however, has important functions relative to the patient's nourishment. It is the nurse who usually finds out what the patient's food preferences are and learns about his appetite and food consumption.

The amount of food that patients eat and the amount of fluids they drink are sometimes very important therapeutically. It is the nurse who observes how much he eats and drinks and who has the responsibility for communicating this knowledge to other members of the health team. Many hospitals have a standard form which is kept at the patient's bedside so that fluid consumption can be recorded. Once the record is completed it is usually transferred to the patient's chart.

The nurse is also responsible for helping the patient to prepare for his tray. The patient is offered a bedpan or urinal and is provided with facilities for washing his hands prior to eating. Often a patient who has an unpleasant taste in his mouth will find his appetite is improved if he brushes his teeth before eating.

Some patients like to get out of bed to eat their meals. If this is medically feasible the nurse can help the patient to get up a few minutes before his tray arrives. Patients find it very difficult to eat and to swallow while lying in a dorsal position. If a patient cannot be raised to Fowler's position, he will be more comfortable lying on his side while he eats. A comfortable position with adequate support helps make mealtime a more enjoyable experience.

The nurse can also see that the patient is free from pain at mealtime and that he is not subjected to unpleasant treatments immediately before and after meals. Enemas and dressing changes should be carried out at a time when

---

[7]Lowenberg et al., op. cit., p. 97.

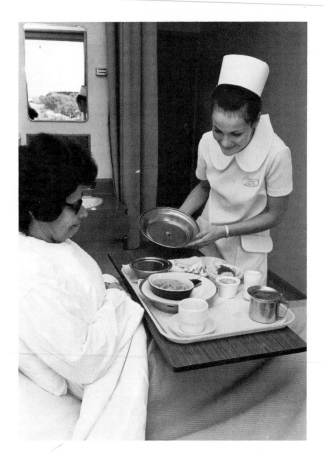

An attractively arranged tray can often help to stimulate a patient's appetite.

they have little effect upon a patient's appetite.

The environment at mealtime should be clean and tidy. The air should be free from unpleasant odors and the patient's unit free from unpleasant sights. Bedside treatment trays are neatly covered and any unnecessary equipment is removed.

Some patients prefer company at mealtime; pleasant conversation with visitors or members of the nursing staff often relaxes the patient so that the meal is more enjoyable and his appetite and digestion are augmented. If the nurse stops to talk with a patient she should be guided by the patient's wishes regarding the subject of conversation.

TRAY SERVICE

In spite of the fact that dining-room service for patients is gaining increas-ing popularity, the majority of patients in hospitals still receive their food on trays in their rooms. Patients are not always physically able to go to a dining room and not all hospitals have dining-room facilities for their patients as yet.

The nurse needs to be aware of good standards for tray service and see that these are adhered to.

1. The tray should be large enough to hold the dishes and utensils needed for the patient's meal and, at the same time, small enough to be accommodated on the patient's overbed table or bedside table.

2. Food must be served at the proper temperature; that is, hot food should not be allowed to cool and cold food should not be allowed to warm.

3. Food should always be covered when it is being carried to the patient's bedside. Covering food helps not only to maintain the proper temperature but also to prevent drying out, which affects

the flavor, texture and appearance of food.

4. Food should be served as attractively as possible in arranged portions, with garnishes to give color appeal. Small portions are more stimulating to the appetite than large portions.

5. The napkins, dishes, utensils and the tray itself should be spotlessly clean.

6. The arrangement on the tray should be neat and organized. Any spilled food should be replaced.

7. China and utensils should be attractive and in good condition.

8. The patient should always get the right tray with the right diet. Each tray has a card with the patient's name, bed number and type of diet. If the nurse has any doubts as to the correctness of a patient's tray, she can check the physician's orders before leaving the tray with the patient.

FEEDING THE PATIENT

If it is necessary for the nurse to feed the patient, the observance of a few simple rules will make him more comfortable:

1. Whenever possible use the utensils that are normally used for the food being served.

2. Never hurry the patient. Sit down to feed him whenever possible.

3. Offer the patient small rather than large amounts of food.

4. Offer the food in the order that the patient prefers.

5. Note whether any food or liquid is hot and if it is, warn the patient to take only small portions or sips.

6. A straw or drinking cup will often help a patient to take liquids.

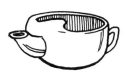

There are several types of drinking cups available commercially which can be useful to people who are ill.

7. If the patient can hold bread or toast, let him manage it himself.

8. Be careful not to spill food. Wipe the patient's mouth and chin whenever necessary. Always protect the patient with a napkin.

After the patient has finished his meal, the tray is removed promptly. A patient is never hurried with his meal. If his fluid intake is to be recorded, the amounts are noted on his fluid sheet. The nurse should be familiar with the amount of fluid contained in the commonly used containers. Estimated volumes of consumed fluids suffice in most situations.

Patients should be provided with facilities for washing their hands and brushing their teeth after meals. This offers a good opportunity for the nurse to teach oral hygiene and the correct method for brushing teeth.

CHANGING FOOD HABITS

It is sometimes necessary for a person to change his food habits because of illness. He may be told by the physician that he can no longer use salt to flavor his food, or he may have to give up eating a favorite dish. The patient may be put on a low-fat diet, or any one of a number of special diets. In these situations, people react differently. Some accept the restrictions of a special diet fairly easily; others are less amenable to change.

One of the most common reasons for failure of a patient to adhere to a diet is lack of understanding of why it is necessary. Another underlying cause may be fear resulting from the loss of a familiar food. The person who has been used to eating pasta all his life and for whom this represents a basic security food, will find it difficult to adjust to a diet on which this is banned. An individual may rebel against being told what to eat or may resent the loss of personal choice in the matter.

The nurse should remember that merely imparting knowledge to the patient does not ensure that dietary instructions will be followed.[8] Explaining the reasons for a specific diet is essential, but there are other factors which must be taken into consideration also. These include socioeconomic factors; the cultural, religious and moral values of the patient; and the matter of control over the purchase and preparation of food in the home.

The most influential member of a household in regard to purchasing and preparing the food that is eaten in the home is, in most instances, the mother. Younger, better-educated homemakers usually have the best nutritional knowledge and are more adaptable, but it is often necessary to work with others who are more resistant to change.

Many older people find it hard to alter the eating patterns they have been used to all their lives, yet often they are the ones on whom dietary restrictions are imposed. Then, too, in most "new American" and "new Canadian" families, it has been recognized that food habits from the homeland are retained long after language, clothing and other aspects of daily living are altered.[9] Often, strong resistance may be encountered to suggested changes involving the removal or alteration of familiar foods.

It is usually better to work within the framework of the individual's existing food habits, and to suggest modifications wherever possible rather than complete change. The old age pensioner's protein intake may be increased, for example, by the addition of cheese to his lunch of tea and toast. Supplementing a familiar diet of beans and rice by the addition of meat and milk may be accepted more readily by the Puerto Rican family than the suggestion of a completely different way of eating.

Another important item to consider is the effect of the patient's diet on other members of the family. Can the family afford to buy the special foods that are required for the patient? What problems may develop as a result of the need for preparing a different meal for one individual? If, for example, the patient is placed on a low-salt diet, this may involve cooking meat and vegetable dishes for him separately from those for the rest of the family, an additional chore for the homemaker.

In her role as teacher, the nurse must coordinate her efforts with those of the physician and the dietitian. The nurse's knowledge of the patient, his family and his home conditions can contribute much to ensuring the success of a teaching program.

[8]Lowenberg et al., op. cit., pp. 115–121.
[9]Ibid.

GUIDE TO ASSESSING NURSING NEEDS

1. What kind of diet is the patient on?
2. Does he understand the purpose of his diet?
3. Does the patient need extra fluids?
4. Does he need help with his meals?
5. Are there foods the patient needs to avoid or to eat?
6. Does the patient have cultural or religious values concerning food which conflict with his dietary needs?
7. Does the patient or his family require information regarding his diet in the future? For example, do food patterns need to be changed?

GUIDE TO EVALUATING THE EFFECTIVENESS OF NURSING ACTION

1. Is the patient eating his meals?
2. Does he enjoy them?
3. Is his intake of food and fluids adequate to meet his daily requirements?
4. Is the patient able to select foods that are compatible with his prescribed diet from the diet menu?

STUDY
VOCABULARY

Amino acid	Catabolism	Metabolism
Anabolism	Glycerol	Nutrient
Basal metabolic rate	Glycogen	Pathology
Calorie		

STUDY
SITUATION

Mr. John Smith is in the hospital and you are assigned to look after him. He is obese and the physician has placed him on a low calorie diet. Mr. Smith underwent surgery three days ago and his dressing needs changing four times a day. Although he is on a low calorie diet, he eats very little and complains that he is not hungry.

1. Why might Mr. Smith's appetite be poor?
2. What measures could the nurse take to improve Mr. Smith's appetite?
3. Mr. Smith wants extra sugar for his coffee. What should the nurse say?
4. At what hours are Mr. Smith's dressings best changed?
5. What is a low calorie diet? What food is likely to be restricted on such a diet?
6. Why is it particularly important that Mr. Smith have nourishment?

BIBLIOGRAPHY

Burgess, Anne, and R. F. A. Dean (eds.): *Malnutrition and Food Habits.* New York, The Free Press, 1963.

Department of National Health and Welfare, Nutrition Division: *Healthful Eating.* Ottawa, Information Canada, 1970.

Di Laura, Ann: The Nutritionist and the Team Approach, *Hospital Progress,* 46:130, 132, February, 1965.

Food Customs for New Canadians, Toronto, Toronto Nutrition Committee, 1967.

Guyton, Arthur C.: *Function of the Human Body.* Third edition. Philadelphia, W. B. Saunders Company, 1969.

Lowenberg, Miriam E., et al.: *Food and Man.* New York, John Wiley & Sons, Inc., 1968

Mitchell, H. S., et al.: *Cooper's Nutrition in Health and Disease.* Fifteenth edition. Philadelphia. J. B. Lippincott Company, 1968.

Olson, Edith V., et al.: The Hazards of Immobility. *The American Journal of Nursing,* 67:780–797, April, 1967.

Ritchie, Jean A. S.: *Learning Better Nutrition.* Rome, Food and Agriculture Organization of the United Nations, 1967.

Stare, Frederick J.: Good Nutrition from Food. Not Pills. *The American Journal of Nursing,* 65:86–89, February, 1965.

University Hospital. *Diet Manual.* Third Edition. Saskatoon, Saskatchewan, 1970.

15 THE SAFETY NEEDS
OF THE PATIENT

The nurse should be able to:

Name principles from the biophysical and social sciences
   basic to accident prevention
List common causes of mechanical trauma in hospital
Describe measures to prevent accidents of this type
Describe various safety devices used to protect people who
   are ill in bed
Outline safety measures taken by health agencies to protect
   the patient from errors in the administration of medi-
   cations
Name common causes of hospital fires
List fire prevention measures usually taken in hospitals
Describe types of fire extinguishers
Outline the nurse's responsibilities in the event of a fire
Describe methods of removing patients from a fire area,
   including four basic carries

INTRODUCTION

Safety is important to all people in society, but especially to those who are ill. The sick person is particularly prone to accident and injury by virtue of the illness itself. He is often physically weak and impaired in his ability to carry out normal daily activities. As a result he may fall while walking or easily lose his balance on an uneven surface. He also may have a low resistance to infections and be particularly susceptible to virulent microorganisms in the environment. Virulence refers to the ability of microorganisms to produce disease. The prevention and control of infection are discussed in Chapter 16.

The protective senses of the sick person, for example, his sight, may be so impaired that he cannot perceive dangers to himself. Moreover, the anxiety that is concomitant with illness may interfere with an individual's ability to make judgments, and thus expose him to injury.

An accident has been defined as "an event occurring by chance or from unknown causes."[1] In common usage, an accident is any event which has the potential to cause injury. With this definition in mind, many health agencies require that all accidents, that is, all events which did or could have resulted in injury to a patient, a visitor or a staff member, be reported so that remedial measures may be instituted. For example, if a patient receives an incorrect medication, notification of the nursing supervisor or the physician permits the initiation of measures to prevent a recurrence of this error.

Another purpose of reporting accidents is to guide the safety committee of an agency in its preventive program. The findings of these committees can be used as the bases for changes in medical and nursing practices and as indications of the need for the education of patients and personnel.

In nursing, a knowledge of safe nursing practices is essential. This involves not only a sound knowledge of the nursing and allied sciences, but also a knowledge of preventive nursing measures. To recognize circumstances which could result in an accident and to intervene effectively are essential. The nurse therefore needs to be alert to any activity which could cause injury and to any evidence of potential accident. Her observation should encompass the patient's total environment, in which she can look for such hazards as dangling electric cords, misplaced footstools and slippery floors, in short, any situation that could result in an accident.

SAFETY IN HOSPITALS

A hospital is generally thought of as a place where the sick and injured come

---

[1] *Webster's Seventh New Collegiate Dictionary.* Springfield, Mass., G. & C. Merriam Company, 1963.

RIVERSIDE HOSPITAL OF OTTAWA
CASUALITY OR COMPLAINT REPORT
DETAILS OF CASUALTY OR COMPLAINT

NOV 4 71

BLACK   GRACE   SP 1242
451 TOLL RD   OTT 234-7566-600
BLACK   GEORGE   HUS
SAME
8.30.71 1PM F 36 M SURG   RC
    420   1

casualty complaint

Date of Casualty
or complaint_____Sept 2/71_____

Time of Casualty
or Complaint_____7³⁰_____ (A.M.) P.M.

Examined by Doctor(name)____White_____

Date of Examination _Sept 3/71_ Time _8¹⁵_ (A.M.) P.M.

Attending Doctor Notified   Yes [✓] No. [ ]

On entering Mrs Black's room (212) I found her sitting on the floor between her bed and an armchair. She stated she had wanted to go to the bathroom and felt dizzy on getting ooo. — She didn't want to fall so she sat on the floor and grabbed the foot of the bed & her left hand. She is complaining of left wrist being sore. — no signs of swelling or bruising. Patient is allowed up and about as desired. She received no sedation at nurse bedtime. Call-bed attached to pillow & bed lowered to floor. Supervisor & doctor notified).

Ward___4N____ Date _Sept 2nd_ 19_71_ Signature _W Stratton, Reg N._

REPORT OF INVESTIGATION

_____No evidence of Nursing neglect — patient allowed to be up and about without assistance_____

Date _Sept 2_ 19_71_   Signature of Investigator _E Able_   Position _Supervisor_

NOTE: SEND THIS FORM, WHEN COMPLETED, TO NURSING
OFFICE IMMEDIATELY

2-8750

RIVERSIDE HOSPITAL OF OTTAWA

DOCTORS CASUALITY REPORT

Date of Casualty _Sept 2/71_ TIME _7³⁰_ AM

Date of Examination _Sept 2/71_ TIME _8¹⁵_ AM

NOV 4 71

BLACK   GRACE   SP 1242
451 TOLL RD   OTT 234-7566-600
BLACK   GEORGE   HUS
SAME
8.30.71 1PM F 36 M SURG   RC
     420   1

NATURE OF CASUALITY:

Patient apparently tried to go to the washroom and felt dizzy when she got up - slipped to the floor.

PHYSICAL FINDINGS ON EXAMINATION OF PATIENT

- _No signs of swelling a discolourization_
- _Complaining of left wrist being sore_

DATE OF X-RAY EXAMINATION   _Sept 2/71_   TIME _10²⁵_ (A.M) P.M.

X-RAY FINDINGS: _NIL_

Ward _4N_   Date _Sept 2/71_   _A. White_   M.D.

(To be filled out by the Doctor and forwarded to the Office of the Administrator of the Department of Nursing, immediately on completion.

To be filled on patient's chart on discharge.

for care; it is seldom thought of as a place where people are injured. Yet a national survey has indicated that the average frequency of accidents in hospitals was higher than in most industries.[2]

The problem of safety in hospitals is diverse; the hospital administrator is concerned with the safety of hospital patients, personnel and the visiting public. Each group presents unique problems in regard to safety practices. For example, hospital personnel work with equipment and pharmaceutical preparations which, if not used correctly, can be dangerous to both the patient and the staff. The visiting public is constantly changing and thus needs continuous orientation to hospital safety practices.

Many hospitals are making concerted efforts to prevent accidents. One study of hospital accidents in pediatric units indicated that falls from cribs or beds accounted for over one-half of the total accidents; medication errors were the next most common cause. The report, which was prepared after a study of the circumstances surrounding the medication errors, indicated that the provision of an isolated area in which the nurse could prepare medications might lower the incidence of error. It further recommended that orders for medications be highly specific and that pediatric dosages of commonly used medications be stocked.[3] Hopefully, the initiation of these recommendations would result in safer patient care.

The nurse is intimately involved in preventing accidents and injuries. She is one of the people most concerned with providing the patient with an environment that is therapeutically conducive to health. By definition, such an environment must be safe. Furthermore, nurses carry out many measures at the patient's bedside, and it is in this area— actually within a radius of 10 feet of the patient's bed—that 65 per cent of patient injuries take place.[4]

PRINCIPLES BASIC TO ACCIDENT PREVENTION

Basic to safe nursing practices and accident prevention are the following concepts, which can guide the nurse in many of her functions.

Many body structures serve as defenses against harmful agents. The skin and mucous membranes act as defenses against injury from many sources. If mechanical, chemical, thermal or bacteriological agents penetrate these defenses, injury to internal structures may result. Nursing measures to protect the integrity of the skin and mucous membranes are therefore of vital importance. The maintenance of good oral hygiene, the use of emollient and protective creams for skin care, and proper positioning, exercise and other measures to prevent the formation of decubitus ulcers are but a few examples of the ways in which the nurse helps to preserve the integrity of the patient's skin and mucous membranes. Other body structures serve to protect internal organs; for example, the ribs serve to protect the chest organs from mechanical pressure. The blood also acts as a defense, by providing agents that fight infection, by helping to regulate body temperatures and by transporting nourishment to tissues.

Normally functioning body senses inform the individual about his environment. Through the senses of sight, hearing, taste, smell, touch and temperature an individual can often identify potential dangers and take measures to protect himself. The person who is recovering from an anesthetic is not able to identify potential dangers and thus needs added safety measures, as for example, siderails on his bed to protect him from falling. The elderly patient

---

[2]George H. Lowrey: The Problem of Hospital Accidents to Children. *Hospital Topics*, 42:91, August, 1964.
[3]Ibid., pp. 92–94.

[4]Gustave L. Scheffler: The Nurse's Role in Hospital Safety. *Nursing Outlook*, 10:681, October, 1962.

may have impaired senses, and as a result his ability to perceive his environment and to protect himself from injury is decreased.

The psychosocial status of an individual can affect his ability to identify dangers and protect himself from harm. Through education and trial and error, individuals learn to identify harmful and potentially harmful situations. Children often encounter situations about which they have not yet learned and which could prove harmful were it not for suitable guidance. Likewise, an adult in a strange environment encounters situations for which he has no frame of reference, and as a result he may make judgments which could be harmful to him. A good orientation for patients, which includes showing them where bathrooms, showers and other facilities are located, helps to familiarize them with their surroundings. It also helps to minimize some of the anxiety of being in a new situation.

Physical disorders and emotional stress can affect an individual's ability to protect himself from harm. A person whose mental faculties are functioning abnormally or whose normal body defenses are impaired is less able to protect himself from injury. The emotionally upset person may rush blindly into danger; the unconscious patient is completely unaware of danger. Similarly a person who is worried, preoccupied or emotionally distressed is often less able to make judgments compatible with his physical and psychological health. These patients require extra vigilance on the part of the nursing staff. Many agencies will permit family members to stay with the confused patient if they wish to do so.

ACCIDENT PRONENESS

It is generally recognized that some people are accident prone; that is, they are more likely to have accidents than the average person. For example, some children always seem to have more bruises and scrapes than their brothers and sisters. Some people may drive a car for 20 years without an accident, while others have one accident right after another. It is believed that emotional disturbances underlie accident proneness. Tension of any kind is more likely to make an individual susceptible to accidents by impairing his critical functions and exhausting his defenses.

A person who has a history of being accident-prone will need extra safety precautions when he is ill. The nurse's alert observation of potential hazards is an important measure to prevent accidents, as is provision of adequate support to the patient—when he needs help with walking, for example. Efforts to minimize anxiety should also be made. Sometimes accident-prone people need psychiatric assistance to learn to cope with their problems.

THE PREVENTION OF MECHANICAL TRAUMA

Among the most frequently occurring types of mechanical accidents are falls. Falling from beds, from chairs or while walking is not uncommon, but it is often preventable. A person who is weakened by illness can lose his balance and fall while simply leaning toward a table that is out of reach. Nurses can prevent many accidents of this kind by being alert to potentially dangerous situations and remedying them. For example, beds that can be raised or lowered can be left in the low position when the nurse is not present. At this level the patient will be able to get in and out of bed more safely. Also patients who have been in bed for several days or who are weakened by illness can be helped to recognize their need for assistance in getting about.

Slippery floors can be dangerous not only to patients, but to people in any situation. To minimize this danger non-slippery materials are used on the floor surfaces of hospitals. Also, since any material spilled on a floor is likely to make it slippery, it should be mopped up before someone slips on it. Floors should be washed and polished at a time when there is little traffic upon them, . . . signs should be prominently placed to notify people that the floor is wet and slippery.

Untidyness can also contribute to accidents. People can trip over electric cords, footstools, bed gatches and equipment that is left on the floor. Walkways, such as areas from patients' beds to bathrooms, can be particularly hazardous when they are not kept clear. Patients have fallen from their beds while reaching for articles on their bedside tables or while looking for a misplaced call light. The nurse can help the patient to arrange these items so that they are within easy reach.

Other possible causes of falls are movable wheelchairs or stretchers. So often, just as a patient is about to sit in a wheelchair it moves out of place. Today most movable equipment is furnished with locks for the wheels. These locks should be set when the equipment is to be used and released only after the patient is secure.

When a patient first becomes ambulatory after a period of time in bed, he often requires some physical support. If he is unsteady while walking he can be supported by a piece of linen, such as a bath towel which encircles his waist and is held at his back by the nurse. With this type of support the patient can be pulled back against the nurse and gently lowered to the floor if he loses his balance. Many hospitals and other health agencies have rails in the halls to guide and support patients while they are walking. These, as well as rubber treads on stairs, can prevent many falls.

A procedure which is chiefly a threat to people working within the hospital is the discarding of broken glass and sharp instruments. Most institutions have special containers for glass, razor blades and the like in order that they can be disposed of separately from other materials. In this way there is less danger of injuring hospital personnel. It is the policy of many hospitals that an employee who is injured at work should report to the employees' health clinic or to a physician for care. In addition, a written report is usually required.

Safety Devices

In her concern for her patient's safety, the nurse may employ specific safety devices. In most institutions these devices are used either upon the request of the attending physician, or when, in the judgment of the nurse, they become necessary. Policies vary from place to place, however, and the nurse should be familiar with the practice in the institution in which she works.

Siderails. Siderails on beds can stop the patient from rolling off the bed. They do not deter the patient from climbing out; rather, they serve merely as reminders to the patient that he is in bed and should exercise care. Most hospitals have policies regarding the use of siderails; it is not uncommon to require them on the beds of patients who are blind, unconscious or sedated or who have muscular disabilities or seizures. Some hospitals require that the beds of all patients over the age of 70 years have siderails. A number of hospitals have adopted a policy of using siderails on the beds of all patients, particularly at night.

It is important when siderails are in use that both rails be up. For example, when the patient's bed is against the wall both rails should be used; the wall does not serve as a good replacement for the rail. When caring for the patient whose bed has siderails, the nurse normally takes down the siderail on the side at which she is working. She should go no further than an arm's length from that side of the bed without returning the siderail to its "up" position. Many patients dislike the use of siderails; they may find them an embarrassing reminder of their childhood crib. Some people are fearful of them, while to others, siderails signify a loss of independence and control over their situation. An explanation of the purpose for using siderails often helps such patients to accept them. Generally siderails will not keep a patient in bed against his will; if a patient needs restraining, a safety jacket should be used.

Safety Jacket and Posey Belt. Patients who are confused sometimes try to climb over the siderails of the bed. They are frequently unaware of their surroundings; they just want to leave the bed. These patients can be restrained comfortably in bed by means of a safety jacket or Posey belt. The jacket is an inconspicuous sleeveless garment which has long crossover ties in front that can be attached to the frame on either side of the bed. The ties are secured to the frame out of the reach of the patient. The Posey belt performs the same function as the jacket. It is secured around the patient's body, and ties are attached to the bed frame. Both the safety jacket and the Posey belt allow the patient to move relatively freely in bed, yet restrain him from climbing over the siderails and possibly falling to the floor.

Arm and Leg Restraints. Occasionally it is necessary to apply arm or leg restraints to patients in bed. Generally this is an undesirable nursing care measure because it limits a patient's movements, and this in turn often causes anxiety, increasing restlessness and subsequent fatigue. It is a particularly dangerous practice to restrain only one side of the body (as, for example, the right arm and leg). This practice tends to increase the patient's restlessness, and he may injure himself as he tries to move the arm and leg that are restrained. Few patients like to be tied down, regardless of how irrational they are. Their reaction is usually to struggle against whatever is hampering their movement and they may become quite agitated. Injury to the tissues of the wrists and ankles may result from the friction engendered by rubbing against the restraints. Occasionally, leather restraints may be used. Many agencies will not permit their use except on a doctor's order. There is a greater possibility of both adverse patient reaction to leather restraints and injury to patient from them.

A physician may order an arm restraint during an intravenous infusion. Its chief purpose in this instance is to remind the patient to keep his arm immobilized during the treatment.

Arms and legs should not be restrained any longer than is absolutely necessary,

and at least every four hours the restraints are loosened and the limbs are exercised. There is a danger that a patient's circulation may be restricted if a restraint is tight or if a limb is restrained in an abnormal position. At any sign of blueness, pallor, cold or complaints of tingling sensations in the extremity, the restraint is loosened and circulation restored by exercise and massage. A limb is best restrained in a slightly flexed position.

Mittens. Mittens are indicated for patients who are confused or semiconscious and may pull at their dressings and tubes. The mittens are often used, for example, for a patient with a head injury or for a patient who has had a stroke. They have the advantage of not permitting the patient to grasp such objects as dressings, tubing or bedrails, but they do not limit movement. A mitten is like a soft boxing glove which pads the patient's hand. Commercial mittens are available, or mittens may be made using dressing pads, gauze bandage and adhesive tape. One method of making mittens is as follows.

Before applying a mitten the patient's hand is placed in a naturally flexed position. This allows unrestricted circulation and places little strain upon muscles. A soft rolled dressing is grasped by the patient so that his thumb approximates his fingers. The soft pad permits the patient to flex his hand while the mitten is in place. All skin surfaces are separated to avoid irritation. The patient's wrist is padded with a dressing to avoid rubbing bony prominences.

Two dressings are then placed over the patient's hand; one medial to lateral, one dorsal to ventral. Large, 8 by 16 inch dressings are suggested. These are secured by a gauze bandage applied in figures of eight (Chapter 22).

To secure the dressings a stockinette is fitted over the hand and secured by adhesive tape just beyond the wrist pad. A double fold of stockinette open at one end suffices.

Mittens need to be removed at least once every 24 hours. At this time the patient washes his hand and exercises it, or the nurse may do this for him. Mittens should not be so tight as to impede circulation, but they must be secure and pad the patient's hand well.

THE PREVENTION OF CHEMICAL TRAUMA

Accidents involving chemicals generally result from the incorrect use of pharmaceutical preparations. Physicians and nurses are well aware of the dangers incurred through errors in the administration of medications. Many institutions have special policies and rules that are designed to prevent errors of this nature. Thus, medicines are generally kept in locked cupboards in special areas away from patients and busy nursing-unit offices. Medicines for topical use are separated from medicines administered orally or parenterally. Drugs that are poisonous are well marked. Usually narcotics such as codeine and morphine are kept in a separate double-locked cupboard, and they are counted at the end of each nursing shift and the tally recorded in a special book. Medicines that are provided for use at home are labeled with complete instructions as to dosage and frequency of administration. It is becoming fairly common practice for the name of the drug to be included on the label of medications for home use so that patients will not inadvertently take the wrong drug or one to which they are allergic.

It is common practice for medications which a patient brings in with him from home to be picked up by the nurse who admits him to the nursing unit. The nurse should ascertain the nature of the drugs contained in these medications. She should also notify the attending physician of any medications the patient is using that were prescribed by another doctor. For example, the patient may be under the care of a surgeon while in hospital and yet have an eye condition for which his ophthalmologist has prescribed twice daily eye drops. The attending physician (in this case, the surgeon) should be alerted to the medication the patient is receiving for his eye condition.

In addition to these generally accepted practices, many agencies require that the nurse have her computations of doses checked by another nurse before the drug is actually prepared. In this way any errors in arithmetic are found before a patient can be harmed. Most hospital pharmacies try to provide nurses with the exact dosage ordered by the physician in order that arithmetical calculations and the division of prepared medicines can be avoided.

Many hospitals now use drugs which are packaged in individual dosages. This practice makes the administration of medications both easier and safer; there is less chance of error. In an increasing number of agencies, medications are delivered from the pharmacy directly to the patient's room, where they are administered by the nurse. This practice helps to reduce the possibility of giving a medication to the wrong patient, another potential hazard in the administration of medications.

Specific orders by the physician help to avoid errors due to ambiguity and misinterpretation. This does not mean that a nurse does not require a thorough knowledge of the pharmaceutical preparation that she is administering. She needs this knowledge in order to protect the patient from harm, to make intelligent observations and to give intelligent nursing care.

If an error is made in the administration of a medicine, it should be reported immediately to the nursing supervisor and to the patient's physician. In this way steps can be taken to protect the patient from injury. Hospitals usually require that a written account of the error be submitted subsequently. The nurse's responsibilities in the administration of medications are further discussed in Chapter 21.

THE PREVENTION OF THERMAL TRAUMA

Thermal accidents involve the presence of harmful levels of heat or cold. The most common sources of thermal injuries are fire, hot appliances or any electrical circuit which is improperly functioning. It is generally a hospital policy that electrical appliances be regularly checked and adequately maintained in order to prevent injury. As an added precaution, patients are often required to have their radios, electric razors and other appliances checked by the hospital maintenance staff before they use them in hospital. Hot water bottles, heating pads and infrared lamps are also possible sources of thermal injury. Heat that is applied to a patient is generally regulated well within the safety limits for that patient.

Fire is a constant threat in institutions. Even though modern construction materials have lessened the danger of the actual building catching fire, there are many materials within a hospital that are highly combustible. For example, oxygen supports combustion and substances such as ether are highly inflammable.

In a study of the causes of 200 hospital fires it was found that 20 per cent were due to carelessness with matches and cigarettes, 10.7 per cent were electrical fires in fixed installations, 8.7 per cent were due to spontaneous ignition and 6.3 per cent were rubbish fires. The remainder of the fires were due to miscellaneous causes.[5]

For a fire to start there must be three elements present: a combustible material, heat and oxygen. A combustible material is anything that will burn. Among the most common materials involved in hospital fires are: paper, as in wastebasket or garbage chute fires; textiles, such as patient's bedding or oily rags; flammable liquids, such as ether or other liquid gases (for example, those used as anesthetic agents); and electrical equipment. Heat sufficient to ignite the combustible material may come from such sources as a lighted match, a live cigarette, a spark or friction. There is usually enough oxygen in the atmosphere to support combustion if the other two elements are present. Fire prevention is usually directed, therefore, toward controlling the first two elements, that is, the combustible materials and heat; fire extinguishing measures toward the reduction of heat (as by water cooling) and the exclusion of oxygen.

Fire Prevention

Most hospitals have active programs in fire prevention. Education of the patients, the personnel and the public in safe practices is an essential part of such programs. Some of the areas that are included in the fire control programs of hospitals are discussed in the following paragraphs.

Smoking Regulations. Usually smoking is prohibited in certain areas of the hospital and these areas are well marked. The no smoking rule is enforced within 12 feet of equipment for administering oxygen, in operating rooms where combustible gases are used and in places where combustible materials are stored.

Patients who do smoke require ashtrays which do not easily tip and which are so constructed that if a cigarette is left burning it will fall into the ashtray. Some patients, for instance, those who are confused or under the influence of a sedative or hypnotic drug, should not smoke unattended. It may be necessary to keep matches and cigarettes locked in a cupboard if the patient is confused.

Scrupulous Housekeeping. Thorough housekeeping and adequate maintenance of equipment lessen the likelihood of fires. For example, oily rags, paint and solvents are stored carefully in a special area so as to prevent spontaneous combustion.

Adequate Storage and Distribution of Volatile Liquids and Gases. Generally ether in large quantities should not be kept in patient areas because of the danger of fire. Volatile gases and liquids are distributed to the various areas under strict control and all the necessary fire precautions are observed.

[5]*Hospital Safety Manual.* Chicago, American Hospital Association and National Safety Council, 1954, p. 9.

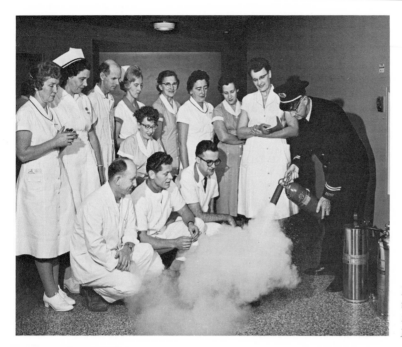

In many health agencies one of the functions of a fire marshal is to teach the staff how to use fire-extinguishing equipment.

Fire Prevention and Fire Extinguishing. In an active fire prevention program all employees must be educated in fire prevention and fire extinguishing.

Types of Fires and Fire Extinguishers

There are basically three classes of hospital fires. Class A fires involve paper, wood and similar solid combustible materials. Class B fires involve flammable liquids, for example, anesthetics. Class C fires involve electrical equipment.

Many kinds of fire extinguishers are available and the nurse needs to know how to operate the ones used at the agency in which she works. Five widely used extinguishers are:

Soda and Acid Extinguisher. This extinguisher, which supplies water under pressure, can be used to put out rubbish or mattress fires (Class A). It is not used for electrical fires, because water conducts electricity. To operate the extinguisher it is turned upside down. The sulphuric acid mixes with the bicarbonate to produce hydrogen, which in turn releases the water under pressure. To stop the flow, the extinguisher is turned right side up.

Water Pump Can. This extinguisher also provides water under pressure, and it also can be used for nonelectrical fires (Classes A and B). To operate this extinguisher the nurse merely has to pump the handle up and down, directing the stream of water with the nozzle.

Carbon Dioxide Extinguisher. This extinguisher is used for compressed-gas fires and electrical fires, as well as fires involving grease (Classes B and C). In order to operate the extinguisher the nurse presses the trigger, directing the horn toward the root of the fire so as to exclude the oxygen from the source of the fire.

Water or Antifreeze Extinguisher. This extinguisher stores water under pressure. It has a pressure gauge which indicates its readiness for use. To operate the extinguisher the nurse pulls the pin and squeezes the handle. It is used for class A and class B fires.

Dry Chemical Extinguisher. This extinguisher contains bicarbonate of soda, dry chemicals and carbon dioxide gas. It contains no water and operates on the principle of blanketing the burning substance to exclude air. It is used on electrical fires (Class C) and is also effective on Class A fires. To operate the extinguisher, the nurse pulls the pin and opens the valve (or presses the lever) and squeezes the nozzle valve.

Fire extinguishers must be accessible to personnel. Generally they are kept in obvious places in all patient and service areas. The kind of extinguisher that is placed in a specific area depends upon the type of fire most likely to occur there. Part of a safety program is the regular inspection and maintenance of fire extinguishers.

In addition to having fire extinguishers, nursing units and other departments of a hospital are usually equipped with fire hoses, and personnel are instructed in their use. In the event of a small fire, it may be easier and quicker to use material near at hand, for example, to smother the fire with a blanket or mattress pad, or to pour a pitcher of cold water over it.

The Nurse's Responsibilities in the Event of Fire

If a fire does occur in a nursing unit the nurse should make sure that the following steps are carried out.

1. Remove patients from the immediate danger area.

2. Notify the local fire department.

3. Shut off the fire area and decrease the ventilation to the area.

4. Employ available extinguishing equipment.

In some health agencies it is accepted practice to telephone the fire department directly, reporting the exact location of the fire. Other agencies have a fire alarm system which when set off causes an alarm to ring in the fire station. A third method of reporting a fire is to telephone the operator at the central hospital exchange, who then notifies the fire department. When reporting a fire, it is important that the nurse give the exact location of the fire clearly.

The Removal of Patients. When a fire occurs, the nurse in charge of the nursing unit assumes the responsibility for directing the activities of the hospital personnel until the firemen arrive. All fire doors should be closed. Patients in immediate danger must be moved to safety quickly. Generally, ambulatory patients are assisted in walking to safety. In moving immobilized patients, the entire bed is wheeled to a safe area. When it is not feasible to move the entire bed, a portable stretcher can be employed to move immobilized patients. The nurse may occasionally find it necessary to carry a patient in order to remove him from danger. Four basic carries are:

PACK STRAP CARRY. With the patient in a sitting position in bed, the nurse faces the patient and grasps the patient's wrists, the right wrist in the left hand and the left wrist in right hand. The nurse then pivots and slips under the patient's arm so that the patient's chest is against her shoulders and the patient's arms are crossed on the nurse's chest. With one leg forward for balance the nurse then rolls the patient off the bed and on to her back.

HIP CARRY. The patient lies on her side near the edge of the bed. The nurse faces the head of the bed and puts her arm that is nearest the patient around the patient's back and under the armpit. She then turns so that her hips are against the patient's abdomen and puts her other arm around the patient's thighs and under her knees. The patient is then drawn up on the nurse's hip and the nurse carries her from the bedside.

SWING CARRY BY TWO NURSES. One nurse stands on each side of the patient. The patient's arms are extended around the nurses' shoulders and each nurse grasps one of the patient's wrists with the arm that is farthest from the patient. Each nurse then reaches behind the patient's back with her free arm (nearest the patient) and grasps the other nurse's shoulder. The patient's wrists are then released. Each nurse reaches under the patient's knees and grasps the other's wrist. The patient is then in a sitting position between the nurses.

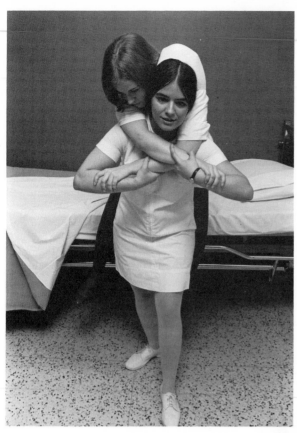

Position for the pack strap carry.

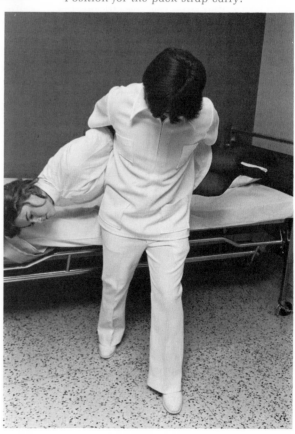

Position for the hip carry.

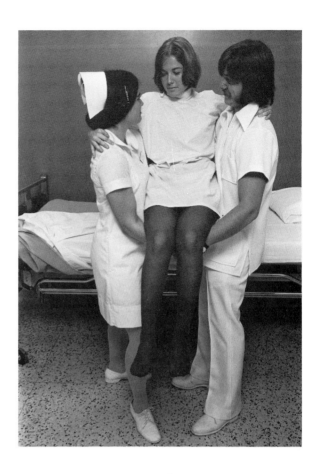

Position for the swing carry.

THREE MAN CARRY. (See Chapter 11, page 125.)

As part of any fire prevention and fire extinguishment program all agency personnel require information about specific policy and practice. Demonstrations in the use of fire equipment, practice in moving patients and a knowledge of the established practice to be followed upon the discovery of a fire are important. It is only through a continuous in-service educational program in fire prevention and extinguishing methods that the safety of all is safeguarded.

SAFETY PROGRAMS

A safety program is an endeavor to control the physical environment in such a manner that accidents can be prevented. In order to be effective a program must involve all the people who are concerned with the agency. Many hospitals have safety committees whose job it is to plan a safety program for the institution. Nurses are frequently members of these committees.

The committee's function is to conduct a continual analysis of the kind of accidents that occur in the hospital and their causes. On the basis of this analysis an active program is developed. Continual assessment of hospital practices and continual education of employees are important. Another part of a safety program is the regular inspection of agency facilities; for example, fire extinguishers are checked as often as recommended by the manufacturer. To be effective, a safety program must motivate all employees to accomplish the purpose of the program, for it is only through the active cooperation of all the people in an agency that accidents can be prevented.

GUIDE TO
ASSESSING
NURSING NEEDS

1. Is the patient alert, conscious and in full command of his mental faculties?
2. Does he require additional safety precautions because of his age, his physical condition or his mental state?
3. Is the patient receiving medications that impair his senses?
4. Does the patient require restraints of any sort?
5. Does he smoke?
6. Is electrical equipment in use in the patient's room? Does the patient have electrical appliances at his bedside?
7. Is heat used as a therapeutic agent in the care of this patient?
8. Are there any information or safety practices which can help the patient to avoid injury or accident?

GUIDE TO
EVALUATING THE
EFFECTIVENESS OF
NURSING ACTION

1. Are nursing measures safe and are possible accidents foreseen and steps taken to prevent them?
2. Is the patient safe from mechanical injury, such as may result from falls?
3. Is the patient safe from thermal injury, such as heating pad burns?
4. Is the patient safe from chemical injury? For example, does he take the medicines as ordered?
5. Do the restraints, if the patient is restrained, permit maximal movement compatible with health?

STUDY
SITUATION

Mrs. R. Ross, who is 73 years old, is in the hospital because she has a fractured femur. The physician has ordered that she sit in a chair for 15 minutes twice a day. Mrs. Ross walks with considerable difficulty and requires support.

1. What factors should the nurse be aware of in providing a safe environment for Mrs. Ross?
2. Give six specific measures that the nurse should take to prevent mechanical injury to Mrs. Ross.
3. If there is a fire in this patient's room, what should the nurse do? How should this patient be moved?
4. By what criteria can the safety of Mrs. Ross's environment be evaluated?

BIBLIOGRAPHY

Development of Fire Emergency Programs. Chicago, American Hospital Association, 1951.
Hospital Safety Manual. Chicago, American Hospital Association and National Safety Council, 1954.
Kummer, Sylvia B., and Jerome M. Kummer: Pointers to Preventing Accidents. *The American Journal of Nursing,* 63:118–119, February, 1963.
Lowrey, George H.: The Problem of Hospital Accidents to Children. *Hospital Topics,* 42:91–94, August, 1964.
McGrath, Robert: *Emergency Removal of Patients and First-Aid Fire Fighting in Hospitals.* Chicago, National Safety Council, 1956.

Scheffler, Gustave L.: The Nurse's Role in Hospital Safety. *Nursing Outlook*, *10*:680–682, October, 1962.
Webster's Seventh New Collegiate Dictionary. Springfield, Mass., G. & C. Merriam Company, 1963.

16 THE PREVENTION AND CONTROL OF INFECTION

The nurse should be able to:

Define infection

Name potential sources of infection in a health agency

List methods by which microorganisms may be transferred in a hospital or other health agency

Describe modes by which infection is spread in a hospital or other health agency

Describe nursing responsibilities in the collection of specimens for microbiological examination

Name principles from the biophysical and social sciences relevant to the prevention and control of infection

Describe a basic procedure for cleaning equipment

Differentiate between disinfection and antisepsis

Describe methods for the sterilization of equipment used in health agencies

Differentiate between medical and surgical asepsis

Describe handwashing techniques used in medical and surgical asepsis

Describe techniques for masking and gowning

Describe barrier technique

Describe nursing measures to help patients with their reaction to barrier technique

INTRODUCTION

Although pathogens (disease-producing microorganisms) are always present in the environment, community programs in environmental sanitation and preventive medicine generally keep down the incidence of disease. Nevertheless, microorganisms in the environment are of concern to people in many activities, for example, to those operating restaurants, hotels and schools. But wherever there are sick people, pathogenic organisms present a more serious threat to health, since the average patient is highly susceptible to infection because of his generalized debility. Moreover, since some patients have particularly serious infections, their close proximity to other patients on a nursing unit produces situations conducive to the transfer of microorganisms. Thus, in every instance of patient care, members of the health team are concerned with the presence of disease-producing microorganisms in the environment.

An *infection* is an invasion of the body by pathogenic organisms and the body's subsequent reaction to these organisms. The bacteria which are common causes of infection are gram-negative bacilli, such as *Escherichia coli* and *Pseudomonas pyocyanea*, and the gram-positive cocci, such as *Staphylococcus aureus*, as well as many viruses. These microorganisms, as well as many others, can cause infections when they come in contact with broken skin or mucous membrane, or when they are inhaled or ingested.

Microorganisms are found in the air, on the floors, on equipment and furniture, and on articles which come in contact with a person who has an infection. They can be spread through the air and by such vectors as linen, dishes and even a nurse's hands. Health team personnel sometimes unknowingly act as carriers of microorganisms. When handwashing techniques break down, for example, microorganisms are passed on to others. In spite of stringent cleaning practices, hospital personnel are continually working in an environment which harbors many varieties of organisms. Every once in a while a particularly virulent organism is introduced and a worker with an open cut or lowered body resistance becomes infected. An unbalanced diet, fatigue, scratches, cuts or other wounds all predispose any person to infection.

In order to understand the rationale behind nursing measures taken to protect patients and staff from infection, it is important to keep in mind the sources, methods of transfer and modes of spread of microorganisms.

SOURCES OF INFECTION

The most important source of organisms within a health agency is probably the patients themselves. Usually, every patient who comes into a hospital or other inpatient facility is observed for any sign of infection: any boils, fever, septic wounds and the like are reported for further investigation. In most hospitals the charge nurse has the authority to order precautionary technique for a patient if she suspects that he harbors pathogenic organisms which could be spread to other patients and the staff.

A routine measure for most newly admitted patients in a clinic, nursing home or hospital is the chest x-ray. The intent of the x-ray is to detect pulmonary tuberculosis. This is considered particularly important diagnostically for elderly patients. Serological tests for syphilis are done also on all newly admitted patients in many agencies. With the alarming increase of venereal disease among the population in recent years, this is another important diagnostic measure.

As mentioned earlier, people working in a health agency can also be sources of infection. Any person with a fever, diarrhea, nausea, and most certainly, a cold, may be spreading infectious organisms. This is particularly serious in the operating room, the nursery, and the intensive care and coronary units where infection seriously threatens the safety of patients and where the transmission rate is high.

Visitors of patients can also transmit infections, although normally the length of their period of contact is minimal in comparison with that of personnel. Food, vermin and dirt also transmit disease, but they are an unlikely source in a modern institution. Hospital dust is probably heavily laden with pathogenic organisms; however, dryness inhibits their growth and most hospitals have housekeeping policies which eliminate unnecessary moisture and maintain a high standard of cleanliness.

METHODS OF TRANSFER

The methods by which organisms are transferred are diverse, the method or methods applicable in a given situation being dependent on the infecting organism. There are six main methods:

1. *Personal contact.* One child with measles, for example, may give measles to a whole ward full of children. A nurse with a cold may give the cold to a patient.

2. *Aerial routes. Staphylococcus aureus*, which has been the cause of so many hospital infections, is air-borne. The organisms are often transferred by droplet infection from the nose and throat passages of carriers; they may also travel quickly from one place to another by attaching themselves to dust particles in the air. *Staphylococcus aureus* organisms in large quantity have frequently been found on patients' bedding. The nurse must take particular care therefore, when changing the bed linen, not to shake sheets and blankets. Used linen should be put into a hamper (preferably a closed one) as soon as possible after removal from the patient's bed.

3. *Animals and insects.* Rodents may be a concern in cities. They spread the *Salmonella* and *Shigella* organisms. Flies are well-known carriers of microorganisms. Windows in a health agency should always be screened. This is not usually a problem in modern hospitals but may be in a neighborhood health center or a remote nursing station.

4. *Fomites.* Inanimate objects such as needles and syringes are possible sources of infection in health agencies. A number of cases of infectious hepatitis, for example, have been traced directly to contaminated needles or intravenous equipment which has been inadequately cleaned and sterilized. The use of disposable equipment has reduced this hazard, but in agencies where needles, syringes and infusion or drainage sets are reused, cleaning and sterilizing standards must be scrupulously enforced.

5. *Food and drink.* Impure water and contaminated food are known to cause outbreaks of such diseases as cholera, typhoid fever and infectious hepatitis. Although regulations to safeguard the water supply are stringent in most parts of the United States and Canada, there are still remote areas where this is a problem. Contamination of food by workers who are carriers of disease, as for example, the well-known cases of typhoid carriers, is another concern of all institutions, hotels, restaurants and other eating places.

6. *Endogenous spread,* that is, from one area of a person's body to another, as from the skin to an open wound. The maintenance of strict aseptic technique, while doing dressings for example, is important to prevent the endogenous spread of organisms.

MODES OF SPREAD OF INFECTION

Spread from the Respiratory Tract

Masking is practiced under certain circumstances to prevent the spread of microorganisms from the respiratory tract. Masking helps to prevent wound contamination during dressing changes and in the operating room during surgery.

The spread of pathogens from the respiratory tract of patients is thought to be best controlled by teaching safe hygiene practices, which include frequent handwashing under running water. A patient with a pulmonary infection is taught to use several thicknesses of paper handkerchief to cover his nose and mouth when he sneezes or coughs. Also, covered waterproof containers are provided for sputum. Facilities are also made available for the adequate disposal of paper handkerchiefs and sputum containers after they have been used.

Spread from the Gastrointestinal Tract

Microorganisms from the gastrointestinal tract are spread chiefly in feces rather than in vomitus. Many agencies now use bedpans which are used for one patient only and then disposed of when the patient is discharged. The use of paper bedpan covers which are disposed of with the feces is another safety measure. Bedpan disinfectors also eliminate the transfer of organisms via the bedpan. The nurse always washes her hands after handling a bedpan.

Disinfectants are used regularly to disinfect toilets and toilet seats. Since enema tubes and rectal thermometers can also transfer bacteria, viruses and protozoa, they are disinfected after use.

Spread by Direct Contact

People who have open lesions on their skin or who do not wash their hands after contact with sources of contamination, such as feces, can transfer organisms to other people. Any open area on the skin or mucous membrane is a potential site of infection. Personnel who have cuts or open areas on the skin are not only a potential source of infection but they are also especially vulnerable to infection.

Spread from the Blood

Infectious hepatitis is spread from the blood, but other infections are rarely spread from this source. Important in the control of the spread of disease by this route is the disinfection of equipment such as syringes and needles which have been in contact with blood.

Spread by the Aerial Route

Ventilation can reduce the spread of infection by air. If open windows are not feasible, air-conditioning or the recirculation of filtered air should be utilized. Nurses can hold down the level of air contamination by handling bed linen with a minimum amount of movement and by closing doors while making beds.

DIAGNOSTIC TESTS

It is often necessary to obtain various specimens for microbiological examination in the laboratory. Specimens of a patient's secretions and excretions are examined in order to isolate and identify an infecting organism. A *secretion* is a product produced by a gland, for example, bile; an *excretion* is a substance excreted or discharged by the body, for example, feces.

For most specimens a sterile container is required, and precautions must be taken to avoid contaminating the specimen with organisms in the environment. A smear or culture may be needed. If a specimen is required for a smear, clean (preferably new) slides and a sterile, cotton-tipped applicator are needed. The specimen is gathered on the applicator, which is rolled over the center of the slide. The smear is covered with another glass slide. The slides are appropriately labeled and sent to the laboratory.

For cultures, the specimen is placed in a sterile container. Urine, blood, ascitic fluid and the like are usually put in sterile test tubes. For cultures of specimens of wound discharge, many agencies furnish sterile test tubes which are equipped with sterile applicators suspended from the cork that seals the tube. When the cork is removed the applicator is removed with it. The applicator tip is touched to the area of discharge and then returned carefully to the sterile container.

Sputum specimens are collected in wide-necked sterile containers or on Petri dishes. Sputum is collected early in the morning, when the patient is most able to cough up sputum from his lungs.

When stools are sent for culture, it is seldom necessary to send the entire specimen. Normally a sterile applicator dipped in the feces is sufficient. If the feces are to be examined for amebae, the specimen is sent to the laboratory while it is warm and it is examined within 30 minutes after it is obtained. Only a small quantity (approximately 3 cc.) of feces is needed for this examination.

It may be necessary to test a culture for differentiation and sensitivity. *Differentiation* is accomplished by means of Gram's stain, which divides bacteria into two classes: gram-negative organisms stain red; gram-positive organisms stain purple. *Sensitivity* refers to the effect of specific antibiotics upon

bacteria. The organisms are streaked on nutrient plates, various antibiotics are then added to the plates, and the plates are placed in an incubator. The areas where the growth of the bacteria is inhibited indicate the particular antibiotics to which the bacteria are sensitive.

PRINCIPLES RELEVANT TO THE PREVENTION AND CONTROL OF INFECTION

1. *Microorganisms are opportunists that are always present in the environment.* Under suitable conditions these opportunists cause infection.

2. *The integrity of the skin and mucous membranes is a defense which protects the body from bacterial invasion.*

3. *Of the many varieties of microorganisms, only a few are pathogenic.* Some protozoa, viruses, bacteria, yeasts, molds and rickettsiae are pathogenic to man.

4. *Pathogenic organisms are spread by both direct and indirect methods.*

5. *Pathogenic organisms enter the body by one of several routes. The respiratory tract, the gastrointestinal tract and breaks in the skin or mucous membrane* are the portals of entry.

6. *The pathogenic organisms may be destroyed by sufficient heat or by chemical agents.*

7. *Others are affected by the presence of a patient with an infection.* The patient may constitute a threat to the physical and psychological integrity of other patients and hospital personnel.

8. *The psychological equilibrium of the patient is enhanced by a feeling of self-esteem and acceptance by others.*

CLEANING METHODS, DISINFECTION AND STERILIZATION TECHNIQUES

Clean equipment is essential to safe patient care. Many hospitals have a central supply department where all equipment is cleaned and prepared for use. The availability of disposable equipment has contributed greatly to patient safety and has also lessened the amount of time spent by nurses in cleaning and sterilizing equipment. In spite of the increasing use of disposables and the current practice of employing other personnel to clean and prepare equipment and supplies, the nurse is nonetheless well advised to be familiar with standard cleaning methods and disinfection and sterilization techniques to ensure the safety of her patients.

Cleaning Methods

Articles are referred to as *clean* when they are free from disease-producing organisms (pathogens). Dirty or contaminated materials harbor pathogens. An article is said to be *sterile* when it is free of all microorganisms, and unsterile when there are any living organisms on it.

Most utility rooms have a "clean" area and a "dirty" area. The clean area is used for the storage of sterile and clean supplies and the preparation of treatment trays. The dirty area is used for washing and cleaning trays and equipment and for storing used equipment prior to its return to the central supply (or other) department.

A basic cleaning procedure which is applicable to most equipment is the following:

1. Rinse the article in cold water in order to remove any organic material. Heat coagulates protein and thus tends to make blood and pus stick to equipment.

2. Wash the article in soap and hot water. The emulsifying power of the soap, as well as its surface action, facilitates the removal of dirt. The water helps wash the dirt away.

3. Cleanse with an abrasive when necessary.

4. Rinse well with hot water and then dry.

5. Sterilize or disinfect as necessary.

A stiff brush helps in cleaning many types of equipment; it is easier to get into crevices and corners. There are

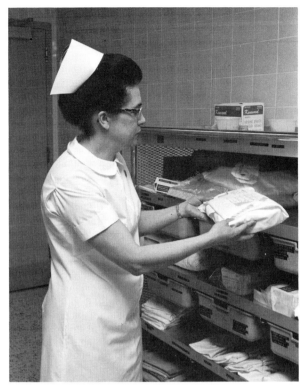

Many health agencies have separate departments in which supplies and equipment are prepared for use. The nurse selects a sterile dressing tray from the central supply cart which has been brought to the service room of a nursing unit.

specially constructed brushes for cleaning the lumina of test tubes, tubing and the like.

Disinfection and Antisepsis

Disinfection and antisepsis are processes by which disease-inducing organisms are killed or their growth is prevented. A *disinfectant* is an agent, usually chemical, which kills many forms of pathogenic microorganisms but not necessarily the more resistant forms such as spores. An *antiseptic* prevents the growth and activity of microorganisms but does not necessarily destroy them. Disinfectants are commonly used to destroy pathogens on inanimate objects such as scalpels, whereas antiseptics are used on the wounds or skin of people. A substance is also spoken of as *bactericidal* if it kills bacteria and *bacteriostatic* if it merely prevents their growth.

Many disinfectants and antiseptics are available commercially. When choosing a disinfectant, five factors are considered:

1. The disinfectant should kill the pathogens within a reasonable time.

2. The disinfectant should not be readily neutralized by proteins, soaps or detergents.

3. The disinfectant should not be harmful to the material on which it is to be used.

4. The disinfectant should not be harmful to the human skin.

5. The disinfectant should be stable in solution.

The choice of the disinfectant for a specific purpose is best made after tests have been made of their conformity to these criteria.

Sterilization

Sterilization refers to the killing of all forms of bacteria, spores, fungi and viruses. It can be accomplished by heat or chemicals. The autoclave is considered to be the most effective method of sterilizing hospital supplies. Generally, it is thought that steam at 15 to 17 pounds per square inch and at a temperature of 121° to 123° C. (250° to 254° F.) for 30 minutes is effective in sterilizing supplies. Prior to autoclaving, the equipment to be sterilized is washed and wrapped in such a way that it will remain protected after it is removed from the autoclave. A piece of autoclave tape which indicates when the sterilization is completed is often put on a package before it is sterilized. One type of tape has white lines which turn dark during the process to indicate that the equipment has been sterilized. Glass indicators are also available for this purpose. A chemical inside the glass changes color upon autoclaving.

When the nurse loads the autoclave for sterilization certain guides are best followed:

1. Place equipment in the autoclave in such a manner that steam circulates freely around each item.

2. Turn bowls and other vessels on their sides so that water will not collect in them.

3. Separate rubber surfaces so that they will not stick together as a result of the extreme heat.

4. Check to be sure that the autoclave is set to sterilize the specific equipment.

Boiling is another method of rendering articles free of microorganisms. It is believed that boiling for 10 to 20 minutes will destroy all pathogens with the exception of spores and the virus of infectious hepatitis. The article to be sterilized must be completely submerged in water during the entire time, the boiling time being counted after the water comes to a full boil.

Dry heat is sometimes used to sterilize supplies. Heating most objects for two hours at 170° C. has been found to be effective for sterilization, but petrolatum and oils require a higher temperature or more prolonged exposure to heat. In the home, an oven can be used to sterilize materials.

Chemical sterilization necessitates the submerging of the object in a sterilizing solution for a specified period of time. Many pharmaceutical preparations are available for this purpose; the choice is dependent upon the article to be sterilized and the kind of microorganism present. The object is soaked for the specified time before it is considered sterile.

Gas sterilization with ethylene oxide has also been found satisfactory in many situations. According to research reports, all microorganisms subjected to a temperature above 43.3° C. (110° F.), a relatively high humidity, and a concentration of ethylene oxide of 440 mg. per liter have been destroyed. Ethylene oxide sterilization has been suggested for plastics, rubber and fabrics. Its effectiveness, however, is reduced in the presence of biological products such as blood.[1]

---

[1]James J. Shull: Ethylene Oxide Sterilization. *The Canadian Nurse*, 58:603–607, July, 1962.

ASEPSIS

The term *asepsis* refers to the absence of all disease-producing organisms. Both medical and surgical asepsis are practiced in patient care. *Medical asepsis* comprises those practices which are carried out in order to keep microorganisms within a given area. For example, if a patient has active tuberculosis, the patient and any articles with which he has had contact are considered to be contaminated with *Mycobacterium tuberculosis* and are therefore able to pass on the infection. In medical aseptic practices microorganisms are kept within a well-defined area, and any articles or materials removed from this area are immediately rendered free of bacteria so that they cannot transfer the infection.

Surgical asepsis refers to practices carried out in order to keep an area free of organisms. It is just the opposite of medical asepsis in that surgical aseptic practices are designed to keep organisms *out of* a defined area. Thus, an operative wound is kept surgically aseptic.

HANDWASHING

Handwashing is an important measure in preventing the spread of microorganisms. Good aseptic technique involves limiting the transfer of organisms from one person to another. By washing her hands after contact with a patient, the nurse can limit the spread of microorganisms to other people, particularly other patients. In handwashing, both mechanical and chemical means are used to remove and destroy organisms. The running water mechanically washes away organisms, while soaps emulsify foreign matter and lower surface tension, thus facilitating the removal of oils, greases and dirt.

For cleansing after contact with a person or an object such as a sputum cup which harbors pathogenic organisms, it is recommended that a two minute wash be done with an alkaline detergent or a bar of ordinary soap. In surgical asepsis, handwashing is indicated prior to working with sterile equipment in order to render the hands as free as possible from bacteria. In either medical or surgical asepsis it is advantageous to wash one's hands at a deep sink where the water can be regulated by a foot or leg control. One procedure for the handwash is as follows:

1. Roll up sleeves above elbows and remove watch.
2. Clean the fingernails as necessary. Disposable sticks are often provided for this purpose.
3. Wash hands and arms to the elbow thoroughly with soap and warm water. Wash in continuously running water, using a rotary motion and taking care to clean the interdigital spaces.
    a. In surgical asepsis, always hold the hands higher than the elbows so that water will flow from the cleanest to the dirtiest area. A surgical scrub brush is sometimes used, although the danger of creating abrasions on the skin needs to be considered.
    b. In medical asepsis hold the hands lower than the elbows while washing in order to prevent microorganisms from contaminating the arms.
4. Rinse hands and arms, allowing water to flow freely.
5. Repeat steps 3 and 4.
6. Dry hands thoroughly with paper towels or a fresh clean towel. Many agencies now use hot air hand driers, which eliminates the use of paper or cloth towels. During the drying process the hands and arms are held higher than the elbows whichever method of drying is used.

When washing her hands, the nurse should take precautions to protect her uniform from getting wet. She should stand so that her uniform does not touch the wash basin and should hold her hands and arms away from her body when she is drying them. When turning off water at a sink that does not have foot

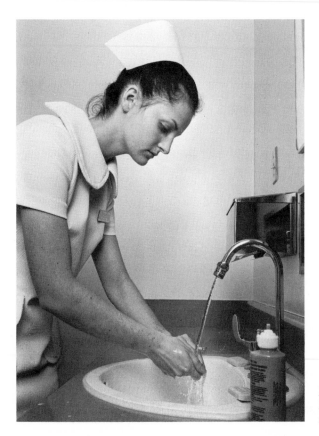

During a handwash for medical asepsis, the hands are kept lower than the elbows to keep microorganisms away from the elbows.

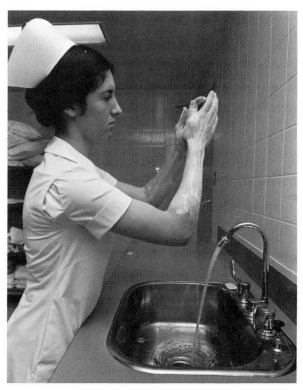

The hands are held higher than the elbows during a surgical asepsis handwash so that the water will flow from the hands to the elbows, i.e., from the cleanest to the dirtiest areas.

or leg controls, a dry towel is used to handle the taps; they are considered grossly contaminated. The basin is considered contaminated also. If a break in technique occurs—for example, if the nurse accidently touches the side of the basin during or after the hand-wash—the wash should be repeated from the beginning. It is important that the nurse keep the skin on her hands in good condition. Hand lotions or creams should be used frequently.

MASKING

Masks are used in a variety of situations. Their general purpose is to limit the spread of microorganisms. Putting a mask over one's mouth and nose serves to filter both inspired and expired air. In some situations visitors and patients wear masks, for example, to protect an open wound.

Masks may be made of cotton, gauze or glass fiber, although disposable paper masks are increasingly being used. Generally a mask should be worn only once, then discarded. It is a violation of technique to hang a mask around one's neck when it is not in use. Masks are changed when they become wet, since moisture facilitates the passage of bacteria through the mask.

In surgical asepsis, masks are generally worn by personnel to keep equipment sterile or a wound free from microorganisms. It is inadvisable to cough or to sneeze while masked, and one talks only when necessary. Although the mask acts as a barrier, bacteria can escape around the sides of the mask and through the material itself, particularly during forceful respirations. Masks should be changed frequently. Although the length of time a mask is effective has not been precisely determined, LeMaitre and Finnegan suggest that a mask should be worn no longer than two to three hours in the operating room even for the same case.[2]

When doing dressings or other treatments for a number of patients, it is good practice for the nurse to don a new mask for each patient.

Policies on the use of masks in medical asepsis vary from place to place. It is sometimes indicated for hospital personnel to wear masks in order to protect themselves from the pathogenic organisms of patients.

GOWNING

Gowning is indicated if there is any possibility that the nurse may contaminate her uniform while she is attending a patient with an infection. The gown is long enough to cover the nurse's uniform completely, and generally it is not worn outside the boundaries of the patient's unit.

The simplest and safest practice is to use a clean gown each time it is necessary to protect one's uniform. The gown is put on so that the uniform is completely covered, and when it is taken off it is discarded in a container within the patient's unit. Care is taken that the outside of the gown, which is contaminated, does not touch the nurse's uniform. The nurse washes after she has discarded her gown.

If it is not possible to use a clean gown each time, then the nurse removes the gown *after* she has washed. When she takes it off she hangs it in such a way that the clean side is protected from contamination and the gown can be safely and easily put on later. The neck ties are kept against the clean side so that they do not become contaminated. The next time the nurse uses this gown, she picks it up by the clean side and ties the neck ties before she contaminates her hands on the outer side of the gown.

For visitors' use, many agencies now provide disposable gowns. These are used once and thrown away.

BARRIER TECHNIQUE

In situations in which the presence of pathogens is suspected or has been

---

[2]George LeMaitre and Janet Finnegan: *The Patient in Surgery.* Second edition. Philadelphia, W. B. Saunders Company, 1970, p. 90.

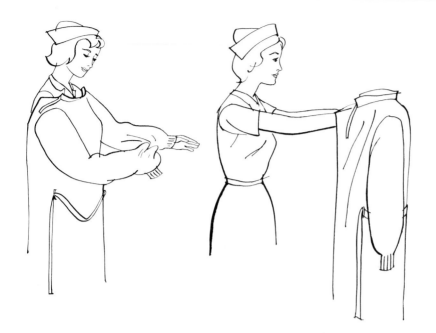

When taking off a contaminated gown that is to be discarded, the nurse keeps her "dirty" hands and the contaminated side of the gown away from her.

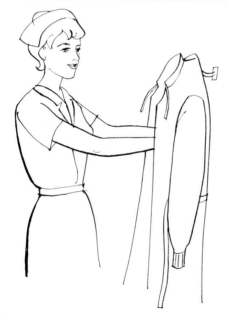

When reusing a contaminated gown, the nurse slips her clean hands inside without contaminating herself with the gown.

proved, medical aseptic practices are observed in order to control their spread and contribute to their destruction. Such medical aseptic practices are called *barrier technique*. The exact technique employed in a particular situation depends upon the portal of exit, the method of transfer and the portal of entry of the particular pathogen.

In barrier technique, mechanical barriers are established to confine the organisms within a given area. The boundaries in a hospital or at home can be the patient's unit or a single room, but all equipment within the designated area is considered contaminated. Barrier technique has the psychological advantage of reminding people of the existence of the pathogenic organisms and the physical advantage of a separate room, which decreases the transfer of organisms by air.

In the past, barrier technique was known as *isolation*. The very word "isolation" describes what can happen to a patient who has an infection. It has been observed that hospital personnel and other patients tend to actually isolate such patients, who then become lonely and feel that they are nuisances. In many instances the words "dirty," "contaminated" and "isolated" have a moral significance for the patient, causing him to feel unworthy and unaccepted. Patients for whom barrier technique is necessary should not be psychologically isolated from others;

indeed, physical isolation is often unnecessary when proper precautions are taken. The importance of explanations and support is paramount for these patients; consequently the nurse needs to understand both her own attitudes and the practices which contribute to her own safety and that of the patient.

Reverse Barrier Technique

A development of recent years is the reverse barrier technique, in which the patient is protected from pathogens in the environment. Instead of keeping pathogens within a defined area, as in barrier technique, the organisms are kept outside the defined area. This is done in a variety of ways, one of which is to place a plastic enclosure around the patient. All air reaching the patient is filtered, and all equipment entering the enclosed area is free of pathogens. Reverse barrier technique is used for patients who are particularly susceptible to infections, for example, people who have severe burns or leukemia. Since these patients do not have normal resistance to pathogenic microorganisms, they are protected within barriers which permit an aseptic environment to be established.

Care of Equipment and Supplies

The increasing use of disposable equipment and supplies has simplified the practice of barrier technique. The wide range of disposables currently available includes dishes, cutlery, medicine cups, syringes, needles, treatment trays, gloves, intravenous sets, drainage sets, bedpans and bedpan covers. When these articles are used for a patient who requires barrier-technique nursing, concurrent disinfection is considerably easier. There are still some aspects of patient care, however, for which disposables are not applicable. Disposables are also costly and may not be used in all situations. The nurse should, therefore, be familiar with measures that may be used in

concurrent and terminal disinfection to control the spread of microorganisms.

Concurrent disinfection refers to the ongoing measures taken to control the spread of infection while the patient is considered infectious. Pathogenic organisms are destroyed continually while the patient requires barrier technique. Measures for concurrent disinfection are detailed later in this section. *Terminal disinfection* comprises those measures which destroy pathogenic organisms after a patient leaves an examining room or a hospital or when he no longer requires barrier technique. In terminal disinfection all equipment within the patient's room is rendered free of pathogenic organisms by appropriate means; for example, the walls and floor are washed with a disinfectant, and linen is wrapped and sent to the laundry to be disinfected. If the patient is to remain in the hospital, he usually takes a shower and then goes to another bed unit with clean equipment. The tub or shower is also cleaned with a disinfectant after use.

Equipment. All equipment used for a patient who has an infection is rendered clean immediately after it is taken from the patient's unit. Equipment such as glass medicine containers, artery forceps and stainless steel bowls can be autoclaved and thus rendered safe easily and quickly. Many hospitals place such equipment in two heavy paper bags in such a way that the outer bag remains clean. The bag is marked "infectious" and is then autoclaved. If equipment is wet the inner bag should be made of waxed paper in order to contain the moisture and the organisms.

If equipment cannot be rendered safe by autoclaving, it can be exposed to ultraviolet light or soaked in or wiped with a disinfectant solution. Gas sterilization may also be used for some articles. The exact method depends upon the organism of infection and the type of equipment.

Laundry. Linen bags are generally placed in the patient's unit to hold contaminated linen. When linen has accumulated in the bag, a designated person brings in a clean linen bag, and

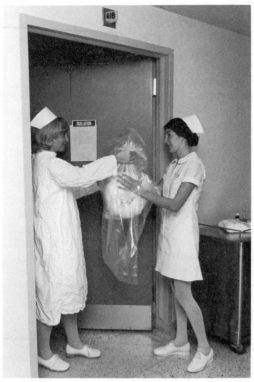

Concurrent disinfection includes the safe disposal of contaminated linen. These nurses are using a "double bagging" technique for the linen which has been taken from the patient's room.

the contaminated bag is placed in it carefully in order to avoid contaminating the outside of the clean bag. In this way the linen can be transported without danger of contaminating other personnel or equipment. The outer bag is marked "infectious."

The washing methods used in most hospital laundries render most contaminated materials clean. If it is necessary to take special precautions, as with spore-forming bacteria, linen is usually autoclaved prior to laundering.

Dishes. After a patient who has an infection has eaten, his dishes are removed to the bathroom, where the uneaten foods and fluids are disposed of (in the same manner as excreta; see following section); the dishes are then either replaced on the tray and taken to the dishwasher or they are double-bagged and autoclaved prior to washing.

Many health agencies have automatic dishwashers which render dishes free of pathogens.

If an autoclave or dishwasher is not available, dishes can be boiled after they have been rinsed or they can be soaked in a disinfectant solution. The latter method is the least desirable, because of the difficulty of immersing the dishes completely and because of the errors that can occur. For example, organic material left on dishes can protect pathogens sufficiently for them to remain active after the normal soaking time.

Disposal of Excreta

Most contaminated excreta can be safely disposed of in the general sewage, where it is subsequently rendered harmless by the sewage treatment facilities of the community. In areas where the treatment of sewage is not considered satisfactory for a particular infectious organism, excreta must be rendered safe before disposal into the sewage system. One method of doing this is to treat the excreta with a prescribed disinfectant, such as chloride of lime, for the time necessary to destroy the pathogens.

PATIENT REACTION TO BARRIER TECHNIQUE

Patients for whom barrier technique is being maintained often have special needs for emotional support. They are frequently physically isolated from other patients, and the hospital staff tends to ignore them, to "leave them until the last." Some patients attach a moral significance to their disease; they feel unworthy and think they are creating extra work for the nurse. If a nurse hesitates in full view of the patient before she enters his room and if she puts on a gown reluctantly or as if it is a bothersome duty, she will only enhance his feeling of unworthiness and lowered self-esteem.

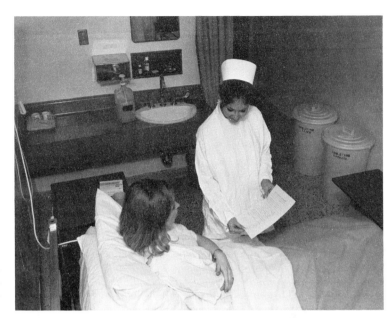

Patients for whom barrier technique is required need an explanation of the various measures involved.

Often a patient will want some recreational activity. Such activities should be designed so that they do not interfere with barrier technique, yet still meet the patient's needs. Materials such as magazines or woodcraft sets can be made safe after they are removed from the contaminated area. Magazines can usually be destroyed, and wood can be sterilized. With a little ingenuity the nurse can usually provide materials which can be either destroyed or sterilized after they have been used.

The explanations provided to a patient who requires barrier technique are crucial to his care. Most people want to participate in their own therapy; moreover, the success of medical asepsis and barrier technique is largely dependent upon the patient's willingness to help. The nurse should be guided in her explanations by the needs of the patient within the context defined by the physician. Words such as "dirty" and "contaminated" are avoided whenever possible, because of the danger of misinterpretation and the value judgments that the patient may attach to them.

The nurse needs to understand what an infection means to the patient. Frequently a patient acquires an infection as a complication of another disorder after admission to the hospital. Such a complication means a lengthened hospital stay, increased financial cost and perhaps a real threat to life. Some patients react to these stresses with aggression and hostility directed toward the hospital in general or perhaps toward the nursing staff and the doctors. The nurse can offer support by providing an accepting environment in which the patient feels free to work through his feelings. She can also instruct patients in the possible sources of infections. For example, many people acquire infections because of the manner in which they carry out their daily activities, and some are reluctant to see how their faulty hygienic practices could be contributing factors.

The patient with an infection or a communicable disease has, in addition to nursing needs related to his role as a patient, others made necessary by his physical illness. Many of these, for example, those associated with fever and wounds, are discussed in other chapters.

GUIDE TO ASSESSING NURSING NEEDS

1. Why is barrier technique used for this patient?
2. What is the specific organism causing his infection?
3. What is the portal of entry, method of transfer, mode of spread and portal of exit for this organism?
4. What special precautions are indicated to prevent the spread of the patient's infection and why should these be taken?
5. Does he have the contact he wishes with his family, hospital personnel and other patients without endangering their health?
6. Does he have the knowledge and skills he requires to prevent the spread of his infection and to participate actively in his care insofar as he is able?

GUIDE TO EVALUATING THE EFFECTIVENESS OF NURSING ACTION

1. Is the barrier technique keeping the organisms within defined areas? Would cultures reveal this?
2. Are other people in the environment free of the infection?
3. Does the patient have misconceptions about his infection?
4. Does the patient indicate in any way that he feels isolated? For example, does he complain verbally or show signs of depression?
5. Does he get exercise adequate to meet his needs?
6. Does he demonstrate an active interest in and is he encouraged to participate in his care insofar as he is able?
7. Does he have diversionary materials that interest him?
8. Do the people in the environment know and take the appropriate precautions to prevent their infection?

STUDY VOCABULARY

Antiseptic	Infection
Bactericidal	Isolation
Bacteriostatic	Medical asepsis
Barrier technique	Pathogens
Clean	Secretion
Concurrent disinfection	Sensitivity
Differentiation	Sterile
Disinfectant	Sterilization
Endogenous spread	Surgical asepsis
Excretion	Terminal disinfection

STUDY SITUATION

Mrs. R. Jackson is admitted to a hospital for an operation to remove an ulcer on her left leg. Three days after her surgery, Mrs. Jackson's wound appears reddened and has a purulent discharge. The patient requires a wound culture to identify the infecting organism. Barrier-technique nursing is commenced.

Mrs. Jackson, who is 54 years old, is in a room that has four beds and a shared bathroom. Her physician suggests that she move to a private room on the same floor where she will have her own bathroom.

1. What factors would you consider prior to explaining barrier technique to this patient?

2. What should you include in your suggestion to Mrs. Jackson that she move to a single room?
3. Why might she not want to move?
4. Why would it be advantageous for the patient to move?
5. The infecting organism is found to be *Staphylococcus aureus*. What do you need to know about this organism in order to establish a safe environment?
6. Mrs. Jackson's wound is dressed at least twice a day. After this measure what is done with the (a) old dressing, (b) linen drapes, (c) artery forceps and (d) unused disinfectant?
7. "The safety of an environment is related to the number of pathogenic organisms in it." What measures in medical asepsis are based on this principle?

BIBLIOGRAPHY

Benson, Margaret E.: Handwashing—an Important Part of Medical Asepsis. *The American Journal of Nursing,* 57:1136–1139, September, 1957.
Blair, Esta H.: Oh, for a Mask—Effective, Comfortable, Inexpensive and Disposable. *Nursing Outlook,* 7:40–42, January, 1959.
Colbeck, J. C.: *Control of Infections in Hospitals.* Chicago, American Hospital Association, 1962.
Edgeworth, D.: Nursing and Asepsis in the Modern Hospital. *Nursing Outlook,* 13:54–56, June, 1965.
Environmental Aspects of the Hospital, Volume 1, Infection Control. Washington, D.C., U.S. Department of Health, Education and Welfare; Public Health Service, 1966.
Foster, Marion: A Positive Approach to Medical Asepsis. *The American Journal of Nursing,* 62:76–77, April, 1962.
French, Ruth M.: *Nurses Guide to Diagnostic Procedures.* Second edition. New York, McGraw-Hill Book Company, Inc., 1967.
Ginsberg, Miriam K., and Maria L. La Conte: Reverse Isolation. *The American Journal of Nursing,* 64:88–90, September, 1964.
Lawrence, C. A., and S. S. Block: *Disinfection, Sterilization, and Preservation.* Philadelphia, Lea & Febiger, 1968.
LeMaitre, George, and Janet Finnegan: *The Patient in Surgery.* Second edition. Philadelphia, W. B. Saunders Company, 1970.
Nahmias, Andre J.: Infections Associated with Hospitals. *Nursing Outlook,* 11:450–453, June, 1963.
Nordmark, Madelyn T., and Anne W. Rohweder: *Scientific Foundations of Nursing.* Second edition. Philadelphia, J. B. Lippincott Company, 1967.
Riley, Richard J., and Francis O'Grady: *Airborne Infection.* New York, The Macmillan Company, 1961.
Safer Ways in Nursing. National Tuberculosis Association, 1962.
Shull, James J.: Ethylene Oxide Sterilization. *The Canadian Nurse,* 58:603–607, July, 1962.
Streeter, S., et al.: Hospital Infection—A Necessary Risk? *The American Journal of Nursing,* 67:3:526–533, March, 1967.

17 THE LEARNING NEEDS OF THE PATIENT

The nurse should be able to:

Explain the importance of meeting the patient's learning
   needs
List principles of learning relevant to the development of an
   effective teaching plan for patients
Describe ways of identifying the learning needs of patients
Cite factors which influence these learning needs
Develop realistic goals for patient learning
Name the three basic types of learning tasks
Describe methods and techniques of teaching suitable for
   each type of learning task
List factors to consider in selecting the time and place for
   teaching patients
Describe methods for the evaluation of patient learning
   suitable for different types of learning tasks

INTRODUCTION

Most people who become ill have learning needs relative to their new situation. They usually want knowledge about tests and examinations, about their disease process and, if they have been hospitalized, about their environment. Some people need help in learning in order to plan for the future, to regain their health, or to cope with physical, psychological and sociological stresses.

Helping to meet the patient's learning needs is an integral part of the nurse's role. In order to meet these needs, the nurse must know something about the learning process; be able to identify patients' learning needs; and be able to select appropriate methods and techniques to facilitate the learning process. She should also be able to evaluate the effectiveness of the patient's learning.

One of the most basic truisms of learning is that we learn what we do. Methods and techniques which encourage active participation on the part of the learner are therefore more effective than those in which the learner plays a passive role. For example, the new mother may need to learn how to bathe her infant. Telling the mother how to give the baby a bath is not a very effective way of teaching her to do this. A more appropriate way would include a demonstration of the procedure and an explanation of reasons for the various steps by the nurse, return demonstration and subsequent practice by the patient. The effectiveness of the learning would be evaluated by the nurse by questioning the mother and observing how she bathed the baby.

THE LEARNING PROCESS

Learning is an active process which continues from birth to death. Throughout his lifetime an individual is constantly learning as he gains information, develops skills and applies his acquired knowledge and skills in adjusting to new life situations. Learning takes place basically in one of two ways —either informally through the ordinary process of living, or formally through a series of selected learning experiences designed to achieve specific goals.

Patients do learn informally about the environment of the hospital and about their disease condition through the actual life experience of being ill. However, there has been a substantial amount of evidence to indicate that many patients' learning needs are not met through informal channels. One of the most frequent complaints of patients is that they do not receive enough information.[1] Yet it has been shown that the better informed the patient is about his condition, the more effective is his therapy. The value of good patient teaching in contributing to the sick person's recovery and his rehabilitation has been well documented. Adequate preoperative instruction has been shown to be a factor in the prevention of many postoperative discomforts, such as pain and vomiting, and a contributing

---

[1]James K. Skipper, Jr.: Communication and the Hospitalized Patient. In *Social Interaction and Patient Care* by James K. Skipper, Jr., and Robert C. Leonard (eds.). Philadelphia, J. B. Lippincott Company, 1965, pp. 61–82.

213

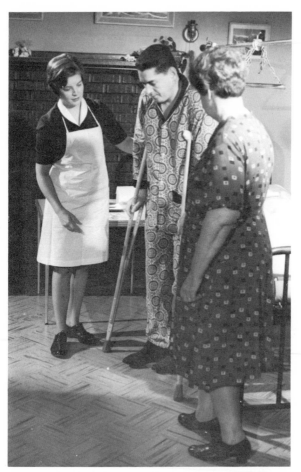

People who are ill sometimes need to re-learn skills that are commonly required in daily activities. The regular visit of the nurse to help with exercises may be the encouragement the patient needs to start walking.

factor in early recovery from surgery.[2] A good teaching program for diabetic patients is accepted as an important aspect of the care of patients with this condition. Many agencies today have a diabetic teaching team whose sole responsibility is to teach patients about their disease.

---

[2]Kathryn M. Healy: Does Preoperative Instruction Make a Difference? *American Journal of Nursing,* 68:1:62–67, January, 1968. See also Lawrence D. Egbert et al. Reduction of Postoperative Pain by Encouragement and Instruction of Patients. *New England Journal of Medicine,* 270:16, April 16, 1964.

The value of good instruction is by no means limited to the care of surgical and diabetic patients. One can justifiably state that all patients have learning needs and a systematic plan for meeting these needs should be incorporated in the nursing care plan for each patient.

Several basic *principles* in regard to the learning process are relevant to the development of a good teaching plan for patients.

1. *Learning is more effective when it is in response to a felt need of the learner.* It is important for the nurse to identify not only what she thinks the patient needs to know but what the patient sees as his learning needs. Most nurses tend to view the patient's learning needs in terms of his disease condition. Often, however, his needs in relation to learning about the hospital are paramount in the patient's mind. His anxiety about this problem may render ineffectual any attempts by the nurse to teach him about his condition. Some patients are not ready, during the acute phase of their illness, to learn everything they need to know, and much teaching may need to be done in follow-up home care programs. For example, the hemiplegic (patient who has had paralysis of one side of his body) may need help with the activities of daily living to be able to cope with feeding and dressing himself, getting in and out of bed, and other common activities after he has gone home from hospital. Much of this follow-up teaching is done in special rehabilitation centers or by public health nurses who visit in the patient's home.

2. *Active participation on the part of the learner is essential if learning is to take place.* Learning takes place *in* the learner and he must be actively involved in the teaching-learning process. Telling the patient what to do or handing him a set of written instructions will not ensure that he will follow these instructions when he gets home. The use of discussion in which the patient takes an active part, problem-solving by the patient and actual practice in performing procedures and handling equipment are much more effective than straight "telling," in which the activity is almost all on the nurse's part.

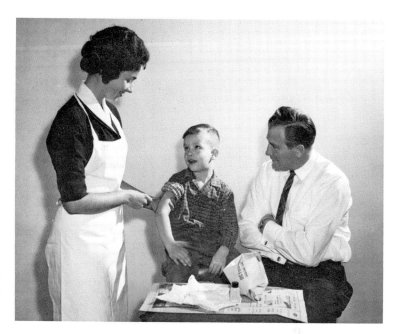

The nurse will teach Father how to give these injections if his son has to continue them indefinitely.

3. *Learning is made easier when material to be learned is related to what the learner already knows.* It is important in this regard to find out what the patient already knows about his condition. Patients today are much more knowledgeable about disease in general and their own health problems in particular than were patients 20 years ago. Medical information is readily available in newspapers, popular magazines, movies, television and public school programs. Moreover, health and illness are now socially acceptable topics of conversation and have become quite popular subjects for television programs. Thus, the average layman of today knows much more about human anatomy and disease than his grandfather ever dreamed of knowing.

4. *Learning is facilitated when the material to be learned is meaningful to the learner.* One can of course learn nonsense syllables, and many experiments have been conducted to see how fast people can learn material which has no meaning. In nursing, however, we are more concerned with the patient's application of his knowledge than his ability to recite facts and figures. A nurse may tell the patient that he needs so many grams each of carbohydrates, fats and proteins in his daily diet, but unless the patient knows the foods which contain these elements and the size of a portion which constitutes so many grams, he is not likely to put the knowledge to use. It is important also to use terms which the patient can understand. The use of technical terminology should be avoided and simple words used wherever possible.

5. *Learning is retained longer when it is put into immediate use than when its application is delayed.* Therefore the diabetic patient who has learned to test his own urine should be allowed to practice this skill immediately and permitted to continue to do so throughout his hospital stay.

6. *Periodic plateaus occur in learning.* The nurse should not become discouraged when the patient seems to lose interest in learning or to be unable to learn at various times. Sometimes a change in teaching method or use of a new technique will help to stimulate further learning. For example, many good audiovisual aids are now available, and these may be used in conjunction with other teaching methods. It is necessary to delay the addition of new material until the patient is ready for it.

7. *Learning must be reinforced.* Questioning the patient about material previously learned and providing for sufficient practice of skills are important ways of reinforcing learning.

8. *Learning is made easier when the learner is aware of his progress.* The patient should be given opportunity to assess his own progress. The nurse can assist the patient by giving encouragement and honest praise. The patient who is learning to walk again finds each new step a challenge, and the nurse's helpful encouragement enables this patient to take pride in his accomplishment. The nurse should be ready, too, to help the patient not to feel discouraged when he does not make as rapid progress as he would like. A recognition that no two individuals are alike and that learning does not take place always in steady progression is helpful in this regard.[3]

ASSESSING THE LEARNING NEEDS OF PATIENTS

Assessing the learning needs of patients is a cooperative endeavor involving the patient, his physician and the nurse. Physicians often have certain teaching regimes which they wish followed for their patients. The nurse may identify needs which are not included in a routine schedule of teaching or there may not be routines established. The patient should be involved as an active participating member of the health team. His perception of his learning needs is sometimes at variance with those views held by the doctor and the nurse.

The patient needs to be given an opportunity to formulate and express his needs. Frequently, his anxiety about his illness lessens his ability to express himself and to make known his needs and wants. Time and encouragement on the nurse's part are required. Patients are often reluctant to ask nurses questions because nurses always seem to be so busy. Nurses usually are busy. However, it is often a matter of establishing priorities for action. A few extra minutes spent with a patient to answer his questions or give him an opportunity to talk often minimizes the number of calls on her time later. A good orientation to the hospital on admission can be extremely valuable in establishing a relationship which permits free communication between patient and nurse. Such an orientation includes welcoming the patient as an individual, describing where he is going and what is going to happen to him, explaining hospital policies in regard to visiting hours, telephone calls, meals and other routines, and answering any questions he may have. It is important also that the nurse take time to talk with the patient's family and gain their cooperation and support in the care of the patient.

The patient's learning needs will vary with the stage of his illness. Initially, the newly hospitalized patient needs to learn about his environment and about his disease process. He will probably be most concerned about the cause of his illness at this point. Later he will want to know about the diagnostic tests that are being performed and the medical plan of therapy. As he convalesces, he begins to think of returning home. His needs will then most likely center around the adjustment to leaving hospital and coping with the exigencies of daily living.[4]

The nurse should always have the rehabilitation of the patient in mind when she is planning a teaching program for him. Her knowledge of rehabilitative measures and understanding of preventive measures help her to identify learning needs which the patient is not always able to perceive. For example, the need for preoperative teaching in regard to coughing and deep breathing may not be apparent to the patient, but the nurse knows that these are important in preventing complications postoperatively and includes this teaching in her planning.

It is important to remember that each patient's needs are different. Teaching plans therefore have to be individualized for each patient. The patient's

---

[3]These principles have been adapted from the list cited in *Adult Education* by Coolie Verner and Allen Booth. Washington, D.C., The Center for Applied Research in Education, Inc., 1964, pp. 89–90.

[4]Patricia Mary Wadsworth: A Study of the Perception of the Nurse and the Patient in Identifying his Learning Needs. Unpublished master's thesis. Vancouver, The University of British Columbia, 1970.

learning needs will depend on a number of factors such as his previous experience with illness, prior hospitalization, and previous experience with his present condition. The patient who is used to repeated admissions to hospital because of a chronic asthmatic condition, for example, will need less orientation to his surroundings than the person who has never been in hospital before. Other factors which influence the patient's learning needs and, therefore, the nurse's teaching plan include age, sex, marital status, education and socioeconomic background of the patient.

DEVELOPING GOALS FOR PATIENT LEARNING

In developing a plan for teaching the patient, the first step is the identification of the patient's needs. The second step is the formulation of goals, or objectives, to be attained. Frequently, these are stated as long-range goals (or primary objectives) and short-term goals (or subobjectives). For example, one long-range goal for the patient with diabetes might be, "The patient is able to control his diabetes through medication and diet." An example of a short-term goal for the same patient could be, "The patient is able to administer his own insulin by hypodermic injection." It is always preferable to state goals in terms of what it is that the patient should be able to do rather than what the nurse is to do. Thus it is better to say, "The patient should be able to..." rather than that the goal of the teaching is "to help the patient to . . . ." Specific goals which can be measured in terms of changes in the patient's behavior make the process of evaluation of the patient's learning much easier. Thus, using the example just given, the patient is either able to administer insulin by hypodermic syringe or he is not.

Goals should be realistic and attainable in terms of the patient's ability to reach them. To expect an elderly patient to be able to progress as quickly as a young person is unrealistic because learning occurs at a slower rate as a person gets older.

For further guidance on the development of objectives, the nurse is referred to Dorothy Smith's article, "Writing Objectives as a Nursing Practice Skill" in the February, 1971, issue of the *American Journal of Nursing.*

THE SELECTION OF METHODS AND TECHNIQUES

After the goals for learning have been established, it is necessary to decide on teaching methods and techniques to facilitate the learning process. This involves an analysis of the tasks to be learned and the selection of appropriate methods to use.

There are three basic types of learning tasks: those that involve the acquisition of information, those that involve the acquisition of skills and those that involve the application of knowledge.[5] Various methods of teaching are particularly suitable for each type of learning task.

The Acquisition of Information

Many of the patient's learning needs come under the heading of a need for information and knowledge. As stated earlier in the chapter, this is the need most frequently expressed by patients. Techniques for giving information include the lecture or short explanatory talk, discussion, the use of programmed

[5]Verner and Booth, op. cit., pp. 75–84.

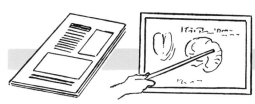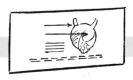

A diversity of teaching aids are available; books, posters, films and charts are all useful at times.

materials and teaching machines and of audiovisual material such as films and film strips. The nurse may find the lecture or explanation useful in some instances, for example, when giving a talk to a group of patients, but these techniques do not involve much participation on the part of the learner. Discussion involving both patient and nurse is usually more effective for the retention of knowledge. Written material is available on a number of different disease conditions, and this literature may be used to supplement other instruction. It is good to vary the teaching technique, for example, by interspersing audiovisual material with talking. An individual's attention span is usually shorter when he is ill than when he is well.

The Acquisition of a Skill

Many times it is necessary for the patient to learn new skills. He may need to learn to administer a hypodermic injection (as in the example just cited); to use crutches for walking; or to change his own dressing. There are any number of instances which could be given of times when patients need to learn skills. Appropriate methods for skill-learning include the demonstration (or lecture demonstration), the return demonstration, and skill practice.

In demonstrating a specific nursing care measure, the type of equipment that the patient will have at home is used whenever possible. Many hospitals, for example, have standard trays of home care equipment consisting of household items. The nurse can use these to advantage in demonstrating nursing measures.

In giving a demonstration, the nurse should first of all explain to the patient what she is going to do and why it is to be done this way. She always stands so that the patient can see exactly what she is doing. For example, the patient should be able to see the numbers on a syringe when measures are explained. An overview of the procedure is given first; then the procedure is broken down into steps. Key points are stressed. The material that is being taught can often

be related to something that is familiar to the patient so that learning can be transferred from the familiar to the new area. The woman who is familiar with the process of preparing jars for jams and jellies can usually learn quite readily how to sterilize equipment when this procedure is shown as a similar process.

The patient should have an opportunity to perform the procedure soon after the nurse has demonstrated it. Sufficient practice sessions should also be arranged so that the patient feels competent before he is on his own.

The Application of Knowledge

Earlier in the chapter it was stated that one of the nurse's primary concerns is that the patient apply the knowledge he has learned. Giving the patient information is not enough; he must learn to apply this information in his day-to-day living. This application involves the integration of knowledge and the use of intellectual processes by the learner. The learner must be actively involved.

The problem-solving method has been suggested by educators as a very appropriate method for learning to apply knowledge.[6] This method has also been suggested for use with patients. The steps in problem-solving include: (1) identification of the problem, or the perception of a felt learning need by the patient (this involves gathering information and pinpointing what the problem is); (2) suggesting possible solutions; (3) selection of one solution to be tried; (4) putting the solution into action; and (5) evaluating the results of this action, reconsidering and possibly trying other solutions.[7]

The nurse's role becomes one of supportive assistant. She helps the patient to identify his problem; to gather information and assess the relative merits of various possible solutions.

---

[6] Ibid., p. 82.
[7] Rosella Denison Collins: Problem Solving A Tool for Patients, Too. *The American Journal of Nursing*, 68:7:1483–1485, July, 1968.

She may help him to select and try out one course of action, and assists him in evaluating this action.

For example, a patient may have been told by his physician that he should stay on a salt-free diet. The dietitian has talked to the patient and instructed him regarding foods that are low in salt, and the patient has been using salt substitutes to flavor his food during his hospital stay. He still seems worried about being able to stay on the diet when he goes home. The nurse may help him to identify the problem by gathering information and helping to pinpoint the difficulty. The patient and his wife are elderly and they live alone. His wife does the cooking. He is afraid that it is going to give her extra work to cook his meals without salt. The nurse helps him to work through possible solutions. Has he talked to his wife about this? In this example, it would seem that the wife, who does the cooking, should be brought into the problem-solving. Together the patient and his wife might examine possible solutions. The patient's food may be cooked separately, in which case there will be two meals to prepare and two sets of pots and pans to wash. Or, food for both may be cooked together without salt, the wife adding salt to hers later. Many people find food tasteless when salt is not added during the cooking, and the wife may not like her food cooked this way. Both alternatives should be explored and a decision reached. The couple may decide to try cooking meals for both together without salt. If this solution does not work, then they can try the alternative.

There are many examples that could be cited of situations in which problem-solving seems the logical method for helping patients to understand their disease processes and make realistic plans to care for themselves. Often the patient's family needs to be included, since many problems related to illness involve adjustments in family living. The family frequently provides excellent resource people to assist in developing and carrying out plans for the patient's care when he goes home from hospital.

SELECTING THE TIME AND THE PLACE FOR TEACHING

All teaching, if it is to be worthwhile, takes time. Much of the nurse's teaching is, as mentioned earlier in the chapter, done incidentally in the course of nursing care, but when specific material is to be taught, sufficient time should be allocated. A time that is suitable for both the patient and the nurse—when neither feels rushed and the patient is not overly tired—should be selected. The choice of time varies, depending upon the patient's daily activities. Often the period in the morning after treatment and care have been completed, or the early afternoon, can be used to advantage for teaching. Teaching periods are kept relatively short because most people, during illness, have a decreased attention span and generally do not feel well, and the nurse is careful not to try to cover too much in any one session.

The place for teaching is most often at the patient's bedside, although some health agencies have separate rooms where patients can come for classes or for consultations with a health worker. It is important that privacy be provided in learning situations which involve personal matters.

Wherever possible, one nurse should initiate and carry through the teaching plan. Patients usually prefer to have the same person teaching them, and the nurse can develop a more effective relationship with the patient if she carries through the complete teaching plan. It also helps to provide for continuity in the teaching-learning situation if there is only one nurse involved. If this is not feasible, however, a team approach in which each nurse is responsible for one aspect of the teaching can be used quite effectively.

EVALUATING THE EFFECTIVENESS OF THE PATIENT'S LEARNING

Evaluation is the assessment of how far along the road toward attainment of the preestablished goals the learner has come. If the goals have been stated specifically in terms of what the learner is expected to be able to do at the end of the teaching program, the task of evaluating the effectiveness of his learning is relatively simple. If, for example, one goal for learning is that the patient should select foods that are low in fat content for his meals, then the extent of his learning would be evaluated through observation of the foods he selects.

Methods of evaluating effective learning will vary with each of the three types of learning task. If the task has been one of acquiring information, for example, learning the danger signals to watch for in patients with a diabetic condition, questioning the patient is a good method of finding out the extent of his knowledge. Can he list the danger signals? Does he understand their significance? Does he know what to do about them?

The acquisition of skills can be assessed by observing the patient's ability to carry out the specific procedures. Can he give himself a hypodermic injection or do his own dressing? Does he know how to prepare the equipment, handle it and maintain good technique while doing it? Questioning the patient while he is performing the procedure helps to ascertain whether he understands the principles involved (or the why's of doing things a certain way).

In assessing the application of knowledge and skills, observing what the patient does in a given situation is probably the only way of measuring this type of learning. In the example just cited, of the patient on a fat-free diet, the only way of assessing whether the patient is applying his knowledge is actual observation of the food he selects and eats. Many times evaluation of the application of knowledge must be delayed until the patient is back in his home situation. This emphasizes the importance of follow-up visits in the home. Indeed one of the most important responsibilities of the public health nurse is teaching the patient and helping him to apply his knowledge in day-to-day living.

SUMMARY

Meeting the patient's learning needs is a primary responsibility of nurses, yet it is one which has not received sufficient attention, particularly in the hospital field, until fairly recently. The topic deserves much more extensive coverage than it has been possible to give in this short chapter. Like the subject of communication, the nurse's role in teaching patients merits a book on its own. The nurse is therefore directed to Pohl's book, *Teaching Function of the Nursing Practitioner*, and Redman's, *The Process of Patient Teaching in Nursing*, for more thorough coverage of this topic. In addition, there are numerous articles in the recent nursing literature and much research is currently being done in the field of patient teaching. A number of articles and reports of research findings are listed in the bibliography.

STUDY VOCABULARY			
	Behavior	Explanation	Teaching
	Demonstration	Learning	Thinking
	Discussion	Practice	Visual aid

STUDY SITUATION

Jimmy Smith, who is eight years old, has an infected cut on his thigh. He is at home and his physician has asked you as the public health nurse to visit his home and teach his mother how to apply hot compresses to the cut. Jimmy's mother is Spanish and speaks very little English.

1. What factors would you consider before initiating any teaching?

2. What methods would best be used for teaching in this situation?
3. What possible factors might inhibit learning?
4. What aids could you use to facilitate learning?
5. How could you evaluate the learning of the patient and his mother?

BIBLIOGRAPHY

Aiken, M.: Patient Problems are Problems in Learning. *The American Journal of Nursing, 70*:9:1916, September, 1970.

Brown, Esther Lucille: *Newer Dimensions of Patient Care, Part II.* New York, Russell Sage Foundation, 1962.

Christman, J.: Assisting the Patient to Learn the Patient Role. *Journal of Nursing Education, 6*:17, April, 1967.

Clark, Vivian V.: Learning Needs of the Patient with Coronary Occlusion About His Illness and Self Care. Unpublished doctoral dissertation, Columbia University, 1967.

Collins, Rosella Denison: Problem Solving A Tool for Patients, Too. *The American Journal of Nursing, 68*:7:1483–1485, July, 1968.

Dloughy, Alico et al.: What Patients Want to Know About Their Diagnostic Tests. *Nursing Outlook, 11*:265–267, April, 1963.

Dodge, Joan: Factors Related to Patients' Perceptions of Their Cognitive Needs. *Nursing Research, 18*:413–421, May, 1968.

Egbert, Lawrence D., et al.: Reduction of Postoperative Pain by Encouragement and Instruction of Patients. *New England Journal of Medicine, 270*:16, April 16, 1964.

Haferkorn, Virginia: Assessing Individual Learning Needs as a Basic for Patient Teaching. *Nursing Clinics of North America, 6*:1:199–209, March, 1971.

Healy, Kathryn M.: Does Preoperative Instruction Make a Difference? *The American Journal of Nursing, 68*:62–67, January, 1968.

Hornback, M.: Diabetes Mellitus—The Nurse's Role. *Nursing Clinics of North America, 5*:3, March, 1970.

Krysan, G. S.: How Do We Teach Four Million Diabetics? *The American Journal of Nursing, 65*:105–107, November, 1965.

Lambertsen, Eleanor: *Education for Nursing Leadership.* Philadelphia, J. B. Lippincott Company, 1958.

Linehan, Dorothy T.: What Does the Patient Want to Know? *The American Journal of Nursing, 66*:1066–1070, May, 1966.

McGrath, Marion E.: Teaching Students to Teach. *Nursing Outlook, 15*:69–71, September, 1967.

Mohammed, Mary F. B.: Patients Understanding of Written Health Information. *Nursing Research, 13*:100–108, Spring, 1964.

Piepgras, Ruth: All Nurses Are Teachers. *Nursing Outlook, 17*:49–51, October, 1969.

Pohl, Margaret: Teaching Activities of the Nursing Practitioners. *Nursing Research, 14*:4–11, Winter, 1965.

Pohl, Margaret: *Teaching Function of the Nursing Practitioner.* Dubuque, Iowa, William C. Brown Company, 1968.

Redman, Barbara K.: *The Process of Patient Teaching in Nursing.* St. Louis, C. V. Mosby Company, 1968.

Skipper, J. K., and R. C. Leonard: *Social Interaction and Patient Care.* Philadelphia, J. B. Lippincott Company, 1965.

Smith, Dorothy M.: Writing Objectives as a Nursing Practice Skill. *The American Journal of Nursing, 71*:2:319–320, February, 1971.

Smyth, Kathleen (ed.): Symposium on Patient Teaching. *Nursing Clinics of North America, 6*:4:571–806, December, 1971.

Verner, Coolie, and Allen Booth: *Adult Education.* Washington, D.C., The Center for Applied Research in Education Inc., 1964.

Wadsworth, Patricia Mary: A Study of the Perception of the Nurse and the Patient in Identifying his Learning Needs. Unpublished master's thesis. Vancouver, The University of British Columbia, 1970.

Weiler, Sister M. Cashel: Postoperative Patients Evaluate Preoperative Instructions. *The American Journal of Nursing, 68*:1465–1467, July, 1968.

Zitnik, Ruth: First You Take a Grapefruit. *The American Journal of Nursing, 68*:1285–1286, June, 1968.

18 THE LEGAL IMPLICATIONS OF NURSING PRACTICE

The nurse should be able to:

State the purpose of nursing practice acts

Differentiate between permissive and mandatory registration for nurses

Differentiate between areas of professional and areas of practical nursing function

Define the following legal terms: *tort, crime, negligence, malpractice, assault, battery, defamation of character, slander, libel*

Explain the legal status of the nurse

List common types of incidents leading to legal suits in which nurses and patients are involved in which negligence is a factor

Explain the status of the nurse in regard to confidential information

Explain the nurse's legal responsibility if she is present at the scene of an accident or gives aid in an emergency

Explain the legal implications of witnessing a will

Explain the implications for nursing practice of statutes controlling narcotic drugs

THE LEGAL IMPLICATIONS 18
OF NURSING PRACTICE

INTRODUCTION

A knowledge of how the law affects both herself and the patient is of increasing importance to the nurse in her day-to-day care of patients. The nurse should be familiar with the laws in her state which concern the provision of health care to the public, and particularly with the acts which control the practice of nursing. She should be aware of her functions and responsibilities as a professional person, both as defined by law and as delineated by her professional nursing associations.

It is important for the nurse to be aware of how the law protects the patient and of her own legal status both as student and as graduate. In recent years there has been an increasing number of legal suits involving nurses, and evidence supports the belief that this trend will continue.[1]

NURSING PRACTICE ACTS

The law in both the United States and Canada is derived from two main sources: the statutes passed by lawmaking bodies such as Congress or Parliament and the decisions of the courts. The latter are collectively known as common law. The law is a reflection of

public opinion and of civic and social movements within a community; the law therefore is not static; rather, it is constantly changing. Changes in the statutes and the decisions of the courts in cases involving nursing reflect the changes in public thinking about the development of nursing.

As nursing has emerged as a profession, there has been an increasing awareness by nurses and by the public of the need to standardize the laws concerning the practice of nursing and to define the functions of both the professional and the practical nurse. The authority to control nursing, together with various other professions and occupations concerned with health and welfare, has been vested in the states (or, in Canada, in the provinces). Thus each state and province has enacted its own laws to control the practice of nursing. These laws are generally termed

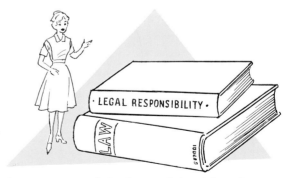

An awareness of the law and the rights of individuals is essential in nursing practice. The law as it affects nursing practice is continually changing, as it reflects changes in society itself.

---

[1] Joseph F. Sadusk (American Medical Association Committee on Nursing): Legal Implications of Changing Patterns of Practice. *The Journal of the American Medical Association,* 190:1135–1136, December 28, 1964.

nursing practice acts, although the exact title of the statute varies in the different jurisdictions. Because each state and province has set up its own law, it is understandable that the statutes vary somewhat. Nevertheless the purpose of these laws is the same, that is, to protect the health of the public through the establishment of minimum standards which a qualified practitioner must meet in order to practice as a nurse.[2]

The majority of the nursing practice acts in both the United States and Canada are permissive registration acts; that is, the nurse may or may not register depending on whether she wishes to have the privileges that accompany registration. These privileges are, in general, that she may designate herself as a licensed nurse and that she may place the initials "R.N." after her name. There is a strong movement currently under way to make the registration of nurses compulsory. In 1970, eight states had mandatory licensing laws for professional nurses, and in 17 other states nursing boards required nurses to be licensed in order to practice.

In addition to the laws controlling professional nurses, most states now have either permissive or mandatory licensing acts for practical nurses. In Canada, the majority of the provincial nursing practice acts are permissive in regard to the registration of nurses. All the provinces except two now have practical nursing laws.

AREAS OF NURSING FUNCTION

The profession of nursing is dynamic and its practice is constantly changing. Anderson states that "Custom and usage primarily determine what functions nurses may perform."[3]

Guidance on what constitutes nursing practice has come principally from two sources, the nursing practice acts and the statements of the professional nursing associations. The opinions of state and provincial attorneys general provide some additional assistance from the legal viewpoint, although these opinions are usually offered in response to requests from governmental agencies and pertain for the most part to specific situations.[4] In some parts of Canada, provincial government agencies have developed guidelines as to the procedures that may be performed by physicians, professional nurses, nursing assistants and other personnel in hospitals.

The Law and Nursing Functions

In their nursing practice acts, some states have defined only the functions of the professional nurse; some protect the title of "Registered Nurse" and do not define her practice; some include a definition of both the professional and the practical nurse. The statutes which define nursing practice for the most part do so in very general terms, usually stating only that the nurse may carry out the physician's orders, apply nursing skills, and supervise others less qualified than herself in the care of patients.[5]

Most medical practice acts are similarly written in broad general terms, giving to physicians the right to make diagnoses and to prescribe for and treat patients. The general nature of the wording in most medical and nursing practice acts has permitted both disciplines to enlarge the scope of their practice without the need for frequent changes in legislation. In many technical areas, there is considerable overlap between nursing and medical practice. The broad definitions contained in the statutes has thus made possible the orderly transfer of many procedural functions from one discipline to the other without changing

---

[2]American Nurses' Association: *Principles of Legislation Relating to Nursing Practice.* New York, Revised, January 1958.

[3]Betty Jane Anderson: Orderly Transfer of Procedural Responsibilities from Medical to Nursing Practice. Nursing Clinics of North America, 5:2:314, June, 1970.

[4]Ibid., p. 313.

[5]Ibid.

the law each time.[6] It was not many years ago that only physicians were allowed to take blood pressures or start intravenous infusions, for example, yet today these are recognized nursing functions.

Recently, there has been a rapid acceleration in the transfer of functions from physicians to nurses and to other newly emerging groups of health workers, such as the "physician's assistant." In some states, the medical and nursing practice acts have been modified to cover the increased delegation of responsibility from physicians to nurses (and others). A number of states have passed additional legislation to regulate the practice of new categories of health personnel. It would be well for the nurse to familiarize herself with the particular laws concerning nursing in the state in which she intends to practice.

Statements by the Professional Nursing Associations

The American Nurses' Association in 1954 issued a statement outlining the functions of the professional nurse.[7] This was followed in 1964 by a statement of the practical nurse's functions.[8] A policy statement issued by the Canadian Nurses' Association in 1967 suggested areas of professional and technical nursing practice.[9]

These statements by the two national nursing associations outline the basic areas of nursing activity. In addition, about one-half of the state nursing practice boards and some of the provincial nursing associations have issued guidelines regarding the additional functions that may be performed by nurses when these are delegated by a physician. Increasingly common also are joint statements issued by various professional groups, such as state medical, nursing and hospital associations, in regard to the transfer of specific functions from physicians to nurses. Although statements made by professional associations lack the authority of legally enacted laws, they are generally persuasive in that they reflect prevailing custom.[10]

Professional Versus Practical Nursing Functions

Creighton considers that "the essential difference between the registered professional nurse and the practical nurse is that . . . the registered professional nurse is obliged to evaluate and interpret facts in order to decide necessary action that may be required."[11] One would infer from this that the professional nurse's practice then encompasses more independent nursing functions, whereas the practical nurse performs more dependent ones, and this is borne out in the statements regarding their functions. Independent nursing functions are those which require the nurse to make independent judgments based on her education, training and experience.[12] An example of an independent nursing function would be the assessment of a patient's condition to determine his need for medical or nursing intervention. Dependent nursing functions are those which are performed under legal medical orders or under the supervision or direction of a physician.[13] When a nurse gives a patient a medication which has been ordered by a doctor, she is performing a dependent nursing function.

[6]Ibid.
[7]American Nurses' Association: Statement of Functions. *The American Journal of Nursing*, 54:868–871, 1130, 1954.
[8]American Nurses' Association: Statement of Functions of the Licensed Practical Nurse. *The American Journal of Nursing*, 64:93, March, 1964.
[9]Canadian Nurses' Association. *Roles, Functions, and Educational Preparation for the Practice of Nursing.* Ottawa, 1967.

[10]Anderson, op. cit., p. 313.
[11]Helen Creighton, *Law Every Nurse Should Know.* Philadelphia, W. B. Saunders Company, 1970, p. 22.
[12]Anderson, op. cit., p. 314.
[13]Ibid.

Professional Nursing Functions. In her book, *Law Every Nurse Should Know*, Creighton outlines the generally accepted areas of the professional nurse as seven:

1. Supervision of a total, comprehensive nursing care plan for the patient
2. Observation, interpretation and evaluation of the patient's symptoms and needs, both mental and physical
3. Carrying out the legal orders of physicians for medications and treatments
4. Supervision of auxiliary help, including practical nurses, student nurses, and other health workers
5. Carrying out nursing procedures and techniques, especially those which require judgment, modification or calculation based on technical information
6. Giving health guidance and participating in health education
7. Accurately recording and reporting facts and evaluations of nursing care[14]

Practical Nursing Functions. Four areas of nursing activity have been suggested for the practical nurse:

1. Environmental and physical management of a patient
2. Factual observation and reporting
3. The execution of prescribed routine nursing procedures and techniques
4. The application and the execution of legal orders of physicians and professional nurses limited by background, scope and subject to an understanding of cause and effect[15]

TORTS AND CRIMES

In addition to understanding her responsibilities as a professional nurse, the nurse should be aware of the types of legal proceedings in which she may become involved either as a witness or as a defendant. Generally speaking, there are two types of court actions in which a nurse can be involved. The first is called a tort. A tort is a legal wrong committed by one person against the person or property of another. The injured party may sue for damages and, if the suit is successful, he is usually awarded money to be paid by the other party. Sometimes this is spoken of as a civil suit, as opposed to a criminal suit.

A crime is also a legal wrong but, in general, it refers to a wrong committed against the public and punishable by the state. The punishment for a crime is either a fine or imprisonment. In a criminal action, the case is designated in the form The People versus Mary Jones, in a tort, John Doe versus James Jones, or Mary Doe versus the Blank Hospital. Acts such as murder, manslaughter and robbery are considered criminal, whereas negligence and malpractice are usually torts.

THE LEGAL STATUS OF THE NURSE

The nurse in her practice can be classed as either an independent contractor or an employee. Private duty nurses, that is, nurses who are engaged by the patient to perform nursing service, come under the category of independent contractors. Nurses who work in hospitals or clinics, in public health agencies, in industry or for private physicians are considered employees. The distinction is a matter of control. On private duty, the nurse works independently; in the hospital, she works under the direction of the employing institution.

Student nurses, when assigned for clinical experience to a hospital or other health agency, are usually considered as employees since they are subject to the control of clinical instructors, head nurses and physicians.[16] In a school of nursing controlled by a hospital, students are generally held to be employees of the hospital insofar as they perform services for the hospital

---

[14]Creighton, op. cit., pp. 19, 20.

[15]Milton J. Lesnik and Bernice E. Anderson: *Nursing Practice and the Law.* Second edition. Philadelphia, J. B. Lippincott Company, 1955, pp. 282–283.

[16]Creighton, op. cit., pp. 56, 57.

and are supervised by its staff. Students in collegiate or other independent schools of nursing may, however, be entirely under the supervision of the faculty of their school while in the practice area. Creighton considers that in these instances "the student would not seem to be an employee of the hospital, but might be held as an employee of the college."[17]

It is well for the student to remember, though, that even though she may be considered as an employee, she is still responsible for her own actions. Anyone who gives nursing care, whether student or graduate, assumes certain duties, and it is expected that these will be carried out with "reasonable prudence" under the circumstances. "Reasonable prudence" is taken to mean that the individual acts with the care that any reasonable person with his or her knowledge, training and experience would take.

The reason for the importance of determining the status of the nurse is that, under the law, not only is an individual liable for his own actions but his employer is also liable under the rule of respondeat superior (Let the master answer). Thus if a nurse is negligent and a patient is harmed, both the nurse and her employer can be sued by the patient.

In some states, charitable institutions and government hospitals, such as municipal or country hospitals, are exempt from the rule of respondeat superior and may not be sued; however, the employee of such an institution who performs a negligent act may still be sued. The law is somewhat different in various states in this regard.

Nor is the nurse absolved of responsibility for her actions simply because she is carrying out the orders of a physician. The law states that the nurse must understand the cause and effect of the treatment that she undertakes. If she carries out an order which she knows is wrong, she is guilty of negligence. At all times the patient's safety must be paramount.

If the nurse undertakes work that she knows is beyond the scope of her professional training— for example, if she performs some action or treatment which is defined as being within the province of medical practice—she may again be considered negligent or guilty of malpractice.[18]

NEGLIGENCE AND MALPRACTICE

It has already been noted that each individual is responsible for his own actions and that a nurse can be held liable for her own negligent actions. Negligence on the part of nurses has been defined by the courts as "the failure to exercise that degree of skill, care, and diligence exercised by professional nurses in light of the present state of nursing science in comparable situations."[19] As a general rule, nursing negligence usually results when the nurse fails to take the appropriate action to protect the safety of the patient.[20] Thus, if the nurse does not carry out a physician's order correctly, as, for example, if she gives a wrong medication, she may be considered negligent. Similarly, failure to put up siderails on the bed of a confused patient could also be considered negligence on the nurse's part.

Malpractice has been defined as "any professional misconduct, unreasonable lack of skill or fidelity in professional or judiciary duties, evil practice, or illegal or immoral conduct."[21] Thus, it would appear that negligence implies more the failure to do something, whereas malpractice implies a more positive act of wrong-doing. A nurse who participates knowingly in an illegal operation could be considered to be guilty of malpractice.

---

[17]Ibid., p. 101.

[18]Kenneth G. Gray: Law and Nursing. *The Canadian Nurse,* 60:546, June, 1964.

[19]Anderson, op. cit. p. 315

[20]Ibid., p. 317

[21]Ibid.

In civil court actions, there appears to be little distinction made between willful wrong-doing, as opposed to negligence, with regard to damages or blame. Many courts use the terms "negligence" and "malpractice" interchangeably. Some courts have held that the term "malpractice" should be used in connection with only the two professions of medicine and the law.[22] The term is, however, being more widely applied now to other professional groups, including nurses.

Common Acts of Negligence

Professional nurses may be called upon to testify in a legal proceeding in regard to some matter pertaining to their work. The most common types of incidents leading to legal proceedings involving a hospital patient and a nurse are those in which negligence is a factor. Some of the more common of such acts of negligence which have resulted in suits for damages are:

Overlooked Sponges. In any operative procedure care must be taken that no sponges are left inside the patient. Counting sponges is a nursing responsibility in most instances, and the nurse may be held liable if she fails to make a count when it has been ordered or if she makes an error in her count. Many hospitals now require that instruments and needles also be counted both before and after surgery.

Burns. Hot water bottles, heating pads, inhalators, steam radiators, enemas, douches, sitz baths, all are items which can cause a patient to be burned. The nurse may be held responsible if she has neglected to take the usual safety precautions, such as taking the temperature of the water used in a solution administered to a patient or keeping articles that might burn the patient out of his reach.

Falls. Another common type of accident which may result in injury to the patient and subsequently to a suit for damages is falling from bed. The usual

safety precautions include the use of side rails and other restraints. Most health agencies have rules regarding the use of side rails for the beds of postoperative patients and patients under sedation. Many extend this ruling to include the beds of all irrational patients, patients over 70 years of age and children under a certain age.

Wrong Medicine, Wrong Dosage, Wrong Patient, Wrong Concentration. Another common area in which negligence occurs is in giving medications. Labels can be misread or may not be read at all. The nurse may fail to identify the patient correctly and consequently give a medication to the wrong person. Numerous errors are made in giving medicines. With the tremendous increase in the number of medications ordered for patients and the numerous trademarks commonly used for the various drugs, safety precautions assume greater importance in ensuring that the right patient gets the right drug in the proper concentration at the right time and in the proper manner.

Defects in Apparatus or Supplies. Patients can be injured by the use of defective equipment. The nurse is not held responsible if the patient is injured as a result of a hidden defect, but if she uses equipment or supplies that she knows to be faulty, she may be held liable. The use of unsterile gauze for a surgical dressing could be an example of this.

Abandonment. Instances in which patients have been left unattended and have injured themselves as a result, have led to suits for negligence. For example, if the nurse leaves a baby on a table and the baby falls while she is absent, she can be held negligent.

Loss or Damage to a Patient's Property. The nurse is held liable if a patient's property is lost when it has been entrusted to her care. Most hospitals now try to safeguard against suits for lost articles by asking the patient to sign a statement to the effect that he is responsible for items he retains in his possession while he is in hospital. Nevertheless, there are still many instances in which the care of a patient's

[22]Ibid.

property becomes of necessity the nurse's responsibility. For example, when the patient goes to the operating room for surgery, his valuables are placed in safekeeping. The property of the unconscious or irrational patient is also to be safeguarded. Perhaps the most commonly lost items are dentures, although diamond rings, watches and money also seem to disappear quite frequently.

REPORTING ACCIDENTS

The nurse has a moral and legal responsibility to report to the health agency any accidents, losses, or unusual occurrences. Most hospitals have special forms for this purpose. One of the primary reasons for such a report is to ensure that there is a record of the details of the incident and the subsequent action taken, in the event that legal proceedings are instituted. Incident reports are also useful as a source of information in research to improve the quality of care and the effectiveness of policies (see Chapter 15).

THE PATIENT'S RECORD

Patient records can be introduced as evidence in court. This subject is discussed in Chapter 8, under The Patient's Record. Since recording and reporting is an undisputed area of independent nursing function, it follows that the nurse's records about a patient should be accurate and contain all the pertinent information. "Nurses should realize that the removal of portions of a medical record is a serious thing, even though the purpose is to make a correction. . . . It is a good practice to line out incorrect data with a single line in ink."[23] The word "error" may be written, also in ink. The corrected material then follows. The date and the signature of the person making the correction should always be included.

THE NURSE AND CONFIDENTIAL INFORMATION

The question of whether confidential information entrusted to the nurse by the patient is considered to be a privileged communication and therefore inadmissible as evidence in court proceedings has not been definitely settled. A few states have enacted statutes which specifically state that the nurse-patient relationship is a privileged one, and therefore confidential information given to the nurse cannot be used in proceedings. In instances in which the doctor-patient communication is considered privileged, the ruling has been held to extend to nurses when they are acting as agents of the physician. In Canada, the rule of privilege for confidential information is not absolute. Although the nurse and the physician should not disclose confidential information entrusted to them, they may be directed to do so, if this is justified by public policy or if the law requires reporting of the matter.[24] In the United States, a witness cannot be required to give evidence which would tend to incriminate him, whereas in Canada the law requires that a witness answer all questions that are relevant whether or not the answer tends to incriminate him. He can, however, invoke the protection of the Canada Evidence Act in certain cases.

ASSAULT AND BATTERY

In some instances, nurses have been involved in legal proceedings as a result of a charge of assault and battery by a patient. Assault refers to threats to do bodily harm to another. Battery is "the application of force to the person of another without lawful justification."[25]

---

[23]Helen Creighton: On the Witness Stand. *The American Journal of Nursing*, 57:1595, December, 1957.

[24]Helen Creighton: *Law Every Nurse Should Know*. Philadelphia, W. B. Saunders Company, 1970, p. 218.

[25]Ibid., p. 145.

Assault and battery are considered criminal offenses as well as torts. The law protects every individual against bodily harm by another person and also against any form of assault due to interference with his person. Therefore a person cannot take a blood sample from a patient without his consent. Nor may a person be operated on for any condition unless he has given his consent to the procedure and understands the significance of the procedure. Autopsy without the consent of relatives may be considered assault and battery.

Most hospitals have standard forms which the patient signs to grant permission for the treatment and operative procedures deemed necessary during his hospitalization. The nurse obtains the patient's permission for operation before the patient is sedated for surgery, because consent obtained while the patient is under sedation can be questioned. Some religious beliefs forbid the use of certain treatments, for example, blood transfusions; however, in any case in which treatment is a matter of life and death and the patient is unable to give his consent, it has been ruled that consent is implied.[26] In the case of children, either parent can give consent. In the case of mentally incompetent persons, it is necessary to obtain the permission of the patient's legal guardian for treatment and surgery. Except in emergencies, restraints should not be used unless they are ordered by the physician; at all times undue force is avoided in handling patients.

GOOD SAMARITAN LAWS

The majority of states (and some provinces) have enacted legislation designed to protect the professional practitioner from malpractice suits arising from care given to the injured at the scene of an accident or other emergency. Some of these statutes cover physicians only; others, all practitioners of the healing arts. These laws are usually referred to as "Good Samaritan"

laws and are intended to encourage qualified people to give aid in an emergency. In general, these laws protect the individual who renders emergency care from civil liability for this care, unless he, or she, is guilty of gross negligence or extreme malpractice in giving the care.

In some states, there is specific legislation to the effect that no one may leave the scene of an automobile accident without first giving aid to those injured in the accident. In the absence of such a law, there is no legal compulsion for the nurse, or anyone else for that matter, to give assistance in an emergency. If aid is given voluntarily, the person giving the aid is under an obligation to give the best care possible under the circumstances, commensurate with his knowledge, training and experience. Most medical practice acts contain a waiver to the effect that, in an emergency, a volunteer who is not medically qualified may perform procedures to "save life or limb" that ordinarily lie within the scope of medical practice. In doing so, the volunteer is not considered guilty of practicing medicine without a license.

If a nurse is present at the scene of an accident, or finds herself in an emergency situation and feels morally obligated to give assistance, she should first of all ascertain that she is the best-qualified person there to give aid. She should also make sure that a state of emergency truly exists. The nurse should then render the care that is necessary and transfer the patient as soon as possible to a medically qualified practitioner for continued treatment. In such a situation, the nurse is expected to act as any other nurse of equal training and experience would act under the same or similar circumstances.[27]

DEFAMATION OF CHARACTER

Another area of the law of which the nurse should be aware is that of suits

[26]Lesnik and Anderson, op. cit., p. 312.

[27]Harvey Sarner, *The Nurse and the Law*, Philadelphia, W. B. Saunders Company, 1968, pp. 86–88.

arising from defamation of character. The term "defamation of character" means that a person's reputation is damaged by written or spoken words which tend to lower his esteem in the eyes of other people. If written, as in a letter to a third party, or in a cartoon which causes the person to be the subject of ridicule or contempt, the term "libel" is used to describe the action.[28] "Slander" is the term used for defamation of character through spoken words, as, for example, if one speaks badly of someone in conversation with another person. The nurse should always be careful not to discuss patients except with others who are concerned with their care. Not every mention of a patient is slander or libel, of course; these terms are used only when there is a threat to the individual's reputation. For example, most courts consider it defamatory to let other people know that an unmarried woman is pregnant, or that a patient has venereal disease. To state that a patient had a broken leg would not ordinarily be considered defamatory. If, however, one added that the reason for the broken leg was that the patient was intoxicated and fell down the stairs, this might be considered to be defamation of character.

MALPRACTICE INSURANCE

Because of the increase in the number of malpractice suits generally, and against nurses in particular, many authorities now recommend that each nurse carry her own malpractice insurance to cover the cost of lawyers' fees and possible damages. The American Nurses' Association and several of the provincial nursing associations in Canada have made malpractice insurance available to their members at a reasonable cost.

Many nurses are under the mistaken belief that, because they are employees, their employer will carry the burden of responsibility for their negligent actions.

This is not so; the nurse can be sued as an individual.

WILLS

Nurses are often asked to witness the will of a patient. A will is a declaration of an individual's wishes regarding what is to be done with his property after his death.[29] The individual making the will is called the *testator*. A will must ordinarily be in writing and must be signed by the testator. The law usually requires the signature of two or three competent witnesses in addition. An individual who may expect to benefit from a will should not act as a witness to the signing of that will. The family and close friends of a patient are naturally reluctant, then, to be witnesses, and the nurse is frequently called upon to act in this capacity since she is a disinterested party. The nurse should not agree to act as a witness, however, if she is a minor. Minors, that is, persons under the legal age as defined by the law of the particular state or province, are not usually acceptable as witnesses.

In most jurisdictions, it is required that all witnesses be present at the same time and that they sign the will in the presence of the person making it. The witness should see the testator sign the will before signing it himself. If, however, the will has already been signed, the witness should either ask the testator to sign again or to declare that this is his will and he has signed it. In affixing his signature to a will, the witness indicates that he has either seen the person sign the document or that the testator has declared to him that he has signed it, and that the testator was competent to sign.[30] It is not necessary for the witness to know the contents of the will, nor in most jurisdictions it is necessary for the witness to be told that the document is a will.

For a will to be valid, the person making it must be capable of understanding what he is doing. If the patient dies and

---

[28]Creighton, op. cit., pp. 149–152.

[29]Ibid., p. 191.
[30]Sarner, op. cit., p. 108.

the validity of the will is questioned, a nurse may be called upon to testify in court as to the mental capacity of the individual at the time the will was made, whether or not she acted as a witness to the will. If the nurse is aware that a patient has made a will while in hospital, it is a good practice for her to note on the patient's record the fact that a will was made, the date and time that it was signed, and the nurse's observations regarding the mental state of the patient at the time the will was made.[31]

NARCOTICS LEGISLATION

Another area of law in which the nurse is involved is the control and administration of narcotic drugs. In the United States, there are both federal and state laws controlling narcotics. The principal federal law is the Harrison Narcotic Law, which was enacted in 1941. In addition, almost all the states also have their own laws regarding narcotics, and most have adopted the Uniform State

---

[31]For a more detailed discussion about wills, the nurse is referred to: Creighton, op. cit., pp. 191–195, and Sarner, op. cit., pp. 107–112.

Narcotic Act. Both federal and state laws affect the nurse in her nursing practice.

In Canada, the federal drug act controlling narcotics is called the Opium and Narcotic Drug Act, enacted in 1960. Violations of this law are dealt with by the Royal Canadian Mounted Police. The Opium and Narcotic Drug Act of Canada is similar to the Harrison Narcotic Law in the United States, but the former is broader in scope in that it includes the control of barbiturate drugs. These laws control the use of such drugs as opium, coca leaves and any compound, salt or derivative or preparation of them, and isonipecaine. In the United States, marijuana has been added to this list in some states.

Under the Harrison law, the nurse can give narcotics under the direction or supervision of a duly licensed physician or dentist, but it is unlawful for her to have narcotic drugs in her possession. The attempt to obtain narcotic drugs by fraud or deceit is a violation of the law. Penalties for violation include fine or imprisonment or both. The nurse must be careful when handling narcotics to see that they have been ordered in writing by a duly licensed physician and that careful records of their use are kept.

STUDY VOCABULARY	Assault	Liable	Prudence
	Battery	Libel	Slander
	Crime	Malpractice	Testator
	Defamation	Negligence	Tort

BIBLIOGRAPHY

American Nurses' Association: Statement of Functions. *The American Journal of Nursing*, 54:868–871, 994–996, 1130, 1954.

American Nurses' Association: *Principles of Legislation Relating to Nursing Practice.* New York, Revised, 1958.

American Nurses' Association: Statement of Functions of the Licensed Practical Nurse. *The American Journal of Nursing*, 64:93, March, 1964.

Anderson, Betty Jane: Orderly Transfer of Procedural Responsibilities from Medical to Nursing Practice. *Nursing Clinics of North America*, 5:2: 311–319, June, 1970.

Canadian Nurses' Association: *Roles, Functions and Educational Preparation for the Practice of Nursing.* Ottawa, The Association, 1967.

Creighton, Helen: On the Witness Stand. *The American Journal of Nursing*, 57:1593–1595, December, 1957.

Creighton, Helen: *Law Every Nurse Should Know.* Second edition. Philadelphia, W. B. Saunders Company, 1970.

Donahue, J. C. (ed.): Symposium on the Nurse and the Law. *Nursing Clinics of North America,* 2:1:115–197, March, 1967.

Fillmore, Anna: The Visiting Nurse Service and the Law. *Nursing Outlook,* 12:28–32, June, 1964.

Gray, Kenneth G.: Law and Nursing. *The Canadian Nurse,* 60:545–548, June, 1964.

Hershey, Nathan: As Society's Views Change, Law Changes. *The American Journal of Nursing,* 67:2310–2312, November, 1967.

Hershey, Nathan: The Doctrine that Helps the Patient. *The American Journal of Nursing,* 68:120–121, January, 1968.

Hershey, Nathan: The Changing Law. *The American Journal of Nursing,* 69:120–123, January, 1969.

Hershey, Nathan: License Revocation, the Board of Nursing, and the Court. *The American Journal of Nursing,* 69:567–569, March, 1969.

Hershey, Nathan: Patient Record. Incident Reports. *The American Journal of Nursing,* 69:1931, September, 1969.

Lesnik, Milton J., and Bernice E. Anderson: *Nursing Practice and The Law.* Second edition. Philadelphia, J. B. Lippincott Company, 1955.

Sadusk, Joseph F.: Legal Implications of Changing Patterns of Practice. *The Journal of the American Medical Association,* 190:1135–1136, December 28, 1964.

Sarner, Harvey: *The Nurse and The Law.* Philadelphia, W. B. Saunders Company, 1968.

19 SUPPLEMENTARY NURSING FUNCTIONS

The nurse should be able to:

Name three component parts of a complete physical examination

List types of information usually included in the case history

Outline the nurse's responsibilities in assisting with the physical examination itself

Name nursing functions relative to the collection of specimens

Outline general responsibilities of the nurse when assisting with medical procedures—before, during and after the procedure.

Describe the purpose and procedure of each of the following diagnostic or therapeutic measures:
1. Lumbar puncture
2. Paracentesis
3. Thoracentesis
4. X-rays
5. Special x-ray examinations
6. Basal metabolic rate
7. Electrocardiography
8. Electroencephalography

Outline specific nursing responsibilities in assisting with each of these measures

List criteria for the evaluation of the effectiveness of nursing measures

234

INTRODUCTION

In some functions the nurse acts as an assistant, supplementing the services of other members of the health team, such as the dietitian, the radiologist and the pathologist. These specialists contribute their particular talents to patients' care, but their presence on the nursing unit tends to produce a fragmentation of therapy which can be confusing and anxiety producing to patients. The nurse performs an integrative function relative to these various services; she helps the patient to participate in tests and she supplements and assists other health team members.

Examinations and diagnostic tests create a good deal of anxiety in many people. Frequently this anxiety is most directly concerned with the results of the tests, which can mean life or death to the patient. In present ethical practice, the nurse does not give the patient the results of his examinations or tests. This is a function of the physician. The nurse, however, can provide the patient with explanations and reassurance before, during and after many procedures so as to allay fear and lend emotional support.

In a study of what patients want to know about their diagnostic tests, it was found that knowledge of what the results meant in terms of treatment and prognosis was of paramount importance.[1] Patients also wanted to know the reasons for the test and when they would know the results. The nurse can lend support by reiterating what the physician has said about the "whys" of the test and by giving the patient general information which he feels he needs. Thus, she can explain how the procedure is carried out in terms that patients understand and find helpful. She can also assist them in their need to help by explaining what they can do before, during and after the test in order to facilitate the procedure. Moreover, the nurse can communicate her understanding of the patient's need to have confidence in the members of the health team.

THE PHYSICAL EXAMINATION

A physical examination is generally carried out by the doctor in an office, clinic or hospital. Although most people have had a physical examination at some time, it should not be assumed that patients do not require any explanation from the nurse. If a patient does not know the physician, he may be unduly fearful; in such instances the nurse can introduce the doctor and the patient and perhaps explain why the patient requires an examination at this time. Also, since the patient is often fearful about what the physician will find when he examines him, support and understanding from the nurse at this time is particularly important.

There are usually three parts to the examination: the case history, the physical examination itself and special tests. The *case history* includes both the

---

[1] Alice Dlouhy et al.: What Patients Want to Know About Their Diagnostic Tests. *Nursing Outlook,* 11:265–267, April, 1963.

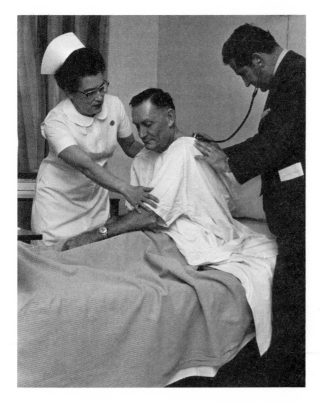

One of the nurse's functions during a physical examination is to provide the reassurance and assistance that the patient requires.

personal and medical history of the patient. The physician will want to know about the patient's present complaints as well as previous illnesses. The personal history is investigated without using interrogation. It includes the patient's social, religious, educational and economic backgrounds as well as his feelings of achievement and frustration. Habits of nutrition, sleeping patterns, bowel habits, and, for women, the nature of the menstrual cycle are usually included in the history taken by the physician. Habits such as drinking alcohol and smoking may also be relevant.

The patient's family history can also be pertinent to his present illness. Some diseases are inherited and some tend to recur in families. Also, with the recognition of psychosomatic illness and an understanding of the reactions of the body to stress, the neuropsychiatric history of the patient has become important (see Chapter 3).

The *physical examination* proceeds from the head to the feet of the patient,

with the findings being described in some detail. For the physical examination the physician requires the following equipment: stethoscope, otoscope (for examining the ears and nose), ophthalmoscope (for examining the eyes), percussion hammer, tongue blades, scales, tape measure, sphygmomanometer cuff and dial, and a clinical thermometer. Usually these instruments are kept in a central place in the nursing unit of the hospital.

The responsibilities of the nurse involve assisting both the patient and the physician with the physical examination. Most patients need some explanation about the examination and its purpose. The patient must undress and may require assistance putting on the gown provided; the gown is removed during parts of the examination. In a hospital, where the patient generally lies in bed for the examination, a bath blanket is put over him. Patients require privacy and warmth.

Generally, the nurse does not stay during the entire physical examination;

however, she should know whether the patient wants her to stay or whether she will be needed to drape the patient. Many agencies and physicians ask that a female nurse always be present during a vaginal examination of a female patient. The reason for this is twofold: it contributes to the comfort of the patient and eliminates the possibility of unjust accusations against the physician.

The physical examination includes the taking of vital signs, observation of the general physical and emotional status, and a general inspection of posture, skin, head, eyes, ears, nose, mouth, throat, neck (including thyroid gland and lymph nodes), chest and lungs, heart, breasts, abdomen, genitalia, extremities, back and spine, nervous system and rectum. When the physician examines the external genitalia and rectum of the male patient, the nurse (if female) usually leaves.

As part of the physical examination the physician may need to carry out a rectal examination or a vaginal examination. For a rectal examination the patient assumes the Sims position and is draped so that only the rectal area is exposed (see Chapter 13). The physician needs a rectal glove, lubricant and kidney basin. He inserts his lubricated gloved finger into the patient's rectum, palpating for abnormalities such as hemorrhoids and fissures. For a vaginal examination the physician requires rubber gloves, lubricant, a vaginal speculum, kidney basin and a good light. This equipment is sterilized after use in order to prevent the transmission of infection. The patient assumes the lithotomy position with or without stirrups (see Chapter 13). The drape permits the exposure of only the perineal area. The physician may also want a tongue blade and a microscopic slide in order to take a sample of the cervical secretions, which are then sent to the laboratory for examination for abnormal cells. This is called a Papanicolaou smear.

The third aspect of the patient's examination comprises the *special tests* and examinations that the patient requires in order to augment the findings of the general physical examination.

THE COLLECTION OF SPECIMENS

Frequently, the nurse is responsible for collecting specimens from patients. These may include specimens of blood, urine, sputum and drainage from wounds. For these tests, patients usually need explanations as to what they can do to help. Most patients like to be able to assist, and often the success of a test is dependent upon the patient's willingness to provide a specimen or perform some activity at a particular time.

When the nurse collects specimens, her functions include:

1. Explaining to the patient and gaining his cooperation
2. Collecting the right amount of specimen at the correct time
3. Placing the specimen in the correct container
4. Labeling the container accurately (This usually includes the patient's full name and registration number, the date, the physician's name, and if in a hospital the number of the nursing unit.)
5. Completing the laboratory requisition (This specifies what tests are to be carried out and gives pertinent data about the patient.)
6. Charting anything unusual about the appearance of the specimen

GUIDES TO ASSISTING WITH MEDICAL PROCEDURES

Before the Procedure

1. Prepare the patient.
   a. Explain the procedure beforehand.
   b. Explain how the patient can help with the examination.
   c. Be guided by the physician in discussing the significance of the test.
   d. Provide privacy.
   e. Drape the patient for his comfort and to facilitate the test.
   f. Help the patient to assume the best position for the test.
2. Prepare the equipment.

PLEASE INDICATE [X]
TEST REQUIRED BY

RIVERSIDE HOSPITAL
OF OTTAWA

LAB. NO.

NOV 4 71

NORTH   JANE   SP 1249
223 TREE RD   OTT   234-7566-600
NORTH   RICHARD   HUS
SAME
1.9.71 1PM   F 30 M SURG   RC
      420   1

☐ CBC
INCLUDES Ht, WBC,
DIFFERENTIAL AND R B C
MORPHOLOGY

☒ HEMOGLOBIN *12* g%   ☒ HEMATOCRIT *39* %

☒ WBC COUNT *7,000*   X 1000/CU MM

☐ DIFFERENTIAL

☐ RBC MORPHOLOGY

PROVISIONAL DIAGNOSIS *Cataract Extraction*

STABS, BANDS _____ %
NEUTROPHILS _____ %
LYMPHOCYTES _____ %
MONOCYTES _____ %
EOSINOPHILS _____ %
BASOPHILS _____ %
_____ %
_____ %
_____ %

☒ SED RATE *10*   mm/h

☐ INDICES   MCV   cµ
RBC COUNT   MCHC   %
         10⁶/cu mm   MCH   µµg

☐ RETICULOCYTE COUNT   %

☐ PLATELET COUNT   X1000/cu mm

☐ PROTHROMBIN TIME
PATIENT_____ SEC. _____ %
CONTROL _____ SEC. _____ %

☐ BLEEDING TIME _____ min.
☐ CLOTTING TIME _____ min.
☐ CLOT RETRACTION _____

☐ FLUIDS _____
RBC   POLYS   %
WBC   LYMPHS   %

☐ PARTIAL THROMBOPLASTIN TIME
PATIENT _____ SEC.
CONTROL _____ SEC.

DR. PIERRE FOURNIER, CHIEF
DEPT. OF PATHOLOGY   DATE *Sept 2/71*

HAEMATOLOGY REPORT   6100

A sample laboratory report for routine blood examination. (Courtesy of the Riverside Hospital of Ottawa.)

a. Obtain all the equipment for the test.
b. Maintain the sterility of equipment before and during the test as necessary.
c. Obtain the containers necessary for specimens and label them.
3. Prepare the environment.
   a. Close the windows and eliminate drafts.
   b. Provide privacy.
   c. Place equipment so that it is convenient for the doctor.
   d. Provide a chair for the doctor when indicated.

During the Procedure

1. Provide emotional support for the patient and help him to cooperate in the test.

2. Provide physical support for the patient while he is maintaining a position.
3. Assist the doctor with the equipment as necessary.
4. Observe the patient for his reactions to the test.

After the Procedure

1. Carry out nursing care measures for the patient's comfort and to prevent complications.
2. Observe the patient closely for untoward reactions.
3. Chart the necessary information in the patient's record.
4. Send labeled specimens to the laboratory.
5. Clean and dispose of equipment as necessary.

LUMBAR PUNCTURE

A lumbar puncture is the introduction of a needle into the subarachnoid space for diagnostic or therapeutic purposes. Frequent diagnostic purposes of the lumbar puncture are to obtain a specimen of cerebrospinal fluid for examination, to measure the pressure of the cerebrospinal fluid and to inject air or dye into the subarachnoid space preparatory to taking x-rays of the brain and spinal cord. Therapeutically a lumbar puncture is done either to remove cerebrospinal fluid and thereby to reduce the pressure, or to inject medications or anesthetics directly into the subarachnoid space.

The site of the lumbar puncture is usually between the third and fourth or the fourth and fifth lumbar vertebrae. This level is below the spinal cord, and therefore there is no danger of injury to the cord upon the insertion of the needle.

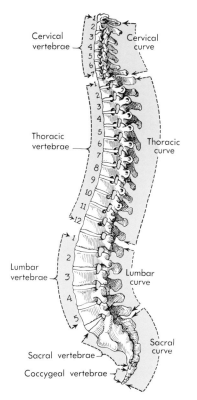

The sites for a lumbar puncture are the third or fourth intervertebral lumbar spaces.

The subarachnoid space normally contains cerebrospinal fluid, which is a clear colorless liquid. The fluid formed, chiefly by the choroid plexuses in the ventricles or the brain, circulates between the ventricles, the cisterna around the brain and the subarachnoid space. Almost all the cerebrospinal fluid is absorbed into the blood stream through the arachnoidal granulations which project into the subarachnoid spaces. The normal cerebrospinal pressure is between 70 and 200 mm. of water when the subject is in a horizontal position. A person usually has approximately 100 ml. of fluid, which is normally sterile.

In helping a patient prepare for a lumbar puncture, the nurse explains what the patient can expect and what he can do to facilitate the procedure. Since the patient is often anxious about a lumbar puncture, the nurse can reassure her that there is usually very little discomfort. The physician uses a local anesthetic at the site of the entry in order to decrease discomfort. Most frequently the patient is asked to lie on her side with her back near the edge of the bed. Her knees are brought up to her chest in order to accentuate the lumbar curve, thus enlarging the intravertebral spaces. It is important that the patient does not move during the procedure because of the chance of dislodging the needle.

The lumbar puncture is a sterile procedure. The equipment that the physician requires usually includes sterile sponges, disinfectant, syringes, needles (Nos. 21 and 24), local anesthetic, mask, sterile gloves, lumbar puncture needles (Nos. 18 and 24, 2 to 5 inches long), specimen tubes as necessary, manometer to measure spinal fluid pressure, adaptors for needles and a discard container.

The patient is draped for comfort prior to the procedure. Many doctor's offices and health agencies have sterile fenestrated drapes which the physician puts over the lumbar area, thereby exposing only the site for the puncture. During the procedure itself the nurse can help the patient to maintain the

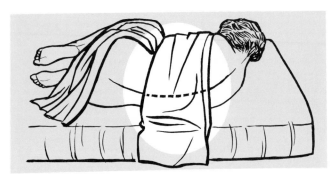

The position for a spinal puncture. Note the curvature of the lumbar region to increase the size of the intervertebral spaces.

proper position by placing her arms at the back of the patient's neck and behind the knees.

The physician applies a disinfectant and local anesthetic to the area. He then inserts the lumbar puncture needle into the intravertebral space. Usually the physician attaches the manometer to the spinal needle in order to obtain a spinal fluid pressure reading. The physician may also perform a Queckenstedt's test. To assist in this test, the nurse firmly compresses the internal jugular veins on both sides of the patient's neck. Normally the manometer will register a high pressure, because the

spinal fluid flow is impeded temporarily. In conditions in which there is already blockage of the canal, there will be no change in the spinal fluid pressure.

During a spinal puncture the patient is observed for signs of shock, nausea and vomiting. Shock can be demonstrated by sudden facial pallor, accelerated pulse rate, excessive perspiration and perhaps loss of consciousness. These can occur as a result of the lowering of the spinal fluid pressure or upon the administration of a drug intrathecally (into the spinal canal).

After the spinal puncture the doctor advises the patient about what position to maintain. It is not unusual to have the patient stay in a recumbent position for anywhere from one to 24 hours. There is a difference in medical opinion as to how long it takes to reestablish normal spinal fluid circulation.

A complication of a lumbar puncture that is seldom seen today is the spinal headache. If the patient does complain of a headache, the physician usually orders an analgesic for it.

After the lumbar puncture the nurse records in the chart the time; the procedure; the name of the doctor; the amount, color and consistency of the

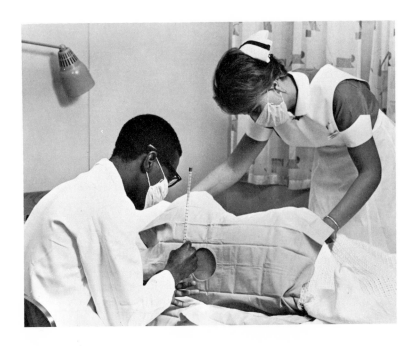

During a spinal puncture a manometer can be used to ascertain the spinal fluid pressure.

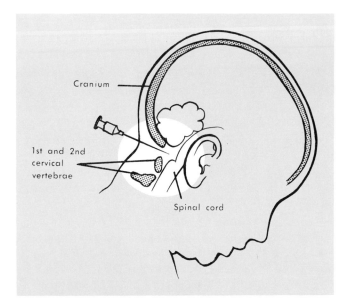

The site for a cisternal puncture is between the foramen magnum and the first cervical vertebra.

fluid; the initial and final pressures; the administration of medications and her observations of the patient.

The *cisternal puncture* is a variation of the lumbar puncture in which the physician inserts a needle into the subarachnoid space at the cisterna magna. The procedure is similar to the lumbar puncture except that the patient's neck is acutely flexed to permit insertion of the needle between the rim of the foramen magnum and the first cervical lamina. A cisternal puncture is sometimes done for a ventriculogram, which requires the injection of an opaque medium in order to visualize the ventricles of the brain on an x-ray. The nursing care measures are similar to those involved in a lumbar puncture.

PARACENTESIS

An abdominal paracentesis is the removal of fluid from the peritoneal cavity. When a large amount of fluid accumulates in this cavity, the condition is called ascites and the fluid is called ascitic fluid.

An abdominal paracentesis can be done for either diagnostic or therapeutic purposes. Diagnostically it is performed to obtain a specimen of fluid, which is sent to the laboratory for examination to detect abnormal cells and disease organisms. Evidence of abnormal cells may indicate the existence of a malignancy; the presence of disease organisms may indicate the etiology of an infectious process. In therapeutic paracentesis, fluid is usually removed from the peritoneal cavity in order to relieve pressure on the abdominal organs and the diaphragm.

Normally the peritoneal cavity contains just enough fluid to keep the peritoneum lubricated so that the surfaces are not irritated and friction does not result between the peritoneum and other surfaces. The fluid is normally sterile.

Prior to an abdominal paracentesis, the patient requires an explanation of what he can expect and what he can do to help. Most physicians explain the purpose of the test to their patients, and the nurse can be guided by his explanation in what she says about the purpose of the test. An abdominal paracentesis is usually not a painful procedure, but most physicians use a local anesthetic to minimize discomfort. Before the treatment is started the patient voids in order to empty his bladder. Failure to do this could result in puncturing the bladder with the trochar. If the patient cannot void, the physician should be told in advance of the procedure.

The best position for an abdominal paracentesis is a sitting position so that the force of gravity and pressure from

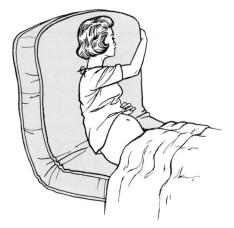

The patient assumes the Fowler's position for an abdominal paracentesis.

the abdominal organs can assist the outward flow of ascitic fluid. The usual site for the paracentesis is halfway between the umbilicus and symphysis pubis on the midline of the abdomen. An incision to either side is likely to puncture the colon. The patient is screened for privacy and draped for comfort.

Many hospitals have abdominal paracentesis sets which contain all the equipment that is needed for the procedure. The equipment usually includes local anesthetic and a syringe with No. 24 and No. 22 needles, trochar and cannula, rubber tubing which attaches to the cannula and guides the fluid to the container, sterile gloves, mask, disinfectant, sterile gauze sponges, suture material and containers for the specimens. The equipment must be sterile.

After the physician has painted the area with the disinfectant, he anesthetizes the place of entry with a local anesthetic. A small incision is then made and the trochar and cannula are inserted. The rubber tubing is attached to the cannula, the trochar is removed and the fluid is allowed to drain into the container provided (usually a large drainage bottle).

During the paracentesis the nurse observes the patient closely for any signs of shock, such as pallor, sweating, rapid pulse or syncope. These can occur particularly when the fluid drains quickly. Many physicians ask that a

stimulant such as Adrenalin be on hand during the procedure.

After the paracentesis is completed, a small dressing is placed over the incision. The wound may or may not be sutured. If the patient feels faint an abdominal binder can be applied after the procedure to provide support and comfort. The patient is observed frequently for several hours for any signs of shock, and if these do appear they are reported to the physician.

The nurse records in the patient's chart the time; the treatment; the name of the physician; the color, consistency and amount of fluid that was obtained; and the condition of the patient.

THORACENTESIS

A thoracentesis is the aspiration of fluid from the pleural cavity. Normally there is just enough fluid present to lubricate the pleura so that the lungs can move freely. Pleural fluid is serous. The pleural cavity is a potential space which under normal conditions does not contain any fluid or air except the few milliliters of pleural fluid. The pressure in the pleural cavity is normally negative (−4 mm. of mercury), and because of this the lungs are kept from collapsing.

A thoracentesis may be indicated for either diagnostic or therapeutic purposes. In a diagnostic thoracentesis, a specimen of pleural fluid is obtained in order to identify an infecting microorganism or the presence of abnormal cells. Therapeutically, a thoracentesis is performed to remove fluid which is causing pressure upon the chest organs or to remove air which is inhibiting respirations.

If the patient has not had a thoracentesis previously, he will need an explanation of the procedure beforehand. The patient usually assumes a sitting position so that the fluid collects at the bottom of the pleural cavity. He places his arm over his head or in front of his chest in order to extend the intercostal spaces. The patient is warned not to cough during the procedure, because

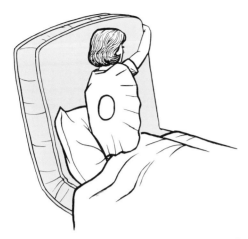

The patient assumes a sitting position with her arm across her chest in order to enlarge the intercostal spaces.

of the danger of the needle's becoming dislodged and piercing his lungs.

The equipment that is required for a thoracentesis consists of an aspirating set, an airtight drainage bottle, tubing, suction machine or pump in order to obtain a negative pressure within the drainage bottle, local anesthetic, syringe, sterile gloves, mask, and discard basin.

Before the doctor begins the thoracentesis the nurse establishes negative pressure in the drainage bottle in order to draw the fluid from the pleural cavity. Because there is some negative pressure within the pleural cavity it is necessary to have greater negative pressure in the drainage bottle before fluid can be drained. It is also essential to prevent air from getting into the pleural cavity because it produces pneumothorax and collapse of the lungs. Pneumothorax is the accumulation of gas or air in the pleural cavity. The thoracentesis needle has an attachable stopcock which can be opened and shut in order to prevent air from getting into the pleural cavity. A syringe can be attached to the stopcock to obtain fluid for laboratory examination.

After the patient assumes a sitting position and is draped comfortably, the physician wipes the area of insertion with disinfectant. The thoracentesis is

done below the surface level of the fluid, often in the frontal plane in line with the crest of the ilium. The doctor determines the level of the fluid by percussion. The area is locally anesthetized and then the long thoracentesis needle is inserted through the intercostal space into the pleural cavity. The tubing is connected to the stopcock and to the source of negative pressure, and upon a signal from the doctor the valves are opened to let the fluid flow into the drainage bottle.

During the procedure the nurse watches the patient carefully for any signs of respiratory distress, for example, cyanosis or dyspnea. If the fluid is removed quickly the patient may faint. Puncturing a blood vessel with the needle is a complication which can result in a lung hemorrhage.

After the needle is withdrawn, a sterile dressing is applied to the site. The patient is observed frequently for several hours after the thoracentesis for any signs of respiratory embarrassment. Damage to the lungs may be indicated by the presence of frothy, blood-tinged sputum (hemoptysis).

The nurse records on the patient's chart the time; treatment; name of the doctor, amount, color and consistency of the fluid obtained; and the condition of the patient. If the thoracentesis is successful therapeutically, the patient will probably find breathing easier because the fluid is no longer present to exert pressure upon his lungs.

X-RAYS

X-rays are used as diagnostic and therapeutic measures on almost every system of the body. In this century, with radiation such a highly publicized word, some people are afraid that x-rays are injurious. The nurse can safely reassure people that the amount of radiation received in an examination is limited. The nurse herself should be aware that radiation in excess can be dangerous, but it is unusual for patients to receive enough radiation to destroy tissue unless this is done therapeutically. The unit of measurement of x-ray dosage is the roentgen (R).

There are four methods of x-ray examination: visualizing a part of the body on photographic film, visualizing a part of the body on a fluoroscope screen, a combination of these two methods, and cinefluorography.

One of the important factors in taking x-rays is the position that the patient assumes. His position must be such that the part to be visualized is clearly outlined on the film. The nurse can help the patient to prepare for an x-ray examination by explaining that he may find it necessary to assume difficult and perhaps uncomfortable positions for short periods of time.

To x-ray some parts of the body, it is necessary to use a contrast medium so that cavities become radiopaque and thus show on the film or the fluoroscope screen. For the gastrointestinal tract, barium sulfate is the contrast medium used. To visualize the esophagus, stomach and duodenum, the patient drinks the barium; to visualize the colon and rectum, the barium is given as an enema.

For x-rays of the ventricles of the brain, oxygen is injected into the spinal canal; organic soluble iodides are used to visualize the gallbladder, urinary tract and blood vessels.

In preparing for abdominal x-ray examinations, it is frequently necessary for the patient to clear his gastrointestinal tract of fecal material. Usually the physician orders castor oil the night before, to be followed by a cleansing enema the day of the examination. Patients are generally asked not to take food or fluids after midnight of the night before an examination. Special attention should be given to expulsion of the barium after the x-ray studies are completed. An enema or cathartic may be ordered for the patient following the x-ray series.

SPECIAL X-RAY EXAMINATIONS

Intravenous pyelogram. The contrast media, for example, Diodrast, is injected intravenously and when it is excreted by the kidneys it outlines the kidney pelvices, calices, ureters and urinary bladder.

Retrograde pyelogram. The contrast media is introduced through ureteral catheters into the kidney pelvis to outline the urinary tract.

Cholecystogram. An x-ray examination of the gallbladder in which a radiopaque contrast media such as Telepaque is used.

Pneumoencephalogram. An x-ray examination of the ventricles and meningeal spaces of the brain in which air or oxygen is used as the contrast medium.

Ventriculogram. An x-ray examination of the ventricles of the brain in which air or oxygen is used as the contrast medium.

Myelogram. An x-ray examination of the subarachnoid space of the brain in which a contrast medium such as air is used.

Bronchogram. An x-ray examination of the bronchial tree in which an iodized oil is used as the contrast medium.

Hysterosalpingogram. An x-ray examination of the uterus and fallopian

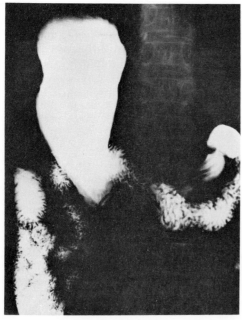

An x-ray showing barium sulfate filling the stomach and the first portion of the small bowel.

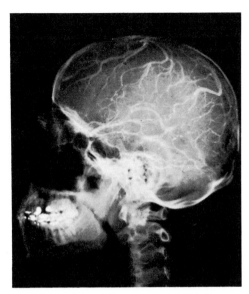

Cerebral angiogram. A radiopaque contrast medium shows the blood vessels of the brain. (J. L. Curry and W. J. Howland: Arteriography: Principles and Techniques. *Philadelphia, W. B. Saunders Company, 1966.)*

tubes in which a radiopaque contrast medium such as Lipiodol is used.

Cardioangiogram. An x-ray examination of the heart and great vessels in which a catheter introduced into one of the great vessels is used to administer contrast medium such as Hypaque.

Angiogram. An x-ray examination of the blood vessels in which a contrast medium such as Hypaque is used.

BASAL METABOLIC RATE

The basal metabolic rate (B.M.R.) as a test to reflect thyroid function is gradually being replaced by other tests of thyroid activity, such as the iodine uptake test in which I^{131} or radioactive iodine is used. Nevertheless basal metabolic rate tests are carried out in some clinical situations, and therefore people may need to be prepared for them.

The objective of the basal metabolic rate test is to determine the energy expended by the body at rest. In order to do this, oxygen consumption is meas-

ured; oxygen consumption is directly related to the rate of cell metabolism. In this test the patient is at rest both physically and psychologically. He does not take food after 9 P.M. or fluid after midnight the night before. Furthermore, he does not smoke prior to the test and he remains in a restful inactive state.

During the test the patient lies down and breathes in oxygen, which is usually provided through a mask. The amount of oxygen that he uses in a designated time is used in calculating the B.M.R.

ELECTROCARDIOGRAPHY

An electrocardiogram is a graphic representation of electrical impulses emitted by the heart. Although electrocardiography is a painless procedure, the idea of heart disease is anxiety producing in many people. Therefore, frequent reassurance and an explanation are necessary.

Electrocardiography is carried out in hospitals and doctor's offices by a technician or a doctor. Small electrodes are strapped on the patient's body in order to pick up the electrical impulses of the heart. A paste is used between the skin and the electrodes to facilitate the transfer of impulses.

ELECTROENCEPHALOGRAPHY

An electroencephalogram is a graphic representation of electrical impulses from the brain. Electroencephalography is similar to electrocardiography in principle, but it is usually done in a hospital laboratory. It is generally a painless procedure, but the patient is often sedated beforehand.

The patient assumes a resting position. Tiny electrodes are attached to his scalp, and to a machine. These electrodes pick up the electrical potentials produced by the brain cells and record them on a graph. Electroencephalography is a diagnostic measure to determine the presence of brain disease.

GUIDE TO ASSESSING NURSING NEEDS

1. What tests or examinations have been ordered for this patient?
2. What information should the patient have about these tests or examinations? What other preparation does he need?
3. Is the patient anxious about the test?
4. Does the family of the patient require reassurance or explanations about the tests?
5. What equipment is required for the test?
6. Are there specimens to be collected?
7. Is there a possibility that emergency equipment may be needed?
8. Are there measures to be followed after the test? Does the patient need instructions regarding these measures?

GUIDE TO EVALUATING THE EFFECTIVENESS OF NURSING ACTION

1. Is the patient comfortable?
2. Was the test or examination carried out successfully?
3. Were all specimens sent to the laboratory? Were they correctly labeled and in appropriate containers?
4. Has the test or examination been recorded on the patient's chart? Were pertinent observations noted?
5. Have all after-care measures been instituted? For example, should the patient be in a recumbent position?

STUDY VOCABULARY

Abdominal paracentesis	Lumbar puncture	Pneumothorax
Cisternal puncture	Manometer	Roentgen
Electrocardiogram	Ophthalmoscope	Subarachnoid
Electroencephalogram	Otoscope	Thoracentesis

STUDY SITUATION

You are a nurse in a doctor's office. A patient, Mr. Dawson, has been told by the doctor that he needs to have x-rays taken of his upper and lower gastrointestinal tract before his illness can be determined. Mr. Dawson does not appear to understand the doctor and, apprehensively, he asks you to explain.

Mr. Dawson is 37 years old, has had an eighth grade education and works on a fishing boat. For the past two weeks he has had periods of acute vomiting and diarrhea, which caused him to stop working and come to the doctor. He has a wife and four children at home.

1. What factors about this patient would you consider pertinent to your explanations?
2. What might Mr. Dawson need in the way of an explanation?
3. What should you explain about the x-ray examination?
4. How could you perhaps relieve some of his apprehension?
5. How could you evaluate whether your help has met Mr. Dawson's needs?

BIBLIOGRAPHY

Bonnell, G. E.: Urological Investigative Procedures. *Canadian Nurse*, 59: 825–828, September, 1963.

Dlouhy, Alice, et al.: What Patients Want to Know About Their Diagnostic Tests. *Nursing Outlook*, 11:265–267, April, 1963.

French, Ruth M.: *Nurse's Guide to Diagnostic Procedures*. New York, Blakiston Division, McGraw-Hill Book Company, 1962.

Garb, Solomon: *Laboratory Tests in Common Use*. Fourth edition. New York, Springer Publishing Company, 1966.

Guyton, Arthur C.: *Textbook of Medical Physiology*. Fourth edition. Philadelphia, W. B. Saunders Company, 1971.

Harmer, Bertha, and Virginia Henderson: *Textbook of the Principles and Practice of Nursing*. Fifth edition. New York, The Macmillan Company, 1960.

Specialized Diagnostic Laboratory Tests. Los Angeles, Bio-Sciences Laboratories, 1965.

Sutton, Audrey Latshaw: *Bedside Nursing Techniques in Medicine and Surgery*. Second edition. Philadelphia, W. B. Saunders Company, 1969.

20 HEAT AND COLD AS THERAPEUTIC AGENTS

The nurse should be able to:

List principles from the biophysical sciences relevant to the use of heat and cold as therapeutic agents

Explain reasons for the application of heat

Explain reasons for the application of cold

Describe the physiological effects of heat and cold on the body

Describe measures commonly used for the local application of heat to the body

Describe measures commonly used for the local application of cold to the body

Differentiate between irritants and counterirritants and give an example of each

INTRODUCTION

Applications of heat and cold as therapeutic measures are probably well known to the student before she commences her nursing education. Applying a hot water bottle or a heating pad to cold feet is a comfort familiar to many, particularly to those who live in cold climates. The application of ice as a means of stopping epistaxis (nosebleed) is a common therapeutic measure carried out in the home. In addition, rubbing the chest with a decongestant ointment or a liniment is a long-standing remedy for the treatment of colds in many families. Thus the student herself has probably already had firsthand experience with many of these therapeutic measures.

Generally speaking, applications of heat and cold are used in the hospital and the home as therapeutic measures. In the hospital, these measures are carried out at the direction of the physician. Occasionally heat and cold also serve as comfort measures. If this is the sole reason for their use, it is often left to the judgment of the nurse and patient whether and how to apply them. The nurse therefore needs a knowledge of the physiological reactions resulting from these measures and of the untoward reactions which may occur. If the nurse is ever in doubt about the use of heat or cold, she should consult the physician before she applies these measures.

Applications of heat and cold are also used in the course of physical medicine as part of rehabilitation programs. In these instances physical therapists use such measures as paraffin baths and whirlpool baths on the advice of the physician.

TYPES OF APPLICATIONS

Many different types of hot and cold applications can be used as therapeutic measures. Both heat and cold can be applied as dry treatments or as moist treatments, and the source can be varied according to the purpose. Moreover, irritants and counterirritants are not dissimilar in action to applications of heat. An irritant is a substance which, when applied to a patient's skin, produces a local inflammatory reaction through its chemical action. An irritant becomes a counterirritant when the purpose of its application is a reflex action in underlying tissues, that is, when the purpose of the treatment is to initiate a physiological reaction in tissues underlying the skin. Mustard is a common example of a counterirritant that has long been used in a local application (mustard plaster) to relieve congestion in the chest.

The choice of the kind of application that is to be used is dependent upon a number of factors:

1. The purpose of the application
2. The age of the patient and the condition of his skin
3. The general physical health of the patient

4. The area of the body that is affected
5. The duration of the treatment
6. The availability of equipment

PRINCIPLES RELATED TO THE APPLICATION OF HEAT AND COLD

The following principles serve as guides to the use of hot and cold applications:

1. Heat is distributed throughout the body by the circulating blood and by direct conduction throughout the tissues.
2. Heat is lost from the body chiefly through radiation and evaporation at the surface of the skin.
3. The amount of heat that is lost from the body is directly proportional to the amount of blood that is circulating close to the surface of the skin.
4. The amount of blood that circulates close to the surface of the skin is influenced by the dilatation and constriction of peripheral arterioles.
5. Applications of heat and cold influence the dilatation and constriction of peripheral blood vessels.
6. Moisture conducts heat better than air.
7. People vary in their ability to tolerate heat and cold. People at both extremes of the age spectrum, that is, the very old and the very young, are particularly sensitive to heat and cold.
8. People become less sensitive to repeated applications of heat and cold.
9. The length of time of exposure to extremes in temperature affects the body's tolerance of the temperature.

The temperature at the surface of the skin of the torso is generally 33.9° C. (93° F.). Applications at this temperature are usually undifferentiated as either cold or hot, but applications that are 11.1° C. (20° F.) below or 8.3° C. (15° F.) above this level excite cutaneous nerve fibers. Local tolerance is thought to range between 4.4° C. (40° F.) and 43.3° C. (110° F.). Generally any application that is above or below these levels can be the cause of tissue damage.

REASONS FOR THE APPLICATION OF HEAT

Heat is applied to the body for any of several reasons. It can be applied to produce a local or systemic effect or both. A local effect is one that is specific to a defined area of the body, for example, to relieve local muscle spasm. A systemic effect is one that is reflected in the body as a whole, for example, general warmth felt throughout the body.

Heat is known to relieve pain. Thus pain that is caused by the contraction of muscle fibers is relieved when the muscle spasm is reduced by heat. Heat also increases circulation to an area and can thereby relieve the pain of ischemia (lack of blood). Sometimes the collection of fluid in an area can cause pain because of the increased pressure. By applying heat, blood circulation is increased and the pain is relieved as fluid absorption is hastened. Toxins and waste products are also thought to be causes of discomfort which can be relieved by an increase in blood circulation to the irritated tissues.

The fact that heat helps to alleviate many types of pain does not mean that it is indicated for all instances of pain. Heat can hasten the suppurative (pus-forming) process, and in the case of an inflamed appendix it could cause the appendix to rupture. Although the physician supplies the directions regarding the application of heat, the nurse must always be aware of the purpose of the treatment and alert to possible untoward actions. There is, for instance, always a danger that a burn may result from the local application of heat, or that deeper-lying tissues may be affected and, for example, an inflammatory process may be aggravated. Inflammation is the reaction of tissues to injury; it is characterized by pain, swelling, redness and local heat.

Heat increases circulation to the area of the body to which it is applied. It therefore can be applied to improve the oxygenation and nourishment of tissues, thus aiding tissue metabolism and subsequent healing. For example, heat applied to an infected surgical incision not only hastens suppuration, but it increases the nourishment of the tissue cells and the healing process. Improved circulation in this case also enhances the elimination of toxic and waste substances via the blood stream.

Swelling can also be reduced by the application of heat. As blood circulation improves, fluid is more easily absorbed from the tissues and consequently swelling or edema is reduced. Frequently hot applications to a swollen area, such as the ankle, are alternated with cold applications, because heat and cold are most effective while the temperature of the area is changing. The cold in this instance reduces the flow of fluid to the swollen area.

A hot drink is known to have the effect of intensifying peristalsis. Peristalsis is the wavelike contraction of the muscles of the digestive tract which propels its contents along. This increased peristalsis can be utilized to help a patient establish regular defecation habits. For example, one-half hour after drinking coffee for breakfast the patient is encouraged to try to defecate so as to utilize the mass peristalsis stimulated by the hot fluid.

Another purpose of applying heat locally is to soften exudates. An exudate is a discharge produced by the body tissues. Sometimes the discharge from an open wound forms hardened crusts over the area. Hot moist compresses are often used to soften these crusts so they can be easily removed. It has already been mentioned that heat is also used as a comfort measure. It can be used to promote the relaxation of skeletal muscles and thereby to promote general comfort and rest.

REASONS FOR THE APPLICATION OF COLD

Cold is applied to the body for both systemic and local effects. For systemic purposes, cold is applied to slow the basal metabolic rate. This is indicated in certain kinds of heart surgery, because a low basal metabolic rate results in a lessened demand of the body tissues for oxygen and nourishment and thus decreases the work of the heart. For a similar reason a patient's limb may be packed in ice prior to amputation. The cold slows the speed of the circulation of the blood and thus enables the surgeon to control bleeding more easily during the operation.

Cold can also be applied to stop hemorrhage, since it constricts the peripheral arterioles and increases the viscosity of the blood, in addition to contracting the muscles and depressing cardiac action. The nurse often sees ice bags applied routinely to patients after a tonsillectomy as a prophylactic measure against hemorrhage.

Cold applications slow the suppurative process and the absorption of tissue fluids. They also reduce swelling, such as that in epididymitis (an inflammation of the epididymis), and slow other inflammatory processes, for example, inflammation of the eye.

Because cold contracts the peripheral blood vessels, it raises the blood pressure. This is more usually a side effect rather than the sole reason for cold applications.

Pain can also be relieved through the use of cold applications. Cold restricts the movement of the blood and tissue fluids; therefore it relieves pain caused by an increased amount of fluid moving into the tissues, as in the case of a sprain. In addition, intense cold numbs pain receptors. As a result cold is used as a local anesthetic. There is, however, a danger in the prolonged use of intense cold: it interferes with the supply of oxygen and nourishment to the tissues and may result in tissue death.

THE PHYSIOLOGICAL EFFECTS OF HEAT AND COLD

Heat and cold are relative degrees of temperature dependent to some extent upon the perception of the individual. The temperature at the surface of the skin of the torso is generally 33.9° C. (93° F.). It is thought that a temperature of 8.3° C. (15° F.) or more above this level stimulates the thermal nerve endings in the skin.

Temperature is perceived in gradations: cold to cool, indifferent and warm to hot. Different areas of the body have varying sensitivity to changes in heat and cold. For example, the back of the hand is not particularly sensitive to changes in temperature. Also, people perceive the temperature more acutely when the temperature of the skin is changing. That is why a hot bath feels hotter at first than it does after the skin becomes adjusted to it. Extremes in temperature, both hot and cold, are perceived as painful (see Chapter 28).

Effects of Heat

Heat is transferred by conduction, convection and radiation. Conduction is the passage of heat from molecule to molecule as through a metal. Convection refers to the transfer of heat in the same manner but through liquid or air. Radiation requires no medium; it is the passage of heat in the form of electromagnetic waves through space; the transfer of heat by radiation may be perceived by holding one's hands in front of an open fire. An insulator is a substance which inhibits the transfer of heat; for example, clothes act to keep the heat of the body from escaping.

When heat is applied locally to the skin surface, it stimulates receptors in the free sensory nerve endings. Impulses are then initiated which travel via the lateral spinothalamic tracts to the preoptic centers in the anterior hypothalamus, from which they are relayed to the cerebral cortex. The anterior hypothalamus acts to decrease the amount of heat production and increase the amount of heat loss.

Heat production is decreased by slowing the metabolic rate and decreasing the muscle tone. Heat loss is increased by stimulating the sweat glands and promoting vasodilatation of the arterioles near the skin surface. Vasoconstriction of the surface arterioles is inhibited through impulses from the posterior hypothalamus.

Not all impulses from the skin surface go to the brain; some make a reflex arc at the spinal cord and return to the skin. This reflex action accounts for some vasodilatation and sweating at the place of the application of heat.

As a result of these physiological reactions, reddening of the skin and sweating are observed. Through the stimuli to the cerebral cortex, the patient becomes aware of the heat applied to his body; however, he becomes less sensitive to heat if its application is prolonged. This can be dangerous, for the patient may be unaware of tissue damage because his sensitivity to the heat is dulled.

Because of local vasodilatation the blood is often diverted from an underlying vital center. This explains why some people feel faint (syncope) when they get into a hot bath; the blood is diverted from the brain to the skin surface.

The application of intense heat (over 45°C.) to the body causes pain. This calls forth a generalized alarm reaction —the body's response to any stimulus perceived as threatening (see Chapter 3). As a result, there is a vasoconstriction of the surface blood vessels and the nurse will observe a whiteness of the skin due to this vasoconstriction.

Effects of Cold

Bierman, in his article, "The Therapeutic Use of Cold," has suggested four degrees of cold:[1]

Tepid	26.2–33.9° C.	80–93° F.
Cool	18.3–26.7° C.	65–80° F.
Cold	12.8–18.3° C.	55–65° F.
Very cold	Below 12.8° C.	Below 55° F.

The application of a moderate degree of cold to the skin surface stimulates the cold receptors in the skin. These

[1]William Bierman: Therapeutic Use of Cold. *The Journal of the American Medical Association,* 157:1189, April 2, 1955.

stimuli travel via the lateral spino-thalamic nerves to the posterior hypo-thalamus and then are relayed to the cerebral cortex. In this latter area the awareness of the cold takes place.

As a reaction to the application of cold, the body endeavors to increase heat production and decrease heat loss. Heat production is increased by con-traction of the muscles. Even the erector pili muscles of the skin contract to cause the goose flesh seen in a person who is cold. Muscle contraction increases heat production by increasing the basal metabolic rate. The decrease in heat loss is accomplished by vasoconstric-tion of the arterioles. The skin takes on a bluish white appearance due to vaso-constriction and the subsequent venous congestion. The skin surface feels cooler not only at the site of application but also at remote areas. The patient's skin also becomes less sensitive and he complains of a numbing sensation. Cold therefore has anesthetic value, which is put to use during minor surgery, as when portions of tissue are frozen by means of ethyl chloride.

The application of cold decreases the rate of tissue metabolism, thus decreas-ing the demands upon the heart for food and oxygen. Cold also increases the viscosity of blood and as a result slows its rate of flow.

LOCAL APPLICATIONS OF HEAT

Heat can be applied to a patient as radiant heat, conductive heat or con-versive heat. Radiant heat is heat whose wavelength is in the infrared portion of the electromagnetic spectrum.[2] Conduc-tive heat is heat transferred by direct application, for example, by a hot water bottle or hot compresses. Conversive heat is heat converted from primary sources of energy, for example, from short wave or ultrasound wave energy.

---

[2]Howard A. Rusk: *Rehabilitation Medicine.* Second edition. St. Louis, The C. V. Mosby Company, p. 79.

The application of this latter type of heat is classified as medical diathermy; it is utilized to provide heat to deep tissues. Radiant and conductive heat provide heat to the superficial tissues only.

Both moist and dry forms of heat can be applied to the skin or mucous mem-branes. Usually it is necessary to apply superficial heat for 20 to 30 minutes in order to obtain the desired effect. Dry heat up to 58° C. (135° F.), as in the form of a hot water bottle, can be ap-plied safely to the skin of most adults, provided that circulation and sensation are intact. For patients who are debili-tated, who have impaired circulation or who are unconscious, 50° C. (120° F.) is considered safe. Because children's tissues are more easily damaged than are the tissues of adults, 50° C. (120° F.) is also considered desirable for chil-dren.

Since patients become accustomed to heat after prolonged applications, they should be cautioned against turning up a heating pad or refilling a hot water bottle without checking the tempera-ture. All patients are observed closely for any untoward reactions to heat ap-plications, such as a prolonged eryth-ema (redness), blister formation or discomfort.

The Hot Water Bottle

The hot water bottle has long been a vehicle for applying dry heat to the body. It is used as both a therapeutic and a comfort measure, although thera-peutically its use is being surpassed by the electrical heating pad.

The water for a hot water bottle is tested for its exact temperature. It has already been explained that 58° C. (135° F.) is generally considered to be a desirable temperature for an adult whose sensations and circulation are intact. A temperature of 50° C. (120° F.) is considered safe for children and for adults who are unconscious or debili-tated or who have impaired circulation. The water for a hot water bottle can usually be obtained from the hot water tap; its temperature is checked by the thermometers that most hospitals provide for measuring the temperature of unsterile solutions.

The hot water bottle is filled one-half to two-thirds full, and the air is expelled from the remainder of the bottle by pressing the sides together before the top is applied. In this way the hot water bottle remains fairly light and is easily molded to the patient's body.

After the outside of the hot water bottle has been dried, it is tested for leakage and then placed in a cloth cover before it is taken to the patient. The cover slows the transmission of heat, absorbs perspiration and thereby lessens the danger of burning. The stopper of the hot water bottle is well covered, because it can become sufficiently hot that on direct contact it will burn a person's skin.

The hot water bottle is placed on the desired area and molded to the patient's body. If the hot water bottle is given to a person who burns easily, it is wise to place a sheet or blanket between the person and the bottle. When continuous heat is to be applied, it is usually necessary to change the hot water bottle every one and a half to two hours in order to maintain the desired temperature.

When hot water bottles are not in use they are hung upside down with the top unscrewed. This allows the bottle to dry inside and prevents the sides of the bottles from sticking together.

The Electric Pad

Electric pads and electric blankets are becoming increasingly popular as a means of providing dry heat. They have the advantages of being light, of being easily molded to the patient's body and of providing constant heat. Their disadvantages are related to cleaning and to the danger of short circuits, particularly when they are used with oxygen equipment. The heating pads that are used in hospitals are frequently covered with a plastic material that can be easily and effectively cleaned. It is often pos-

sible to lock the mechanism for setting the temperature of the heating pad so that it cannot be changed without the nurse being aware of it.

The Infrared Lamp

The infrared lamp, which supplies radiant heat, is used to provide heat to a localized area of the body. Infrared radiation penetrates 3 mm. of tissue at the most; thus it provides surface heat only.

The action of infrared heat is to increase blood circulation (hyperemia), thereby increasing the supply of oxygen and nourishment to the tissues. An infrared lamp is frequently ordered by the physician in the treatment of decubitus ulcers. It is also often used in obstetrical and gynecological cases to promote the healing of a suture area on the perineum.

Before applying heat from an infrared lamp, the nurse observes that the patient's skin is dry and clean. This lessens the danger of burning the skin. A small infrared lamp is placed 45 to 60 cm. (18 to 24 inches) from the area of skin that is to be treated; a larger lamp is placed 60 to 75 cm. (24 to 30 inches) away. The heat is provided for from 15 to 20 minutes, but the patient is checked after the first five minutes to make sure that he is not being burned. At the end of the treatment the patient's skin is generally moist, warm and pink.

The danger in the use of the infrared lamp is that the patient will be burned. The nurse should frequently observe the patient's reaction to the application of infrared heat and terminate the treatment at the first sign of reddening or pain. In addition the patient should be warned that the lamp will become hot after it has been on for a few minutes. Placing an infrared lamp under the bedclothes is inadvisable because of the danger of fire.

The "Baker" (Heat Cradle)

The "baker" is another means of providing radiant heat. In this case the heat is less localized; it is often applied to large areas, such as the abdomen, chest or legs. The baker is a metal cradle into which are installed several electrical sockets for luminous bulbs. The metal acts to reflect the heat from the bulbs toward the patient. Often the baker is covered by the top bedding in order to hold in the heat and to prevent cooling by the circulating air. The temperature of the baker shoud not exceed 52° C. (125° F.).

Steam Inhalations

In the care of patients with respiratory conditions, steam inhalations are frequently used to loosen congestion and to help liquefy secretions. Both hot and cold steam are used. The topic of inhalations is discussed in Chapter 25, The Care of Patients Who Have Dyspnea.

The Hot Compress

Hot compresses, which utilize the principle of heat conduction, can be either sterile or unsterile moist applications. Generally gauze is soaked in the solution designated by the physician, the excess fluid is wrung out of the gauze and then the gauze is applied to the specified body surface. The compress should be moist but not so wet that the solution drips from it. Sterile precautions are indicated when the compress is to be applied to an open wound or to an organ such as the eye. In such cases, sterile gauze is soaked in a sterile or antiseptic solution, and sterile forceps or sterile gloved hands are used to wring out the compress. The compress is applied at the hottest temperature that the patient can tolerate. Frequently an insulating waterproof cloth is placed over the compress in order to hold in the heat. In some situations heating pads or hot water bottles are placed over the compress to provide additional heat.

Hot compresses are often indicated to hasten the suppurative process and to improve the circulation of blood to the tissues. Normal saline and antiseptic solutions are frequently ordered by the physician.

Compresses generally retain heat poorly, the length of time that they remain hot being somewhat dependent upon the thickness of the material, the temperature of the solution, and the use of insulating materials. Ordinarily compresses are ordered every hour or every two hours; however, if constant applications of hot moist compresses are ordered, the nurse or the patient should change them every 10 to 15 minutes.

The Hot Pack

A hot pack, which is sometimes referred to as a hot fomentation or foment, is a piece of heated moist flannel that is applied to a patient's skin in order to provide superficial moist heat. Because intense heat can be applied in this manner there is a danger that the patient may be burned. This danger is minimized if the hot pack is sufficiently dry that water does not drip from it.

A hot pack can be prepared by boiling or steaming pieces of flannel or by heating commercially prepared packs. If the flannel is boiled it is necessary to wring it out before applying it. There are hot pack machines available which steam the flannel to prepare it for application. Once the foment has been heated it is applied directly to the patient as hot as he can tolerate it. If the hot pack is shaken slightly before it is applied there is little danger of burning the patient and it is more comfortable for him. Sometimes petrolatum is applied to the skin beforehand to serve as a protective coating and to slow the transfer of heat. The hot foment is covered with an insulating waterproof material and then secured to the patient with a towel or binder. Often a hot water bottle or heating pad is applied over this to provide additional heat.

A hot pack usually keeps hot for 10 to 15 minutes. Once it has cooled it is removed and, if continuous heat is required, it is replaced with another pack. If the patient does not need another application for some time, his skin is dried.

Hot packs are frequently indicated to relieve muscle spasm, as when a patient has poliomyelitis. They are also applied to hasten the suppurative process and to decrease muscle soreness.

Upon the application of a hot pack, an erythema of the skin is to be expected as a result of the vasodilatation of the local blood capillaries. Blistering of the skin should be avoided.

Body Soaks

Body soaks and arm and foot soaks are therapeutic measures ordered by the physician to provide warmth or to apply a solution to cleanse an area of the body. Generally they are indicated to hasten suppuration, to cleanse an open wound or to apply a medicated solution to a designated area.

Special portable containers, including both arm and foot baths, are available commercially for this purpose. These containers can be sterilized in order to provide a sterile environment when one is indicated, as when burned areas need to be soaked.

The solution for a body soak is ordered by the physician. Often sterile normal saline or sterile water is used. The temperature of the solution should be 47.2° C. (115° F.) unless otherwise ordered by the physician for a specific reason.

The patient's dressings are removed and his limb is immersed gradually into the solution. The dressings may need to be soaked before removal to avoid trauma to the tissues. The limb is immersed slowly in order to acclimatize the patient to the temperature of the solution. The patient assumes a comfortable position during the treatment to avoid fatigue and muscle strain. The length of the treatment is usually 20 minutes. The temperature of the solution is checked every five minutes, and additional solution is supplied when necessary. After the soaking is completed, the patient's limb is dried and dressings are replaced as necessary.

If the patient has an open wound, aseptic technique is carried out. The container, the solution and the towels are sterile. In some agencies, the nurse wears a mask when carrying out this procedure. Sterile dressings are applied after the soak (see Chapter 22).

During and after soaking an area of the body the nurse observes the condition of the patient's wound and the amount and character of any discharge. It is expected that the heat of the solution will cause some vasodilatation and erythema and that the solution itself will cleanse and soften exudates. These observations are then recorded.

The Therapeutic Bath

Therapeutic baths are provided to supply warmth, to cleanse and to apply a medication. They are indicated chiefly for people who have skin diseases or who have had certain kinds of perineal or rectal surgery.

The solutions that are used are ordered by the physician; the most common are saline, tap water, sodium bicarbonate, starch and oatmeal. The last three, often called colloid baths, can now be purchased commercially in special preparations.

The temperature for the therapeutic bath can vary from 4.4° C. to 47.2° C. (40° F. to 115° F.). The temperature ranges of the baths are generally classified as follows:

Hot bath	40.6–47.2° C.	105–115° F.
Warm bath	38.9–40.6° C.	100–105° F.
Tepid bath	36.7° C.	98° F.
Cold bath	4.4–21.1° C.	40–70° F.

The temperature of a therapeutic bath is generally about 36.7° C. (100° F.) unless it is otherwise ordered by the physician or is uncomfortable for the patient.

A bathtub contains approximately 30 gallons of fluid when it is two-thirds full. The nurse may need this information in order to calculate the correct amount of medication to be added to a bath. For example, a normal saline solution requires 40 gm. of sodium chloride to 4 liters of water (1½ ounces to 1 gallon). The following quantities of medication are for a bathtub two-thirds full.

Medication	Amount or Strength
Sodium bicarbonate	250 gm. (8 ounces)
Potassium permanganate	1:20,000
Sodium chloride	1200 gm. (45 ounces)
Tar	60 cc.

Once the patient's bath is drawn, the ordered medication is added and the temperature is checked. Then the patient is assisted into the tub. Generally a male patient prefers an orderly or male nurse to help him. Usually the patient remains in the bath for 15 minutes, and he is checked regularly for any untoward reactions. If the patient complains of vertigo (dizziness) or syncope (fainting) the bath should be terminated at once. The water should be drained off and the patient assisted from the tub as soon as he is over the attack. The nurse should not attempt to move the patient when he is feeling dizzy or faint. She should always obtain assistance as needed to ensure the patient's safety.

The patient's skin is patted dry with a soft towel after a medicated cutaneous bath. If dressings are necessary, new ones are applied.

The *sitz bath* is a special bath the purposes of which are chiefly to provide warmth, to cleanse and to provide comfort to the patient's perineal area. It is often indicated after rectal or perineal surgery.

There are several commercially manufactured sitz baths available. Some models fit over toilets, on chairs or on beds. There are also comfort seats that can be placed in bathtubs, as well as separate sitz bath units.

The sitz bath is generally ordered with saline solution or tap water. The temperature is 38° to 41° C. (100° to 105° F.), and the patient stays in it for 10 to 20 minutes. The nurse observes that the perineal region of the patient is immersed if he is seated in a bathtub or that his perineal area is being irrigated if he is seated in a commercial sitz bath.

Usually patients who require sitz baths have recently had rectal or perineal surgery and therefore comfort is an important concern. Adequate support during the bath is also essential. The patient may require help during the bath, particularly if there is any doubt about his ability to tolerate the bath. The patient's pulse is taken five minutes after the start of the bath; if it is unduly accelerated or irregular, he should return to bed, and the nurse then reports this to the physician.

In recording a sitz bath on the patient's chart, the nurse records the appearance of the patient's wound, the amount and character of the discharge and any untoward reactions experienced by the patient, as well as the time of the treatment and the treatment itself.

Diathermy

Medical diathermy is the provision of heat to the deep tissues of the body by transforming certain kinds of physical energy into heat in the deep tissues. It is usually done in a physiotherapy department under the direction of a physician.

Various types of high frequency currents are used: short wave, microwave and ultrasound. The treatment is painless, the patient's chief perception being one of warmth. It is used for much the same reasons as superficial heat.

The Ultraviolet Lamp

Ultraviolet radiation is also used clinically to treat wounds and skin diseases. The sun is a natural source of ultraviolet light, but artificial sources are used therapeutically. The hot quartz mercury lamp, the carbon arc lamp and, of course, the sun lamp are all used.

Generally, ultraviolet radiation is carried out in a special department, such as the physical therapy department. The normal skin reaction produces an erythema, tanning and a proliferation of the cells of the epidermis.

If the patient needs ultraviolet treatments the physician generally orders them every other day for maximum effect. Fair skinned people are more sensitive to ultraviolet radiation than dark skinned people. Sulfanilamide medications increase this sensitivity.

LOCAL APPLICATIONS OF COLD

The Ice Bag

The ice bag or ice cap and the ice collar are commonly used means of applying dry cold to the body. An ice collar is a long narrow rubber or plastic bag which fits around the neck.

Ice bags are usually made with an opening through which small pieces of ice are inserted. Once the ice bag is filled the air is expelled before the top of the ice bag is secured. The air is removed in order that the ice bag can be molded to the patient's body.

Before the flannel cover is put on, the bag is dried. The cover retains cold for more gradual application and it absorbs the water formed by atmospheric condensation. The bag is placed on the area of the body to be cooled.

Generally, ice bags need to be refilled when all the ice has melted or upon the physician's order. If continuous ice applications are ordered, the ice bag is checked once an hour to see that the cold is maintained.

When an ice bag is in place the pressure of the bag should not occlude circulation. At the first sign of tissue numbness and a mottled bluish appearance, the bag should be removed and the physician notified. These signs could be the result of either the cold or pressure upon the tissues.

Cold applications are often alternated with hot applications, or the cold applications are spaced in such a way that the tissue warms between applications. The alternate contraction and dilatation of the blood vessels is a highly effective method of inducing hyperemia and increasing tissue fluid absorption.

When ice bags are not in use they are stored with the tops removed so that the air will dry the inside and prevent the sides from sticking together.

The Ice Compress

Moist cold can be applied by means of ice compresses. These are frequently used to terminate an epistaxis (nosebleed) or to supply moist cold to the eye.

An ice compress is usually made of gauze or other cloth material. The gauze is cooled over ice chips, wrung out and then applied. It is replaced as it becomes warm. Another method of applying a moist cold compress is to place some chipped ice in a cloth bag, which is then placed directly over the area to be cooled. The disadvantage of this is that as the ice melts the water drips on the patient.

Just as in the application of the ice bag, the patient's skin is observed for any signs of untoward effects of the cold. Prolonged vasoconstriction can result in venous congestion and subsequent tissue anoxia. If the patient's skin maintains a bluish, mottled appearance for several hours there is danger of permanent damage to the cells.

Most hospitals have ice making machines and ice crushers to break the ice into small pieces. The chips of ice are used in ice applications because they mold easily to the body and are more comfortable.

The Ice Pack

Ice packs are used occasionally to lower the body temperature or to lower the temperature of a patient's limb prior to surgery. Hypothermia refers to lowering the body temperature artificially. It is done in some types of open heart surgery, and it is usually carried out in the operating room.

On a hospital nursing unit the nurse occasionally sees a patient's limb packed in ice in preparation for amputation. A special container is available commercially for this purpose. The patient's leg is wrapped in cloth and placed in the container. Chips of ice are then packed around the limb. It is important that the patient be given the explanation of the procedure that he requires and that the ice be kept around the limb for the prescribed length of time. Hypothermia blankets containing an alcohol coolant are also used to lower body temperature for a variety of reasons, including heart surgery. The topic of hypothermia is discussed further in Chapter 23, The Care of Patients Who Have Fevers.

APPLICATIONS OF IRRITANTS AND COUNTERIRRITANTS

Many kinds of preparations are available for administration as irritants. The purpose of some irritants is merely to cause hyperemia through surface vasodilatation (rubefacients), whereas others have been used to produce blisters (vesicants) or abscesses (pustulants). The latter two kinds of irritants are rarely used today.

An irritant is applied gently to the designated surface area. Following its application the area is observed every five minutes, the irritant being left on for 20 minutes unless otherwise specified. Irritants are washed off gently with warm water and soap and the skin is patted dry.

An irritant becomes a counterirritant when its primary purpose is to relieve underlying congestion or pain. Goodman and Gilman state that the afferent nerve impulses from the skin area upon which the counterirritant is applied are relayed via the cerebrospinal axis to efferent vasomotor fibers that supply the internal organ. As a result there is a relief of congestion of the internal tissues by redirection of the blood toward the surface. It has also been suggested that the pain of internal sources is relieved because of interference by the local surface pain stimuli which travel over the same fibers.[3]

Of the many counterirritants that were used in the past—for example, the linseed poultice and the flaxseed poultice—the mustard plaster is the one still used occasionally today. The mustard plaster (mustard sinapism) is a mixture of mustard, flour and warm water. Hot water is not used because it inactivates enzymes in the mustard. The proportions vary according to the age of the individual:

Infant: 1 part mustard, 12 parts flour
Child: 1 part mustard, 8 parts flour
Adult: 1 part mustard, 3 parts flour

The skin is observed after the application has been on for five minutes; if it is reddened it is removed. At the end of the treatment (20 minutes) the skin should appear reddened but not blistered. People with fair skins tend to burn easily. After the mustard plaster has been removed and the patient's skin has been washed and dried, petrolatum or olive oil is applied to the skin to soothe it.

Mustard plasters can be purchased commercially. The precautions just mentioned should also be followed when using these preparations.

---

[3]Louis S. Goodman and Alfred Gilman: *The Pharmacological Basis of Therapeutics*. Third edition. New York, The Macmillan Company, 1965, pp. 981–983.

GUIDE TO ASSESSING NURSING NEEDS

1. Does the patient understand the purpose of the treatment?
2. What precautions need to be taken to protect the patient from harm?
3. Is he aware of the dangers?

4. Does the patient require added safety precautions because of his age, his general physical condition, the condition of his skin or his mental state?
5. Is the patient able to participate in his treatment? Is this desirable?
6. Are there specific skills that the patient (or his family) needs to learn or knowledge that he needs to gain in order to carry out the treatment at home?

GUIDE TO EVALUATING THE EFFECTIVENESS OF NURSING ACTION

1. Is the patient safe during the application?
2. Is he comfortable?
3. Is the hot or cold application producing the desired physiological effect, for example, increased circulation to the part, or relief of pain?

STUDY VOCABULARY

Conductive heat	Erythema	Hypothermia
Conversive heat	Exudate	Inflammation
Counterirritant	Hyperemia	Irritant
Epistaxis	Hyperthermia	Ischemia

STUDY SITUATION

Mrs. J. Watson has an infected cut on her right hand. She is at home and the physician has ordered hot soaks for her hand. As the public health nurse you have been asked to assist Mrs. Watson. This patient is 75 years old and she has poor blood circulation.

1. What are the specific needs of this patient in relation to her infected cut?
2. What factors should you take into consideration in helping to plan this patient's care?
3. What physiological reactions are to be expected as a result of the hot soaks?
4. How could the effectiveness of the soaks be evaluated?
5. What specific precautions should be taken? Why?
6. Outline the objectives and a plan of care for this patient.

BIBLIOGRAPHY

Abel-Sayed, W. A., et al.: Effect of Local Cooling on Responsiveness of Muscular and Cutaneous Arteries and Veins. *American Journal of Physiology, 219*:1772, December, 1970.

Bierman, William: Therapeutic Use of Cold. *The Journal of the American Medical Association, 157*:1189–1192, April 2, 1955.

Copeland, B. E.: Heat to Dilate Veins. *New England Journal of Medicine, 283*:209, July 23, 1970.

Goodman, Louis S., and Alfred Gilman: *The Pharmacological Basis of Therapeutics.* Third edition. New York, The Macmillan Company, 1965.

Guyton, Arthur C.: *Textbook of Medical Physiology.* Fourth edition. Philadelphia, W. B. Saunders Company, 1971.

Harmer, Bertha, and Virginia Henderson: *Textbook of the Principles and Practice of Nursing.* Fifth edition. New York, The Macmillan Company, 1955.

Nordmark, Madelyn T., and Anne W. Rohweder: *Scientific Foundations of Nursing.* Second edition. Philadelphia, J. B. Lippincott Company, 1967.

Rosenthal, S. M., et al.: Influence of Temperature on Swelling Following Experimental Thermal or Tourniquet Trauma. *American Journal of Physiology, 219*:131–135, July, 1970.

Rusk, Howard A.: *Rehabilitation Medicine.* Second edition. St. Louis, The C. V. Mosby Company, 1964.

Sutton, Audrey L.: *Bedside Nursing Techniques in Medicine and Surgery.* Second edition. Philadelphia, W. B. Saunders Company, 1969.

21 MEDICATIONS AS THERAPEUTIC AGENTS

The nurse should be able to:

Describe methods commonly used in health agencies for recording and communicating physicians' medication orders for patients

Name basic principles related to the administration of medications

List general safety precautions the nurse observes in the preparation and administration of medications

Identify common routes for the administration of medications

Compare the advantages and disadvantages of administering medications via the oral, subcutaneous and intramuscular routes

Describe the preparation and administration of medications to be given by the oral route

List criteria for selecting an injection site for medications to be given by the subcutaneous route

Describe the preparation and a basic technique for the administration of medications to be given by this route

List criteria for selecting an injection site for an intramuscular injection

Compare the advantages and disadvantages of commonly used sites

Describe the preparation and technique of administration of medications by this route

262

INTRODUCTION

The use of medications as therapeutic agents has been known throughout history. In recent years, however, the number of different medicines that are manufactured commercially for distribution has increased enormously. Although hundreds of new drug products are introduced each year, relatively few of these are new chemical substances. Most new preparations are actually new dosage forms, new combinations of drugs or new forms of previously marketed drugs.[1] Nurses are continually challenged to keep up to date with these constantly changing products.

Sources of information available to nurses about new drugs include the agency pharmacy department, physicians, the professional nursing and medical journals, and information put out by the commercial drug firms. In many health agencies, the pharmacy department maintains an up-to-date *formulary* which lists and describes drugs currently used in the agency. Copies of the formulary are usually distributed to all nursing units, where they are readily available for reference. In addition, many charge nurses like to keep a drug file on their nursing units with information about new drugs. The pharmacist is, of course, an excellent reference source, and the nurse should not hesitate to request information from

him. Physicians too are usually very willing to explain the nature and purpose of new drugs they have prescribed for patients. With the multitude of new drug products constantly appearing on the market, it is difficult for anyone to keep informed about them all. The nurse should be aware of the sources of information available in her agency about new drugs and should make use of these.

Many drugs are marketed under their trademarks; however, one drug can have as many as four names; its trademark, official name, chemical name and generic name. A *trademark* is given a drug by the manufacturer. Consequently some drugs may have many trademarks, since the same drug may be manufactured by several companies, each one giving it a different trademark. The *official name* of a drug is the name under which it is listed in one of the official publications: *The Pharmacopeia of the United States of America, The Homeopathic Pharmacopoeia of the United States* or *The National Formulary*.[2] The *chemical name* of a drug is a description of its chemical constituents. The *generic name* is the one given a drug before it becomes official. The generic name can be used internationally, since it is not protected by law.

An increasing number of health agencies are adopting the practice of using the generic or official names of drugs

---

[1]Ralph G. Smith: The Development and Control of New Drugs. *The American Journal of Nursing*, 62:56, July, 1962.

[2]Canadian equivalents of official publications listing drugs are *The Vademecum International of Canada* and *The National Formulary*.

for patient prescriptions. This practice not only eliminates much confusion about the nature of the drug prescribed, but means too that products of different drug companies can be used alternatively.

Drug standards provide for identification, purity and uniformity of the strength of drugs. The *Pharmacopeia of the United States of America* (U.S.P.) lists drugs and defines the standards according to which a pharmacist in the United States must fill a prescription. The *Vademecum International of Canada* does the same for pharmacists in Canada. In this way the physician can always be assured of the uniform purity and potency of the medications that he orders. In 1951 the World Health Organization published the *Pharmacopoia Internationalis* (Ph. I.), a major step toward establishing international standards for drugs.

The administration of medications is a therapeutic nursing function which is chiefly dependent upon the orders of the physician. Some medication orders state the exact time for administration; others leave the time of administration to the nurse's judgment. For example, it is not unusual for ferrous sulfate to be prescribed three times a day after meals, whereas an order for ¼ gr. of morphine subcutaneously is often written so that the nurse can give it when in her judgment the patient requires an analgesic.

ORDERING AND RECORDING MEDICATIONS

Medications, then, are given upon the order of the physician. Generally this is a written order that is dated and signed by the physician, although some health agencies permit physicians to telephone orders to the nursing staff. In such cases, the physicians are usually required to countersign their orders within a definite number of hours. In an emergency situation medications are given on a verbal order that is later written and countersigned as needed. Generally speaking, written orders are considered to be the safest practice.

There are two types of written orders: the self-terminating order and the standing order. Self-terminating orders have a time limit on them. A stat. order is a self-terminating order that is to be carried out only once and immediately, for example, Demerol 100 mgm. I.M.

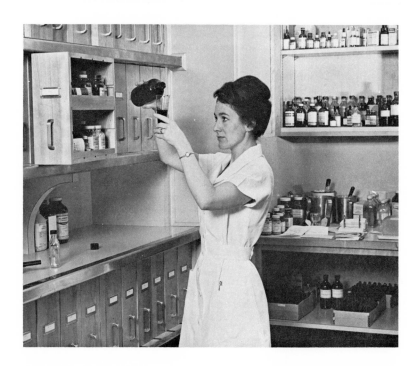

Medications are prepared by the pharmacist.

stat (I.M. refers to intramuscularly). It is not repeated unless there are specific instructions to that effect. Another type of self-terminating order is an order in which the time limit is actually specified; for example, the physician writes, aspirin gr.$\bar{x}$ q.4.h. for six doses, or digitalis gr.$\overline{\text{iss}}$ June 12th and 14th. Sometimes a self-terminating order is dependent upon the condition of the patient as when an order is written, aspirin gr.$\bar{x}$ q.4.h. until temperature has remained below 37.8° C. (100° F.) for 24 hours. Some institutions have policies which place a time limit on orders regardless of how they are worded. For example, it is not unusual for a narcotic order to be effective for only three days, after which it is automatically discontinued unless the physician writes another order.

Standing orders are orders which are carried out indefinitely; for example, vitamin C 500 mgm. q.4.h. Some standing orders contain the direction "p.r.n." which means "as necessary." The administration of a drug under a p.r.n. direction is left to the nurse's judgment. An example of this type of order is Demerol 100 mgm. I.M.q.4.h.p.r.n.

An order should always include the name of the drug, the exact dosage, the route of administration and the frequency of administration. If the physician wishes a medication to be given at a time other than the accustomed distribution time, this should also be specified. The nurse has an obligation to question any order that is ambiguous or which she feels is unsafe for a patient. In health agencies it is a customary practice for all of a patient's orders to be written on a doctor's order sheet, which may be kept in the patient's chart or in a central book. Hospitals employ different ways of flagging charts to indicate that a patient has new orders. The orders are then usually copied in the nursing unit Kardex system or nursing care plan and a medication card may be filled out. A medication card has the patient's full name, the name of the drug, the dosage, the route of administration (in some hospitals if the route is oral it is omitted), the frequency of the

administration and the times of administration. Frequently, the room number or location of the patient is also written on the medication card. If the drug is ordered q.i.d., the exact times are added, for example, 8 A.M., 12 noon, 4 P.M. and 8 P.M. Medication cards are kept in a central place in the nursing unit and are frequently grouped so that they are easily selected at the time of administration.

Although different methods of posting medication orders are used in various agencies, the nurse should remember that the original written order is the primary source of information. Whenever orders are copied, whether onto a Kardex file, a nursing care plan or a medicine card, the possibility of error is present. The nurse who administers medications should always check the original orders to make certain that communication tools are accurate.

Agencies have different methods of indicating that a medication has been discontinued. In hospitals it is common practice for "discontinued" to be imprinted across the physician's order once it is no longer in force and for the medication card to be discarded. In a public health agency the notation "discontinued" and the date are entered on the nursing care record. Communication tools such as medication cards and nursing care records should be regularly checked against the original orders in order to keep them up to date. In hospitals where orders change frequently this is generally done at least once a day.

Medications are recorded in the patient's chart immediately after they have been administered. They should be recorded by the nurse who administered them. The recording includes the name of the drug, the time it was administered, the exact dosage, the method of administration and the signature of the nurse administering the drug. Some agencies also require that the status of the person administering the drug also be designated.

When a p.r.n. order has been administered a notation is also made as to why the patient took the medicine at that particular time. Recording should also include observations of the effect of the medication when these are, or should be, apparent. In some hospitals the nurse also indicates on the doctor's order sheet that stat. dosages have been administered.

The administration of narcotics and, in some places, barbiturates is not only recorded on the patient's chart, it is also recorded on a special form which is kept separately. Narcotics and barbiturates are kept in locked containers in hospitals and their distribution is closely governed. The forms upon which narcotics are recorded vary from place to place, but usually the nurse records the name of the patient to whom the narcotic was administered, the drug and dosage, the date and time, the name of the physician ordering the drug and the signature of the nurse administering the drug. Any narcotics that are wasted are also recorded with a notation that the drug was wasted. Narcotics and barbiturates are counted at specific times—for example, at the end of each shift—and the number distributed plus the number remaining on hand must tally with the number assigned to the nursing unit or agency. This count is usually done by two nurses, the one coming on duty and the nurse who is "handing over" to her. This practice helps to protect both nurses. Narcotics and barbiturates are under strict Federal control. Any losses or inconsistencies in the count must be reported immediately.

PRINCIPLES RELATED TO THE ADMINISTRATION OF MEDICATIONS

The type of drug preparation often governs the method of administration. Medications are distributed in a variety of preparations and each type usually requires a specific method of administration. It may be that one preparation can be administered in several ways, but this is specified on the medication label. More often a preparation of a drug has only one method of adminis-

tration, and if the drug must be administered by some other route, another preparation is required. Drugs are administered only by the route ordered by the doctor and specified on the medication label. For example, penicillin tablets are taken orally, but a special solution of penicillin is given intramuscularly.

The route of administration of the drug affects the optimal dosage of the drug. The optimal dosage of a drug administered by mouth may not be the same as the optimal dosage when the drug is administered subcutaneously. For example, portions of drugs taken orally are excreted through the digestive tract instead of being absorbed into the cells.

The safe administration of medications requires a knowledge of anatomy and physiology as well as a knowledge of the drug and the reason it has been prescribed. A knowledge of anatomy and physiology is particularly important when medications are administered intramuscularly or subcutaneously. For example, when administering a drug intramuscularly, large blood vessels and nerves could be damaged if they are accidentally punctured.

A knowledge of the drug and its effects also helps safeguard against the administration of a medication which could harm a patient. For example, if a patient has very slow respirations (e.g., 10 per minute), morphine can be contraindicated, because it can depress the respirations even more. This knowledge helps the nurse to make intelligent observations which assist in the assessment of the effectiveness of both the medication and the nursing care.

An understanding of the total plan of care for each patient and the desired therapeutic effect of the medications prescribed for him is essential. The nurse should know why the individual patient is receiving each medication so that she knows what to observe in that patient.

The method of administration of a drug is partially determined by the age of the patient, his orientation, his degree of consciousness and his disease.

It is important for the nurse to report any difficulties that are encountered when administering a medication. Perhaps the disoriented patient refuses to swallow his oral medication, or the nauseated patient vomits his medicines after he has taken them. The unconscious patient is unable to take a medication orally, and a child might be too young to swallow a capsule. These observations should be reported to the physician in order that he can assess the specific needs of the individual.

The element of error is a possibility in all human activity. Errors in the administration of medicines can be serious and, because the possibility of error is always present, special precautions are taken to avoid mistakes. If a nurse is ever in doubt about her activity, she should always consult a reliable source before going ahead. Most agencies have literature to which the nurse can refer, and physicians and pharmacies can also be consulted.

If an error is made it is reported immediately to the physician or to the nurse in charge so that immediate steps can be taken to protect the patient from injury. Most hospitals also have accident forms which the nurse fills out to inform the agency administration of the details of the error (see Chapter 15).

Each patient has his own needs for explanations and support with respect to the administration of medications. Medications are given to people, and the nurse will find, as in all of her nursing care, that each individual is different. Some people want to know about their medications; others prefer not to know about them. The amount of knowledge that a person requires is highly dependent upon individual circumstances. For example, the person taking a drug at home needs a knowledge of the correct dosage, how and when to take the medication, the action of the drug and indications of untoward reactions. The seriously ill patient in a hospital, on the other hand, might be too ill to care about any knowledge of the drug. The information that each person should have is dependent upon his intelligence, age, education, illness and emotional needs. The nurse is guided by both the patient and the physician as to the amount of information she provides.

GUIDES TO NURSING ACTION

The administration of medications is a nursing function in most health agencies. At some hospitals the nurse administers all intravenous injections, but in others it is the physician's responsibility to administer specific medications such as ergotamine, which is used to contract the uterus.

There is, then, a wide variety in the medication policies which guide nursing action. But, regardless of policy, before the nurse administers any medicament she must be sure that her action is safe for the patient. A sound basis for safe nursing practice is knowledge.

Traditionally the "five rights" have served as guides to the administration of medicaments: the right drug, the right dose, the right route, the right time and the right patient. These rights are no less true today than they were years ago; however, sound nursing function involves more than just a knowledge of these. The nurse's information should extend to an identification of the individual nursing needs of the patient and how she can help the patient meet these needs. For example, will assisting a patient to change his position and the provision of physical support augment the action of an analgesic?

An adjunctive to the administration of many medications is the provision of nursing care measures which serve to augment or supplement the action of a drug. For example, giving the patient a back rub and straightening his bed might increase the effectiveness of a sedative, and drinking fluids can help prevent the crystallization of some antibiotics in the kidneys.

People vary in their reactions to specific drugs. The patient's reaction to any drug is important and should be recorded. Patients often require information about what reactions to report to the nurse or the physician. This is particularly true for the person who is taking medicine at home and does not have constant contact with health personnel.

A knowledge of the significance of a drug and its prescribed dosage is a need of some people. It is not infrequently heard that "If one tablet is good for me, two tablets are twice as good." Some people also require assistance in order to understand the value of a prescribed dose and its action as well as a realistic explanation of the anticipated results. This is not only a need of hospitalized patients, but it is often important for people who take medicines in their homes.

Another area of nursing practice is concerned with idiosyncratic reactions to medications, overdoses of drugs and the ingestion of poisonous materials. Many medical centers provide immediate information to laymen and physicians about the antidotes and emergency measures for the common poisons. An up-to-date list of the poison control centers can be obtained from the Superintendent of Documents, U.S. Government Printing Office, Washington, D.C. A list of poison control centers in Can-

ada is contained in the *Vademecum International of Canada: Pharmaceutical Specialties and Biologicals* (updated each year) and also the *Compendium of Pharmaceuticals and Specialties of Canada.*

It is also a part of the nursing function to assist the physician to evaluate the effectiveness of a medication and often to make a judgment as to when a specific medication should be given. In order to make this evaluation the needs of the patient are considered, as well as the purpose of the therapeutic agent itself.

The need of a patient for some medications varies from time to time and, of course, needs vary from patient to patient. One patient may require frequent sedation, whereas another requires none. The intent of the physician depends upon the needs of the patient and the effect on his prescribed therapeutic regime. For example, the physician may want to give a patient a drug that prevents vomiting because of the strain of vomiting upon a freshly sutured wound.

A knowledge of pharmacology includes the actions of drugs, usual dosages and factors which affect dosages,

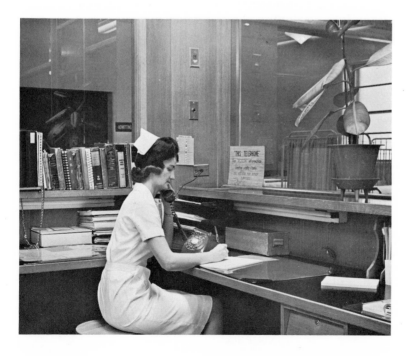

The poison control center is a source of information about the composition, action and antidotes of poisonous materials. Its services are available to everyone in the community.

untoward reactions, methods of administration, drugs that counteract or react with each other and correct methods of administration. The nurse will find it advantageous, when learning about drugs, to group them according to their systemic action. Many related medicines have similar actions and reactions.

Medications and the Patient

One of the most important factors in the administration of a medication is the identification of the patient. Any method which accurately identifies a patient is satisfactory. Some hospitals provide each patient with an identification band. Other institutions suggest asking the patient his name before administering a medication. If this is the case, the nurse should not say, "Are you Mr. Smith?" nor should she rely on the patient answering to his name. In both situations, the patient may reply with an automatic "yes." It is better to say, "What is your name?" The habit of

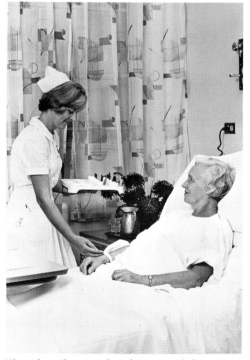

The identification band is one of the means by which a patient's identity can be ascertained.

relying upon bed numbers and even room numbers in order to identify people is also dangerous, for patients' rooms are changed and patients move to other units. In situations in which patients are continually reassigned to new rooms, identification is especially difficult.

After the nurse has accurately identified a patient, his need for any explanation and support must be met. Often, simple explanations are reassuring to the patient; they can often enhance the effectiveness of the drug and are considered to be more helpful than refusing to give him any information. At this time the nurse can also provide him with information about the action of the medication as he will perceive it. Patients usually like to feel they are participating in their therapy and have some control over situations. If the physician does not want the patient to receive information about a medicine from the nurse, it can be suggested that he confer with the physician about this subject.

If the administration of a drug is contingent upon some factor, such as the patient's pulse, this is assessed first. With few exceptions the nurse stays with a patient until his medication has been completely administered. The exceptions are drugs which have been ordered to be left with a patient, for example, a drug which the patient has for immediate use as needed (such as nitroglycerin for cardiac pain), a cough medicine or a drug which is contained in an intravenous infusion for gradual administration.

Sometimes people refuse a medication, and often their reasons are valid. If a patient does refuse, the nurse should find out why. Some of the possible reasons are:

1. The medicine is nauseating and makes him vomit.

2. He is allergic to the medicine. A record of the patient's allergies should be noted on admission. Sometimes this is not possible, however, as, for example, if the patient has been brought in when he was unconscious.

3. The medicine does not help him.

4. He thinks it is the wrong medicine.

5. He believes the physician has changed the order.

6. The needles with which the medicine is administered hurt him.

7. The medicine has an unpleasant taste.

8. He does not want it because of religious or cultural beliefs. For example, a patient of the Hindu religion may refuse a hormonal preparation that contains extracts from cattle; a patient who belongs to the Jehovah's Witness sect may refuse a blood transfusion. Many people who believe in naturopathic remedies will refuse any medicine prepared from inorganic chemicals.

9. He does not understand and is afraid it will harm him.

10. The nurse wants to administer the medication at an inconvenient time, for example, when his visitors are present.

The reason a patient refuses a medicine can often be satisfactorily dealt with by the nurse; for example, if it has an unpleasant taste it can usually be administered in a vehicle such as orange juice. The physician's order should be checked if the patient questions it. Perhaps there is a new order in the chart which has not been transcribed to his medication card. A patient's refusal to take a medication should always be reported to the physician or to the nurse in charge and recorded in the patient's chart. Under some circumstances it is best to notify the physician at once, particularly when a patient's condition is seriously affected by the omission of the medication, as when a patient with heart disease does not take his digitalis.

Observing and Reporting

Immediately after a medication has been administered, it is recorded on the patient's chart. The recording includes the date, the time, the name of the medication, the exact dosage, the route of administration and the nurse's signature (and status). If the drug was administered at the nurse's discretion, then the reason for the administration is also charted.

After the administration of any therapeutic agent, the nurse observes the patient for his reaction. The criteria by which the nurse judges the effectiveness of a drug vary. It can be the alleviation of pain, the reduction of fever, a decrease in swelling or even orange-colored urine. These results are anticipated results and they reflect the effectiveness of the particular medication. The observations are recorded in detail on the patient's chart. Sometimes patients experience untoward reactions as a result of a medication, for example, nausea and vomiting, diarrhea or a skin rash. If a reaction is severe, that is, if the patient is acutely uncomfortable or essential body functions are impaired, the physician is notified immediately so that he can institute measures to counteract the adverse symptoms. For example, in severe allergic reactions the tissues of the throat may become so edematous that breathing is difficult. Prompt intervention at the earliest sign of an allergic reaction is required. These reactions are also recorded in detail on the patient's chart.

THE PREPARATION OF MEDICATIONS

The first step in the preparation of any medication is to get the complete order and make sure it is understood. Sometimes agency policies or the orders themselves govern the administration of a specific drug or the special nursing measures which accompany its administration. For example, an order might read "withhold drug if pulse is below 60 beats per minute."

Before administering drugs, the nurse washes her hands to minimize the transfer of microorganisms and then she gathers the equipment she needs. In a hospital all the necessary equipment is usually kept in a medication room near the nursing unit office yet separate from it in order that medications can be prepared without disturbance. In the home, such equipment is generally kept in one place, usually in a cupboard which is out of reach of small children. Some hospitals use medication carts to deliver the medicines; others use trays, often with special slots so that the medicine card stands upright and can be easily read.

A hospital medication cupboard is usually locked, the key being kept by the charge nurse or in a designated place in the nursing unit. Adjacent to the medication cupboard are usually a locked narcotic cupboard and a refrigerator. Drugs which lose their potency unless kept cold are kept in the refrigerator.

The nurse selects the medicine that was ordered by the physician. Drugs kept in a hospital are either stock or private (prescription). The former are the more commonly used medicines; the latter are especially prepared for a patient. Stock drugs are frequently grouped according to action; for example, all vitamin preparations are kept together. Another method is to group the drugs alphabetically according to their generic or trade names. Either method facilitates finding a specific preparation quickly.

It has become an accepted safety practice in the preparation of medications to read the label three times on a bottle, tube, package, envelope, or the like. It is read before the container is taken off the shelf, before it is opened and just before it is placed back on the shelf. Reading includes the name of the drug and its strength. Particular attention is paid to the route of administration by which the particular medicine is designed to be given.

Medications come in a variety of preparations; capsules, Spansules, lozenges, tablets and liquids can all be given orally. A capsule contains a powder, oil or liquid within a gelatinous covering, a tablet is a compressed powdered drug. Troches are oral preparations which are sucked. Vials and ampules contain either powdered or liquid medications for injection. A vial is a glass container with a rubber stopper, whereas an ampule is a sealed glass container. A suppository is a medication which is molded into a firm base in order that it can be inserted into a body orifice or cavity. An ointment is a semi-solid mixture which is applied topically to mucous membranes or skin.

A medicine must be administered in the exact dose that is ordered by the physician. If small doses are required, for example, for children, the usual practice is to have these doses prepared accurately by a pharmacist. In situations in which the dose must be calculated, the safest practice is for a second nurse to check the calculation made by the first. The nurse should not estimate a dosage on her own initiative; for example, it is not a safe practice to break an unscored tablet to get a dosage. The dose of a drug is ordered by the physician in consideration of the weight, age, sex and physical condition of the patient. Thus, approximating dosages can be a dangerous practice.

In order to avoid errors the nurse who prepares a medication should administer it herself immediately after she has prepared it. If prepared medicines are left unattended, the chances of the drug being misplaced or taken by another patient are increased. More to the point, the nurse is legally responsible for the medications she administers, and only if she has prepared a medication herself can she testify to the actual constituents of the medication and to its strength. The identification of a medication just by its appearance is a dangerous practice. If it happens that medications are distributed while a patient is in another department, his medication can be returned to the nursing unit and locked in the cupboard with the medication card which serves to identify it.

When a nurse is preparing a variety of medications for a group of patients, the medicines for one patient are separated from the medicines for another. Generally all medicines that are administered by the same route for one patient can be placed in the same container, except for specific drugs whose administration is dependent upon some specified criterion. For example, if digitalis gr.$\overline{\text{iss}}$ is to be withheld when the patient's pulse is below 60 beats per minute, then this drug is put in a separate container from the other oral medications for that particular patient.

Only a pharmacist should label a container of drugs. Therefore when the nurse finds an unlabeled container or a label which has been partially obscured, the entire container is returned to the pharmacy for clarification. It is also considered a safety practice not to return medications to a container once they have been removed; they should be disposed of by flushing down a toilet or hopper. Some agencies require that a witness be present when narcotics (and sometimes other drugs as well) are disposed of. Drugs should not be transferred from one container to another. The reason for these precautions is that the danger of committing an error is too great.

METHODS OF ADMINISTRATION OF MEDICATIONS

The most common method of administering medications is by mouth. Not only is it simple but it is also the most economical way. Capsules, liquids, tablets, powders and troches are all administered by mouth. Troches are usually sucked for their local effect. *Sublingual administration* involves placing the drug, for example, nitroglycerin, under the patient's tongue, where it is slowly dissolved and absorbed.

Parenteral refers to the administration of drugs by a needle. Intramuscular, intradermal, subcutaneous and intravenous injections are common means of parenteral therapy. Intracardiac, intrapericardial, intrathecal (intraspinal), and intraosseous (into bone) injections are less common methods which may be used by physicians. All parenteral therapy involves the use of sterile equipment and sterile, readily soluble solutions. Generally drugs that are administered parenterally are readily absorbed by the body.

Inhalation is the administration of a drug into the respiratory tract. Once the drug is inhaled it is almost immediately absorbed. Volatile and nonvolatile drugs can be inhaled, the latter by means of a vehicle such as oxygen.

Instillation is a method of putting a drug in liquid form into a body cavity or orifice, for example the ears, the eyes and the urinary bladder. Liquid medications can be instilled with a dropper (into the ear), or with a syringe (into the urinary bladder).

Medications are also applied to the skin and mucous membranes; this process is called *topical application*. Antiseptics, astringents and emollients can be applied as liquids or ointments.

Drugs are generally administered for either their systemic or local effect. *Systemic effect* refers to the actions of the drug upon the entire body, whereas *local effect* is the effect upon one specific area, such as that of an ointment upon a particular area of the skin. Sometimes drugs that are administered for their local effect have systemic actions; for example, an untoward reaction such as a fever may result from the topical application of an ointment to an incision.

A *suppository* is used for insertion into a body cavity or orifice, such as the rectum or vagina. As the suppository gradually dissolves at body temperature, the drug is released and is absorbed through the mucous membrane. Although a suppository is sometimes used to administer drugs when a systemic action is desired, as, for example, a sedative, it is not considered as efficient as a medication administered by other routes. Suppositories are therefore used principally for their local action. They may be used, for instance, to administer an analgesic to the rectal area, or to stimulate peristalsis and bring about a bowel movement.

Oral Administration

Oral medications are absorbed chiefly in the small intestines, although they can also be absorbed in the mouth and the stomach. Medications administered sublingually are absorbed through the capillaries under the tongue. Drugs in liquid form, either upon administration or upon dissolution within the stomach, are absorbed through the gastric mucosa. Absorption is slowed by the presence of food in the stomach as well as by the administration of a concentrated drug. Dilution, an alcoholic base, and an empty stomach facilitate absorption.

Advantages and Disadvantages. The oral administration of medications has the advantages of convenience, economy and safety. It is convenient in that it is a simple method of administration; it is economical in that oral preparations usually cost less to manufacture than many other preparations; it is safe in that its administration does not involve breaking through any of the body defenses—for example, the skin—as is necessary with injections.

The chief disadvantages of the oral administration of medications are their taste, gastric irritation, effect upon teeth, inaccurate measure of absorption and limited use. Drugs which are decidedly *unpleasant tasting* can stimulate nausea and vomiting. Drugs in liquid or partially dissolved form activate the taste buds more than drugs in tablet or capsule form; however, since cold is less stimulating than warmth, the taste buds can be partially desensitized by giving cold fluids or ice chips.

Some medications are particularly *irritating to the gastric mucosa*; others are destroyed by the gastric secretions. The latter are usually manufactured with an enteric coating so that they either do not dissolve in the stomach, or are given by parenteral administration. Irritation of the gastric mucosa can be minimized by administering a drug after a meal, while food is still in the stomach. Also the more diluted the medicine the less irritating it is to the mucosa. A medicine which is particularly irritating can sometimes be given in conjunction with another drug or with food, such as bread, in order to modify its undesirable effect.

Some medications are *harmful to the teeth.* Drugs such as hydrochloric acid damage enamel, and liquid iron preparations often discolor the teeth. These undesirable effects can be avoided by giving highly diluted forms and by using a straw in order that the teeth do not come in contact with the liquid. It is also wise to have the patient rinse his mouth with water or a mouthwash after he takes these medicines.

Another disadvantage of the oral administration of medications is the relatively *inaccurate measure* of their absorption in the gastrointestinal tract. Certain disorders affect absorption; for example, accelerated peristalsis will decrease absorption because of the drug's speedy propulsion through the gastrointestinal tract. Moreover, some medications are destroyed to a variable extent by gastrointestinal secretions, and the adequacy of the circulation of the blood to the tract affects the rate of absorption. If a person vomits after he has ingested a medicine, the amount of drug retained in his body is questionable. Generally the physician is consulted when this happens in order that he can assess the patient's need for a repeated dose of the medicine.

Oral medications are *limited in use* to patients who are able to swallow and retain them. The unconscious patient, the patient who is unable to swallow and the vomiting patient are unable to take these medications. Patients who are restricted to taking nothing by mouth (N.P.O) cannot be given oral medications. Some patients cannot take oral medications because of gastric suction and some find swallowing difficult because of surgery or paralysis. Frequently it is the nurse who first becomes aware that a patient has difficulty in swallowing a medicine, and her communication of this fact to the physician can result in a change in the order to a more easily consumed drug. Tablets can be crushed and a scored tablet can be broken for easier administration, but the protective coverings of capsules or enteric-coated pills should not be removed to facilitate administration.

Preparation. In the preparation of oral medications for distribution, the nurse follows the general guides outlined earlier in this chapter. Oral drugs are generally distributed in disposable containers. Liquid medications are often given in plastic or waxed paper medication containers. The advantages of using disposable containers are obvious: their cleanliness is assured and washing and sterilizing are eliminated. Medications should not be handled indiscriminately with the fingers; it is considered a cleaner practice to drop a tablet into the bottle cap or into an empty medicine container before transferring it to the container that the patient uses. If there is any doubt about administering a specific drug, the drug is kept separately from the other tablets for a specific patient.

When pouring liquids, the dose is measured from the bottom of the concave meniscus. Some liquids separate after standing in a bottle and need to be shaken before they are poured. Minims and drops are not interchangeable measures; special minim droppers or glasses are used when doses are indicated in minims.

Administration. After the patient is appropriately identified, the nurse gives him his medications and stays with him until they have been taken. Sometimes the patient needs assistance to sit up or to turn on his side to swallow without choking. Usually people find it easier to take oral medicines with water or juice. If the consistency of a liquid is unpleasant, as, for example, mineral oil, patients often find it easier to take if the medicine has been chilled. With few exceptions drugs are not left at a patient's bedside in hospitals.

Subcutaneous Injection

Advantages and Disadvantages. Some medications are best administered into the subcutaneous tissue by a needle. This route has the advantage of almost complete absorption, providing the patient's circulation is good; therefore an accurate measure of the amount of the drug absorbed is possible. Medicines administered in this manner are not affected by gastric disturbances (although it should be remembered that the medicines may themselves cause gastrointestinal disturbances), nor is their administration dependent upon

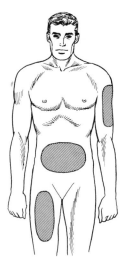

Three sites which are commonly used for subcutaneous injections are the outer aspect of the upper arm, the loose abdominal tissue and the anterior aspect of the thigh.

the consciousness or rationality of the patient.

The chief disadvantage of this method is that by introducing a needle through skin one of the body's barriers against infection is broken. It is therefore important that aseptic technique be used for all needle injections.

The Site of Injection. The subcutaneous tissue is just below the cutaneous tissue or skin. It is areolar tissue which has fewer pain receptors than the skin itself; therefore once a needle is through the skin an injection is relatively painless. Some drugs sting upon injection, but an isotonic solution can usually be administered painlessly. Isotonic refers to a concentration that is the same as a normal saline solution.

The exact site for a subcutaneous injection is dependent upon the need of the specific patient and to some extent upon the policy of the institution. Since drugs administered subcutaneously (hypodermically) are usually given for their systemic effect, the site is irrelevant with respect to any local effect. Areas in the upper arms, anterior and lateral aspects of the thigh and the lower ventral abdominal wall are suggested.[3] The

[3]Martha Pitel: The Subcutaneous Injection. *The American Journal of Nursing,* 71:1:79, January, 1971.

skin and subcutaneous tissue should
be in good condition, that is, free of
irritation such as itching and free from
any signs of inflammation such as redness, heat, edema, tenderness or pain.
Areas where there is scar tissue should
not be used. A common practice is to
choose the outer aspect of the patient's
upper arm about one-third of the distance down between the shoulder and
the elbow. Other sites are the anterior
aspect of the thigh, the loose tissue of
the abdomen and the subscapular region of the back. Actually the subcutaneous tissue in any area can be injected provided that it is not over bony
prominences and is free of large blood
vessels and nerves. If a patient is receiving a series of injections the sites
are rotated and the site is charted each
time so that two consecutive doses are
not given in the same area. Sometimes
a map is drawn on the patient's skin to
indicate the sites for rotating injections,
or a chart may be attached to the nursing
care plan for the patient.

Equipment. Subcutaneous   (hypodermic) injections involve the use of
sterile equipment and supplies. These
include a syringe, a needle, the medication and a swab and disinfectant to
cleanse the skin. Syringes vary in size
from 1 cc. to 50 cc. The 2 cc. syringe,
commonly used for subcutaneous injections, is calibrated in cubic centimeters and minims. For the administration of insulin, special 1 cc. syringes are
often used. Insulin syringes usually
have an 80 unit scale and a 40 unit scale
to correspond to the strength of the
particular insulin. They are calibrated
in units.

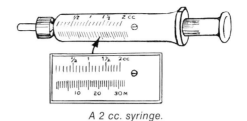

A 2 cc. syringe.

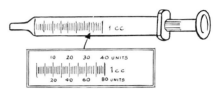

*An insulin syringe. Note the 40 unit scale
and the 80 unit scale.*

A syringe has two parts, the barrel or
outer part and the plunger or inner part.
Most syringes are manufactured so that
their parts are interchangeable, but if
they are not they bear corresponding
numbers on the plunger and barrel.

Syringes are made of glass or plastic.
The latter, which are usually disposable,
are increasingly being used in hospitals,
offices and clinics. A 2 cc. syringe is
usually used for subcutaneous injections. The maximum volume of solution
which can be given comfortably by this
route is thought to be 20 minims. Certainly anything greater than 2 cc. (30
minims) will cause pressure on surrounding tissues and therefore be painful.

A needle has a hub and a stem or
cannula. The hub is the larger part that

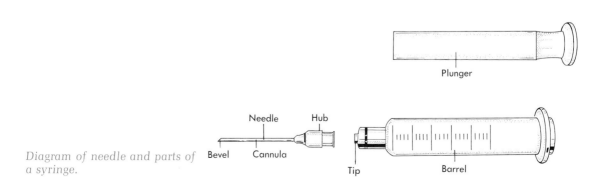

*Diagram of needle and parts of
a syringe.*

connects to the barrel of the syringe; the cannula is the long narrow part. At the end of the cannula is the bevel or slanted portion where the fluid is ejected. A short or small bevel is used when there is a danger that a larger bevel would become occluded, as in intravenous injections in which the bevel could rest against the side of the vein. The longer bevel provides the sharper needle and is used for subcutaneous and intramuscular injections.

The needle used for a subcutaneous injection is usually 24, 25 or 26 gauge. The larger the number the smaller the diameter of the needle. The length that is required varies anywhere from $3/8$ inch to 1 inch, depending upon the obesity and hydration of the patient. A longer needle is needed for the obese patient, a shorter needle for the dehydrated person. Generally a No. 24 needle $5/8$ inch in length is used for the average adult.

The needle used for any injection should be straight and sharp. As disposable needles are increasingly being used, the problem of the bent or dull needle is disappearing. If disposable needles are not used, the needles are checked for sharpness and the presence of barbs before they are sterilized. A needle may be checked for the presence of barbs by passing the tip lightly over a piece of absorbent cotton. If the needle does catch on the cotton, it may have a barb and will be uncomfortable for a patient. Needles that are bent should not be used, because of the danger that they will break off in a patient. The weakest point in a needle is where the cannula joins the hub.

A word of caution on the use of disposable needles and syringes: After use they should be discarded in the designated containers, never where they can be obtained by addicts. Disposable needles and syringes should be bent after use so that they cannot be used again. These practices also help to protect the housekeeping staff from injury.

Two variations to the traditional means of administering injections subcutaneously are the injector syringe equipped with a spring which releases the needle for rapid insertion, and the jet injector by which the medication is introduced into the subcutaneous tissue by means of high pressure rather than through a needle. Although these methods are preferred in some instances, they have not replaced the usual subcutaneous injection by hypodermic syringe.

Preparation. Medications for injection come in tablet, liquid and powder forms. All these forms must be kept sterile during preparation and administration. If a drug in tablet form is to be administered subcutaneously, it is first dissolved in a sterile solution. The safest method is to carefully drop the tablet into a sterile container, draw up a measured amount of sterile solution into the syringe (sterile normal saline is less painful to the patient than sterile water), add the solution to the tablet to dissolve it and, finally, draw up the measured amount of medicated solution into the syringe ready for administration. Another method which is being used increasingly is to mix the tablet and the solution directly in the syringe.

Medications in a liquid form generally come in single dose ampules or multiple dose vials. To open an ampule, the nurse first taps it to shake all the medication to the bottom and then obtains a sterile cotton ball which she holds behind the neck of the ampule. Some ampules open directly upon pressure at the neck; others require filing. The cotton ball is used to protect the nurse's fingers when breaking the glass. After the ampule is opened, the needle is carefully inserted, the ampule is inverted, and the solution is drawn into the sterile syringe.

Multiple dose vials of medication have a sealed rubber cap at the top which makes them airtight. The cap is first wiped off with an antiseptic solution, the plunger of the syringe is drawn back to a point which indicates the volume of solution to be withdrawn and then the needle is inserted through the rubber cap. Air is injected into the vial to equalize the pressure and thus facilitate the removal of the solution. The vial is held upside down with the syringe at eye level in order to obtain an accurate measure of the drug. Incorrect holding of the vial may result in air being drawn into the syringe.

Injectable drugs that come as powders are dissolved in sterile solution before they are administered. Generally there are directions on the label as to the amount and kind of solution that is to be added to a vial. In order to maintain normal pressure inside the vial, air is removed in a volume that corresponds to the amount of solution that is inserted. If a large vial is used, it is often easier to insert a second sterile needle through the rubber cap to allow the free flow of air out of the vial as the fluid flows in.

Some drugs are now being prepared commercially in two-compartment vials. One compartment contains the powdered medication and the second contains the sterile liquid for dissolving the drug. The insertion of a sterile needle or pressure upon a rubber diaphragm releases the liquid to mix with the powder, which is then ready for injection. Some drugs are packaged this way because they are more stable in a dry state and thus can be kept for a longer period of time than the same drug in liquid form.

Whenever a powder or tablet is prepared for injection it should be completely dissolved before it is drawn into the syringe. Rotating a vial between one's hands is an effective way of mixing a powder and a liquid without creating bubbles on the top of the solution. Bubbles can make it difficult to ascertain an accurate measure of the drug.

Administration. When a subcutaneous injection is to be administered, a site is selected and cleansed with an antiseptic solution. The type of antiseptic used depends on the policy of the agency. Isopropanol in 70 per cent solution is used in many hospitals. The antiseptic solution is allowed to dry on the skin surface prior to insertion of the needle to prevent local irritation at the site of the injection.

When the skin is dry, air is expelled

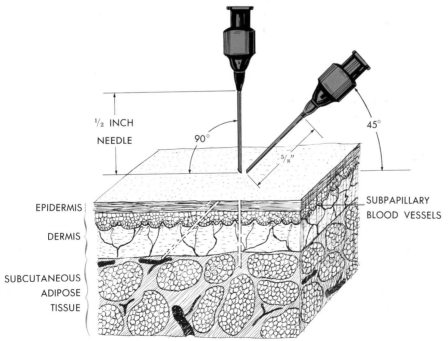

For a subcutaneous injection the needle enters the skin at a 90 degree angle if a ½ inch needle is used, at a 45 degree angle if a ⅝ inch needle is used. The bevel of the needle is uppermost. The needle is inserted deeply into the subcutaneous tissue.

from the needle. The needle is then inserted through the skin. The angle of insertion depends on the size of the needle used. It is recommended that the injection should be given deeply into the subcutaneous tissue. Therefore, if a ½ inch needle is used, it is inserted at a 90 degree angle, that is, perpendicular to the skin surface. Injections with a ⅝ inch needle are inserted at a 45 degree angle. Recent research indicates that the skin should not be drawn taut, pinched or pulled into a skin fold for the injection. Rather, it should be left in its natural state.[4] The nurse will find it easier to give the injection, however, if she lightly holds the area around the injection site.

After the needle is inserted the plunger is drawn back in order to determine whether the needle is in a blood vessel. If no blood appears in the syringe, the solution is injected slowly, after which the needle is quickly withdrawn. If blood does appear in the syringe, the needle is immediately withdrawn and another medication prepared. After the needle is withdrawn the area is massaged gently with an antiseptic sponge to facilitate dispersion of the solution. If there is any sign of bleeding from the site of the injection, firm pressure over the area for a few minutes will usually stop the bleeding and thus prevent bruising.

Recording. A subcutaneous injection is recorded on the patient's record as is any medication but, in addition, the word "subcutaneous" or the abbreviation "H" follows the dosage of the drug to indicate the route. Sometimes the site of the injection is also recorded.

Intramuscular Injection

Advantages and Disadvantages. Intramuscular injection is the method of choice for the administration of some medications. Drugs which are irritating to subcutaneous tissue are often given by this route. In addition, a larger amount of fluid can be given into mus-

cle tissue than into subcutaneous tissue. Absorption through a muscle is faster than through subcutaneous tissue because of the vascularity of the muscle area. The danger of damaging nerves and blood vessels, however is greater.

The Site of Injection. The selection of an area for an intramuscular injection depends on a number of factors: the size of the patient and the amount of muscle tissue available for injection, the proximity of nerves and blood vessels, the condition of the skin around the area, and the nature of the drug to be administered. The site should be anatomically safe; that is, an area should be chosen where the danger of hitting a nerve or large blood vessel is minimal. The tissues in the area should be free of bruising or soreness. There should be no abrasions on the skin, and areas with hardened tissue (such as scar tissue) should be avoided.

Various sites are suitable for intramuscular injections; areas in the buttocks, the thigh and the upper arm are used most frequently. Generally it is best to rotate the areas when a series of injections is to be given. The gluteal muscles are thick and permit the injection of larger quantities of fluid. Also, the use of these muscles in many normal daily activities aids in the absorption of drugs administered by this route. Two sites in the gluteal muscles are commonly used: the dorsogluteal site and the ventrogluteal site.

The *dorsogluteal site* uses the gluteus maximus muscle. The site may be located by dividing the buttock into quadrants. The crest of the ilium and the inferior gluteal fold act as landmarks for describing the buttock. The injection is given in the upper outer quadrant of the buttock, 2 to 3 inches below the crest of the ilium. By using this area, large blood vessels and the sciatic nerve are avoided. Another method for locating a safe gluteal site is to draw an imaginary line from the posterior superior iliac spine to the greater trochanter of the femur. This line runs lateral and parallel to the sciatic nerve, and consequently an injection lateral and superior to it is in a safe area.

---

[4]Ibid.

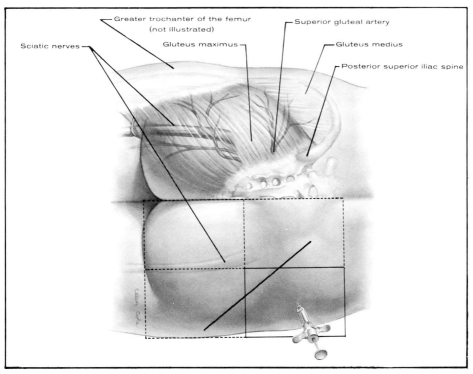

Intramuscular injection. With the patient lying in a prone position, the nurse can establish the dorsogluteal site as indicated. (Courtesy of Wyeth Laboratories, Philadelphia, Pa.)

When the *ventrogluteal site* is used the injection is made into the gluteus minimus and the gluteus medius muscles. To locate the ventrogluteal area, the nurse has the patient lie on his back or his side. She then places her hand on the patient's hip with her index finger on the anterior superior iliac spine, and stretching her middle finger dorsally, palpates the crest of the ilium and presses below the iliac crest. The injection site is the triangle that is formed by her index finger, middle finger and the crest of the ilium. The ventrogluteal site is being used increasingly because there are no large nerves or blood vessels in the area; also there is usually less fatty tissue than in the buttocks. If the patient's gluteal muscles are tense, he can flex his knees to relax them for the injection.

The *vastus lateralis* muscle on the lateral aspect of the thigh is also being used more frequently for intramuscular injections. The area is free of major blood vessels and nerve trunks, and the vastus lateralis muscle provides a good long area when numerous injections have to be given. The muscle extends the full length of the thigh from mid-anterior to mid-lateral and is approximately 3 inches wide. The site of injection may be anywhere from approximately 4 inches above the knee to approximately 4 inches below the hip joint.

The *deltoid muscle* of the arm is also used for intramuscular injections. This site is two to three fingerbreadths down from the acromion process on the outer aspect of the arm. In most people this is a smaller muscle than the gluteal muscle and therefore is not capable of absorbing as large a volume of medicine comfortably. The essential danger in this area is that of harming the radial nerve.

Equipment. The equipment required for an intramuscular injection is similar to that used for a subcutaneous injection. The quantity of solution to be administered varies from 2 to 10 cc.

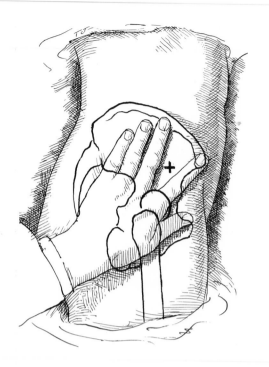

Locate the triangle for injection by placing the left index finger on the anterior iliac spine and the middle finger just below the iliac crest. (From What's New. Abbott Laboratories, No. 211, Spring, 1959.)

Four sites used for intramuscular injections are the deltoid muscle, the ventrogluteal site of the gluteus minimus and gluteus medius muscles, the dorsogluteal site of the gluteus maximus muscle, and the vastus lateralis muscle on the lateral aspect of the thigh.

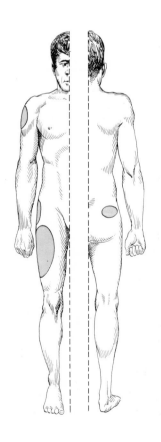

In many agencies, however, nurses are permitted to inject no more than 5 cc. in any one injection; therefore, if more than 5 cc. is ordered, the amount is given in two injections. A 2 cc., 5 cc. or 10 cc. syringe is used with a No. 19 to 22 needle, 1 to 2 inches in length. The gauge of the needle to be used depends on the viscosity of the drug and the sensitivity of the patient. The length of the needle depends on the size of the patient's muscle and the amount of adipose tissue that is present. It is desirable to inject the drug into the center of the muscle. A No. 22 needle 1½ inches long is commonly used for an adult.

Preparation. The drug is prepared for administration in the same way as for a subcutaneous injection. Some authorities recommend that a small air bubble be left in the syringe to force the last of the drug out of the needle into the muscle and thus prevent any solution from being left in the subcutaneous tissue when the needle is removed. There is probably considerable merit to this practice, particularly with drugs that are known to be irritating to subcutaneous tissue.

Administration. For an intramuscular injection to the gluteal muscle, the patient lies in a prone position with his toes internally rotated in plantar flexion. In this position the gluteal muscles are relaxed and there is good visualization of the injection site.

The selection of the area for an in-jection is determined by four factors: Is it anatomically safe? free of bruises or sore areas? free of hardened areas? free of abrasions on the skin?

The muscle is palpated and the skin is wiped as for a subcutaneous injection. The skin is held taut and the needle is inserted at a 90 degree angle to the distance required to reach the center of the muscle. When the needle is inserted smoothly and firmly, this is a relatively painless procedure. The skin is then released and the plunger is withdrawn in order to make sure the needle has not entered a blood vessel. Keeping the needle in place, the solution is injected slowly into the muscle tissue. The needle is then removed quickly and the area massaged gently with the disinfectant sponge to aid in dispersion of the solution.

In the air bubble method mentioned, it is common practice to draw a small bubble of air into the syringe before the solution is injected. The bubble rises to the top of the solution when the syringe is inverted for the injection. The air then helps to clear the needle of fluid before the needle is withdrawn. This prevents dripping of the fluid as the needle is being withdrawn through the subcutaneous tissue.[5]

---

[5] Audrey L. Sutton: *Bedside Nursing Techniques in Medicine and Surgery.* Second edition. Philadelphia, W. B. Saunders Company, 1969, pp. 79–80.

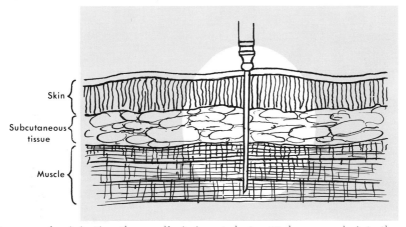

Skin

Subcutaneous tissue

Muscle

For an intramuscular injection the needle is inserted at a 90 degree angle into the center of the muscle.

When administering particularly irritating drugs into muscle tissue, the **Z** track method is used. In this method the site is selected and then the skin is pulled firmly toward the lateral aspect of the buttock. The injection site is reassessed, cleansed with disinfectant solution and then the needle is inserted at a 90 degree angle to one-half the desired depth. The needle is then moved slightly to the side and inserted the rest of the way, the nurse continuing to hold the syringe at a 90 degree angle to the skin surface. When the needle has been inserted the full way, the skin is released, the plunger is drawn back and then the solution is injected slowly. After injecting the solution, the nurse restretches the skin laterally, waits 10 seconds and withdraws the needle. The skin is then released, and the area is massaged with a cotton ball. This method helps keep the drug in the muscle and away from the subcutaneous tissue.

With careful technique, complications from intramuscular injections can be avoided. Abscesses, nerve injuries, cysts and necrosis of tissue do occur as a result of intramuscular injections; however, the use of aseptic technique, individual establishment of landmarks for injection sites and the alternating of sites help to avoid these unpleasant results.

As more research is done in the field of intramuscular injections, the nurse may well find traditional techniques being modified in many agencies in the light of new research findings.

Recording. After the administration of an intramuscular injection, the drug, dosage and method of administration are recorded. The abbreviation "I.M." is frequently used to indicate the route. The site of administration is often recorded also.

Intradermal Injection

An intradermal injection is the injection of a small amount of fluid into the dermal layer of the skin. It is frequently done as a diagnostic measure, as in tuberculin testing and allergy testing. The areas of the body commonly used are the medial aspect of the forearm and the subscapular region of the back.

A 1 cc. syringe (or a tuberculin syringe) and a 26 gauge needle ⅜ inch in length are commonly used. A tuberculin syringe is calibrated in tenths and hundredths of a cubic centimeter in order that minute doses can be measured. The needle is inserted at a 15 degree angle with the bevel up, and the fluid is injected to produce a small bleb just under the skin.

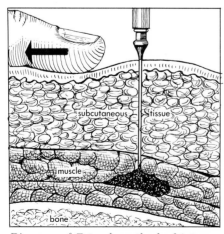
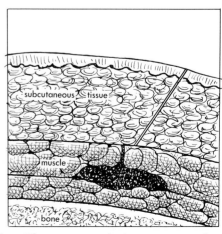

Diagram of Z track method of intramuscular injection. The correct technique converts the needle track into a zig-zag which prevents leakage into tissues.

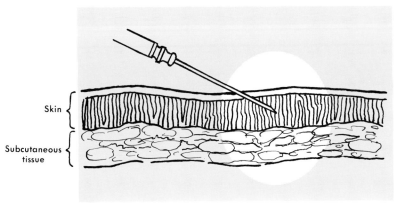

For an intradermal injection the needle is held at a 15 degree angle, bevel upward, and inserted into the dermal layer of the skin.

TOLERANCE AND ADDICTION

When some medications are taken over a long period of time, the effect of the drug diminishes and the patient requires continually larger doses. This reaction to a medicine is called tolerance. Narcotics are among the drugs for which patients frequently develop such a tolerance.

Addiction refers to the habitual use of a drug. Usually the person is physically and psychologically dependent upon the drug. Addiction is a serious problem with many drugs. It may become a problem when people are ill and receive narcotics or barbiturates over a prolonged period of time.

An awareness of which drugs are most likely to result in tolerance and addiction is important. At the first indication that a drug is not acting as it did previously, or at the first indication of dependency upon a particular medication, the physician should be notified. Often alternative medicines can be administered as a preventive measure.

GUIDE TO ASSESSING NURSING NEEDS

1. Does the patient have any allergies?
2. What medications have been prescribed for the patient?
3. Why is the patient receiving these medications?
4. What observations should the nurse make relative to the effect of these medications on the patient?
5. Are there specific nursing measures indicated because of the action of drugs contained in these medications?
6. How are the patient's medications to be administered?
7. What precautions should be taken in administering these medications? Are there special precautions that should be taken because of the patient's age, physical condition or mental state?
8. Do any of the medications require special precautionary measures in their administration?
9. Does the patient have learning needs relative to his medicinal therapy?
10. Does the patient or his family require specific skills or knowledge in order to continue medicinal therapy at home?

GUIDE TO EVALUATING THE EFFECTIVENESS OF NURSING ACTION

1. Is the patient taking the medicines that have been prescribed?
2. Have the medications been administered safely?
3. Does the patient exhibit signs or symptoms which indicate that the medications are effective (or ineffective)?

4. Has the administration of the medications been accurately charted on the patient's record? Have pertinent observations been recorded and reported to appropriate personnel?

<table>
<tr><td>STUDY
VOCABULARY</td><td>Addiction
Ampule
Inhalation
Intradermal
Intramuscular</td><td>Isotonic
Minim
Oral
Parenteral</td><td>Subcutaneous
Sublingual
Topical
Vial</td></tr>
</table>

STUDY SITUATION

Mrs. J. Sloskey is a patient in a large metropolitan hospital. She is 67 years old and has a heart disease. Her physician has ordered an intramuscular injection of Mercuhydrin 2 cc. daily, digitalis gr. 1½ daily if her pulse is above 60 beats per minute and nitroglycerin gr. 1/150 p.r.n. for chest pain.

Mrs. Sloskey was born in Europe. She has been in this country only two years and does not understand English. She lives with her son and three grandchildren. This is her first time in the hospital.

1. What factors would you consider when explaining to this patient about her medicines?
2. How could you explain about the nitroglycerin if it is to be left for her to take when it is necessary?
3. Draw up a sample teaching plan for this patient.
4. What observations should you make regarding the effectiveness of the medications?
5. What should be charted relevant to this patient's medications?
6. What difficulties could you anticipate in regard to helping this patient with her medicinal therapy?
7. If Mrs. Sloskey is to continue to take her digitalis when she returns home, what additions to the teaching plan would you make?

BIBLIOGRAPHY

Bergersen, Betty S., and Elsie E. Krug: *Pharmacology in Nursing.* Tenth edition. St. Louis, The C. V. Mosby Company, 1966.

Dann, T. C.: Routine Skin Preparation Before Injections—Is it Necessary? *Nursing Times,* 62:1121, 1966.

Falconer, Mary W., Mabelclaire R. Norman, H. Robert Patterson and Edward A. Gustafson: *The Drug, The Nurse, The Patient.* Fourth edition. Philadelphia, W. B. Saunders Company, 1970.

Friedrich, H.: Common Sense in Intramuscular Injection. *Nursing Clinics of North America,* 1:333, 1966.

Goodman, Louis S., and Alfred Gilman: *The Pharmacological Basis of Therapeutics.* Third edition. New York, The Macmillan Company, 1965.

Hanson, Daniel J.: Intramuscular Injection Injuries and Complications. *The American Journal of Nursing,* 63:99–101, April, 1963.

Hershey, Nathan: Question That Drug Order. *The American Journal of Nursing,* 63:96–97, January, 1963.

Hershey, Nathan: The Nurse Wasn't Liable. *The American Journal of Nursing*, 67:1875, 1967.

Kernicki, J.: Needle Puncture: Health Asset or Menace? *Nursing Clinics of North America*, 1:269, 1966.

Nordmark, Madelyn T., and Anne W. Rohweder: *Scientific Foundations of Nursing*. Second edition. Philadelphia, J. B. Lippincott Company, 1967.

Pitel, Martha: The Subcutaneous Injection. *The American Journal of Nursing*, 71:1:76–79, January, 1971.

Pitel, M., and M. Wemett: The Intramuscular Injection. *The American Journal of Nursing*, 64:4:104–109, April, 1964.

Smith, Ralph G.: The Development and Control of New Drugs. *The American Journal of Nursing*, 62:56–58, July, 1962.

Sutton, Audrey L.: *Bedside Nursing Techniques in Medicine and Surgery*. Second edition. Philadelphia, W. B. Saunders Company, 1969.

22 THE CARE OF PATIENTS WHO HAVE WOUNDS

The nurse should be able to:

Define terms commonly used to classify wounds

Describe the three stages of wound healing

Differentiate between healing by first, second and third intention

List factors which affect wound healing

List factors predisposing to the development of infection in a wound

Name microorganisms frequently found in infected wounds

Describe localized and general symptoms of wound infection

Accurately record and report her observations about wounds using appropriate medical terminology

List principles from the biophysical sciences relevant to wound care

Describe a safe technique for carrying out a sterile dressing

Explain the purpose of binders; list types commonly used, principles relevant to their application and problems associated with their use

Explain purposes for which bandages are used; name materials commonly used in their manufacture and principles relevant to their use

Describe five turns used in bandaging

286

CLASSIFICATION OF WOUNDS

A wound by definition is a break in the continuity of any body structure, internal or external, caused by physical means. Wounds can be classified in three ways; according to the presence or absence of microorganisms, according to the presence or absence of a break in the surface tissue and according to the cause of the wound.

A wound is said to be clean, contaminated or infected. A *clean* wound does not contain pathogenic (disease-producing) microorganisms, whereas *contaminated* and *infected* wounds do contain these organisms. Normally a wound that is made under aseptic conditions, for example, a surgical incision, is considered to be a *clean* wound; wounds that occur as a result of accidents are considered *contaminated* until they are proved to be clean. If the pathogenic microorganisms in a contaminated wound are sufficiently virulent (capable of producing disease) and present in sufficient quantity, then an infectious process becomes apparent. The wound is then referred to as an *infected* wound. Frequently the terms "contaminated" and "infected" are used interchangeably although, in the strict sense of the meanings of these words, the two are not the same.

No wound is ever completely sterile. The skin and mucous membrane harbor some microorganisms as normal inhabitants. These are not normally pathogenic; their lack of virulence and their sparsity usually serve to prevent the development of an infectious process.

Wounds are also classified according to the presence or absence of a break in the surface covering. In a *closed wound* there is no break in the skin or mucous membrane. Such wounds are frequently caused by direct blows, traction or deceleration, a twisting or bending force or direct muscle action. A common example of a closed wound is the fractured femur which so often results when an elderly person pivots or falls. *Open wounds* involve the destruction of skin or mucous membrane, thus exposing the underlying tissue to open air. Cuts, punctures and surface abrasions are examples of open wounds.

Wounds are classified according to their etiology. A *traumatic* or accidental wound is one which occurs by accident. Since it happens under septic conditions, its chances of becoming infected are considerable. An *intentional* wound is one that is produced for a specific purpose, usually under aseptic conditions. For example, the wound made during an operation, generally under ideal sterile conditions, is an intentional wound.

Wounds are further described according to the manner in which they occur.

An *abraded wound* occurs as a result of friction or scraping. It is a superficial wound in which the outer layers of the skin or mucous membrane are damaged or scraped off. An example is the scrape a child gets when he falls on his knees on a cement sidewalk.

287

A *contused wound* occurs as a result of a blow from a blunt instrument, such as a hammer, without breaking the skin.

An *incised wound* occurs as a result of a cut by a sharp instrument. An example of an incised wound is one made by a scalpel during surgery; the wound edges are smooth.

In a *lacerated wound* the tissues are torn apart and remain jagged and irregular. An example of a lacerated wound is a cut by a saw.

A *penetrating wound* occurs as a result of an instrument which penetrates into the deep tissues of the body. An example is a bullet which enters the chest and lodges in the lung.

A *puncture or stab wound* is a wound made by a pointed instrument such as a nail or wire. The scalpel is occasionally used by the physician to make a puncture wound so as to promote drainage from tissues. The term "puncture wound" is also used to describe an open wound resulting from a break (or puncture) of the skin surface and underlying tissues by the bite of an animal or the sting of an insect.

THE INFLAMMATORY PROCESS

A wound, by definition, implies that there has been damage to body tissues. Whenever body tissues are damaged, an inflammatory reaction occurs at the site of the injury. The injury may have been caused by bacterial, chemical, thermal or physical means; the localized response of tissues in the damaged area is the same. In order to understand wound healing, it is first of all necessary to discuss the nature of the inflammatory process.

When body tissues are damaged, an increased supply of blood is always diverted to the area and certain substances are released by the injured cells to promote the repair and regeneration of the tissues. Among these substances are *leukotaxine* and *necrosin*. Leukotaxine draws white blood cells to the area, where they help to destroy and remove foreign substances such as bacteria and decaying tissue cells. Necrosin increases permeability of the capillary walls, which allows the fluids, proteins and white blood cells to move into the area. Necrosin also activates the clotting mechanism so that the fluids clot and serve to "wall off" the injured area.[1]

Typically, there are five observable results from the inflammatory process: heat, redness, pain, swelling and limitation of function. The redness is due to the local dilation of blood vessels and consequent increase in the supply of blood to the part. The heat of the area is also the result of the increased blood supply. The swelling results from the exudative process, in which serum and leukocytes leave the blood stream to invade the area. The pain is believed to result from the stimulation of pain receptors in the area by certain substances released by the damaged cells and possibly also by the pressure of accumulated fluid (see Chapter 28). Limitation of function is usually due to the swelling and the pain.

THE PROCESS OF WOUND HEALING

The process of wound healing can be divided into three phases: the lag phase, the fibroplasia phase and the phase of contraction.

In the *lag phase*, as a result of the injury to the cells, the capillaries become dilated in the injured area. The volume of blood in the area is increased but the speed of the flow of blood is slowed. The blood brings leukocytes and plasma which form an exudate in the injured area. At this time the injured cells disintegrate and there is some swelling due to the plugging of the lymphatics by fibrin. During this phase, the wound is usually covered lightly by a scab or

[1]Arthur C. Guyton: *Function of the Human Body.* Philadelphia, W. B. Saunders Company, 1969, p. 100.

fibrin network which is later absorbed.

In the *fibroplasia phase* there is an ingrowth of new capillaries and lymphatic endothelial buds in the wounded area. Fibroplasia results in the formation of granulation tissue (a connective tissue); subsequently there is epithelization. The wound appears pink, owing to the new capillaries in the granulation tissue, and the area is soft and tender.

In the third phase, that of *contraction*, there is cicatrization or scar formation by the fibroblasts after the cessation of fibroplasia. The capillaries and lymphatic endothelial buds in the new tissue disappear, and the scar then shrinks.

Open wounds require the formation of more granulation tissue, fibrous tissue and epithelial tissue than closed wounds. During the first five or six days there is little strength in a healing wound; however, during the next 10 days the tissue becomes stronger and better able to withstand tension.

Types of Healing

Healing by First Intention. In healing by first intention the sutured wound heals without infection or separation at the edges. There is minimal granulation tissue present and thus a small scar results. In most surgical incisions, the edges of the wound are sutured closely together and healing occurs by first intention.

Healing by Second Intention. In healing by second intention the edges of the wound are not approximated. As a consequence a large amount of granulation tissue is formed during the healing process, and the scar that results is usually large. The healing of decubitus ulcers illustrates healing by second intention. The crater of the ulcer must be filled in by the growth of new tissue. The process is a slow one and the resultant scar is large.

Healing by Third Intention. This is a combination of the two previously mentioned types of healing. Either the wound is initially left open and later sutured or it breaks open after an original suturing and has to be resutured.

There is considerable granulation tissue formed in this type of healing.

Factors Which Influence Healing

Many factors influence the speed and the character of the healing process:

Extent of the Injury. The process of repair and regeneration is naturally longer when tissue damage is extensive.

Nutrition. Nutritional status, specifically the protein and vitamin C levels, affects the healing process. Protein is necessary for the formation of new tissue; vitamin C is involved in the maturation of the collagen fibers (the fibrous tissue) during the later stages of healing.

Age. Healing is more rapid in children than in elderly persons. There are many factors which are felt to retard the healing process in the aged. These include a lessened efficiency of the circulatory system, particularly to surface areas of the body, and an increased likelihood of poor nutritional status among older people.

Blood Supply. The blood supplies the products used in healing. Hence any factor which restricts blood circulation to a wound area interferes with healing. Edema, restrictive bandages and damaged arteries can slow the healing process.

Hormones. It has been demonstrated that large doses of the adrenocortical hormones slow wound healing; for example, cortisone decreases the formation of collagen. This has implications in situations in which prolonged stress stimulates the release of these hormones.

Infection. Infectious processes result in tissue destruction, which in turn results in a longer healing time. Foreign bodies also interfere with healing.

Edema. Gross edema hinders healing by inhibiting the transport of the building supplies to the area. There is some evidence, however, that a small amount of edema enhances fibroplasia.

Irradiation. It has been shown that five to six days after irradiation, the healing process is slowed.

THE INFECTED WOUND

An infected wound is one in which an active infectious process is present. All wounds contain organisms; many organisms are present in the air and thus, immediately after a wound is opened, it can be expected to harbor organisms. But the mere presence of bacteria in a wound does not mean that an infection will necessarily ensue. Other factors are involved in the development of an infection:

The Virulence, Number and Types of Organisms. Certain types and strains of microorganisms are more likely to produce a disease than others. Also the fewer the number of pathogenic organisms, the less likely they are to produce an infection.

Devitalized Tissue. Unhealthy tissue is less resistant to infection than healthy tissue. Poor circulation, inadequate nutrition and dehydration all contribute to devitalization of tissue.

Local and General Immunity. Some tissues have a greater immunity than others. Highly vascular tissue is less prone to infections than tissue nourished by a more limited circulation. Also there is a variability in the general resistance of the tissues of individuals.

Nature of the Wound. The occurrence of infection depends to some extent upon the presence of foreign bodies and organic contamination. Infection is also more likely in extensive wounds and in areas where local resistance is low, for example, in the perineal area. Generally the tissue of the face and neck have high resistance and heal well.

General Condition of the Patient. Anemia, dehydration, etc., lower resistance and make any wound more prone to infection.

Organisms Causing Infection

There are several organisms which are commonly found in wound infections. Of the gram-positive group, *Staphylococcus aureus* and *S. albus* are found most commonly. These are spherical asymmetric bacteria that are normally found in the nose, skin and feces. The α- and β- hemolytic streptococci are also the cause of many infectious processes. It has been stated that 8 per cent of all people carry these bacteria in the nasopharynx.

The toxigenic clostridia are anaerobic spore-forming bacilli. They thrive in airless conditions, being found in the intestinal tracts of animals, in dust and in soil. *Clostridium tetani*, the cause of tetanus, is a well known member of this family; many physicians automatically give prophylactic doses of tetanus antitoxin to patients whose wounds have come in contact with soil.

Of the gram-negative bacteria, *Escherichia coli*, *Aerobacter* and *Alcaligenes* are frequently found in wounds. These, together with *Proteus* and *Pseudomonas*, are the principal inhabitants of the intestine. They can also often be isolated in the anogenital area, and are frequent causes of urinary tract infections.

Symptoms of Infected Wounds

The patient who has an infected wound is likely to present local and general symptoms of infection. The local symptoms of wound infection are due to an aggravation of the inflammatory process. Typically the wound area is more reddened, swollen, hot to the touch and painful than it should be in the normal healing process. In addition there may be purulent drainage from the wound.

The generalized signs and symptoms of an infection are fever, lethargy, headache, anorexia (loss of appetite), nausea and possibly chills. General symptoms frequently occur when the invasive bacteria emit toxins in the body. The degree to which a person exhibits some or all of these symptoms is highly dependent upon the severity of the infection and the resistance of the body.

OBSERVATION OF WOUNDS

When a wound is examined, for example, while a dressing is changed, certain features of the wound itself and the discharge from it are carefully observed. The wound is observed for the approximation of the edges. Some wounds are closed by sutures or skin clips, others by the pressure of a bandage or butterfly tape. A butterfly tape can be made from a strip of adhesive tape narrowed in the middle and placed across the wound so that the adhesive part of the tape sticks to the patient's skin on both sides of the wound and draws the edges of the wound together. The adhesive side of the tape directly over the wound is usually covered so that it will not adhere to the wound itself. Gaping in a sutured or taped wound could delay healing and should be reported. Some wounds are not closed deliberately but are left to close naturally by second intention. A wound is also observed for signs of inflammation and infection, such as redness, swelling, pain, heat and limitation of function of the part of the body afflicted.

The amount of discharge that is considered normal is dependent upon the site, size and type of wound. Normally it is not unusual for a wound to exude some *serous drainage* postoperatively. (Serum is the clear portion of the blood). A wound in the anogenital area can be expected to have more serous discharge than a wound of the face. Serous discharge is amber in color and contains water, blood cells and some cellular debris.

Sanguineous drainage is red. "Sanguineous" refers to blood. Bright sanguineous drainage is composed of fresh blood; dark sanguineous drainage is composed of old blood.

Infected wounds often have a *purulent discharge.* "Purulent" is defined as containing pus. Pus can be white, yellow, pink or green, often depending upon the infecting organism. It is usually thick and may have a distinctively unpleasant odor. Other than the three basic kinds of wound discharge there are combinations, which may be described as serosanguineous, seropurulent and purosanguineous for example.

An accurate description of a wound's discharge must include the amount. Traditional descriptions, such as gross, moderate and small, are highly subject to individual interpretation and often relative to the site and type of wound. For example, the amount of drainage that would be considered moderate after perineal surgery would usually be considered abnormally large after an appendectomy. Because the use of these adjectives can be misleading, more exact measures are used. It is the policy in some agencies to describe the amount of drainage by the number of dressings that are soaked and the exact measure of the spread of the drainage upon the dressing. An example of this kind of descriptive charting would be "serosanguineous drainage 3 inches in diameter soaked through two gauze dressings."

In addition to a description of the wound and the drainage other signs and symptoms are recorded, for example, stabbing pain near the wound or evidence of fever, headache or anorexia.

PRINCIPLES RELEVANT TO THE CARE OF WOUNDS

Skin and mucous membranes normally harbor microorganisms. In order to decrease the transfer of organisms to a wound, handwashing is indicated before and after attending a patient. In addition, the use of a disinfectant upon and around a wound decreases the number of microorganisms and thus lessens the danger of infection.

Microorganisms are present in the air. Sometimes a wound is left exposed, particularly if it is a superficial one which has closed itself. The majority of surgical incisions, however, and wounds involving deeper-lying tissues are protected by a sterile dressing. When the dressing is changed, precautions are usually taken to keep the time the wound is exposed as short as possible and the circulation of the air in the room at a minimum. These precautions have a twofold purpose: to protect the wound from possible contamination by airborne bacteria in the atmosphere and to minimize the convection of microorganisms from the wound to the circulating air. When a wound is infected, or there is possibility that pathogenic bacteria (as, for example, *Staphylococcus aureus*) are present in the atmosphere, these precautions are particularly important.

Moisture facilitates the growth of microorganisms. Dressings that are wet with drainage are more likely to foster the growth of organisms than dry dressings. Often dressings are changed whenever they become soaked through to the top. If there is no order to change the dressing, it can be reinforced with additional dry sterile dressings to inhibit the transfer of organisms from the outside to the wound until the physician has been notified.

Moisture facilitates the movement of microorganisms. When a dressing becomes soaked through to the outside, the movement of microorganisms toward the wound is facilitated because the moisture provides a vehicle for their transport. Because the outside of a dressing is generally highly contaminated, the movement of organisms from the outside inward must be prevented. Maintaining dry dressings inhibits the multiplication and the transfer of organisms.

Fluids flow downward as a result of gravitational pull. In a draining wound the area of greatest contamination is, in all probability, the lowest part, where the drainage collects. If it is desirable to promote drainage, a drain or packing is usually placed in the lowest part of the wound by the doctor.

The respiratory tract often harbors microorganisms which can be spread to open wounds. When an open wound is exposed, measures are taken to prevent the spread of microorganisms from the respiratory tract. It is common practice in many agencies for nurses and physicians to wear masks while dressing wounds, and in some instances patients also wear masks. In any case, as a precautionary measure against contamination, it is advisable not to talk while a wound is exposed.

The blood transports the materials that nourish and repair body tissues. When dressing and bandaging a wound, care is exercised to ensure that circulation to the area is not restricted in any way. Bandages and dressings are never made restrictively tight, and they are applied starting at the distal portion of the body and proceeding to the proximal portion as a means of promoting venous flow.

Skin and mucous membranes can be injured by chemical, mechanical, thermal and microbial agents. The disinfectants and medications used to cleanse and treat a wound and the surrounding tissue should be strong enough to be effective, but they should not irritate healthy tissue. Protective ointments such as sterile petrolatum can be used to protect the skin when it is necessary to use irritating disinfectants, such as Dakin's solution, upon open wounds.

To avoid mechanical injury at bony prominences which are to be bandaged, padding is provided to prevent irritation due to friction. Adhesive tape must be removed carefully; often, to avoid trauma, specially prepared solvents can be used to loosen the adhesive. Thermal injury can be avoided by the use of solutions at a temperature which is noninjurious to tissue. Room temperature is generally considered to be safe for most tissues.

Microbial injury can be largely avoided by practicing sterile technique in the care of wounds. All solutions, dressings and equipment that come into contact with an open wound should be sterile.

Fluids move through materials by capillary action. Loosely woven fabrics such as gauze provide a good surface for capillary action. The fluid is absorbed through the material as each thread in the material conducts the fluid away from the wound by the action of the surface tension of the fluid and the forces of adhesion and cohesion. Adhesion and cohesion refer to forces which draw together.

GENERAL WOUND CARE

Just as there is considerable variety in the kinds of wounds so there is variety in the care that they require. A wound may be closed by sutures, with no drainage resulting. This type of wound is often left with the original dressing in place until it is completely healed. Sometimes wounds are sprayed with a clear plastic material which seals the wound and eliminates the need for any dressings.

Operative wounds are normally sutured with black silk or wire sutures or they may be held together by metal clips. These wounds do not heal over for the first four or five days postoperatively, and they may or may not require attention. If a wound is expected to drain excessively, a drain or packing is inserted by the physician to facilitate this process. Soft and firm rubber drains as well as plastic drains are used for this purpose. Packing is usually made of a long strip of gauze, often impregnated with a disinfectant or antibiotic. Drains and packing are sometimes withdrawn a little each day to encourage healing from the depth of the wound toward the surface. Considerable drainage can be anticipated from wounds of this nature. Some drains are sutured in place, whereas others are freely movable. Soft rubber drains (Penrose drains) often have a sterile safety pin attached to the distal portion of the drain to prevent it from slipping completely inside the wound.

Wounds that are draining need to be changed whenever the dressings are wet. The drainage is not only frequently irritating to the skin, but it also serves as a likely site for infection. Wounds that drain urine, feces or gastric and intestinal secretions necessitate the use of ointments, such as zinc oxide or petrolatum, on the surrounding skin as a protection against irritation. The skin around these wounds should also be cleaned regularly with a mild soap or disinfectant to remove the irritating materials.

DRESSINGS

The frequency with which dressings are changed is dependent upon the needs of the patient and to some extent upon the orders of the physician. An order might state that a wound is to be dressed at regular intervals, for example, twice a day, or it might leave the frequency with which a dressing is to be changed to the nurse's judgment. In the latter situation the dressing is changed when it is wet, but never more often than necessary, because each time a wound is exposed the chance of initiating an infection is increased.

Preparation of the Environment

When a wound is to be exposed to the open air, every effort is made to decrease the number of microorganisms which could possibly come in contact with it. Consequently windows and doors are closed to eliminate drafts, and curtains are drawn around the patient to provide privacy.

The bed unit is arranged for the convenience of the person changing the patient's dressings. Usually the bedside table or overbed table is cleared beforehand so that the nurse can put the dressing tray in a convenient place. Before wound care, the nurse washes her hands to reduce the number of microorganisms which are normally on her skin (see Handwashing, Chapter 16).

Preparation of the Equipment

The specific equipment required depends upon the kind of wound. It is considered that the safest aseptic technique is that carried out by using individual trays containing only the materials and equipment which can be discarded or sterilized after the wound is dressed. By not taking bottles and the like from one patient to another the transfer of microorganisms by such vectors is eliminated.

For changing most wound dressings it is necessary to have a receptacle for the old dressings and gauze sponges (wax paper bags permit such contaminated materials to be covered and disposed of easily while the wax keeps the moisture inside the bag), a container of disinfectant, two or three forceps (tissue and

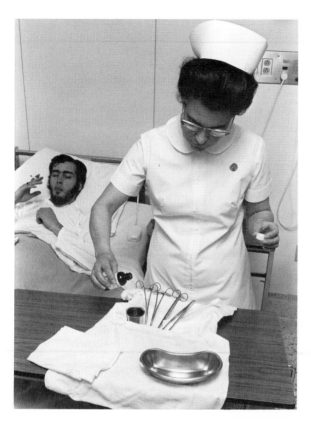

The nurse prepares the dressing tray at the patient's bedside.

artery forceps are often used), sterile dressings and gauze sponges. For the care of some wounds it is also necessary to have sterile scissors either to shorten drains or to shape the dressings. The nurse will usually need adhesive tape as well.

After this equipment has been placed on a tray and protected from contamination, for example, by covering it with a sterile towel, it can be safely transported to the patient. Some agencies have standard sets ready for use; it is then necessary only to add the disinfectant and any additional equipment needed by a particular patient. If a mask is to be worn, it is usually put on before the equipment is arranged, and it is kept on until the wound care has been completed.

Preparation of the Patient

Prior to the dressing of a wound, the needs of the patient for information about the procedure are determined. If the patient will be seeing his wound for the first time, he may want some information about its appearance and what will happen during the dressing change. The details of the explanation depend upon the patient's needs. Often a wound has a meaning for the patient other than the obvious; for example, he might be worried about the appearance of a scar.

The patient can assist by lying still during the procedure in order that the wound and the equipment do not accidentally become contaminated. Some patients need to be advised not to talk and to keep their hands away from the wound area so that sterile technique is maintained. During the explanation, words such as "infection," "contaminated" and "dirty" are used with caution, since they may make the patient feel that something is wrong or may stimulate him to speculate about future complications.

Inexperienced people often ask whether changing a dressing or removing drains and sutures is painful. These people are frequently worried about their ability to cope with pain in a socially acceptable manner. Generally all of these measures are painless, with the exception of removing dressings that adhere to the skin surface. Dressings that do stick to the skin because of dried discharges can usually be removed with little discomfort by soaking them with sterile normal saline or sterile water.

Another possible source of discomfort is the use of a disinfectant with an alcohol base. Such applications may feel cold to the patient and may possibly sting when they come in contact with an open wound. The use of a disinfectant without an alcoholic base is often advisable. If the procedure is going to be uncomfortable, patients are usually better able to cope with it if they have been given some warning so that their responses can be structured in advance.

Prior to the changing of a dressing the patient assumes a position which is convenient and comfortable for him. It may be necessary to provide drapes for adequate warmth and privacy.

Procedures for Changing the Dressing

The equipment is arranged in a manner such that it is not necessary to pass soiled dressings and sponges over the sterile field. Some health agencies advocate the use of sterile gloves for changing a dressing and cleansing a wound; others suggest that sterile forceps technique be used. Whichever method is practiced it is important that all equipment coming in contact with an open wound be sterile.

Generally the old dressing is removed with sterile forceps, the old dressing is dropped into the wax paper bag and the forceps are then placed in a discard container. The wound is then cleansed with a disinfectant. Four rules for cleansing a wound are:

1. Use a sponge only once, cleansing from the top of the wound to the bottom, and then discard the sponge. The cleanest part of the wound is at the top, where there is the least amount of drainage.

2. After cleansing the wound itself, work away from the wound to a distance of about 2 inches. The wound is the cleanest area; the surrounding skin contains more microorganisms.

3. When not wearing sterile gloves, keep the tips of the forceps lower than the handle. Ungloved hands contaminate the handle of the forceps and the solution on the tips will run down to the handle if the tips are held up; then upon lowering the tips the contaminated solution returns to the tips, contaminating the entire instrument.

4. Do not carry contaminated sponges over sterile areas. There is a danger that the contaminated solution will drop on sterile equipment.

After a wound has been cleansed, it is irrigated if this has been ordered. Normally about 500 cc. of a sterile solution at room temperature is used for wound irrigation. If the irrigating solution is irritating to the skin, the surrounding areas should be protected beforehand by an ointment such as sterile petrolatum. During irrigation, the patient lies so that when the nurse administers the irrigating solution with a sterile syringe it flows freely over the wound and then into a receptacle. After an irrigation, the skin is patted dry with sterile sponges.

The new sterile dressing is placed over the wound with sterile forceps. It should be dropped in place rather than moved over the skin so as not to transfer microorganisms from the skin to the center of the wound and to avoid mechanical injury to the wound. When wet dressings are used, they are soaked in the prescribed solution, wrung out with artery forceps and then placed on the wound. The outer dressings should extend at least 2 inches beyond an open wound as a precaution against later contamination should the edges be accidentally turned back.

The dressings can be secured by adhesive tape, elasticized tape, waterproof tape, adhesive ties (Montgomery straps), binders, bandages or plastic tape. The type of material and the method by which it is secured depend upon the site of the wound and the specific needs of the patient. For the patient who is allergic to adhesive tape, some other type of commercially prepared adhesive bandage can be used. Plastic tape is frequently used on the face because of its nonirritating quality. Waterproof tape keeps a wound dry; thus it is especially useful next to a draining area. Adhesive ties are used when frequent dressing changes are necessary, since only the tie part needs to be undone when the dressing is changed; the adhesive portion does not have to be removed from the skin unless the tape becomes soiled.

When a dressing is to be secured by adhesive tape, painting the patient's skin with tincture of benzoin beforehand serves to protect the surface epithelium. It is also more comfortable for the patient when areas that have hair are shaved so that the tape does not stick to the hair on removal. Adhesive tape can be readily removed by using a solvent such as acetone to loosen the gum of the tape. Ether and benzene can also be used, but they are highly flammable and for this reason are not often kept near patients.

BINDERS

Binders can be used to retain dressings, to apply pressure, to support an area of the body and to provide comfort. Binders are generally made of a heavy cotton material which is strong and durable. Scultetus binders are occasionally lined with flannel, which absorbs moisture and provides additional comfort. When the purpose of the binder is to provide support to abdominal muscles, a two-way-stretch type of girdle is sometimes used for women patients.

Principles Relevant to the Application of Binders

1. Binders are applied in such a manner as to provide even pressure over an area of the body.

2. Binders should support body parts in their normal anatomical position, with slight joint flexion.

3. Binders are secured firmly so that they do not cause friction and thereby irritate the skin or mucous membrane.

Types of Binders

There are five basic types of binders: T binder, straight abdominal binder, scultetus (many tailed) binder, breast binder and triangular binder.

The T Binder. This binder is made of two strips of cotton attached in the shape of a T. The top of the T serves as a

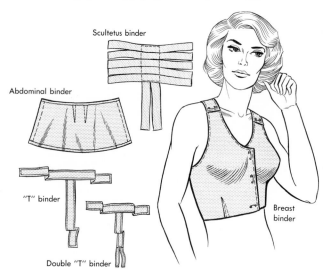

Scultetus binder

Abdominal binder

"T" binder

Double "T" binder

Breast binder

Types of binders.

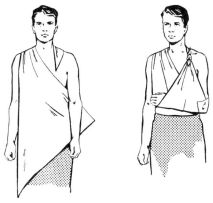

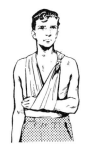

A small arm sling.

A large arm sling.

band which is then placed around the patient's waist. The stem of the T is passed between the patient's legs and is then attached to the waistband in front. In some T binders the cotton strip that goes between the patient's legs is split into two tails about 9 inches from the end. These tails provide wider support to the perineal area and add to the comfort of the male patient particularly.

T binders are used chiefly to retain perineal dressings. Because of the profuse drainage that often occurs from this area, they are usually changed frequently.

The Straight Abdominal Binder. The straight abdominal binder is a rectangular piece of cotton from 6 to 12 inches wide, and long enough to encircle the patient's abdomen and overlap at least 2 inches in front. This type of binder is used to retain abdominal dressings

or to apply pressure and support to the abdomen.

The Scultetus Binder. Also known as the many-tailed binder, the scultetus binder is a rectangular piece of cotton, usually 9 to 12 inches wide and 15 inches long, with perhaps 6 to 12 tails attached to each side. It is usually used to provide support to the abdomen, but it can also be used to retain dressings. It can be applied to the chest as well as the abdomen. The advantage of the scultetus binder is that it fits the contours of the body closely.

The Breast Binder. This binder is a rectangular piece of cotton shaped roughly to the contours of the female chest. It usually has straps which fit over the shoulders and pin to the binder in front. Breast binders are used to retain dressings and to apply pressure to the breasts, as when drying up breast milk after the birth of a baby.

The Triangular Binder (Sling). Various forms of the triangular binder are used to support a limb, to secure a splint (as a first aid measure) and to

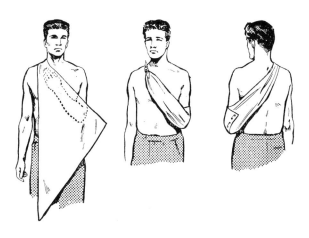

A triangular sling.

secure dressings. The triangular binder is made of heavy cotton, is triangular in shape and has two sides approximately 40 inches in length. It can be applied as a full triangle or, after it has been folded, in a variety of ways.

As a full triangle, the binder is used frequently to make a *large arm sling*. Folded into a broad bandage, it can be used as a *small sling* to support the patient's wrist and hand. A triangular binder can also support a person's arm in such a manner as to elevate the hand. This is called a *triangular sling*.

Triangular binders can also be used to retain dressings on the elbow, hand, shoulder, hip, knee and foot. For details on the application of binders the nurse should consult a bandaging or first air book. There are also a number of multimedia aids now available to assist students to develop skills in applying binders and bandages.

Problems Related to the Use of Binders

Binders are most often used for large areas of the body, and since they are not secured to skin surfaces, they have a tendency to slip out of position. A binder should be changed or reapplied as often as necessary to maintain its intended function of support, comfort or the application of pressure. Soiling is also a problem with binders. Because a dirty binder can be a source of both irritation and infection, it is essential to see that soiled binders are changed promptly.

When a binder is applied it should be secured firmly, but the nurse should be careful that there is no interference with normal body functioning. An abdominal or breast binder that is too tight, for example, can restrict movements of the chest wall and interfere with respiration. In postoperative patients this could lead to serious complications. The nurse should be alert for signs of impaired respiration, such as shallow breathing, which could indicate that a binder is too tight and should be loosened.

BANDAGING

A bandage is a piece of material that is used to wrap a part of the body. The purposes of applying a bandage are:

1. To limit movement
2. To apply warmth, for example, to a rheumatoid joint
3. To secure a dressing
4. To keep splints in position
5. To provide support, for example, to the legs to aid venous blood flow
6. To apply pressure in order to control bleeding, promote the absorption of tissue fluids or prevent the loss of tissue fluids

The type of bandage that is used most frequently in hospitals, physicians' offices and clinics is the roller bandage. This is a strip of material from 2 to 8 yards in length and varying in width from ½ to 6 inches. A roller bandage has three parts: the initial or free end, the body or drum and the terminal or hidden end.

Materials Used in Bandaging

Gauze is one of the most frequently used materials for bandaging. It is a soft, woven cotton that is porous but not bulky, light in weight and readily molded to any contour. Although gauze does not wash well and frays with repeated use, it is inexpensive and easily disposed of. The gauze is sometimes impregnated with various ointments such as petrolatum. Gauze is frequently used to bandage fingers and hands and to retain dressings on draining wounds.

Kling is gauze which has been woven in such a manner that it will stretch and thus mold to the body contours. It has a crepelike texture and tends to cling to itself, an attribute which helps keep it in place after it has been applied.

Flannel makes a soft and pliable bandage. It is heavy and keeps in the heat of the body; therefore it can be used to apply warmth to body joints.

Crinoline is a loosely woven gauze, coarse in texture and strong. Crinoline is impregnated with plaster of paris for use as a base for applying casts. It is impregnated with petrolatum for application to an open wound.

Muslin (factory cotton) is a strong, heavy cotton that is not pliable. It is used to provide support, as for splints, or to limit movement.

Elasticized bandages made of cotton with an elastic webbing (Ace bandages) are often used as tensor bandages to apply pressure. They are expensive but can be washed and reused. Patients who require support for their legs immediately following surgery for varicose veins often use tensor bandages.

Elastic adhesive (Elastoplast) is a woven bandage with an adhesive side. It is applied to give support, for example, when dressings are being secured.

Plastic adhesive is a waterproof bandage with an adhesive side. It is somewhat elastic and can be used to apply pressure and at the same time keep an area dry.

Principles Relevant to Bandaging

Microorganisms flourish in warm, damp and soiled areas. A bandage is applied only over a clean area; if it is to be placed over an open wound, the wound is dressed aseptically beforehand. Skin surfaces are dry and clean and are not pressed together when bandaging. Adjacent skin surfaces may be kept separated by inserting a 2″ by 2″ piece of gauze between them. Bandages are removed at regular intervals and the skin surfaces are washed and dried. Soiled bandages are never reused.

Pressure exerted upon the body tissues can affect the circulation of blood. A bandage is applied from the distal to the proximal part of the body to aid the return of the venous blood to the heart. Bandages are always applied evenly so that they do not restrict circulation. They should be checked frequently to make certain that there is no interference with blood supply to the part.

Friction can cause mechanical trauma

to the epithelium. A bony prominence of the body is padded before it is bandaged, so that the bandage does not rub the area and cause an abraded wound. Skin surfaces are separated to prevent friction and maceration.

The body is maintained in the natural anatomical position with slight flexion of the joints to avoid muscle strain. Bandages are applied with the body in good alignment to avoid muscle extension, which is fatiguing and produces strain. In particular, adduction of the shoulder and hip joints is avoided.

Excessive or uneven pressure upon body surfaces can interfere with blood circulation and therefore with the nourishment of the cells in the area. Bandage evenly and if possible leave the distal portion of a bandaged limb exposed so that any restriction in circulation can be detected. Signs and symptoms of restricted circulation are pallor, erythema, cyanosis, tingling sensations, numbness or pain, swelling and cold.

When a bandage is applied over a wet dressing, allowances are made for shrinkage, as the bandage becomes wet and subsequently dries.

Fundamental Turns in Bandaging

There are five fundamental turns in bandaging, and it is these turns that are used to make up the variety of bandages applied to the various parts of the body.

The *circular turn* is used to bandage a cylindrical part of the body or to secure a bandage at its initial and terminal ends. In a circular turn, the bandage is wrapped about the part in such a way that each turn exactly covers the previous one. Two circular turns are usually used to initiate and to terminate a bandage. For comfort the initial and terminal ends are not situated directly over the wound.

The *spiral turn* is used to bandage a part of the body that is of uniform circumference. The bandage is carried upward at a slight angle so that it spirals around the part. Each turn is parallel

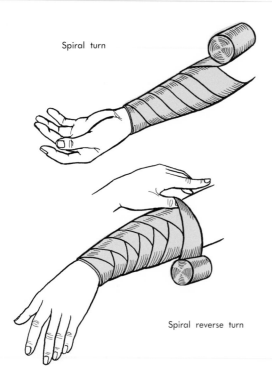

Spiral turn

Spiral reverse turn

to the preceding one and overlaps it by two-thirds of width of the bandage. A spiral turn is used on parts of the body such as the fingers, arms and legs.

The *spiral reverse turn* is used to bandage cylindrical parts of the body that are of varying circumference such as the lower leg. To make a spiral reverse turn, the thumb of the free hand is placed on the upper edge of the initial turn, the bandage being held firmly. The roll is unwound about 6 inches and then the hand is pronated so that the bandage is directed downward and parallel to the lower edge of the previous turn, overlapping it by two-thirds of the width. The roll is then carried around the limb and another reverse is made at the same place so that the turns are in line and uniform.

The *figure of eight* is usually used on joints but may also be used for the entire length of an arm or leg bandage. It consists of repeated oblique turns that are made alternately above and below a joint in the form of a figure of eight. After the initial circular turns are made over the center of the joint, the next turn is superior to the joint and the next is inferior to the joint. Thus the turns are worked upward and downward, with each turn overlapping the previous turn by two-thirds of the width of the bandage.

The *recurrent turn* is used to cover distal portions of the body such as the tip of a finger or the toes. After anchoring the bandage with a circular turn, the roll is turned and brought directly over the center of the tip to be covered. It is

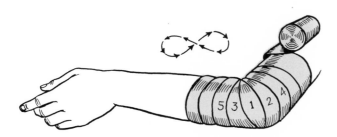

Figure-of-eight turn on the elbow.

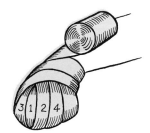

Recurrent turn on the hand.

then anchored inferiorly, and alternate turns are made, first to the right and then to the left, over the original turn covering the tip so that each turn is held above and below. Each turn overlaps the preceding one by two-thirds of its width. The bandage is secured by circular turns which gather in the ends.

Generally speaking, bandages for the hands, arms and feet are made with circular, spiral and spiral reverse turns. Bandages for the joints are made with figures of eight, and bandages for the distal portions of the body are done with recurrent turns.

In addition, there are many special bandages, such as the thumb spica, ear and eye bandages and skull bandages. It is suggested that the nurse consult a bandaging text for more detailed information.

Guides to Bandaging

1. Face the person who is being bandaged.

2. Start a roller bandage by holding the roll of the bandage upward in one hand, the initial end in the other hand.

3. Bandage from the distal to the proximal and from the medial to the lateral.

4. Do not initiate or terminate a bandage directly over a wound or an area where the patient is likely to exert pressure, as for example, the posterior side of the thigh.

5. Bandage evenly and firmly, overlapping the preceding turn by two-thirds of the width of the bandage.

6. Use the bandage material which best serves the purpose of the bandage.

7. Cover a dressing with a bandage that extends 2 inches past each side of the dressing.

8. Separate the skin surfaces and pad bony prominences and hollows to prevent friction and to apply even pressure.

9. Check the bandage and look for any signs of restricted circulation.

10. A bandage should be safe, durable, neat, therapeutically effective and economical.

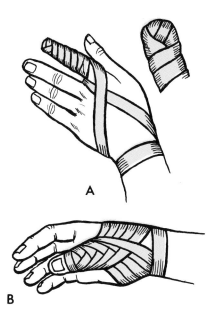

A, Finger bandage with the tip covered; B, thumb spica.

GUIDE TO ASSESSING NURSING NEEDS

1. What type of a wound does the patient have?
2. What phase of healing would you judge this wound to be in?
3. Is the wound healing normally?
4. Are there factors which might delay healing of the wound? For example, is the patient in poor nutritional status? Does he have an infection?
5. Does the patient show localized or generalized symptoms that would indicate the wound is infected?
6. How would you describe the wound?
7. Does the wound require dressing? If so, how often? Are there special precautions to be taken or additional equipment required for doing the dressing?
8. Does the patient need a binder or bandage? If so, for what reason? What is the best type to use for this patient's needs?

GUIDE TO EVALUATING THE EFFECTIVENESS OF NURSING ACTION

1. Is the dressing, binder or bandage accomplishing its purpose?
2. Are there signs and symptoms to indicate its effectiveness? For example, is there a decrease of redness or evidence of healing?
3. Is the patient concerned about the wound? Is his anxiety allayed?
4. Is circulation to the area unrestricted?
5. Is safe sterile technique maintained?
6. Is each measure performed as comfortably as possible?

STUDY VOCABULARY

Anorexia	Infected wound	Serous
Clean wound	Purulent	Virulence
Contaminated wound	Sanguineous	Wound

STUDY SITUATION

Mrs. R. S. Brown has just had an infected appendix removed. Upon her return to the nursing unit of the hospital, she has two separate dressings over the lower right quadrant of her abdomen. Her chart indicates that she has two wounds; the larger one is the suture line from the appendectomy, the smaller one is a stab wound in which is inserted a soft rubber drain to facilitate drainage. The larger wound is covered with waterproof adhesive tape. The physician's orders for Mrs. Brown include:

1. Change dressings as necessary.
2. Apply scultetus binder to abdomen.
3. Cleanse wounds b.i.d. with tincture of Zephiran 1:1000.
4. Serve high protein diet.
5. Force fluids.

Mrs. Brown had been very anxious before her surgery; she was concerned that the operation would leave a scar, which would mean she could not wear a bathing suit to enter a modeling contest.

1. What should you consider in the provision of support to Mrs. Brown?
2. Why are Mrs. Brown's wounds dressed separately? Which wound should be cleansed first?
3. How often should the dressings be changed?
4. The drainage from Mrs. Brown's stab wound is pinkish white. Describe this in medical terms.
5. Give a sample of the charting after changing Mrs. Brown's dressings.
6. What nursing measures would facilitate wound healing?
7. Describe the stages of wound healing.
8. Why does Mrs. Brown need a scultetus binder?
9. Why is Mrs. Brown taking a high protein diet and forced fluids?
10. Could this wound have a meaning for the patient other than the obvious? Explain.
11. Outline the principles which serve as guides to cleansing Mrs. Brown's wounds and changing her dressings.
12. By what criteria could you judge the effectiveness of Mrs. Brown's care?

BIBLIOGRAPHY

Beland, Irene L.: *Clinical Nursing: Pathophysiological and Psychosocial Approaches.* New York, The Macmillan Company, 1965.

Belilios, Arthur D., et al.: *Handbook of First Aid and Bandaging.* Fifth edition. London, Bailliere, Tindall & Cox, 1962.

Davis, Loyal: *Christopher's Textbook of Surgery.* Ninth edition. Philadelphia, W. B. Saunders Company, 1968.

Guyton, Arthur C.: *Function of the Human Body.* Philadelphia, W. B. Saunders Company, 1969.

Harkins, Henry N., et al.: *Surgery: Principles and Practice.* Second edition. Philadelphia, J. B. Lippincott Company, 1961.

LeMaitre, George D., and Janet A. Finnegan: *The Patient in Surgery: A Guide for Nurses.* Second edition. Philadelphia, W. B. Saunders Company, 1970.

Manual of Preoperative and Postoperative Care by the Committee on Preoperative and Postoperative Care. American College of Surgeons. Second edition. Philadelphia, W. B. Saunders Company, 1971.

Nordmark, Madelyn T., and Rohweder, Anne W.: *Scientific Foundations of Nursing.* Second edition. Philadelphia, J. B. Lippincott Company, 1967.

Warren, Richard: *Surgery.* Philadelphia, W. B. Saunders Company, 1963.

Wolff, LuVerne: Problems with Surgical Dressing. *The American Journal of Nursing,* 57:1463–1464, November, 1957.

23 THE CARE OF PATIENTS WHO HAVE FEVERS

The nurse should be able to:

Define fever

Use correct terminology to record and report observations concerning patients with fever

Explain the primary factors affecting heat production in the body and the processes by which heat is lost from the body

Describe the normal activities and physiological factors that may cause an elevation in temperature and list the common pathological conditions that may give rise to fever

Describe the manifestations of fever that may be observed in patients

Identify the nursing needs of the febrile patient

Describe appropriate nursing action, including measures to reduce heat production and facilitate heat loss, and measures to minimize the effects of heat on the body

Establish criteria for evaluating the effectiveness of nursing action

THE CARE OF PATIENTS WHO HAVE FEVERS 23

INTRODUCTION

Usually the heat-regulating mechanisms of the body maintain a precise balance between heat production and heat loss. In this way the internal body temperature is kept within a very narrow range, usually varying not more than a degree or so in a day. Many people who are ill, however, have an elevated temperature. An elevated temperature is one of the cardinal symptoms of illness, and it is often one of the first observable indications that there is a disturbance of body function.

The patient with a fever presents the typical picture of an ill patient as visualized by the layman. His face is flushed and warm to the touch, he complains of feeling hot and uncomfortable, he is thirsty and he may be restless or drowsy. If the fever is not checked the patient may also become delirious (subject to a mental disturbance) before prostration ensues. Prostration is defined as extreme exhaustion.

Fever is an elevation of the body temperature due to abnormal processes within the body. As discussed in Chapter 7, the normal body temperature taken orally ranges between 36.1° and 38° C. (97° and 100.4° F.), but 37° C. (98.6° F.) is usually considered the average oral temperature for a normal healthy adult.

The rectal temperature is usually 0.6° C. (1° F.) higher than the oral temperature, and the temperature taken by axilla is 0.6° C. (1° F.) less, although this varies from person to person. Most individuals show a daily rhythmic change in body temperature with a variation of about 0.6° C. (1° F.) at different times during the day. The daily variation may be as much as 1.1° to 1.65° C. (2° to 3° F.) in some individuals. The body temperature is usually lowest during the early morning hours before a person wakens and reaches its maximum after 6 P.M.[1] In people who work at night and sleep during the day, the daily temperature pattern may be reversed.

A term that is frequently used synonymously with fever is *pyrexia*. *Hyperpyrexia* and *hyperthermia* are used interchangeably to designate an abnormally high fever, that is, 40.6° C. (105° F.) or over. *Habitual hyperthermia* refers to a condition in which the average daily temperature is slightly above normal limits. *Hypothermia* is an abnormally low body temperature.

Although prolonged fevers are not seen as commonly today as in the years before antibiotics, it is well for the nurse to know the technical terms used for different types of fevers. The terms are descriptive and explain the nature of the fever.

An *intermittent* or *quotidian* fever is one in which the temperature rises each day but falls to normal sometime during the 24 hour period, most usually during

---

[1]William A. Sodeman and William A. Sodeman, Jr. (eds.): *Pathologic Physiology: Mechanisms of Disease.* Fourth edition. Philadelphia, W. B. Saunders Company, 1967, pp. 202, 203.

the early morning hours. A *remittent* fever is one which shows marked variations in the temperature readings during a 24 hour period, the lowest reading, however, being always above the patient's normal level. In a *relapsing* fever, the patient's temperature may be normal for one or two days, then elevated for varying periods. These periods of normalcy are interspersed irregularly throughout the course of a relapsing fever. The term *hectic* or *septic* may be used to describe an intermittent fever in which there are wide fluctuations in daily temperature readings. It is not unusual for the temperature to vary as much as 2.2° C. (4° F.) within a 24 hour period in this type of fever. Another type of fever is called a *constant* fever. In this type, the patient's temperature remains at essentially the same level over a period of days or weeks.

Fever can also be described according to its onset, course and termination. The onset refers to the initial period of the fever; it can be either gradual or sudden. During the course of a fever the high point is called the fastigium or stadium caloris. A fever terminates either by lysis or by crisis. Crisis refers to the rapid fall of an elevated temperature, usually over a period of a few hours. The patient's temperature usually reaches normal in 12 to 24 hours, and he shows an improvement in his general condition. Lysis is the gradual fall of an elevated temperature over a period of several days to a week. The patient's temperature often falls in an irregular manner, and he shows a gradual improvement in his condition.

THE PHYSIOLOGY OF FEVER

Body temperature is the result of the balance between the heat produced and the heat eliminated by the body. In the average man, 58 Calories[2] of heat must be added to the body in order to raise the temperature 1° C. or 1.8° F.

---

[2] 1 Calorie = 1000 calories.

Heat Production

Five primary factors affect heat production in the body.

Basal Metabolism. The higher the basal metabolic rate, the greater the amount of heat that is produced within the body.

Muscular Activity. The amount of heat produced by the muscles varies markedly. When a person shivers the rate of heat production can be increased as much as two to four times that of normal. Exercise also increases heat production.

Thyroxine. Thyroxine has a direct effect upon the cells of the body by increasing the rate of metabolism and thus increasing heat production. Since thyroxine is produced by the thyroid gland, any factors which increase thyroid activity increase heat production.

Epinephrine and Sympathetic Activity. Both epinephrine and stimulation of the sympathetic nervous system have a direct effect on the cells of the body. They increase heat production through an increase in the rate of cell metabolism.

Body Temperature. A rise in body temperature in itself stimulates the cells to increase the rate of heat production and metabolism. For each 1° C. rise in temperature, the rate of heat production increases 13 per cent. As a result, an increased temperature by itself tends to heighten a fever.

Heat Loss

Heat is lost from the body by means of four processes:

Radiation. Radiation is the transfer of heat from warm objects to cool objects in the form of electromagnetic waves. About 60 per cent of body heat loss is the result of radiation.

Conduction. Conduction is the transfer of heat from a warmer to a cooler substance by direct contact. The body loses only a minimal amount of heat by direct conduction to objects, as for example, through contact of the body with a bed or a chair. Direct transfer of heat from the body surface to the air immediately surrounding it, however, accounts for a sizeable proportion of the body's heat loss.

Convection.   Convection is the movement of air. Convection currents around the body carry away heat that has been conducted to the air from the body surface. In a normally comfortable room without gross air movement, about 12 per cent of body heat loss results from conduction of heat from the body to the air and subsequent convection away from the body.

Evaporation.   Evaporation of water from the body surface and respiratory tract reduces body heat. Approximately 20 per cent of body heat loss results from the evaporation of sweat. This figure is greatly increased by increased perspiration, as occurs in hot climates or as a result of exercise.

Sweating is therefore an important factor in the loss of heat from the body. It is produced when stimuli from the anterior hypothalamus excite the sweat glands. The rate of sweating varies according to the amount of exercise, weather and emotional factors. Among other things, sweat is composed of sodium and chloride ions, whose loss can alter the electrolyte balance of the body.

THE ETIOLOGY OF FEVER

Fever may be the result of excess heat production in the body, inadequate heat loss, or a combination of both. Under conditions of good health, a number of normal activities and physiological processes affect body temperature. These include: exercise, the digestion of food, changes in the environment, emotions, the menstrual cycle and pregnancy. In exercise, muscular activity increases body temperature as a result of heat production by the body muscles. Heavy muscular exercise may increase the body temperature by as much as 2.2° to 2.7° C. (4° to 5° F.).[3] Usually an elevated

temperature due to exercise quickly returns to normal with the cessation of exercise.

The digestion of food is also thought to increase body temperature. This elevation is believed to begin 30 minutes after food intake and to reach its peak after 90 minutes.

The environment has a pronounced effect upon body temperature. Not only permanent changes, such as those encountered when moving to a hot climate, but temporary changes, such as a brief hot spell, affect the body by raising its temperature. The body's ability to withstand high environmental temperatures is dependent on the humidity of the atmosphere. When the air is dry and there are sufficient air currents to carry away heat from the body by convection, an individual can stand very high temperatures with little or no increase in body temperature. If on the other hand, the humidity is high, body temperature begins to rise very quickly. This explains why one feels so uncomfortable on hot, "muggy" days. Similarly, a cold environment decreases body temperature. These changes are most obvious in infants and elderly people.

During the menstrual cycle it has been observed that there is a fall in the early morning temperature of most women just after the onset of menstruation. The temperature remains at this lower value until ovulation takes place. Then there is an abrupt rise of 0.3° to 0.4° C. (0.5° to 0.75° F.) which continues until the start of the next menstrual period.

Early in pregnancy there is a slight rise in the temperature of most women, which continues until about the fourth month. There is then a gradual fall in the temperature, which usually remains slightly below normal levels throughout the remainder of the pregnancy.

Strong emotions, such as anger, may also raise the body temperature owing to the production of epinephrine. The term "feverish with excitement" may thus be an accurate one. One notices this particularly in children, whose body temperatures are more labile

[3]Sodeman and Sodeman, op. cit., p. 203.

(susceptible to change) than those of adults.

In addition to the normal processes which cause fluctuations in body temperature, there are certain pathological conditions of which fever is a typical manifestation. The most common of these are infections, diseases of the central nervous system, neoplasms and metabolic disorders. The prolonged use of some drugs, among them morphine and LSD, may also give rise to fever.

The physiological mechanisms responsible for fever in all disease processes are not known. It is generally felt that it may be caused by abnormalities in the brain itself or by toxic substances that affect the heat-regulating mechanisms.

It has long been recognized that the regulatory centers of body temperature are located in the hypothalamus. There is evidence to suggest that the supraoptic and preoptic areas in the hypothalamus are excited by an elevated temperature. The centers in the posterior hypothalamus are excited when the body temperature falls below normal. When one of these centers is activated, the other is depressed.

It is felt that a number of stimuli may activate the hypothalamic centers. Important among these are the substances called *pyrogens* which are secreted by toxic bacteria or released by degenerating tissue. It is believed that these substances stimulate the release of a second substance, *leukocyte pyrogen*, from the leukocytes which have been drawn to the diseased area. The leukocyte pyrogens then act on the thermoregulatory centers.[4]

There is evidence to support the belief that fever caused by pyrogens has some beneficial effects in helping the body to combat infection. It is felt that the fever acts in two ways: (1) It creates an undesirable temperature for the survival of bacteria; and (2) the increased rate of metabolism in the cells increases their production of immune bodies and also their ability to phagocytize foreign bodies, thus preventing bacterial invasion.

Dehydration can also affect the hypothalamic centers directly so that the temperature rises to febrile levels. Part of the elevation is due to lack of fluids for sweating, which deprives the body of one of its principal mechanisms for losing excess heat.

Fever may occur postoperatively owing to any one of a number of causes. It may be due to excessive heat production, as in the case of pathogenic infection, but is usually felt to be due to inadequate heat elimination.[5]

Fever frequently accompanies a head injury and is often seen in patients with spinal cord injuries. In these cases, it is felt to be caused by pressure on, or injury to, the hypothalamus or the tracts leading to and from the heat-regulating centers.[6]

Heat stroke, a condition of severe prostration, may be caused by prolonged exposure to high environmental temperatures. It is most frequently seen in the elderly and is believed to be due to failure of the heat regulatory centers in the brain. The condition is characterized by fever, coma and the absence of sweating.

SIGNS AND SYMPTOMS ACCOMPANYING FEVER

The signs and symptoms that accompany fever occur in response to the physiological processes that are occurring within the body. There are three distinct stages to a fever: (1) the onset, or period of rising temperature; (2) the course of the fever, when the temperature is maintained at an elevated level; and (3) the termination, or period when the temperature falls to normal. During

---

[4]Arthur C. Guyton: *Textbook of Medical Physiology.* Fourth edition. Philadelphia, W. B. Saunders Company, 1971, pp. 836, 840.

[5]American College of Surgeons: *Manual of Preoperative and Postoperative Care.* Philadelphia, W. B. Saunders Company, 1967, p. 266.

[6]Cyril M. MacBryde and Robert S. Blacklow (eds.): *Signs and Symptoms: Applied Pathologic Physiology and Clinical Interpretation,* Fifth edition. Philadelphia, J. B. Lippincott Company, 1970, p. 462.

the three stages, different sets of mechanisms are operating, giving rise to the signs and symptoms characteristic of each stage.

The Onset

During the onset of a fever, it is felt that there is a resetting of the body's internal "thermostat" at a higher level.[7] This may be due to the presence of pyrogenic substances, or to any one of the other causes listed in the section on the etiology of fever. The resetting of the internal thermostat brings the body's heat-producing mechanisms into play as an attempt is made to bring the temperature up to the "desired" level. The person experiences what is known as a *chill*. Muscular activity is increased, in the form of shivering, which may vary in severity from merely a feeling of being cold, with slight shivering, to violent muscular contractions (shaking chills).

At the same time as the shivering mechanism is induced, there is increased secretion of epinephrine and norepinephrine into the blood stream. This accelerates the rate of cellular metabolism. As metabolism increases, the waste products of metabolism, carbon dioxide and water, are greater. The increased carbon dioxide level in the blood stimulates the respiratory center and the person breathes faster and more deeply. This leads to extra fluid loss, and the patient feels thirsty. Also as metabolism is accelerated, there is an increased demand by the cells for more oxygen and glucose. The heart beats more rapidly (in response to this demand), and the nurse will note that the patient's pulse rate is higher than normal.

Concomitantly, heat-conserving mechanisms are instituted. Vasoconstriction occurs and blood is drawn from surface vessels to minimize the amount of heat lost through conduction and convection. The patient becomes pale, and his skin is cold to the touch. He also feels cold and may ask for extra blankets. Often, there is a "goose-flesh" appearance to the skin as "pilo-erection" takes place. Pilo-erection means that the hairs "stand on end." In animals with long fur, this mechanism serves to entrap a layer of warm air next to the skin. In human beings, the mechanism is not so effective in providing insulation, but it occurs nonetheless. There is usually a cessation of sweating to reduce the amount of heat lost through evaporation of water from the body surface.

During the chill phase, the rectal temperature rises steadily, although the elevation is usually not evident by oral thermometer until the end of a chill. Body temperature may be increased by as much as $1.1°$ to $4°$ C. ($2°$ to $7°$ F.).[8] A chill may last for a few minutes or as long as an hour. In mild cases of fever, such as one sees with the common cold or in light cases of influenza, the chill phase is usually brief.

The Course of a Fever

During the second stage of a fever, or when the fever is "running its course," the temperature has reached the preset level and there is a balance between heat production and heat loss. The patient usually no longer feels hot or cold. Because of the increased body temperature, however, the skin feels warm to the touch and there is usually a generalized flushing of the skin. The increased metabolic rate required to maintain the elevated temperature puts heightened demands on the body for more oxygen and glucose. The heart and respiratory rates remain high, and water loss through respiration increases the patient's feeling of thirst. The elevated temperature also increases nervous irritability. Headache, photophobia (sensitivity to light), and restlessness or drowsiness or both are not uncommon symptoms. An abnormally high fever is often accompanied by a state of mental confusion, termed *delirium*. The patient becomes disoriented as to time and

---

[7]Guyton, op. cit., p. 841.

[8]MacBryde, op. cit., p. 460.

place. He may not know where he is or, often, what day it is. Sometimes the patient may have *hallucinations*, that is, disturbances of sensory perception. For example, the patient may think he hears someone calling to him although there is no one there. The patient may become quite irrational and combative. Finally, prostration (collapse) may ensue. In young children, a convulsion not infrequently accompanies fever, usually at the outset.

The maintenance of an elevated temperature is very debilitating to the patient. During the first week or so of a fever, there is always some destruction of body protein and albuminuria is usually noted in the laboratory findings of the febrile patient.[9] The patient often complains of a generalized weakness and he is not inclined to much activity. Aching of the muscles and joints is also frequently present. In addition to the destruction of tissue protein, it is felt that the parenchyma of many cells begins to be damaged when the body temperature rises above 40° C. (105° F.).[10] In sustained high fevers there may be permanent damage to nervous tissue, since this tissue does not regenerate. The upper limit for survival has been estimated by various experts to be a body temperature of 46° C. (114. 8° F.).[11]

Febrile patients usually lose weight. Although the increased metabolic rate maintained during the course of a fever increases the body's need for nourishment, most patients have little interest in food. This loss of appetite (anorexia) may give way to nausea and vomiting as the fever progresses. The combination of increased need for food and lack of interest in it leads to a loss of weight.

Usually, during the course of a fever, the temperature does not remain at a constant level but tends to fluctuate. Thus, periods when body temperature is rising are usually interspersed with periods when it is falling, even though the lowest temperature reached may be always above normal. When the temperature is falling, mechanisms for ad-

ditional heat loss are dominant. Vasodilatation occurs and the skin becomes flushed and warm as the body attempts to rid itself of excess heat by circulating more blood to the surface of the body where it is cooled by conduction and convection. Sweating (diaphoresis) is usually present to maximize heat loss through evaporation. The body thus loses more fluids, and the possibility of dehydration presents a problem.

When fever is prolonged, the problem of dehydration is more likely to occur. This is due to a number of factors including the greater loss of water through increased respirations and the further loss of fluids from sweating during periods when the body temperature is falling. There is often a lessening in the output of urine as more than the usual amount of fluid is lost through the skin and lungs. Other evidences of dehydration may be noted. The skin and mucous membranes may appear parched and dry. The patient's lips may become cracked and sore, and lesions may occur at the corners of the mouth. These lesions are termed *herpes simplex,* but are often referred to as "fever blisters" because they are so frequently seen in patients with fever. The nurse may note other signs and symptoms of dehydration, as discussed in Chapter 29. It is well to remember that young children, in particular, become dehydrated very quickly if there is a sustained fever.

The Termination of a Fever

When the cause of the elevated temperature has been removed, as for example, when antibiotics have "taken hold" and removed the cause of infection, the body's thermostat is reset at its original level. The mechanisms for increased heat production cease to operate, and mechanisms for increased heat loss are instituted. These are the same mechanisms which have already been described as operating during the course of a fever when the temperature is fluctuating and there is a temporary drop. There is increased flushing of the skin, and profuse diaphoresis may occur.

[9]Guyton, op. cit., p. 842.
[10]Ibid.
[11]MacBryde, op. cit., p. 456.

Hence, there is an increasing possibility of dehydration at this stage. The patient's temperature may drop to normal quickly, over a period of hours (by crisis), or gradually over a period of days or weeks (by lysis).

ASSESSING THE NURSING NEEDS OF THE FEBRILE PATIENT

An evaluation of the patient's condition to determine the need for medical or nursing intervention is of prime importance in the case of the febrile patient. Any elevation in body temperature is significant. An abnormally high temperature is considered a medical emergency, and efforts to lower the body temperature should be instituted as quickly as possible.

It is important to observe all patients for the signs and symptoms of fever. Many agencies have specific policies in regard to the taking of temperatures. Some institutions require that all patients have their temperature taken once, or sometimes twice, a day to screen for fever. If once a day, it is usually considered that early evening is the best time, since in most individuals, the temperature does not reach its maximum until 6 P.M. If temperatures are taken in the morning, it should be an hour or so after the patient wakens and the body temperature is stabilized. When a patient has a fever, the temperature should be taken at more frequent intervals. If it is abnormally elevated, as often as every 15 minutes is sometimes indicated. All newly admitted patients should have a temperature taken, as well as all preoperative and postoperative patients. Postoperatively, the temperature is usually taken every four hours for the first 48 hours. In addition to these general guidelines, the nurse should be alert to signs and symptoms indicating the presence of fever and should take the patient's temperature if, in her judgment, it should be taken. The temperature should be evaluated in relation to such factors as: the patient's usual normal temperature, the time of day, the environmental tempera-

ture and the normal physiological processes that may affect body temperature. Details on the methods of taking body temperature are given in Chapter 7.

The pulse and respirations should be checked, both for rate and quality. The color of the patient's skin should be noted, since it is relevant to heat elimination. The amount of blood circulating to the body surface is proportional to heat loss. Hence, a reddened, flushed appearance indicates a high proportion of blood near the surface. It is usually seen when a fever is established and the body is attempting to rid itself of excess heat. On the other hand, pallor may indicate the onset of a chill and a rising body temperature. The nurse should note if the patient complains of any physical symptoms such as headache, malaise or other discomfort.

An accurate assessment of the patient's nutritional status is important. In this regard, the nurse should determine the patient's ability to tolerate food and fluids. The patient should also be observed for signs of weakness and fatigue.

The nurse should be alert to signs of dehydration in the patient. She should note the presence or absence of sweating. Both the amount and the color of the urine should be observed. When there is an inadequate intake of fluids, or an excessive amount is being lost through sweating or other means, the body attempts to balance this through the excretion of a more highly concentrated urine. The urine may then be scanty in amount and darker (more brown) in color than normal, straw-colored urine.

The nurse should also be alert to the patient's mental condition. The patient who has a fever may be irritable. He may complain about the details of his care and manifest anxiety and irritation in ways which are often annoying to nursing personnel. His need to be understood and to be helped in handling his anxieties must be recognized by the nurse. In patients with a high fever there may be mental confusion. The nurse should be alert to the increased need to protect the safety of these patients.

PRINCIPLES BASIC TO THE CARE OF PATIENTS WITH FEVER

The maintenance of a temperature above normal level requires the expenditure of an increased amount of energy by the body.

Body cells are damaged by excessively high temperatures.

A high body temperature may in itself stimulate further heat production.

Heat is lost from the body through the mechanisms of radiation, conduction, convection and evaporation.

OBJECTIVES OF NURSING INTERVENTION

The principal objectives of nursing intervention in the care of the febrile patient are twofold:

1. To reduce the amount of heat produced within the body and to facilitate heat elimination from the body
2. To minimize the effects of fever on the body

MEASURES TO REDUCE HEAT PRODUCTION AND FACILITATE HEAT LOSS

In determining priorities for nursing action, the nurse must assess the severity of the febrile condition. If the patient's temperature is abnormally high, there is an immediate need to lower it. The patient should be put to bed, if he has been up and around, and the physician notified promptly. There are a number of measures which may be used to bring about a rapid reduction in body temperature. These include the use of antipyretic drugs which have a systemic action and various techniques for "surface cooling" of the body.

Antipyretic Drugs

Antipyretic drugs, such as aspirin, are often ordered to reduce a patient's fever. These drugs have a specific action on the heat-regulating centers, but do not eliminate the cause of the fever. Their administration may be designated at specific times or the order may leave the time of their administration to the nurse's judgment. It is not unusual for antipyretic drugs to be given when a patient's temperature reaches 38.9° C. (102° F.). When a patient who has a fever is receiving antibiotics, these are usually administered at regular intervals in order to maintain a therapeutic drug level in the patient's body. The use of antibiotics for patients with infections reduces the fever by eliminating the cause of it, that is, the infection within the body.

Tepid Sponge Bath

When it is considered desirable to lower the patient's temperature rapidly, a tepid sponge bath may be given. This is a simple and reliable nursing measure that can be employed either in a home situation or in the hospital. It is carried out on the order of a physician. The technique is based on the principle that the body loses heat through the mechanisms of conduction to a cooler substance, in this case the tepid water, evaporation of water from the surface of the body, and convection of the heat away from exposed body surfaces during the bathing process.

Prior to the bath, the temperature, pulse and respirations are taken. These observations are important for the subsequent evaluation of the effectiveness of the bath. There are many ways of giving a tepid sponge. One way is described here.

The equipment required for the tepid sponge bath consists of a basin of water 30° C. to 38° C. (85° to 100° F.), towels, wash cloth, bath blanket and isopropanol rubbing compound. To initiate this nursing care measure the top bedclothes are fan-folded to the foot of the bed, and the patient is draped with his bath blanket. Then his gown is removed and his body is sponged. Heat is lost from the body as water is sponged onto the surface of the body and some of it is permitted to evaporate. Large areas are sponged at a time, for example, one side of the leg, one side of the arm, the chest and the abdomen. Long strokes are used on the legs and on the back. Because the blood vessels are close to the body surface in the axilla, the wrists and the groins, the cooling effect of the bath is enhanced by applying the wet cloths there for an extended period of time, that is, by slowing down the bathing process in these areas. A gentle patting motion is used to dry each area; brisk rubbing increases the activity of the cells and therefore the rate of heat production. The back of the patient is then gently rubbed with the isopropanol rubbing compound before the gown and covers are replaced.

The temperature, pulse and respirations are taken 20 minutes after the sponge bath. The bath is usually repeated until the patient's temperature has reached the level designated by the physician. If the physician's order does not include the temperature at which treatment is to be discontinued, the bath should be stopped before the normal temperature is reached. A further drop in temperature may be expected to occur after it is discontinued.

Sometimes an alcohol bath is ordered, because alcohol evaporates at a lower temperature than water and thus hastens the cooling process. In this case, isopropanol is substituted for the water or, in some instances, may be added to the water. If alcohol is used, the procedure is always terminated before the temperature reaches normal.

A nursing measure which is somewhat similar to the tepid sponge bath is the use of a wet sheet and a fan to increase heat elimination from the body. The patient is covered only by a sheet which has been dampened with water. A fan is so directed that there is constant movement of air over the sheet. This measure promotes evaporation and convection and thereby increases heat loss from the body. It is a rather drastic measure and is used only in exceptional circumstances.

Hypothermia Machines

Many hospitals now have a hypothermia machine which is used for rapid surface cooling of the body. This machine may be used for patients who have temperatures of 39.4° C. (103° F.) and over when it is felt that it is essential to bring the body temperature down quickly or when there has been brain damage to the heat-regulating centers and it is necessary to maintain artificial cooling of the body over a prolonged period of time.

This technique uses the mechanisms of radiation and conduction. The patient is placed on or between cooling blankets which are attached to a refrigerating machine. The blankets contain coils in which a refrigerant circulates. A considerable amount of heat is lost from the body through direct conduction to the cooling substance and through the radiation of heat waves from the body to the cooler blankets.

Because some people shiver in response to the application of the hypothermia blanket, Chlorpromazine is sometimes given to minimize shivering. Patients receiving hypothermia treatment frequently need a great deal of reassurance and explanation about the treatment.

A more detailed account of the procedure for using the hypothermia machine may be found in Sutton's textbook, *Bedside Nursing Techniques in Medicine and Surgery*.[12]

General Measures

The patient who has an elevated temperature needs rest. Rest and inactivity decrease the rate of the metabolic process and also muscular activity and thereby decrease the amount of heat produced in the body. Usually, the patient is restricted to bed in order to curtail his

---

[12]Audrey L. Sutton: *Bedside Nursing Techniques in Medicine and Surgery*. Second edition. Philadelphia, W. B. Saunders Company, 1969, pp. 10–17.

activities. Rest, however, involves more than restriction of physical activity; it also means mental rest. Sometimes the simple act of taking a patient's temperature may itself give rise to anxiety on the part of the patient. An elevated temperature may mean that surgery is postponed, or that a much anticipated return to home and family is delayed. The patient needs to be assured that all is being done for his welfare and that he is in competent hands. Anticipating the needs of the patient assists him to relax. Very often, a simple explanation of procedures and treatments can alleviate many anxieties.

The febrile patient needs a cool, quiet environment. The patient with a fever is often irritable and may be hypersensitive to stimuli. An effort should be made to minimize noise and provide the patient with the opportunity for rest. A cool, comfortable room increases heat elimination and helps the patient to rest more easily. Sometimes a fan is used to increase the circulation of air in the room and facilitate the removal of heat from the body through conduction and convection. Care should be taken, however, that the patient does not become chilled. The bedclothes of the febrile patient should be light and comfortable, since heavy coverings inhibit heat elimination.

MEASURES TO MINIMIZE THE EFFECTS OF FEVER ON THE BODY

The presence of a temperature above the normal level places stresses on the body's adaptive mechanisms. The patient is usually uncomfortable; he is losing more than the normal amount of fluids and using more energy than usual to maintain the elevated body temperature. Nursing action should then be directed toward relieving discomfort, maintaining hydration and maintaining the patient's nutritional status.

Comfort Measures

Good hygiene is important to the patient's health and comfort. Profuse diaphoresis (sweating), a common accompaniment of fever, is uncomfortable. Bathing the patient and assisting him to change his gown and bedding so that he is clean and dry are important con-

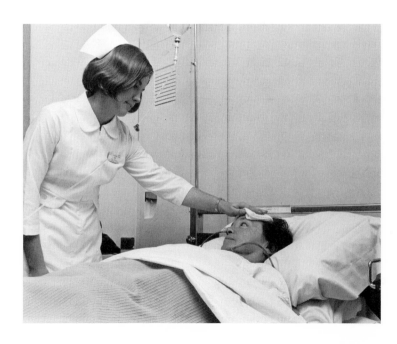

Sometimes a cool, moist cloth on the forehead helps the patient to feel more comfortable when he has a fever.

tributions to his physical well-being. Because sweat glands are more numerous in the axilla and around the genitalia, these areas need particular care when the patient is bathed. Flannelette sheets, because of their greater absorbency, are often used in place of ordinary cotton (muslin) ones on the beds of patients who are perspiring profusely.

Maintaining Hydration

The hydration of the patient is of primary importance. Diaphoresis and the loss of additional fluids through increased respirations increase the amount of fluid eliminated from the body, and this fluid needs to be replaced. In addition, during a fever, there is increased production of metabolic waste products, which must be eliminated. The necessity for removing these products from the body, together with any toxic substances that may be present, emphasizes the importance of fluids. Generally 2500 to 3000 cc. per day is considered a desirable fluid intake. If the patient is unable to take fluids orally or in sufficient amounts, parenteral fluids may be ordered.

An accurate record of the patient's fluid intake and output must be maintained. Intake records should include all fluids taken orally and those given parenterally. In computing output, urine should be measured accurately and a note made of the extent of sweating and the loss of any fluids through vomiting or diarrhea. Suction returns should also be included in the output calculations.

The patient should be observed carefully for signs of dehydration. When a patient becomes dehydrated during the course of a fever, his skin often becomes dry and scaly. The application of creams helps to keep the skin in good condition. Dehydration frequently results also in cracks in the patient's lips, tongue or mucous membrane lining of the mouth. Good oral hygiene is imperative to prevent infection from developing and also to contribute to the patient's comfort. There is a need to cleanse, hydrate and lubricate the mouth and lips. If the patient is unable to clean his own teeth with a toothbrush, he may be helped by the nurse, who uses a toothbrush or a tongue depressor with gauze and mouthwash. If ordinary mouthwash is ineffectual, the nurse may need to use a stronger solution, such as half-strength hydrogen peroxide or milk of magnesia.

Frequent intake of fluids helps to maintain hydration of the oral cavity. Rinsing the mouth with water (or mouthwash) and chewing gum also help to preserve hydration. If the patient is unable to take fluids orally, to rinse his mouth or to chew gum, the nurse may meet this need for the patient by cleaning the mouth with swabs. Glycerin and lemon swabs, or swabs dipped in milk of magnesia, are used in many places for this purpose.

Lubrication may be accomplished by the application of creams or petrolatum to the lips. If the patient is unable to lubricate his own mouth by applying cream, the nurse can meet this need by applying sterile petrolatum to the lips. The petrolatum should be sterile because there are frequently splits or cracks in the lips due to the fever, which provide a portal of entry for infection.

Maintaining Nutritional Status

The old adage of "feed a cold and starve a fever" has been proved wrong. Indeed, because of the body's increased metabolic rate and the increased destruction of tissues that are so often a concomitant of fever, there is a need for both proteins and carbohydrates. Proteins aid in the formation of body tissue; carbohydrates supply the body with much needed energy. Frequently these products are supplied in the liquids taken orally or given parenterally. The patient's weight should be checked at frequent intervals, and the physician should be kept informed of the patient's nutritional status so that appropriate therapy may be instituted.

Rest is essential to minimize the patient's energy requirements. Physical activity should be kept to a minimum. During the convalescent stage, activity should be increased gradually to prevent tiring the patient unduly.

An important function of the nurse is the communication of her observations to other members of the health team. Any elevation in the patient's temperature is considered significant and should be evaluated and reported accurately and promptly. If the temperature is markedly elevated, the physician should be informed immediately so that appropriate therapy can be instituted.

GUIDE TO ASSESSING NURSING NEEDS

1. What is the patient's temperature? His pulse and respiratory rate?
2. Are these abnormal in view of the time of day, the patient's activities and other physiological factors that might cause an elevated TPR?
3. Is immediate nursing or medical intervention indicated?
4. Does the patient show signs that he is having a chill?
5. What is the color of the patient's skin? Does it feel warm or cool to the touch?
6. Is the patient perspiring?
7. Does he complain of any physical symptoms such as headache or fatigue?
8. Is the patient able to tolerate food and fluids?
9. Is the patient losing excessive amounts of fluid through perspiration or increased respirations? Is his urine normal in color and amount?
10. Does he appear dehydrated?
11. Is the patient restless, irritable? Are there signs of mental confusion?
12. What medications have been prescribed for this patient?

GUIDE TO EVALUATING THE EFFECTIVENESS OF NURSING ACTION

1. Has the patient's temperature come down? Is it within safe limits?
2. Is his fluid intake adequate for his needs?
3. Is his nourishment adequate?
4. Is the patient comfortable?
5. Is he getting sufficient rest?
6. Is his skin in good condition? His mouth?

STUDY VOCABULARY

Chill	Hectic fever	Pyrexia
Constant fever	Hyperthermia	Pyrogen
Delirious	Intermittent fever	Relapsing fever
Hallucination	Prostration	Remittent fever

STUDY SITUATION

Mrs. S. James is a 34 year old woman who works as an aide in one of the city hospitals. She is married and has a five year old son. Mrs. James is admitted to the hospital with an elevated temperature of unknown etiology. Her temperature at admission was 39.1° C. (102.4° F.), her pulse 100 and her respirations 24. The patient had a chill during her first evening in the hospital, when her fever rose to 40° C. (104° F.). The following morning she felt improved, but she still perspired profusely and each evening appeared restless and flushed.

The doctor left orders that Mrs. James was to have a tepid sponge bath and aspirin gr. $\bar{x}$ if her temperature rose above 39.4° C. (103° F.). He also asked the patient to drink at least one glass of fluid every hour of the day.

1. What factors are relevant to your explanation of a tepid sponge bath to this patient?
2. How can the patient's production of body heat be minimized?
3. How can the loss of body heat be facilitated?
4. What is the action of aspirin gr. $\bar{x}$?
5. How should you evaluate the effectiveness of the nursing care?
6. Why did the doctor want Mrs. James to drink at least one glass of fluid every hour?
7. What observations would indicate to the nurse that the patient is taking insufficient fluid?
8. Describe an environment which would be therapeutic for this patient.

BIBLIOGRAPHY

Dorland's Illustrated Medical Dictionary. Twenty-fourth edition. Philadelphia, W. B. Saunders Company, 1965.

DuBois, E. F.: *Fever and the Regulation of Body Temperature.* Springfield, Ill., Charles C Thomas, 1948.

Guyton, Arthur C.: *Textbook of Medical Physiology.* Fourth edition. Philadelphia, W. B. Saunders Company, 1971.

Harmer, Bertha, and Virginia Henderson: *Textbook of the Principles and Practice of Nursing.* Fifth edition. New York; The Macmillan Company, 1955.

Keezer, William S.: The Clinical Thermometer. *The American Journal of Nursing,* 66:326–327, February, 1966.

MacBryde, Cyril M., and Robert Stanley Blacklow (eds.): *Signs and Symptoms: Applied Pathologic Physiology and Clinical Interpretation.* Fifth edition. Philadelphia, J. B. Lippincott Company, 1970.

Sodeman, William A., and William A. Sodeman, Jr. (eds.): *Pathologic Physiology: Mechanisms of Disease.* Fourth edition. Philadelphia, W. B. Saunders Company, 1967.

Sutton, Audrey L.: *Bedside Nursing Techniques in Medicine and Surgery.* Second edition. Philadelphia, W. B. Saunders Company, 1969.

24 THE CARE OF PATIENTS WHO HAVE CONSTIPATION OR DIARRHEA

The nurse should be able to:

Define the terms *constipation* and *diarrhea*
Describe the physiology of elimination from the gastrointestinal tract
Explain the etiology of constipation and diarrhea
Describe signs and symptoms that frequently accompany constipation and diarrhea
Assess the nursing needs of patients with these conditions
List principles basic to the care of these patients
Establish goals for nursing care
Determine priorities for nursing intervention
Describe measures to:
    1. Reestablish normal fecal elimination
    2. Relieve distressing symptoms
    3. Maintain fluid and electrolyte balance
    4. Maintain adequate nutritional status
    5. Maintain comfort and hygiene
Establish criteria for evaluating the effectiveness of nursing intervention

INTRODUCTION

Diarrhea and constipation are abnormal variations in the evacuation of feces. Diarrhea is the discharge of loose, watery stools due to excess rapidity in the passage of waste products of digestion through the gastrointestinal tract. Constipation is the passage of hard, dry stools due to undue delay in the evacuation of feces.

The variation in the consistency of feces is explained by the fact that as the waste products of digestion pass through the large intestine, water is absorbed from them. Consequently the consistency of the stool depends to a certain extent on the length of time the food is in the gastrointestinal tract. Normal feces consist of approximately three-fourths water and one-fourth solid materials. In diarrhea, the feces are soft and watery because they move quickly through the gastrointestinal tract, whereas in constipation, the feces are usually hard, that is, there is increased solid content, because they have moved slowly.

There is a wide variation in the normal frequency of evacuation of waste products; consequently diarrhea and constipation must be considered in relation to a person's normal habit. The person who has four or five bowel movements in one day is not necessarily suffering from diarrhea, nor is the person who has one bowel movement every three days necessarily suffering from constipation.

Diarrhea and constipation are not uncommon symptoms of illness, and constipation is a not uncommon discomfort in both the sick and those who are otherwise well. Lack of exercise is an important factor in constipation, particularly in the sick person. Although the constipated person is seldom outwardly ill as a result of his constipation, he is uncomfortable. And because he may be unable to communicate his discomfort verbally, the nurse must be aware of pertinent signs and symptoms which indicate such discomfort. The patient may have had no bowel movements for several days; he may have abdominal distention, and he may be passing large amounts of flatus (gas in the intestines or stomach) by rectum and mouth. On the other hand, if he is able to speak, the patient may explain that he has a bloated feeling, headache, anorexia (loss of appetite) and nausea. These symptoms can be due to improper bowel evacuation.

The patient who has diarrhea is usually more acutely distressed than the patient who is constipated. He complains of abdominal pain of a griping nature and that the frequent passage of stools is usually accompanied by an urgency in the need for defecation (evacuation of feces). If diarrhea is prolonged the patient may suffer a loss of weight and appear thin and emaciated. In addition, he complains of fatigue, weakness and general malaise.

THE PHYSIOLOGY OF CONSTIPATION AND DIARRHEA

The waste products of digestion are passed through the large intestine in wavelike propulsions called peristalsis. In this movement, the part of the colon that is distal to the bolus (waste pro-

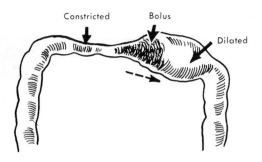

ducts) relaxes while the portion of the colon that is proximal to the bolus contracts. Thus the waste products are propelled forward. Peristalsis occurs in the large intestine at infrequent intervals. It is stimulated by the intake of food and fluids into the gastrointestinal tract. Usually the food or fluid remains in the entire tract from eight to 72 hours after ingestion. When the food enters the duodenum, approximately a half hour after ingestion, there is a mass peristaltic action in the large intestine called the gastrocolic reflex. This is an opportune time for defecation.

Although the rectal reflex is stimulated by the presence of waste products in the rectum, the act of defecation itself is controlled voluntarily. Therefore a person may or may not respond to the stimulus. If he ignores the urge to defecate and the waste products remain within the rectum, he may become constipated. In some patients spinal cord injuries destroy the rectal reflex, which is normally transmitted from the rectum to the sacral area by the parasympathetic nerves. These patients may also lose control of the voluntary muscles concerned with defecation. With special training, however, they can often achieve a certain regularity of bowel habits.

The large intestine, in addition to having its own intrinsic innervation, also responds to stimulation of the sympathetic and parasympathetic nervous systems. The parasympathetic nerves promote peristalsis and increase muscle tone; the sympathetic nerves inhibit peristalsis and decrease muscle tone.

Consequently emotions may affect the functioning of the bowels. For example, anxiety may be mediated either through the parasympathetic nerves, with resultant diarrhea, or through the sympathetic nerves with resultant constipation. This explains the role of emotions as contributing or causative agents in diarrhea and constipation. Sodeman stresses the role of strong emotion in both diarrhea and constipation.[1] He indicates that hostility and defensiveness produce constipation, whereas feelings of inadequacy and fear produce diarrhea.

THE ETIOLOGY OF CONSTIPATION AND DIARRHEA

The numerous causes of constipation and diarrhea may be divided on a physiological basis into three broad categories: those of central nervous system origin; those which result in disturbances in the reflex peristalsis necessary for evacuation; and those caused by mechanical breakdown in the anatomical structures needed for normal, healthy defecation.[2]

[1] William A. Sodeman and William A. Sodeman, Jr. (eds.): *Pathologic Physiology: Mechanisms of Disease.* Fourth edition. Philadelphia, W. B. Saunders Company, 1967, pp. 641–644.

[2] Cyril M. MacBryde and Robert Stanley Blacklow (eds.): *Signs and Symptoms, Applied Pathologic Physiology and Clinical Interpretation.* Fifth edition. Philadelphia, J. B. Lippincott Company, 1970, pp. 381–398.

Constipation

Any factor that causes undue delay in the passage of feces is a cause of constipation. Among those of central nervous system origin, *a breakdown in the conditioned reflex for defecation* is by far the most common. In man, the act of defecation is under voluntary control and is conditioned to time and activity. When the urge to defecate is overcome by voluntary muscle contraction, the rectum adjusts itself to the increased tension or may even return stools to the sigmoid. If this is habitually done, the normal conditioned reflex is lost. This may be due to habits developed in early childhood or to failure on the part of adults to respond to the normal defecation urge because of the pressures of time and daily activities. Pain on defecation, such as that associated with hemorrhoids or rectal surgery will also interfere with the normal conditioned reflex. Hemorrhoids are enlarged veins in the rectal area.

Another common cause of constipation of neurogenous origin is *excessive tone of the circular muscle of the intestines*, which is felt to be due to an imbalance of the autonomic nervous system. Strong emotion, as discussed earlier, is believed to cause constipation through the increased production of epinephrine, with resulting inhibition of peristalsis. Some drugs, among them morphine and to a lesser extent codeine, decrease motility in the small intestine and the colon because of their action on the central nervous system. Constipation may also result from injury to or diseases of the central nervous system.

Disturbances in reflex peristalsis may be due simply to the lack of sufficient bulky foods in the diet. An inadequate intake of foods such as cereals and vegetables may result in insufficient bulk in the residue of waste products to stimulate the reflex for defecation. The excessive use of laxatives may cause constipation, due to over-stimulation of the bowel and a "wearing-out" effect on the nerves initiating the reflex action. People who habitually use laxatives frequently have to change the type taken to overcome this effect. Disease processes, such as inflammation of the pelvic or abdominal viscera, or tumors, may also cause a disturbance in reflex peristalsis.

Mechanical disturbances that cause constipation include weakness of the intestinal muscles as a result of disease processes, old age or lack of essential vitamins (notably the B group) or electrolytes (particularly potassium). Weakness of the voluntary muscles controlling defecation may also cause constipation. The abdominal, the pelvic and the diaphragmatic muscles are all important in initiating and completing defecation. Weakness in any of these will make defecation difficult. Obstruction in any part of the gastrointestinal tract will also delay or prevent the passage of feces. Obstruction may be caused by disease processes or may be due to congenital abnormalities.

Diarrhea

The causes of diarrhea are numerous. Some diarrheas are due to *direct stimulation or irritation of the central or autonomic nervous system*. Diarrhea resulting from tension is an example. In a particularly stressful situation, anxiety may be mediated through the parasympathetic nervous system, with a resultant increase in the motility of the intestine. Diarrhea in these cases may be the most obvious manifestation of anxiety in a stable individual. Pre-examination diarrhea is a fairly common occurrence among students, as is pre-battle diarrhea among soldiers. The action of certain drugs, as for example reserpine (used for the treatment of hypertension), may also cause hyper-motility of the intestine through their action on the autonomic nervous system, with a resultant diarrhea.

Probably the most common set of causes of diarrhea, however, is that group due to *irritation of the gastrointestinal tract*. These result in a reflex type of diarrhea, the reverse of the mechanism that occurs in constipation.

The irritation may be mechanical, as that caused by dietary indiscretions such as eating coarse foods or an excessive amount of seasonings; it may be chemical, as in some food and drug poisonings; or it may be, in some individuals, an allergic reaction to certain foods. Shellfish is a well-known allergen to many people. Inflammation of the intestinal mucosa due to pathogenic infection is another common cause of diarrhea. It is believed that the diarrhea experienced by many international travelers is caused by changes in the normal bacterial flora of the colon. Certain drugs, termed cathartics, cause loose stools through irritation of the intestinal mucosa.

There are a few conditions giving rise to diarrhea which may be considered as due to *defects in the anatomical processes necessary for defecation.* Some disease conditions may cause an increase in the neuromuscular excitability of the intestine. With a decrease in the calcium ion level in the body, for example, as is seen in patients in a uremic state (a toxic condition produced by urinary wastes in the blood) there can be sufficient neuromuscular excitability of the intestine to cause diarrhea. There are also certain "malabsorption syndromes" in which the problem is one of failure on the part of the intestines to reabsorb water as the digestive products pass through it.

SIGNS AND SYMPTOMS
ACCOMPANYING
CONSTIPATION AND
DIARRHEA

Constipation

The person who is constipated may exhibit signs and symptoms other than the passage of hardened feces. Abdominal distention when the bolus remains in the large intestine is frequently apparent in patients who are constipated. The distention is caused by the air which remains in the large intestine and the fluid which moves back into the large intestine when the waste products have been there for a long time. These two, air and fluid, result in abdominal distention. The patient appears to have a swollen abdomen which on palpation feels hard and unyielding.

Flatus results from swallowed air, the consumption of gas-forming foods or bacterial action within the large intestine. The air accumulates in the intestine and often causes generalized discomfort and crampy pain. The patient who is constipated may also complain of headache, nausea and anorexia. These usually disappear upon evacuation of the rectal contents.

Another frequent complaint of the constipated patient is that of *tenesmus,* that is, frequent painful straining in attempts at defecation which are unproductive of stool. If the stool remains in the rectum for a long period of time, it may develop into a large, hardened mass which is difficult to expel. Sometimes there is seepage around the mass, with a resultant discharge of small amounts of liquid stool. This is important to remember, particularly in bedridden patients, because there is the possibility that constipation may be overlooked when it has been noted that the patient has had a bowel movement.

Diarrhea

The person who has diarrhea often complains of generalized abdominal pain. This is usually caused by flatus which distends the large and small intestines. He may also have pains of a piercing, griping nature. These are usually spasmodic and are caused by the strong peristaltic contractions of the intestinal musculature as the waste products are propelled precipitously through the gastrointestinal tract. These pains are frequently accompanied by a feeling of urgency in the need to defecate. Although frequency in the number of stools is not always an indication of diarrhea, it often occurs with diarrhea. Again, as in constipation, there may be frequent, painful straining, which in the case of the patient with diarrhea may produce a small watery discharge rather than formed stool.

If the diarrhea is prolonged, the patient may exhibit signs and symptoms resulting from the loss of fluids and electrolytes. These signs and symptoms are discussed fully in Chapter 29. They include poor tissue turgor, weight loss and thirst. The patient with prolonged diarrhea may appear thin and emaciated. He complains of fatigue, weakness and general malaise. Nausea and vomiting frequently accompany diarrhea and further aggravate the loss of fluids and electrolytes.

ASSESSING THE NURSING NEEDS OF THE PATIENT WITH CONSTIPATION OR DIARRHEA

Through Communication With the Patient

In assessing the needs of the patient with constipation or diarrhea, it is essential to ascertain if the condition is acute or chronic. Initially the nurse needs to know about the bowel habits and the normal patterns of defecation of the individual. People vary in their frequency of defecation, and what is normal for one person may not be normal for another.

Control over defecation and urination is taught in early childhood and may be associated with values of good and bad. In some cultures, control over bladder and bowel functioning is expected early, and there may be much tension and anxiety associated with the early teaching. Moreover, lack of control over urination or defecation represents a loss of independence.

Many people are embarrassed to talk about their elimination problems. In discussing these problems, then, the nurse should ensure privacy, since it is often difficult for patients to talk about their bowel habits in the presence of other people. The nurse, too, may find it hard to ask the personal questions that are necessary. Questions should be phrased in simple, nontechnical language that assists the patient to give pertinent information in his answers and yet maintain his own feelings of personal dignity in doing so.

A knowledge of the patient's pattern of fecal elimination includes the frequency of defecation and a description of the consistency of stools (hard, soft, liquid) as well as their color and odor. Feces may contain foreign matter which the patient may be able to describe, such as blood, worms, pus, or mucus. Most people become anxious if they think there is blood in the stools. Black stools may indicate the presence of old blood, and red stools, fresh blood; however, certain foods and medications can also discolor feces. For example, beets can color feces red and iron (in a medication) can color feces black.

There may be other symptoms of constipation or diarrhea which the patient can communicate verbally to the nurse. The constipated patient may complain of headache, or state that he has a bloated feeling, anorexia (loss of appetite) or nausea. The person with diarrhea often complains of pain and it is important to find out whether it is generalized abdominal pain or pain of a spasmodic griping nature.

The nurse should also determine whether the patient takes laxatives regularly and, if so, what medications are used. It is not uncommon for some people to give themselves a daily enema if they are habitually constipated. On the other hand, some people feel that a "good purge" or "cleaning out" every once in a while is beneficial to the system, and they will use a strong cathartic for this purpose, even if they are not constipated.

Food habits are also pertinent in assessing the needs of the patient with constipation or diarrhea. Failure to ensure that the diet has sufficient bulk may lead to constipation. The ingestion of irritating foods may cause diarrhea. It is important to know then what the individual's dietary intake has been in the immediate past and also what his normal food habits are.

Since emotions play such an important role in the causation of many cases of diarrhea and constipation, it is helpful to determine if the patient has been under any particular stress.

Pertinent Observations

The patient with constipation may not be able to communicate his discomfort verbally to the nurse. She should, therefore, be alert to the signs and symptoms that indicate this discomfort. The patient may have had no bowel movement for several days; he may have abdominal distention, and he may be passing large amounts of flatus by rectum or by mouth. The hospitalized patient is particularly prone to constipation because of lack of exercise and the alterations in daily activity and, often, diet that are imposed by being confined to hospital. These interfere with the normal conditioned reflex for defecation.

In observing the feces of the constipated patient, it is important to note consistency, color, size, shape and odor of the fecal matter. The presence of foreign matter, as described earlier, should also be noted.

Pertinent observations in the case of the patient with diarrhea include the frequency and consistency of the stools as well as their odor and the presence of foreign matter. Undigested food is sometimes present in the feces because of the speed with which it is propelled through the gastrointestinal tract. The nurse should also be alert to the signs and symptoms indicative of loss of fluids and electrolytes as these are described in Chapter 29. Severe diarrhea depletes the body's potassium level and lowers the amount of sodium chloride. The initial effect of this electrolyte loss is acidosis as a result of the loss of base; however, with prolonged potassium loss, alkalosis eventually accompanies a chloride loss. It is essential that an accurate record of the patient's intake and output be maintained. This will include the number of bowel movements and the approximate amount of fluid lost through the feces. The nurse should also note the patient's ability to tolerate foods and fluids.

It is important to determine the patient's nutritional status and to observe signs of weakness and fatigue. Signs of localized irritation around the anus may be present. These include redness and pruritus (itching) which add to the patient's discomfort.

Diagnostic Tests

Among the diagnostic tests for diarrhea and constipation is the laboratory examination of a specimen of feces. It is often the responsibility of nursing personnel to collect the specimen and send it to the laboratory, where it is examined for such substances as blood, microorganisms, fat, undigested food or urobilin. Blood from the lower gastrointestinal tract is usually bright red, whereas old blood from the upper tract may appear black. On the other hand, blood may be present but occult, that is, hidden to the naked eye.

In order to identify microorganisms such as parasites which may be present in the gastrointestinal tract, it is not necessary to keep the specimen warm unless mobile forms, for example, amebae, are suspected. Ova and cysts can be identified in cold specimens.

Excess fat in the stools can be indicative of gastrointestinal disease, as can the presence of undigested food and urobilin. Normally there is a considerable amount of the latter in feces, but in cases of an obstruction in bile flow the feces may be clay colored and negative for urobilin.

X-ray and fluoroscopic examinations of the gastrointestinal tract may also be necessary (see Chapter 19). Usually the patient does not take food or fluids prior to these examinations. For x-rays of the colon and rectum it is not unusual to have a laxative and an enema beforehand.

Sigmoidoscopy is the inspection of the sigmoid portion of the colon with a lighted instrument. After enemas are given, the patient assumes the knee-chest position and the physician inserts the sigmoidoscope in order to visualize the lining of the sigmoid. Usually this examination is embarrassing and uncomfortable. The nurse can assist the patient by draping him comfortably and assuring him that the discomfort is of short duration.

PRINCIPLES BASIC TO THE CARE OF PATIENTS WITH CONSTIPATION OR DIARRHEA

Normal fecal elimination is essential to efficient body functioning.

Fluid and electrolyte balance are affected by disturbances in fecal elimination.

The act of defecation is normally under voluntary control.

Food and fluids can stimulate the gastrocolic reflex.

Control of defecation is an important area of independence to most individuals.

Strong emotions can affect the functioning of the gastrointestinal tract.

OBJECTIVES OF NURSING INTERVENTION

In identifying the nursing needs of patients with constipation or diarrhea and determining objectives for their care, there are five primary areas of consideration:

1. Reestablishment of normal bowel functioning
2. Relief of distressing symptoms
3. Maintenance of fluid and electrolyte balance
4. Maintenance of adequate nutritional status
5. Maintenance of comfort and hygiene

DETERMINING PRIORITIES FOR NURSING ACTION

In determining priorities for nursing action in the care of patients with either diarrhea or constipation, the nurse must take into account the acuteness of the condition. In the severely constipated patient, there may be an immediate need to end the patient's discomfort through bringing about a bowel movement. With the patient who is acutely distressed with diarrhea, nursing intervention will be directed first toward controlling the discharge of stools. There may also be an urgent need to replace lost fluids and electrolytes.

MEASURES TO REESTABLISH NORMAL FECAL ELIMINATION

Constipation

Constipation is a problem for many people, both sick and well. It is almost always a problem for patients confined to bed, and care should be taken to direct nursing action toward its prevention in patients who are ill. Because bowel and bladder habits are learned early in childhood and each individual's pattern of elimination is different, the nurse should develop a plan of care in conjunction with the patient, taking into consideration the individual's previously established pattern.

Important factors to consider in preventing constipation or in overcoming a long-standing problem of constipation include: regularity of time for defecation, prompt attention to the urge to defecate, a diet that contains sufficient laxative foods as well as a sufficient intake of fluids, and exercise.

The gastrocolic reflex is stimulated by mass peristaltic action which occurs most frequently after meals and is believed to be strongest after breakfast.[3] Immediately after the morning meal is therefore a good time to encourage the patient to move his bowels. Affording the patient privacy is important. Sufficient time should be allowed for the process, and the patient should not be

---

[3]Edith V. Olson et al.: The Hazards of Immobility. *The American Journal of Nursing*, 67:4:787, 1967.

hurried. If his condition permits, the individual should be allowed to go to the lavatory to have a bowel movement or to use a bedside commode. Most patients find it awkward to use a bedpan to have a bowel movement. If a bedpan has to be used, the patient should be in a sitting position unless this position is contraindicated.

The patient may need to be helped to increase his sensitivity to the stimulus for defecation. Providing hot fluids helps to activate mass peristalsis, and some people find that a cup of hot tea or coffee, or a glass of hot water (some like hot water with lemon) taken before breakfast helps to stimulate the rectal reflex. The patient should be given an explanation of the process of elimination with stress placed on the importance of responding to the urge to defecate. The individual can sometimes be helped to defecate by massaging the abdomen in a circular motion, moving downward over the descending colon on the left side of the abdomen. Slight pressure on the side of, or posterior to, the anus sometimes helps expel feces. Nursing personnel use cotton gauze or digital pads for this measure.

Through repetition of these measures at the same time each day or as frequently as the patient is in the habit of having a bowel movement, regular habits can often be established. Glycerin suppositories or enemas are also used in some situations to facilitate defecation, particularly when regularity is being established. Their use is then gradually withdrawn as a regular pattern is set. Laxative drugs and stool softeners, such as mineral oil, may also be used sometimes to help in developing regularity, their use again being gradually terminated as the patient gains improved colonic functioning.

The individual may require help also in establishing dietary patterns that give him a sufficient amount of laxative foods and adequate fluids for normal bowel functioning. Fluid intake, it is usually suggested, should be at least 2000 cc. per 24 hour period. The diet should contain sufficient bulk to stimulate reflex activity as well as other foods which the individual finds have a laxa-tive effect on him. Usually, fruits and fruit juices in sufficient quantity have the desired effect. Prune juice is considered to have particularly good laxative effects.

Constipation is aggravated by inactivity and poor muscle tone. A regular program of activity designed to meet the needs of the individual can be planned and the patient assisted to carry it out. Strengthening of the abdominal muscles is particularly important.

Bowel training for patients with spinal cord injuries or for patients who are incontinent of feces for other reasons may be accomplished through systematic and repeated efforts, using the methods just described. Many agencies have developed their own specific regime for bladder and bowel retraining, and descriptions of some of these may be found in the recent nursing literature.[4]

Diarrhea

In attempting to reestablish normal bowel functioning in the patient with diarrhea, it is important to ascertain the cause of the diarrhea. Because the most common cause is irritation of the gastrointestinal tract, removal of the irritant will in most cases stop the symptoms. If the diarrhea is neurogenic in origin, for example, if it is caused by anxiety or tension, medical intervention is usually necessary to help the patient to resolve his problems. Some diarrheas are the result of defects in the anatomical processes necessary for defecation. These conditions require medical therapy.

MEASURES TO RELIEVE DISTRESSING SYMPTOMS

Patients who suffer from constipation or diarrhea are uncomfortable. They

---

[4]Lea L. Tudor: Bladder and Bowel Retraining. *The American Journal of Nursing,* 70:11:2391–2393, 1970. Jean Saxon: Techniques for Bowel and Bladder Training. *The American Journal of Nursing,* 62:9:69–71, 1962.

often have distressing symptoms accompanying their condition such as abdominal distention, excess flatus and pain (see the section on signs and symptoms earlier in the chapter).

The constipated patient is usually relieved of his discomfort and concomitant distressing symptoms when a satisfactory bowel movement is effected. This may be brought about by the administration of a laxative or by the use of a rectal suppository, an enema or a colonic irrigation. At times, manual extraction of feces is necessary. If laxatives are ordered, these are usually given at bedtime so that they will act after breakfast the following morning.

Medications to coat and soothe the lining of the intestines (emulsive drugs) or to reduce muscular spasm (antispasmodic) are often prescribed for patients with diarrhea. Some of these drugs are taken at regular intervals during the day; others are taken after each bowel movement.

Relief of abdominal distention and excess flatus can often be accomplished through the insertion of a rectal tube. Sometimes an enema may be ordered for this purpose also.

Specific nursing measures which are frequently used in the care of patients with disturbances of elimination from the gastrointestinal tract are detailed here.

The Enema

An enema is the injection of fluid into the rectum. Generally its purpose is to aid in the elimination of feces or flatus from the colon. This may be done to relieve constipation or remove fecal impaction, to cleanse the rectum and colon prior to examination, or as a safety measure to prevent possible infection in patients who are undergoing surgery or who are about to deliver.[5] It may, however, be used for other purposes: to reduce fever (ice water enema) or to reduce cerebral edema (magnesium sulfate enema).

Enemas may be divided into three groups according to their mode of action: those that stimulate evacuation by distention, those that stimulate peristalsis by irritation, and those that lubricate.

Cleansing Enemas. Cleansing enemas are given chiefly to remove feces from the colon. There are many kinds of cleansing enema: The *soapsuds enema* usually contains 1000 to 1500 cc. of soap solution. The *saline enema* contains 1000 cc. of normal saline. A third kind of cleansing enema that is often used is the *tap water enema*, which contains 1000 to 1500 cc. of tap water.

These enemas, because of the volume of fluid used, serve to distend the rectum and lower colon, thereby stimulating the evacuation reflex. The soapsuds enema also has an irritating effect, due to the chemicals contained in the soap, and this enhances the action of the enema.

Today, disposable enemas are commonly used in many home and hospital situations. These contain hypertonic solutions, usually of sodium phosphate and biphosphate compounds. Their action is predominantly irritating although the distention produced by the injection of the fluid also helps to stimulate peristalsis.[6]

Oil Enemas. An oil enema may be given in cases in which there is severe constipation or the patient has a painful anal condition. The action of the oil is principally as a lubricant to make evacuation easier. Various oils may be used such as mineral oil, olive or cottonseed oil. The amount given is small, usually 150 to 200 cc., and it is usually intended that the patient retain the enema for approximately an hour. Often a cleansing enema is ordered following an oil retention enema.

Carminative Enemas. The carminative enema is given to help expel flatus from the colon. There are several kinds of carminative enema: The *Mayo enema* contains 240 cc. of water, 60 cc. of white

[5]Betty Tillery and Barbara Bates: Enemas. *The American Journal of Nursing*, 66:3:534–537, March, 1966.

[6]Ibid.

sugar and 30 cc. of sodium bicarbonate. The sodium bicarbonate is mixed with the water and sugar and administered while the solution is still bubbling. The *milk and molasses enema* contains 240 cc. of milk and 240 cc. of molasses. It also is used to remove flatus from the colon. Another type of carminative enema is a *2, 2, 2 enema*. This contains 60 cc. of glycerin, 60 cc. of magnesium sulfate (50 per cent solution) and 60 cc. of water.

Other Types of Enemas. Other enemas are given for a multiplicity of purposes. The *anthelmintic enema*, consisting of 15 cc. of Quassia chips and 250 cc. of water, is used to remove parasitic worms from the colon. The *astringent enema*, one form of which consists of 60 cc. of alum and 1000 cc. of water, is used to contract tissue and to stop hemorrhage. The *emollient enema* is used to coat the mucous membrane of the colon and to soothe irritated tissue; 180 cc. of starch solution is commonly used for this purpose. *Sedative* and *stimulant enemas* are also given. Paraldehyde is commonly used for sedative enemas, whereas 90 to 180 cc. of black coffee is a common ingredient of the stimulant enema. *Magnesium sulfate solution* and *ice water* are also used

for enemas. Magnesium sulfate, 120 cc. of a 50 per cent solution, reduces cerebral edema. Ice water is used as an enema to reduce fever.

Equipment and Supplies. Enema equipment and solutions are obtainable in disposable sets. If these sets are not available the patient requires certain clean equipment. Rectal tubes are usually made of rubber; however, plastic rectal tubes are also available today. Rectal tubes vary in diameter; they are measured on the French scale. A No. 22 or No. 24 French is the size commonly needed by an adult. Also needed are a container for the enema solution, tubing to connect the rectal tube to the container, a small receptacle for extra fluid and a lubricant for the rectal tube. The patient will also need a bedpan if he cannot use a toilet.

Administration. Before the enema equipment is taken to the patient, he will probably require some explanation about this measure. The patient's active help is important to the effectiveness of the enema. For maximum results he should try to hold the solution for 10 minutes. If the patient is in bed the head of the bed is lowered to make the bed level so that the fluid will flow in by force of gravity. It may not always be

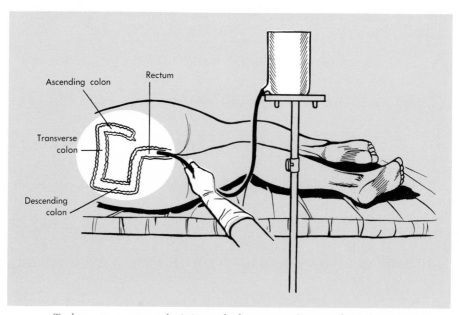

To have an enema administered, the patient lies on the left side.

possible to have the bed completely flat; for example, if the patient is short of breath, the head of the bed should be no lower than is safe for him.

The top bedding is fan-folded to the foot of the bed and the patient is provided with a drape for warmth and comfort. For the administration of the enema, the patient is usually placed on his left side with both knees flexed, the top leg slightly higher than the lower one. It is felt that in this position, the descending colon being on the left side, the injection of fluid is facilitated by the force of gravity. However, this position may be varied according to the patient's condition and his wishes.

The usual temperature of a solution for an enema is 40.6° C. (105° F.). This temperature is not harmful to the mucous membrane lining the colon and rectum. The rectal tube is well lubricated (usually with a water soluble lubricant) in order to facilitate its insertion into the rectum and to lessen the irritation of the mucous membrane. Prior to the insertion of the tube the equipment is connected and a small amount of fluid is run through the tubing to expel the air. Then the tubing is clamped, and the rectal tube is inserted approximately 4 inches into the rectum. The rectum of the average adult patient is 7 to 8 inches in length. If the patient takes a deep breath while the tube is being inserted, the anal sphincter relaxes and the rectal tube can be inserted more easily. If any obstruction to the insertion is encountered, the tube is withdrawn and the physician is notified. A rectal tube should never be forced because it might damage the mucous membrane or aggravate a disease process.

The solution for an enema is released slowly for the patient's comfort and to avoid damage to the mucous membrane. The higher the solution container is held, the greater is the pressure exerted. Hence the solution container should not be more than 2 feet above the level of the bed. For gynecological patients, the container is suspended at the patient's hip level in order to lessen the pressure

on the adjacent reproductive organs. If the patient complains of discomfort while the solution is flowing, the flow is stopped for a few minutes and then recommenced cautiously. Any further discomfort demands the termination of the measure.

Following the administration of the solution, the rectal tube is pinched and removed. The patient retains the enema for 10 minutes if possible. In the case of an oil retention enema, the length of time for retention of the fluid is usually one hour.

When the enema is expelled, the nurse makes certain observations. She observes the color and consistency of the feces, the approximate amount of fluid returned, the general amount of flatus that is expelled (large, small) and the general reaction of the patient. All these observations are recorded in the patient's chart. The nurse also takes particular note of any unusual findings in the enema returns, for example, blood, mucus, pus or worms. Following the expulsion of the enema, the patient is made clean and comfortable. The equipment is then rinsed in cold water and washed in hot soapy water. In hospitals, equipment is sterilized after each use to avoid the transfer of organisms. Disposable equipment is placed in a suitable container for removal.

Siphoning an Enema. If the patient cannot expel the enema within a half hour after its administration, it is usually necessary to siphon off the enema. This is generally a nursing decision. To siphon off an enema is to withdraw the enema solution from the patient by using positive-negative pressures and the force of gravity. The equipment and supplies required include a rectal tube and water soluble lubricant, a small amount of tap water (40.6° C., 105° F.), a receptacle for the enema solution and a funnel.

The patient lies on his right side with his hips drawn to the edge of the bed. In this position the descending colon is uppermost, a situation that facilitates the removal of the enema solution by force of gravity. The receptacle for the enema solution is placed at a level lower than the patient's hips, often on a chair at the side of the bed.

The rectal tube is first connected to the funnel and then well lubricated with the water soluble lubricant. The funnel is then half filled with water while the tubing is pinched to prevent leakage. The rectal tube is inserted into the patient in the same manner as for an enema. The pressure on the tubing is released and a small amount of fluid allowed to run into the rectum. Then the funnel is quickly inverted and lowered over the bedpan. The negative pressure of the fluid in the tube and funnel produces a siphon, which draws the enema fluid from the patient's colon.

After the removal of the enema fluid, the patient may require assistance regarding his comfort and hygiene. The enema fluid is observed for its color and consistency, and these observations are charted on the patient's record.

The Rectal Tube

The purpose of the insertion of a rectal tube is to facilitate the expulsion of flatus. The equipment required for this measure includes the rectal tube, a receptacle for the end of the tube, a lubricant and adhesive tape. The adhesive tape is used to hold the rectal tube in position.

After the patient's need for information about this measure has been met, he lies in the same position as for an enema. The rectal tube is lubricated and inserted 4 inches into the rectum. It is then taped in place, and the free end of the tube is put in a container placed near the patient's buttocks. A rectal tube is usually left in place for half an hour.

After the tube has been removed and the patient has received any needed assistance, the approximate amount (large, small) of flatus that was expelled is noted. Usually the patient can describe this. In addition, since the patient who has flatus usually has a hard distended abdomen, the nurse can palpate his abdomen to note any change.

These observations are then charted on the patient's record.

The Manual Extraction of Feces

The manual extraction of feces is the removal by hand of impacted feces from the rectum. A fecal impaction is a large hardened mass of feces which has accumulated in the rectum, owing usually to prolonged constipation. The equipment required for manual extraction includes a rectal glove, a container for the glove, a lubricant and a bedpan. After the measure has been explained to the patient, he lies on his left side.

The nurse puts on the rectal glove and thoroughly lubricates her second or third finger. She inserts this finger carefully into the rectum and manually breaks the impacted feces. The lubricant is used to facilitate the insertion of the nurse's gloved finger and to protect the rectal mucosa from abrasion. When the feces have been broken, they are removed by hand to the bedpan. The manual extraction of feces is often followed by a cleansing enema. This is ordered by the physician or the nurse in charge. After this nursing measure, the nurse charts the amount, color and consistency of the feces. She also notes the presence of any flatus and the patient's general reaction (pallor, fatigue, and the like).

The Rectal Suppository

A medicated rectal suppository is administered for many reasons: it is used as a local irritant to facilitate elimination, as a vehicle for the administration of a sedative or as an antispasmodic. The equipment needed for the insertion of a rectal suppository consists of a rectal glove, the suppository and a container for the suppository. The patient may need information about the function of the suppository and its insertion as well as the nursing techniques that are involved. The patient lies in the same position as for an enema.

With a gloved hand, the suppository

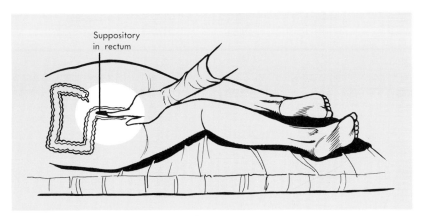

The insertion of a rectal suppository.

is inserted one finger length, approximately 2½ to 3 inches into the rectum. It is usually possible to tell when the suppository is in place because the rectal sphincter "grabs" or "sucks" it in and closes. If the purpose of the suppository is to aid in the expulsion of the rectal contents, the patient should try to retain the suppository for about 20 minutes. If the suppository is administered for other purposes, it is retained indefinitely. When inserting the suppository, care must be exercised to be certain that the mucosa of the rectum is not irritated and that the suppository is not forced when any resistance in the rectum is met.

After the suppository has been administered, this fact is recorded as are the effects of the suppository. These can often be observed 15 to 30 minutes after administration, depending upon the medication.

Care of the Colostomy

Irrigation of a Colostomy. A colostomy is the surgical formation of an artificial anus through the abdomen into the colon. The purpose of a colostomy is usually to divert the feces from the intestinal tract through this artificial opening. A colostomy may be permanent or temporary.

In a permanent colostomy there is usually only one opening (stoma); in a temporary colostomy there may be two. The one closer to the stomach is called the proximal stoma; it is from this opening that the feces are discharged. If there is a second stoma it is farther from the stomach (closer to the anus) and hence is referred to as the distal stoma. There should be some direction in the nursing care plan as to how the nurse may distinguish between the proximal and distal stomas. An irrigation is generally prescribed for the functioning proximal stoma; only occasionally is a solution, an antiseptic solution for example, instilled into a distal stoma.

The purpose of a colostomy irrigation is to cleanse the colon of fecal matter by injecting fluid into the colon through the colostomy opening. The equipment required for this nursing measure is similar to that needed for an enema, with the addition of a small rectal tube, a large glass **Y** connector and unsterile waste gauze. The person who has a colostomy often needs careful instruction with regard to both the colostomy dressing and the colostomy irrigation. Most people can, with guidance, assume the responsibility for carrying out these measures themselves. There are several methods of irrigating a colostomy. One method is detailed here.

The nurse's approach to these nursing measures is extremely important. The patient is often anxious about his adjustment to the change in his life pattern as a result of this surgery, and any revulsion on the part of the nurse could be particularly disturbing to the patient and his family. Patients often feel embarrassed and find the colostomy hard to accept. They may not want to watch the nurse irrigate it at first, or they may be angry that this has happened to them. The nurse may also have strong feelings of dislike at doing this procedure which may show in her facial expression. Her calm acceptance of the situation and her care to protect the patient's feelings of dignity can do much to reassure the patient.

At the commencement of a colostomy irrigation, the patient lies on the side toward which the colostomy opening has been made, or sits upright so that the expulsion of feces is more easily accomplished. If he is in bed, the lower bedding is protected by a waterproof towel and the top bedding is fan-folded down to expose the colostomy opening. A bedpan is placed conveniently at a level lower than the colostomy opening. The container for the irrigating solution is placed not more than 1 foot above the patient's pelvis in order to keep the pressure of the fluid low enough not to damage the mucous membrane of the intestine. A narrow rectal tube is connected to the irrigating container and a small amount of the irrigating solution is permitted to run through the rectal tube in order to expel the air in it.

The rectal tube is lubricated, and then inserted gently into the colostomy stoma. The irrigating fluid is allowed to run slowly into the colon. After a small amount is administered, the intake tubing is clamped and the output tubing is released so that the return flow drains into the bedpan. This process is repeated until the returns from the colostomy are clear.

The returns of the irrigation are observed for color and consistency of the fecal matter. The condition of the operative area is also noted. Throughout this nursing measure the patient should be encouraged to participate actively. Most patients learn to carry out a colostomy irrigation while they are in the hospital so that they can eventually do this independently.

Especially designed for colostomy irrigations are the Binkley and Stockley apparatuses. In essence each has a plastic cup which fits over the colostomy stoma. The cup has a hole for the catheter and a detachable plastic sheath which guides the fluid and feces into a receptacle. One of the advantages of these apparatuses is the complete enclosure of the fluid and feces during the irrigation.

Dressing the Colostomy. The colostomy dressing is a clean procedure rather than a sterile one. The dressing on the colostomy stoma is changed as often as necessary in order to keep the patient clean and his skin free from fecal

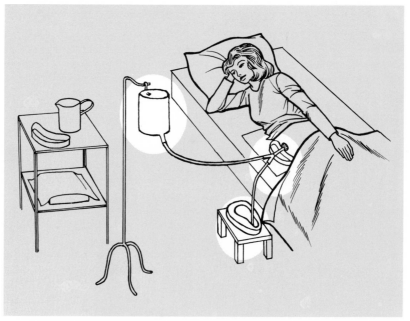

The administration of an irrigating solution to a colostomy by means of a Y tube.

matter. It is important that the skin surrounding the stoma be protected from irritation. Usually a protective lubricant, such as zinc oxide, is used for this purpose.

The equipment that is needed for a colostomy dressing includes unsterile gauze, unsterile dressings, lubricant, a tongue depressor and a container for the disposal of the soiled dressings. Nursing personnel may use rubber gloves if they desire. As with the colostomy irrigation the nurse's approach to this task is important. Most people require considerable reassurance and a calm acceptance of the task. The patient can be helpful; in fact most people learn to change their own dressings. Therefore, each time the nurse dresses a colostomy she should be conscious of the learning needs of the patient.

The patient sits in a comfortable position for his dressing. If he is in bed, the bottom bedding is protected with waterproof material and the bedclothes are fan-folded to expose the colostomy stoma. The patient is draped for warmth and comfort. The soiled dressings are first removed and the skin around the colostomy stoma cleansed with soap and water. A protective substance is then applied generously to the skin around the stoma, and a clean dressing is applied. The first layer of dressing usually consists of gauze, and then unsterile surgical dressings are applied. Adhesive ties are used to hold the dressing in place. The color, the consistency and the amount of fecal matter on the old dressing are charted. The nurse also charts the appearance of the colostomy stoma and the presence of any excoriated areas. (Excoriation is the loss of superficial tissue such as epidermis.)

Plastic colostomy bags are also commercially available. They have attachable, specially designed belts that are worn around the waist or bags that stick directly to the skin. These bags are disposable and are changed whenever they become soiled. The physician usually guides the nurse and the patient in the use of these bags.

Colonic Irrigation

A colonic irrigation (enteroclysis) is a measure designed to wash out the lower colon. Its purpose may be merely to cleanse the large intestine, or it may be to stimulate peristalsis and relieve distention. Other uses of the colonic irrigation are to relieve inflammation and to reduce body temperature. In the latter two instances the temperature of the solution is usually cooler. The equipment required for a colonic irrigation consists of the solution, a solution container, a colonic irrigation tube (No. 30 French is suggested), a lubricant, a catheter (No. 20 French is suggested) and a bedpan.

Initially the colonic tube is marked 2 to 3 inches from the tip; adhesive tape can be used for this purpose. The catheter is marked 5 inches from the tip in the same manner. These marks serve as a guide as to the distance to insert the tubes. The type and temperature of the solution are prescribed by the physician.

This is not a painful measure, but patients usually require information about it. The patient turns on his right side with his hips toward the edge of the bed. This position facilitates the drainage of fluid from the colon. He is provided with drapes. The tubing and the catheter are connected to the solution container and the solution is allowed to run through the tubing before it is clamped. Both the colonic tube and the catheter are lubricated; then the tip of the catheter is placed in the eye on the side of the colonic tube. The other end of the colonic tube is placed in a receptacle at the patient's bedside. Holding the two tubes together the nurse gently inserts them into the rectum up to the 3 inch mark on the colonic tube. Next the catheter is drawn back sufficiently to free its tip from the colonic tube and then is inserted up to the 5 inch mark. The solution is allowed to flow gradually and continuously so that the inflow and outflow are equal. If the patient says he has pain the flow is stopped for a few minutes. If the pain persists, the irrigation is discontinued and the discomfort is reported.

When the irrigation returns are clear, the irrigation is discontinued, but the colonic tube is kept in place until drainage ceases. If at any time the colonic tube becomes blocked it must be removed and cleansed and then reinserted.

The character of the return flow is observed. Particular note is made of the presence of mucus, blood, pus or feces. The observations are recorded on the patient's chart.

MAINTENANCE OF FLUID AND ELECTROLYTE BALANCE

Adequate fluid and electrolyte balance is necessary to normal body functioning. Patients who have diarrhea need extra fluid intake to compensate for the fluid lost through the gastrointestinal tract. In diarrhea, fluids and electrolytes are lost because of hypersecretion of mucus from the membrane (due to irritation) and because of lack of reabsorption by the bowel of fluids ingested and of fluids secreted into the bowel. Normally, 8 liters of fluid are secreted into the bowel in a 24 hour period. Most of this fluid is reabsorbed. Severe diarrhea depletes the body's potassium level and lowers the amount of sodium chloride. The initial effect of this electrolyte loss is acidosis as a result of the loss of base; however, with prolonged potassium loss, alkalosis is eventually accompanied by a chloride loss.

In constipation there is a need for additional fluid intake both as an aid in activating peristalsis and to keep the feces soft. Often merely ensuring that the patient is taking enough fluids is sufficient to relieve constipation.

MAINTENANCE OF ADEQUATE NUTRITIONAL STATUS

Maintaining adequate nutrition can be a particular problem for the patient who has diarrhea. Because the food moves quickly through the gastrointestinal tract, many food constituents are not absorbed. The ingestion of small amounts of nonirritating food at frequent intervals is often helpful in preventing diarrhea and facilitating absorption. Usually a bland diet is ordered to prevent further irritation of the gastrointestinal mucosa.

The constipated patient, on the other hand, may be anorectic and need help to stimulate his appetite. The diet for the constipated patient should be planned to meet his needs for extra bulk and for foods which have a laxative effect. (See section on reestablishment of normal bowel functioning.)

MAINTENANCE OF COMFORT AND HYGIENE

Meeting the comfort and hygiene needs of the patient with elimination problems is a valuable contribution to his sense of well-being. Cleanliness is essential. The sight and odor of fecal material is repugnant, and the high bacteria count in feces is a possible source of contamination. The patient should be given the opportunity to wash his hands after he has had a bowel movement (as he would normally do at home). The rectal area should be cleansed and the patient assisted with this if he is unable to do it himself. Soiled linen should be removed immediately.

Some patients with diarrhea feel more secure if the bedpan is close at hand. In these cases, the pan can be kept covered and placed inconspicuously within reach. Care should be taken that the pan is emptied and cleaned after each use.

After the patient has defecated, his room may require ventilating and freshening to eliminate unpleasant odors. Since such matters can be embarrassing to the patient, the nurse should take the initiative in these measures.

Many patients with defecation problems develop irritation of the skin and mucous membranes in the anal area. Cleanliness is important to prevent infection, and emollient creams help to keep the skin intact and to soothe the irritated area.

An important factor to consider in the care of patients with constipation or diarrhea is the nurse's reaction to these patients and their problems. It is helpful if the nurse can accept her own feelings and not communicate these to the patient.

GUIDE TO ASSESSING NURSING NEEDS

1. Does the patient have constipation or diarrhea? How long has he had this condition? Has he been eating any irritating food?
2. Does he require immediate medical or nursing intervention to relieve these symptoms?
3. What is the patient's normal pattern of defecation? Is he in the habit of taking laxatives or enemas?
4. Is he under stress?
5. What is the consistency of the patient's feces? Their color, odor, and frequency? Do the feces contain foreign matter such as blood or pus?
6. Is the patient able to communicate his discomfort to the nurse? If so, does he complain of accompanying signs and symptoms such as anorexia, headache, abdominal pain or distention? Does he have pain on defecation?
7. Are there signs of fetal impaction as, for example, the passage of small amounts of seepage instead of formed stool?
8. Is the patient's nutritional status satisfactory? His fluid and electrolyte balance normal? Is he taking sufficient exercise?
9. Does the patient's diet contain a sufficient amount of bulky foods to ensure stimulation of the defecation reflex? Is he taking enough fluids?
10. What are the patient's learning needs relative to the reestablishment of a normal pattern of defecation? Relative to hygiene measures in regard to defecation?

GUIDE TO EVALUATING THE EFFECTIVENESS OF NURSING ACTION

1. Is the patient comfortable? Free from distressing symptoms?
2. If the patient has been constipated, has a successful bowel movement been accomplished? If he has had diarrhea, have the stools returned to normal in consistency and frequency?
3. Has a normal pattern of elimination been established?
4. Is the patient aware of his dietary and fluid needs to ensure adequate fecal elimination? Does his selection of foods and his fluid intake indicate this?
5. Does the patient practice good hygiene? For example, does he wash his hands after defecation?

STUDY
VOCABULARY

Cathartic	Feces	Peristalsis
Colostomy	Flatus	Sphincter
Constipation	Impaction	Stool
Defecation		

STUDY
SITUATION

Mr. S. Norris is a 70 year old man living at home who has abdominal pain. He has been retired for five years after an active life as a house painter, and he now spends most of his time watching television. Mr. Norris lives alone in a small house just outside the city. He has three grandchildren who live a few miles away and he visits them on Sundays.

Mr. Norris has been increasingly uncomfortable because of constipation during the past few years. He says he never took medicines when he worked but now has to take a laxative every day. Because he does not like to cook, he generally eats toast and jam. His doctor has asked you to assist Mr. Norris to regulate his bowel habits.

1. What factors should you take into consideration before assisting Mr. Norris?
2. What observations should you make regarding Mr. Norris's bowel habits?
3. For what reasons might Mr. Norris be constipated?
4. Outline the objectives of the nursing care for Mr. Norris.
5. What should you include in your teaching program for this patient?
6. Mr. Norris's physician has ordered saline enemas for the patient. How would you explain this measure to him?
7. Describe the position most desirable for the administration of an enema and why it is desirable.
8. What observations should you record relative to the enema?
9. How would you evaluate the effectiveness of your teaching?

BIBLIOGRAPHY

Beland, Irene L.: *Clinical Nursing: Pathophysiological and Psychosocial Approaches.* New York, The Macmillan Company, 1965.

Elizabeth, Sister Regina: Sensory Stimulation Techniques. *The American Journal of Nursing,* 66:2:281–286, February, 1966.

Guyton, Arthur C.: *Textbook of Medical Physiology.* Fourth edition. Philadelphia, W. B. Saunders Company, 1971.

MacBryde, Cyril M., and Robert S. Blacklow (eds.): *Signs and Symptoms: Applied Pathologic Physiology and Clinical Interpretation.* Fifth edition. Philadelphia, J. B. Lippincott Company, 1970.

Nordmark, Madelyn T., and Anne W. Rohweder: *Scientific Foundations of Nursing.* Second edition. Philadelphia, J. B. Lippincott Company, 1967.

Olson, Edith V., et al.: The Hazards of Immobility. *The American Journal of Nursing,* 67:4:780–797, April, 1967.

Saxon, Jean: Techniques for Bowel and Bladder Training. *The American Journal of Nursing,* 62:69–71, September, 1962.

Secor, Sophia M.: Colostomy Care. *The American Journal of Nursing,* 64:127, September, 1964.

Secor, Sophia M.: Colostomy Rehabilitation. *The American Journal of Nursing,* 70:11:2400–2401, November, 1970.

Sodeman, William A., and William A. Sodeman, Jr. (eds.): *Pathologic Physi-*

ology: Mechanisms of Disease. Fourth edition. Philadelphia, W. B. Saunders Company, 1967.

Thompson, S. M.: Managing the Problems of Elimination. *Nursing Outlook,* 14:58–61, November, 1966.

Tillery, Betty, and Barbara Bates: Enemas. *The American Journal of Nursing,* 6:3:534–537, March, 1966.

Tudor, Lea L.: Bladder and Bowel Retraining. *The American Journal of Nursing,* 70:11:2391–2393, November, 1970.

25 THE CARE OF PATIENTS WHO HAVE DYSPNEA

The nurse should be able to:

Define dyspnea

Use appropriate terminology in recording and reporting observations about the patient with dyspnea

Describe the physiology of respiration, including the five basic processes involved

List factors which may interfere with the normal functioning of these processes

Describe signs and symptoms of oxygen deficiency which may accompany dyspnea

Assess the nursing needs of dyspneic patients

List principles basic to the care of patients with dyspnea

Establish goals for nursing action

Determine priorities for nursing intervention; describe emergency measures that may be used in the case of respiratory failure

Describe appropriate nursing action to:
1. Maintain patency of the patient's airway
2. Increase ventilatory efficiency
3. Ensure adequate oxygen intake
4. Decrease bodily needs for oxygen
5. Minimize the patient's anxiety

Establish criteria for evaluating the effectiveness of nursing action

338

INTRODUCTION

Respiration is one of the body's vital functions. Normal breathing (eupnea) is silent and effortless. A person who is breathing normally is usually not conscious of his respirations. The respiratory rate and its depth can, however, be altered by volition. Eating and drinking, for example, may involve voluntary changes in the breathing pattern. Similarly, speaking and singing require a certain amount of control over respirations. Some people develop considerable skill in adjusting their breathing patterns to produce specific effects with the voice. Singers and actors are usually particularly adept at this. Under normal circumstances, however, most people are not aware of the regular pattern of breathing in (inspiration) and breathing out (expiration) which occurs rhythmically 12 to 18 times per minute in the normal adult.

When a person has difficulty in breathing (dyspnea), he usually becomes acutely aware of his respirations and attempts to control their rate and depth. Dyspnea is a subjective symptom. It is something which the individual feels, and he frequently expresses his distress by such complaints as "I can't breathe" or "I feel as though I am suffocating." Generally, the patient with respiratory problems is an anxious patient. The inability to get oxygen and to control a function which is essential to life can be terrifying. Prompt attention to the patient's needs is imperative, not only because of the vital role of oxygen in sustaining life, but also because the anxiety induced by difficulty in breathing can in itself affect a person's respirations and further aggravate the situation. The competence of the nurse in handling inhalation equipment and helping the patient to feel that he has some control over the situation are important

supportive measures in caring for the patient with respiratory problems.

THE PHYSIOLOGY OF RESPIRATION

The physiology of respiration can be divided into five logical sections:

1. The provision of oxygen from the atmosphere (or from inhalation equipment)
2. The mechanisms which regulate the respiratory process
3. The passage of air from the atmosphere to the alveoli of the lungs and from the alveoli to the atmosphere
4. The diffusion of oxygen and carbon dioxide between the alveoli and the blood and between the blood and the tissue cells
5. The transportation of oxygen to the cells and carbon dioxide away from the cells by the blood stream.

1. Basic to the respiratory process is the availability of oxygen. Normally, the atmosphere supplies all the oxygen an individual requires. The air at sea level contains approximately 20 per cent oxygen and 0.04 per cent carbon dioxide. The provision of oxygen is essential to life. Tissues of the body are differentially sensitive to a lack of oxygen. The cells of the cerebral cortex are damaged after as little as 30 seconds without oxygen, and the medulla of the brain may be irreparably damaged after 30 minutes of oxygen deprivation.[1]

2. A number of factors regulate the respiratory process. The principal mechanism of control is the respiratory center located in the medulla. The respiratory

---

[1]Madelyn T. Nordmark and Anne W. Rohweder: *Scientific Foundations of Nursing.* Second edition. Philadelphia, J. B. Lippincott Company, 1967, p. 49.

center contains both inspiration and expiration centers. Generally speaking, these operate as an "alternating circuit" type of mechanism; when one is active, the other is inactive.

Impulses from a number of specialized receptors in the body are transmitted to the respiratory center to effect changes in respiration. The well-known Herring-Breur reflex is initiated by impulses from *stretch receptors* located principally in the visceral pleura around the lungs. At a specific point in inspiration, these receptors transmit impulses to the respiratory center, which promptly inhibits inspiration and triggers the expiratory phase of respiration. The reverse takes place during expiration. Chemical receptors in respiratory center, aorta and carotid sinuses are called *chemoreceptors*. These receptors are sensitive to changes in the chemical composition of blood and tissue fluid. A lowered concentration of oxygen, a higher concentration of carbon dioxide, a lowered blood pH, or an elevation in blood temperature will all stimulate increased respirations. An alteration in the arterial blood pressure affects *pressoreceptors* in the aorta and carotid sinuses, and these receptors then transmit impulses to the respiratory center. A sudden rise in arterial blood pressure inhibits respirations. Respiration may also be affected by impulses arising from *proprioreceptors* located in the muscles and tendons of movable joints. These receptors are stimulated by movements of the body. Active exercise is a powerful stimulant to respiration.

Emotions also have an effect on the character of respirations. Anxiety, for example, can cause a prolonged state of respiratory stimulation. Pain, fear and anger usually cause an increase in the rate and depth of respirations.

3. The passage of air from the atmosphere to the alveoli of the lungs, the exchange of gases there, and the subsequent return of air to the atmosphere are collectively referred to as *ventilation*. During ventilation, the air passes through the nasal passages, pharynx, larynx, trachea, bronchi and bronchioles to the alveoli and then back. In its passage to the lungs the air is humidified, cleansed of foreign materials and warmed. The respiratory tract is lined with mucous membrane part of which contains cilia and excretes mucus to trap organisms and other foreign material.

4. Once oxygen enters the alveoli of the lungs, it passes into the blood as a result of the difference in the pressures of the gases on either side of the alveolar membrane. Since the partial pressure of oxygen in the inspired air is higher than the pressure of the oxygen in the venous blood, the oxygen passes from the area of higher pressure to the area of lower pressure. The same principle holds in the passage of carbon dioxide from the blood to the alveoli.

5. Once the oxygen enters the blood, it combines with hemoglobin to form oxyhemoglobin and is carried by the arteries to the capillaries throughout the body. From there is is transported via the interstitial fluid to the tissue cells, again because of the difference in the pressures. It is apparent that the delivery of oxygen to the cells is dependent upon the hemoglobin level in the blood plasma and the adequacy of the blood circulation.

THE ETIOLOGY OF RESPIRATORY PROBLEMS

A decrease in the availability of oxygen from the atmosphere can cause serious respiratory problems. The term "anoxic anoxia" is used to describe this condition. At high altitudes, for example, where the pressure of oxygen in the air is low, a person will experience considerable difficulty in breathing until he becomes acclimatized to the rarefied atmosphere. Once acclimatized, his breathing rate may be seven times as fast as at sea level in order to provide him with sufficient oxygen.

The presence of noxious gases in the air will displace the oxygen normally present and lessen the amount available for respiration. In most fires, for instance, suffocation from smoke is usually as great a hazard as bodily injury from the flames. In heavily industrialized areas, a combination of gaseous wastes from industrial plants and the exhaust fumes from automobiles may pollute the atmosphere to a point that is dangerous to health. Many cities now have a pollution monitoring system. When the pollution level reaches a point that is considered dangerous, industries in the area may be restricted in their operations until the pollution level is safe again.

Respiratory problems may also be caused by anything which interferes with the control mechanisms for breathing. A number of different factors may depress or totally inactivate the respiratory center in the medulla. Depressed respirations almost invariably accompany a head injury and are felt to be due to cerebral edema. The edema causes increased pressure within the cranial cavity which depresses the activity of the respiratory center. Drugs and anesthetics which act as depressants on the central nervous system will also depress respirations and may, when administered in large dosage, cause respiratory arrest. Morphine is usually cited as an example of a drug which depresses respirations, although any central nervous system depressant will decrease respirations as well as depressing other parts of the central nervous system.

As discussed earlier in the section on the physiology of respiration, the respiratory center is sensitive to chemical stimuli resulting from changes in the composition of blood or tissue fluids. If a person faints, or voluntarily holds his breath until he faints, the accumulation of carbon dioxide in the blood quickly triggers the mechanism for inspiration and the patient automatically begins to breathe again. A lessened quantity of oxygen in the blood is slower to act as a respiratory stimulant than an increased amount of carbon dioxide. This is because the blood normally carries an amount of oxygen greater than that which is needed for immediate use. It takes a longer period of time for the body to feel the need for

more oxygen and to respond to the oxygen lack. Increased acidity of the blood (a lowered pH) will increase both the rate and depth of respirations as the body attempts to "blow off" acid through the expired carbon dioxide. In patients with a fever, the accelerated rate of metabolism caused by the higher than normal body temperature leads to an increase in the amount of end products of metabolism which are acid in character. The respiratory response is an increase in the rate and depth of respirations.

The passage of oxygen from the atmosphere to the alveoli and the passage of carbon dioxide from the alveoli to the air require an unobstructed airway. Anything which interferes with the patency of any part of the respiratory tract can interfere with the efficiency of respirations. Normally the cough is a mechanism by which the respiratory tract is cleared of foreign materials. Obstructions in the pharynx, larynx, trachea and bronchi can stimulate the cough reflex.

Some patients have difficulty in clearing mucus from the bronchial tree, perhaps because it is painful to cough, because of lack of strength or because of unconsciousness. At any rate, fluids can accumulate and require nursing intervention for their removal. Continual bed rest and maintaining a prone or supine position can contribute to this difficulty by limiting chest expansion and alveolar ventilation. Also, certain drugs and diseases of the nervous system interfere with muscle control and the normal methods of clearing the respiratory system.

Under certain circumstances, oxygen and carbon dioxide are impeded from crossing through the membrane between the alveoli and the blood stream. For example, the distance the gases have to travel may be increased owing to pulmonary edema or inflammation. The successful exchange of gases is dependent on the efficient functioning of the two major pump systems in the body, the lungs and the heart.

Any malfunctioning of the lungs or the muscles of respiration because of injury or disease will interfere with the transfer of oxygen and carbon dioxide. For example, conditions which disturb the balance of the partial pressures of these gases can result from disturbed passage through the airway, as, for instance, in asthma, in which expired air is obstructed in the bronchioles. In addition, any decrease in the elasticity of the lung tissue can impair respiration. For example, in emphysema (a condition common among chronic smokers) extra effort must be made to deflate the lungs because of the inelastic tissue.

The principal muscles concerned with respiration are the muscles of the chest wall and the diaphragm. These include the internal and external intercostals, the sternocleidomastoid, the scalenes, the thoracohumeral and the thorascapular muscles. In addition, in forced breathing, the abdominal muscles may be brought into use. Trauma to any of these muscles, as may result from accidental injury or from surgery, will impair respiration. Similarly any disease process which weakens or paralyzes these muscles, as for example poliomyelitis, will affect the individual's ability to breathe normally.

A great many factors may affect the efficient functioning of the heart. In some conditions there may be inadequate force to pump the blood through the lungs, or there may be an impediment in the return flow of blood from the lungs to the heart, causing a slowing up (stasis) of blood in the small vessels which surround the alveoli. Such conditions will interfere with respiration by disturbing the balance of partial pressures of oxygen and carbon dioxide within the blood circulating through the lungs.

Similarly, any condition affecting the circulation of blood to the tissues can interfere with the transportation of oxygen from the lungs to the cells. This would include all types of heart disease and arterial or venous disorders as well as blood dyscrasias. Since hemoglobin carries the oxygen in the blood stream, a reduction in the amount of hemoglobin, such as in anemia, lessens the amount of oxygen carried to the cells.

SIGNS AND SYMPTOMS OF RESPIRATORY DISTRESS

One of the prominent indications of respiratory distress is the subjective feeling of difficulty in breathing experienced by the patient. This is termed *dyspnea*. The patient's breathing efforts become obvious, and he attempts to control his breathing to overcome the difficulty. In all probability, a change in the rate and character, for example the depth, of the patient's respirations and a general restlessness can be observed. *Orthopnea*, the inability to breathe except when in a sitting position, often accompanies dyspnea.

Cyanosis, a bluish tinge in the skin and mucous membranes, is a frequent manifestation of respiratory (or circulatory) distress. It is attributed to an increase in the amount of reduced hemoglobin in the blood. Cyanosis may appear as a general duskiness of the skin surface, but more frequently it is observed as a bluish tinge in the lips, or around them (circumoral cyanosis), in the earlobes and in the beds of the nails.

When an obstruction occurs in the respiratory tract, coughing is usually stimulated. The cough is a protective mechanism of the body. To *expectorate* is to bring up mucus from the lungs. *Hemoptysis* is the expectoration of blood streaked sputum. *Sputum* consists mostly of mucus which is brought up from the lungs. It usually also contains leukocytes, epithelial cells, secretions from the nasopharynx, bacteria and dirt. Patients with respiratory diseases frequently expectorate sputum. The character of the sputum is often specific to the type of disease the patient has. For example, the sputum of patients with emphysema or chronic bronchitis is usually thick and tenacious, while that from patients with pulmonary edema is usually pink in color and frothy in appearance.[2]

---

[2]Jane Secor: *Patient Care in Respiratory Problems.* Saunders Monographs in Clinical Nursing, Vol. 1. Philadelphia, W. B. Saunders Company, 1969, pp. 40, 41.

Many patients with respiratory problems complain of pain in the chest. The pain may or may not be associated with the act of breathing. Pain may be caused by a number of different factors such as inflammation, the presence of space-occupying lesions, or increased muscular activity as the patient works harder to breathe.

Air hunger is one of the symptoms associated with *hypoxia*, a condition in which there is a reduced oxygen content of the tissues. In air hunger the respiratory rate and the depth of respirations are markedly increased as the body attempts to obtain more oxygen to augment the depleted reserves in the tissues.

Because nervous tissue is very sensitive to oxygen deficiency, the patient with respiratory problems may show signs of impaired brain functioning. An early sign is faulty judgment which may progress to confusion and disorientation. Safety precautions such as using crib sides on the bed should be taken to protect the patient. Other cortical symptoms of oxygen lack include headache, vertigo (dizziness) and drowsiness.

Additional symptoms which may be present are tachycardia, as the heart beats faster in an attempt to keep up with the body's demands for oxygen, and increased blood pressure. Because of the vital role of respiration in total body functioning, other systems may also be affected, and signs and symptoms indicative of their impaired functioning may be present. Because muscular activity, for example, demands increased oxygen consumption, the patient tires easily, particularly with any extra exertion. Distention of the neck veins may also occur.

ASSESSING THE NURSING NEEDS OF PATIENTS WITH DYSPNEA

Difficulty in breathing (dyspnea) is a subjective symptom. It is therefore difficult to assess objectively. The nurse can supplement her observations with information the patient can tell her about

his condition. Pertinent information includes how long the patient has had the problem, the nature and extent of the respiratory distress, and whether it is brought on or relieved by specific factors. Often the patient's family can give assistance in providing background information about the patient's condition prior to his seeking medical care.

Dyspnea must be evaluated in relation to the patient's age, sex, normal pattern of breathing, position, physical activity, emotional state and his disease condition. Any medications which the patient is receiving should also be taken into consideration.[3]

The nurse's alert and astute observations play a very important role in gathering data for assessment of the patient's condition and his needs for medical and nursing intervention. Continuing observations are important for evaluation of the effectiveness of therapy and nursing care measures.

Observations should be directed and purposeful. They are based on the nurse's knowledge of the physiological mechanisms involved in respiration, her ability to identify deviations from the normal and her understanding of the disease process affecting the patient.

Pertinent observations include an assessment of the character of the patient's respirations, his color, his behavior and the presence of pain, cough or sputum, as well as observations related to his general physical status.

In observing the character of the patient's respirations, the nurse should note the rate and rhythm of breathing. The normal rate for adults is 12 to 18 per minute, and normal breathing is silent and effortless. Labored breathing may be observed in the use of accessory muscles for inspiration or expiration and in the flaring of the nostrils on inspiration. Distention of the neck veins may also be present. Difficult breathing is often accompanied by abnormal sounds. For example, *wheezing* is frequently observed in patients with asthma or chronic bronchitis and indicates that

[3]Nordmark and Rohweder, op. cit., p. 57.

the air is passing through a narrowed lumen. *Rales,* short bubbling sounds, are indicative of fluid in the respiratory tract. An obstruction of the upper airway may result in *laryngeal stridor,* a coarse, high-pitched sound which accompanies inspiration.

The nurse should also note the movements of the patient's chest on breathing. Normal respiration results in deep and even movements. Labored respirations may be persistently shallow, or there may be alterations in rhythm and depth. For example, in Cheyne-Stokes breathing there is a regular pattern of gradually decreasing depth to the respirations followed by a cycle of increasing depth. The pattern of inspiration-expiration may be varied also. Normally, the inspiratory phase is shorter than the time for expiration (1.0 to 1.5 seconds for inspiration, 2 to 3 seconds for the expiratory phase). A prolonged expiratory pause is seen in many types of lung conditions.[4]

The patient's color is frequently an important indication of respiratory distress. The presence of cyanosis indicates a large amount of reduced hemoglobin in the circulating blood. Mild cyanosis is sometimes difficult to detect and is best observed in areas where there are numerous capillaries close to the surface, as for example, in the lips, in the tongue or mucous membranes, in the ear lobes or nail beds. Or the nurse may note a general duskiness to the skin.

Cyanosis is not always present in respiratory insufficiency. There are some conditions in which the patient's skin may show an increased reddish tint. This may occur as a result of prolonged anoxia in which there is an increased renal output of *erythropoietin* and a secondary polycythemia develops.[5]

As already noted, the patient's intellectual ability and his behavior may be altered by a lack of sufficient oxygen supply to the brain. The nurse should be alert for signs of mental confusion, drowsiness, or abnormal behavior in the patient. It is important to remember that these symptoms are reversible.

The presence or absence of chest pain should be noted. A description of the pain (for example, sharp, dull, intermittent or steady) should be reported, as should its location and its relationship to breathing.

If the patient has a cough, the nurse's observations should include its frequency and time of occurrence, its relationship to activity (that is, is it present on exertion or when), whether it is productive of sputum, and whether there are specific factors which induce cough or effectively relieve it.

Sputum should be observed for amount, color, consistency, odor and the presence of foreign material such as blood or pus.

Diagnostic Tests

Numerous diagnostic tests are performed in examinations of the respiratory tract. The x-ray, fluoroscopy, bronchography and bronchoscopy are all means by which the lungs may be visualized. In fluoroscopy the chest movements can also be observed.

In *bronchography,* an iodized oil is instilled into the bronchial tree as a contrast medium so that, when a chest x-ray is made, the structures of the lung are visualized. For a bronchogram the patient usually has a local anesthetic sprayed on his pharynx to prevent gagging and coughing. After the procedure the patient should not take any food or fluids until the anesthetic has worn off, because of the danger of aspiration.

Bronchoscopy is the examination of the bronchial tree with a lighted instrument. A local anesthetic is sprayed on the patient's pharynx and he is usually sedated before the examination. In preparation for bronchoscopy, the patient does not take food or fluids for at least six hours beforehand. If he wears dentures, they are removed before the examination.

[4]Marie Kurihara: Assessment and Maintenance of Adequate Respiration. *Nursing Clinics of North America,* 3:1:69–70, March, 1968.

[5]Ibid., p. 72.

The *examination of sputum* is a common diagnostic test. Normally a sterile wide-mouth vial or Petri dish is used to collect the sputum. Sputum is best collected early in the morning, when it is most easily expectorated. The sputum should be coughed up from the lungs, not from the back of the throat. Sometimes a 24 hour specimen of sputum is ordered. If this is the case, the quantity is usually to be measured. The sputum should be collected in a graduated container. If an ungraduated one is used, the nurse can put into the container a measured amount of saline solution. The specimen when collected can then be poured into a graduated container and the quantity of saline subtracted from the total to give an accurate estimate of the amount of sputum in the 24 hour period.

For *nose and throat cultures* a sterile, cotton-tipped applicator is touched to the inside of the nose or throat and then returned to a sterile test tube. Separate swabs and containers are used for the nose and throat.

An important laboratory test that is performed frequently is the measurement of *partial pressures of blood gases.* For this test, a sample of arterial blood is drawn and sent to the laboratory for analysis. The analyses of blood gases reflect the efficiency of ventilation and of the transport system for oxygen and carbon dioxide, and the rate of metabolism in the cells as well as the state of the buffer systems. Normal values for pO_2 are 95 to 100 mm. of mercury and for pCO_2 are 35 to 40 mm. of mercury.[6] The p stands for partial pressure, that is, the pressure of the gas dissolved in the blood. (The particular gas is only a part of the total volume of gases in the blood, hence the term "partial pressures.") It is important that the sample be taken to the laboratory immediately. The container is usually surrounded by ice to ensure that the gases are kept in solution.

There are a number of *tests of pulmonary function* which may also be ordered for the patient. Among those which are commonly done are *maximum breathing capacity* (MBC) and *forced expiratory volume* (FEV).

The measurement of maximum breathing capacity is a good indication of a person's ability to ventilate his lungs. It measures the maximal amount of air a person can breathe in one minute. The normal for adult males is 125 to 150 liters per minute; for females, 100 liters per minute.[7]

Forced expiratory volume measures the volume of expired air which the patient exhales following deep inspiration. This test requires the expenditure of less effort on the patient's part and yields essentially the same information as the MBC. Sometimes the results are given as a ratio to vital capacity or to MBC. A ratio below 75 per cent indicates obstruction in the airway.

For additional information on these tests and other tests of pulmonary function, the nurse is referred to Secor's *Patient Care in Respiratory Problems.*

Nursing responsibilities in regard to diagnostic tests ordered for the patient include explaining the purpose of the test to the patient, giving him a description of the procedure and telling him what is expected of him. Many anxieties and fears can be allayed by a simple explanation in nontechnical terms which the patient can understand. The nurse may also be asked to assist in carrying out these tests. She should know the purpose of the test and the significance of the results. The laboratory findings are important not only in the assessment of the patient's condition but also as an aid in evaluating the effectiveness of therapy.

PRINCIPLES BASIC TO THE NURSING CARE OF PATIENTS WITH DYSPNEA

Oxygen is essential to life.

A patent airway is essential to normal respiratory function.

---

[6]Secor, op. cit., pp. 26–27.

[7]Ibid., pp. 23–24.

The respiratory tract is lined with mucus-secreting epithelium.

Coughing, swallowing and sneezing are mechanisms by which the respiratory tract is cleared of foreign materials.

The average respiratory rate for an adult is 12 to 18 respirations per minute. Respiratory rates under 8 per minute may lead to hypoxemia.

Carbon dioxide concentrations between 3 and 10 percent increase the rate and depth of respirations.

An individual can survive only a few minutes without oxygen. Cells in the cerebral cortex may be damaged by as little as 30 seconds without oxygen. They may be irreparably damaged after five minutes without oxygen.[8]

Difficulty in breathing provokes anxiety.

An insufficient supply of oxygen impairs functioning of all body systems.

Air at sea level contains approximately 20 per cent oxygen; prolonged exposure to high oxygen tension can result in oxygen poisoning.

OBJECTIVES OF NURSING CARE

Principal goals of nursing action in the care of patients who are having difficulty in breathing include the following:

1. Maintaining the patency of the airway
2. Increasing ventilatory efficiency
3. Ensuring that the patient has an adequate supply of oxygen
4. Decreasing the demands of the body for oxygen
5. Minimizing the patient's anxiety

DETERMINING PRIORITIES FOR NURSING ACTION

Difficulty in breathing is a distressing symptom. It always requires immediate attention by nursing and medical personnel. Early and prompt intervention can often minimize attacks and prevent the need for radical measures. The nurse should therefore observe the patient closely for any changes in his condition that indicate increasing difficulty with respiration. These should be reported immediately, and appropriate measures instituted. Severe distress in breathing is a medical emergency. Signs of impending respiratory failure include rapid, shallow breathing; rapid, thready pulse; fear and apprehension; restlessness; and confusion. Restlessness often occurs early and is an important sign to watch for in patients. Cyanosis may or may not be present.

If respiratory failure seems imminent, the nurse should make certain that the patient's airway is clear; institute ventilation by mechanical means; and obtain assistance. Measures for the resuscitation of patients with respiratory failure are detailed in the following section.

EMERGENCY SITUATIONS

Respiratory Failure

Among the several methods of resuscitation for respiratory failure the recently developed mouth-to-mouth method is considered to be the most efficient. The following measures are taken:

1. Place the patient in a supine position.
2. Remove any foreign material from his mouth and throat.

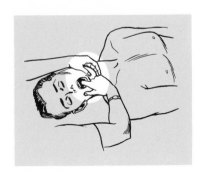

[8]Nordmark and Rohweder, op. cit., p. 49.

3. If an airway such as the Brook airway is available, insert it in the patient's mouth, over his tongue (see section on artificial airways later in this chapter.)

4. If an airway is not available, pull the patient's jaw forward and upward and tilt his head backward.

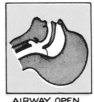

AIRWAY CLOSED   AIRWAY OPEN
(HEAD HYPEREXTENDED)

5. Occlude the patient's nostrils and blow into his mouth by placing your mouth over the patient's.

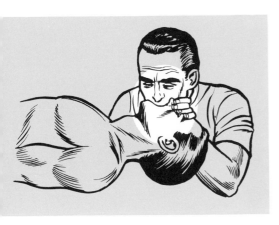

6. Allow the patient to exhale.

7. Repeat this procedure approximately 12 times per minute.

The Holger-Neilson method is an effective manual method of artificial respiration; it is indicated when mouth-to-mouth resuscitation is not advisable, as when there are mouth injuries.

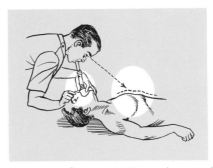

Mouth-to-mouth resuscitation using an airway.

1. Place the patient in the prone position with his hands, one on top of the other, supporting his forehead.

2. Clear any foreign material from the patient's mouth and throat.

3. Kneel with one knee at the side of the patient's head and advance the other leg so that your foot is at the patient's elbow.

4. Place both hands flat on the patient's back with the palms on the shoulder blades, thumbs on the spine and fingers directed toward the patient's feet.

5. Exert a smooth even pressure downward on the patient's back while counting "one, two, three."

6. On the count of "four," rock back and grasp the patient's upper arms above his elbows.

7. Raise and pull the patient's arms to the level of his shoulders and hold for the counts of "five, six, seven."

8. Lower the patient's arms and repeat the entire cycle.

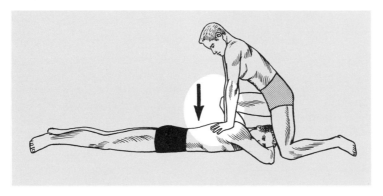

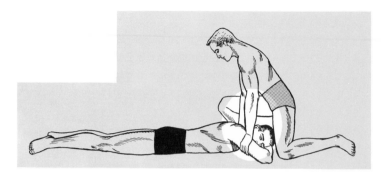

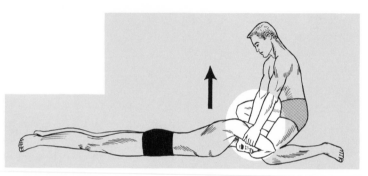

These respirations are continued at the rate of 9 per minute. This method of resuscitation not only ventilates the lungs, but it also stimulates the heart muscle.

MEASURES TO MAINTAIN THE PATENCY OF THE AIRWAY

The maintenance of the patency of the patient's airway is essential to adequate respirations. The conscious, rational patient can tell the nurse when fluids have accumulated in his pharynx and trachea; however, when a patient is unconscious the nurse must rely upon her own observations, and when necessary intervene, for example, with suctioning to clear the patient's air passages. One of the surest indications of partial blockage of air passages by mucus is the sound of "wet breathing"; as the air passes through the secretions it creates a typical gurgling sound.

Suctioning, positioning (for example, the Sims position) and coughing are measures used to maintain the patency of the air passageways. The frequency with which a patient needs suctioning is variable, but if the patient tends to accumulate fluids, a suction catheter should always be near him for immediate use. Suctioning is discussed later in this chapter.

For the conscious patient, medications such as nose drops and aerosol sprays help to liquefy secretions and facilitate their removal from the air passages.

The body position also affects respirations. For the unconscious patient, a semiprone (Sims) position, without a pillow for his head and with the mandible extended forward and up, prevents the tongue from falling back and permits the drainage of fluids from the mouth. For the conscious patient, Fowler's position allows maximum chest expansion and ease of expectoration of sputum. One reason for assisting the patient to change his position every four hours while he is in bed is to permit expansion of all areas of the lungs. Obviously, while a patient is lying on his left side he is not likely to be able to expand his left lung to its maximum capacity.

Coughing is a means by which a person clears his respiratory tract of secretions and foreign material. For the patient who finds it painful to cough, the pain will be eased if the nurse supports the painful area, such as an operative incision, firmly while he coughs.

MEASURES TO INCREASE VENTILATORY EFFICIENCY

The principal factors that impede ventilation are obstruction of the airway and inadequate expansion of the chest. Measures to ensure patency of the airway, as just discussed, are therefore essential to increasing ventilatory efficiency.

Measures which assist in optimal expansion of the chest include positioning of the patient (as already noted) and the alleviation of pain or discomfort associated with breathing. The chest is sometimes splinted to relieve painful respirations, or the physician may leave orders for analgesics. Usually these are given at the nurse's discretion. Coughing may also interfere with respirations. The administration of cough mixtures will usually provide relief from this discomfort. Frequently cough mixtures are left at the patient's bedside to be taken as needed.

Deep breathing at frequent intervals should be encouraged. Exercise helps to improve ventilatory functioning, and active or passive exercise within the patient's level of tolerance should be promoted. Abdominal distention should be prevented by giving the patient small, frequent meals of easily digestable food. Foods that are gas-forming (see Chapter 14) should be avoided. The patient's garments should be loose-fitting and bed coverings should not be tucked in tightly.

MEASURES TO ENSURE ADEQUATE OXYGEN INTAKE

General measures to ensure an adequate supply of oxygen include the provision of fresh air. The patient's room should be kept well ventilated. Many patients with respiratory problems like to have the bed placed beside a window so that they can get fresh air. These patients are often particularly sensitive to alterations in the temperature and humidity of the environment. Atmospheric oxygen may need to be supplemented by means of inhalation aids, such as oxygen masks and oxygen tents. These measures are discussed later.

MEASURES TO DECREASE BODILY NEEDS FOR OXYGEN

The need for oxygen by the body is related to the rate of metabolism of the tissue cells. Factors affecting metabolic rate include physical activity, disease processes and emotional reactions. Although a certain amount of activity is essential to promote optimum ventilation of the lungs, excessive activity should be avoided. The patient's level of tolerance must be carefully assessed and care taken that the patient does not overexert himself.

An elevated body temperature increases the basal metabolic rate and contributes to respiratory distress. Care should be taken then to prevent the patient from developing an infection, and measures taken to keep body temperatures within normal limits.

Emotional tension is also a factor to be considered in patients with respiratory problems. Anxiety, for example, may be mediated through the parasympathetic nervous system and result in constriction of the smooth muscles of the bronchioles. The expression of other emotions such as fear, anger and grief is also closely related to respiration. Strong emotions such as anger and fear initiate responses to prepare the body for action, and respirations become faster and deeper.

MEASURES TO MINIMIZE ANXIETY

Anxiety almost invariably accompanies dyspnea. To be unable to breathe easily and normally is a frightening experience. The person with chronic respiratory problems may live in constant fear that his next breath may be his last one.

The patient's anxiety contributes to his respiratory problems, as noted in several places throughout this chapter. A vicious circle may develop: that is, the patient becomes dyspneic; his dyspnea produces anxiety; the anxiety results in more dyspnea. It is essential that this circle be broken.

Helping to establish the patient's confidence in the care he is receiving is a nursing responsibility and an important factor in alleviating anxiety. Prompt attention to the patient's needs, such as answering his call-light immediately and attending to his wants without delay, can often prevent or minimize an attack of dyspnea. It is important in this regard to remember that anxiety is not always expressed openly. The patient may not necessarily say "I am frightened," but his actions can convey this meaning to the astute and observant nurse. Often, the anxious patient may make a seemingly excessive number of requests, or attempt to keep the nurse engaged in conversation. The physical presence of someone competent who can assist him if need be is reassuring to the patient.

Efficient handling of equipment and skillful execution of procedures contributes to the patient's feeling that he is in good hands. The nurse should be familiar with the equipment used in the care of patients with respiratory problems and should have confidence in her own ability to perform the necessary procedures.

Caring for the patient who has difficulty in breathing can be anxiety-provoking for the nurse. Knowing what measures to take and how to use equipment contributes to her feelings of confidence in giving care.

Measures to ensure the patient's comfort and improve his sense of well-being are also valuable adjuncts in the care of patients with respiratory problems. Good personal hygiene is important, and the patient who experiences dysp-

nea on exertion may need assistance from the nurse in this regard. Many patients with respiratory disorders are "mouth-breathers" and good oral hygiene is needed. Patients who are receiving oxygen therapy, because of the drying effects of oxygen, require special mouth care to maintain hydration of the tissues in the oral cavity and prevent the development of infection or other complications.

Dyspnea is often related to emotional problems. Distressing situations may provoke attacks of difficulty in breathing. The nurse should be alert to conditions which appear to precipitate such attacks and should report these to the physician.

SPECIFIC NURSING CARE MEASURES

Throat Suctioning

Oxygen reaches the alveoli of the lungs by passing through the mouth, the nose, the pharynx, the larynx, and the bronchi and bronchioles. A patent airway is essential to the passage of air through this route. The purpose of throat suctioning is to help a patient to clear his airway by removing secretions and foreign materials from his nose, mouth and pharynx. In most instances, the patient needs an explanation of the procedure. He can be reassured that this is a painless measure that will relieve his breathing so that he will be more comfortable. If the patient can cough while the suction is applied, it will facilitate the removal of mucus.

The equipment required includes a throat suction, a container for cold water and a clean catheter. In hospitals, catheters are sterilized after each use. The catheter has a narrow lumen with a fine tip and several openings along the sides. The openings prevent irritation of the mucous membrane in any one area by distributing the negative pressure of the suction over several areas. Whenever there is any indication

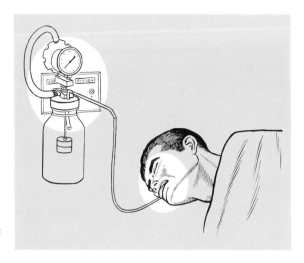

Suctioning a patient's throat to remove mucus that is obstructing the airway.

that a person might require emergency suctioning, this equipment is kept nearby.

The respiratory tract is lined with mucous membrane which can easily be injured by mechanical means; therefore the catheter is never forced against an obstruction. Normally the catheter is inserted by the nurse as far as the pharynx for suctioning; deeper suctioning is generally a physician's procedure.

The catheter is attached to the suction machine and then lubricated with water. Water is drawn through the catheter in order to ensure the patency of the lumen. The patient assumes a position with his head turned to one side, facing the nurse. In this position his tongue falls forward and does not obstruct the entry of the catheter. The catheter is then gently inserted through the nose or mouth into the pharynx, rotated gently and withdrawn. Suctioning is begun when the catheter is in place. This procedure is repeated until the airway is clear. If the patient coughs while the catheter is in place, it helps to remove the mucus accumulations and foreign materials.

A **Y** tube is sometimes used with suction equipment. One stem of the **Y** is closed off with a finger to apply suction through the catheter. When this stem is left open the suction is stopped in the catheter. This method does away with the repeated insertion and removal of the catheter, and thus minimizes

trauma to the mucous membranes of the air passages.

Artificial Airways

An artificial airway is inserted into a patient's throat in order to keep his tongue forward and the airway patent. Artificial airways are usually made of plastic or rubber. There are long and short airways for deep and shallow intubation. In deep intubation the airway extends through the pharynx into the

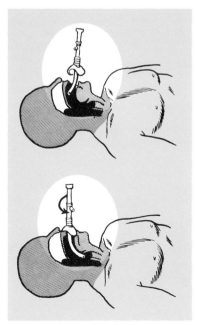

The insertion of a shallow airway.

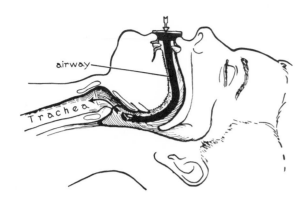

airway

Trachea

An airway in place.

trachea. This type of airway is usually inserted by a doctor. In shallow intubation the airway extends behind the tongue and terminates in the pharynx. This type of airway is often inserted by the nurse.

In shallow intubation the patient's tongue is brought forward and the airway is placed in his mouth with the base of the curve against his tongue. The airway is then turned so that the base of the curve is against the soft palate. It is then in position in the pharynx.

After an unconscious patient has been suctioned, he should remain in a semiprone (Sims) position to facilitate drainage of secretions from his mouth and prevent their accumulation in his pharynx. The approximate amount and the nature of the secretions that were suctioned are recorded on the patient's chart. The appearance of blood should also be reported.

Inhalation Therapy

Steam Inhalation. Some people require steam inhalations for respiratory tract problems. Inhaled steam supplies warmth and moisture directly to the mucous membranes lining the respiratory tract. The warmth increases the local blood supply to the area, increases the transudation of fluid and thereby thins the secretions for easier expectoration. Transudation is the passage of fluid through a membrane. The warmth also relaxes the smooth muscles of the respiratory tract and thus increases the size of the lumen of the passages. The moisture of the steam helps to liquefy secretions and to soothe irritated mucous membranes.

A medication, such as tincture of benzoin, can be administered directly to the respiratory tract by using steam as a vehicle. The steam is passed over the tincture of benzoin, from which it picks up molecules that are then inhaled with the steam.

Many types of steam inhalators are manufactured commercially. Both hot and cold steam inhalators are now available. Whatever kind is used, most patients require some help with the equipment. In the home, an electric kettle can be used to supply steam.

The physician may order continuous steam inhalation or he may order it for one half hour every four hours (steam inhalations ½ hour q.4h)

Nursing care measures relevant to the administration of steam include:

1. Explaining the equipment to the patient and advising him to breathe in the steam deeply

2. Taking safety precautions to protect the patient from burns if a hot steam inhalator is used. The patient should be warned not to touch any of the equipment that may become hot, and the kettle should be kept well out of reach if the patient shows any signs of mental confusion

3. Arranging the steam inhalator so that the steam surrounds the patient's head

4. Preventing drafts which could be chilling

5. Changing linen when it becomes damp

6. Encouraging the patient to expectorate mucus during the inhalations and providing him with a container for the sputum

High Humidity Inhalation. The provision of air that has a high water content is sometimes necessary for patients with respiratory problems. High humidity environments can be established in oxygen tents, in specially constructed plastic hoods and in entire rooms. Humidity is expressed as a percentage, 100 per cent indicating a saturated atmosphere.

High humidity air provides moisture to help liquefy respiratory secretions and to soothe irritated mucous membranes. People receiving high humidity air may become chilled in the dampness if they are not kept warm and dry.

Oxygen Inhalation Therapy. It is necessary under some circumstances to provide the patient with a concentration of oxygen that is higher than that found in the air. The physician orders the method of administration of the oxygen, the liter flow and the length of time that the patient is to receive the oxygen. The latter factor is sometimes left to the nurse's judgment, the order simply stating "oxygen as necessary."

Oxygen is generally supplied in two ways, from tanks or from wall outlets (piped-in oxygen). Oxygen from the latter source is stored in a central storage area. Many newer hospitals employ the piped-in method of supply. In the home, oxygen is supplied in portable tanks.

Oxygen tanks are steel cylinders in which the oxygen is stored under a pressure of more than 2200 pounds per square inch. There are different sizes of oxygen tanks: the larger ones store 244 cubic feet of oxygen; the smaller tanks store less oxygen but are readily portable. Each tank has a pressure reduction valve which enables the oxygen to be released at a pressure lower than that within the tank. An oxygen tank normally has two gauges: one indicates the amount of oxygen in the tank (the pressure) and the other indicates the amount of oxygen being released (in liters per minute).

The oxygen gauges are generally attached to the tank before it is brought to the patient. In large hospitals inhalation technicians usually supply and service the oxygen equipment. The following steps are followed in order to attach the gauges to the tank.

1. Open the cylinder valve slightly and then close it quickly to remove any dust in the outlet. This is known as "cracking the tank." It produces a loud hissing sound which can be frightening when not explained beforehand.

2. Connect the regulator valve to the cylinder outlet and tighten the nut with a wrench.

3. Make sure that the liter flow valve is in the "off" position.

4. Open the cylinder valve slowly until the pressure gauge registers the pressure in the cylinder.

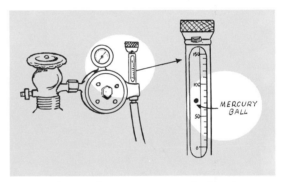

An attachment for an oxygen tank showing the pressure gauge and the liter flow gauge (mercury-ball type).

5. Adjust the liter flow valve to the desired rate of flow.

There are a variety of liter flow indicators. The gauge type and the ball float type are two that are commonly seen.

Piped-in oxygen is usually under low pressure, between 50 to 60 pounds per square inch. Usually only a liter flow valve is needed. To attach the equipment for piped-in oxygen:

1. Make sure that the liter flow valve is in the "off" position.

2. Attach the valve to the outlet. Some valves are attached by a screw nut; others are inserted directly into the wall outlet.

3. Slowly turn the liter flow valve to the desired liter flow.

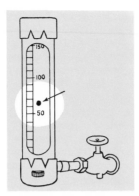

An attachment for an oxygen wall outlet with a mercury-ball liter flow gauge.

FEARS AND PRECAUTIONS IN THE USE OF OXYGEN EQUIPMENT. When nursing a patient who is receiving oxygen inhalations, there are certain precautions, practices and facts with which the nurse needs to be familiar. The administration of oxygen is often a frightening experience for the patient and his family. To many patients, it denotes a serious illness; a surprising number of patients remember a relative or a friend who died while receiving oxygen. Oxygen is essential to life and to have to depend upon equipment in order to live is in itself anxiety producing. This is a situation over which the patient often has little control, and because he is so completely dependent upon others even for the air he breathes, he feels helpless.

Such fears can often be allayed. Explanations about the oxygen equipment are geared to the patient's needs. Some people want to understand in great detail; others are satisfied with a simple explanation. If the patient is well enough to help with his therapy, the nurse can teach him to administer the oxygen himself and thus help him to feel that he has some control over the situation.

Some patients fear suffocation when using inhalation equipment; many dislike the feeling of being enclosed within a tent. Other patients feel isolated from their fellow patients when they are inside a tent. In addition, the necessity of depriving the patient of everyday pleasures such as the use of cigarettes, facial creams and perfumes adds to his feelings of helplessness. Cigarettes are never permitted because a spark could readily start a fire in the presence of concentrated oxygen. Creams and perfumes with an alcohol base are not used because they can contribute to a fire.

When handling oxygen equipment the operator's hands should be free of oils and alcohol, which are highly flammable. Normally the use of electrical equipment around oxygen is restricted to appliances that have been checked and found safe, that is, appliances that will not spark or start a fire.

Lotions and liquids for the patient's use should have a water rather than oil or alcohol base. Special mouth care solutions and back rub lotions that are not flammable must be used in the presence of oxygen equipment.

Principles Relevant to the Administration of Oxygen

Oxygen is a colorless, odorless and tasteless gas that is essential to life. Because oxygen can be neither seen, tasted nor smelled, the equipment gauges are relied upon to indicate that oxygen is being supplied. The concentration of oxygen in a tent can be tested by an analyzer. The patient who is receiving oxygen is interrupted as little as possible in order to decrease oxygen loss and promote rest.

Oxygen dries and irritates mucous membranes. Most patients who are receiving oxygen require special mouth care in order to maintain good oral hygiene. The provision of fluids for the patient is also important; often the patient is dependent upon the nurse for the administration of fluids. Oxygen is often humidified before it is supplied to the patient.

Oxygen supports combustion. It is essential to the patient's safety that there be no smoking within 12 feet of oxygen equipment. This applies to patients and visitors and usually requires continual explanation and enforcement. Oxygen is not explosive, but a spark created in the presence of a high concentration of oxygen can ignite a fire quickly.

Methods of Administering Oxygen.

There are four basic methods of administering oxygen: tent, catheter, mask and nasal inhaler.

THE OXYGEN TENT. The oxygen tents that are used today are made of a clear plastic material that does not permit the diffusion of oxygen or air through it. The motor unit of the tent is usually electrically driven; it circulates the air in the tent and cools it to the desired temperature.

The oxygen tent has the advantage of providing some control of the temperature of the air circulating around the patient. It also enables a high humidity environment to be established if it is desired. Some patients find the tent to be less restrictive and more comfortable than a mask.

The oxygen concentration in a tent can generally be kept between 50 and 60 per cent, although each time the tent is opened oxygen is lost. Oxygen analyzers are instruments which measure the concentration of oxygen inside the tent. These measurements should be done regularly, for example, every four hours.

A temperature between 68° and 70° F. in the tent is comfortable for most people. The ventilation fan can be set at a moderate speed in order to provide sufficient circulation of air. Some patients may desire a specific temperature and ventilation speed. The minimum liter flow of oxygen for the tent is generally 12 liters per minute; however, some patients require a higher liter flow to meet their oxygen needs.

To set up an oxygen tent, the following steps are performed:

1. Turn on the motor and set the liter flow valve to the desired level.
2. Arrange the canopy over the patient's head so that most of the space in the tent is in front of the patient's face.
3. Tuck the canopy under the mattress and secure the canopy over the patient's thighs with a drawsheet folded lengthwise and tucked in on each side of the bed.
4. Make sure that the openings in the tent are securely closed.
5. Flush the tent for two minutes to bring the concentration of oxygen quickly up to 50 per cent. Warn the patient that this makes a hissing noise.
6. Secure the signal light system for the patient. If the signal light is electrically controlled, it is hung over the tent on the outside but within reach of the patient.

Because oxygen supports combustion, precautions are taken to prevent fires. Patients do not smoke in an oxygen tent, nor are any electrical devices used inside the tent, including hearing aids, transistor radios and electrical shavers. "No smoking" signs should be placed on the door of the patient's room and visitors should be counseled not to smoke. The patient in the tent may feel cold because of the circulating air. The temperature can often be raised and extra covers provided. Patients should be discouraged from plugging the oxygen outlet of the tent with towels in order to close off drafts.

Nursing measures for the patient in an oxygen tent are planned so that the tent is entered as infrequently as possible. Each time the tent is opened oxygen is lost, and the patient consequently receives less than the desired concentration of oxygen.

Patients in oxygen tents often feel isolated from fellow patients; however, they have the same needs to communicate and feel a part of a group. Tent motors today are usually so quiet that patients can hear reasonably well inside them. People can normally be heard by the patient if they speak distinctly.

THE OXYGEN CATHETER. Oxygen catheters are made of plastic or rubber. They have a series of six or eight holes on the sides and are about 18 inches long. A No. 14 French catheter is usually used for an adult patient. Because oxygen dries and irritates mucous membranes, the oxygen is passed through water (humidified) before it is administered by catheter.

The advantage of the administration of oxygen by catheter is the freedom of movement that it affords the patient. Patients receiving oxygen by this method can obtain about a 50 per cent concentration of oxygen. The minimum liter flow of oxygen by catheter is generally 6 to 7 liters per minute.

The catheter is lubricated before insertion, preferably with water. An oil base lubricant is dangerous because

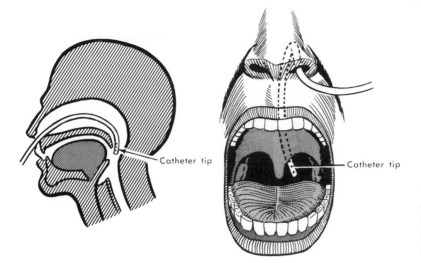

The position of the nasal catheter for oxygen administration. Note that the tip of catheter is opposite the uvula.

it can be aspirated and subsequently irritate the lungs. The catheter is inserted to a distance about equal to the distance from the patient's nose to his earlobe. It is inserted until the tip is opposite the uvula in the oropharynx (seen through the mouth) and is then taped in place as illustrated. It is never forced against an obstruction. In another technique of shallow insertion, a nasal catheter is inserted approximately 3 inches, that is, into the nasopharynx.

Oxygen catheters are removed every eight hours, and a clean catheter is inserted into the other naris. Patients receiving oxygen by catheter require special mouth and nose care. The catheters tend to irritate the mucous membranes, thereby stimulating secretions which must be removed. Water base lubricants will soothe irritated nares.

THE OXYGEN MASK. There are a variety of inhalation masks available for use. The lightweight plastic mask which covers the patient's nose and mouth is

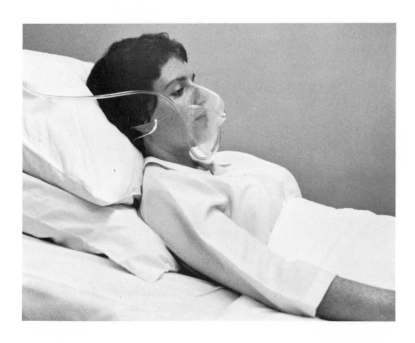

A plastic oxygen mask.

used extensively today. It provides a concentration of oxygen of about 50 per cent with a minimum liter flow of 8 liters per minute. There are also several partial rebreathing masks in use which can provide an oxygen concentration as high as 95 per cent. There are both nasal and oronasal styles available, the latter is used for the patient who tends to breathe through his mouth.

After the liter flow valve is turned on, the mask is applied to the patient's face. Oxygen masks come in different sizes; the mask selected should rest comfortably on the patient's face. Patients who are receiving oxygen by mask are assisted in taking fluids and performing hygienic measures to protect the skin and mucous membrane of the face and mouth from irritation.

Positive-pressure masks are used when oxygen is administered under pressure. The pressure can be applied on inhalation or exhalation or both. There are a variety of positive-pressure masks available. With the meter mask, the concentration of oxygen is regulated by a dial on the mask. The rebreathing mask has a bag below the mask which permits the rebreathing of exhaled air along with the oxygen.

THE NASOINHALER (Nasal Cannula). The nasoinhaler consists of two small plastic tubes which are inserted 1/4 to 1/2 inch into the patient's nose. The tubes are then taped to the patient's

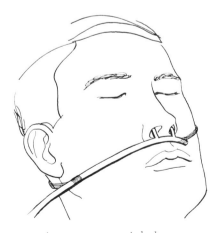

An oxygen nasoinhaler.

face and connected to an oxygen supply. The nasoinhaler supplies an oxygen concentration of 21 to 28 per cent at a flow of 4–6 liters per minute. Oxygen supplied in this way is humidified. The inhaler is changed frequently, and nasal care is provided as needed.

Carbon Dioxide Inhalation. The administration of carbon dioxide at a concentration between 3 and 10 per cent increases the rate and depth of respirations. It is also administered as a treatment for singultus (hiccups).

Carbon dioxide is usually supplied in cylinders in combination with oxygen; this mixture is called carbogen. It is administered by mask. It is generally ordered by the physician for 10 to 15 minute periods several times a day.

In carrying out this treatment the nurse alternates the application of the mask with periods of normal atmospheric breathing during the 10 or 15 minute intervals. That is, the nurse applies the mask for a few minutes, then removes it and lets the patient breathe without it for several respirations, then reapplies the mask. This procedure is repeated during the interval designated for the treatment.

In administering carbon dioxide, the nurse must watch for the signs and symptoms of CO_2 toxicity. At the first indication of vertigo, dyspnea, nausea or disorientation, the treatment is stopped and the condition reported to the physician.

Aerosol Inhalation. Aerosol inhalation (nebulization) is a method by which a nonvolatile drug is inhaled into the respiratory tract. A stream of oxygen is passed over a solution of the drug and picks up small particles to form a spray. The patient breathes in the spray deeply to force the tiny particles to travel deep into the respiratory tract. Different kinds of aerosols are marketed for use, some of which attach to a face mask which the patient wears during the treatment.

A similar spray can be formed by means of a hand atomizer. When the bulb of the atomizer is squeezed air passes over the medicine and picks up

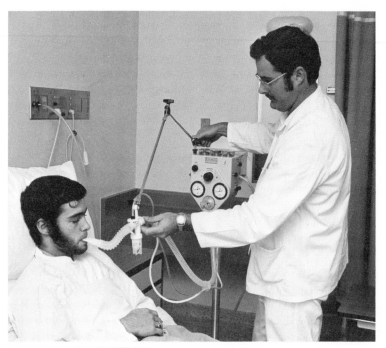

A patient receiving a treatment with a Bennett respirator. The inhalation therapist is assisting the patient.

small particles to form the spray which the patient inhales. The particles formed by the hand atomizer are usually larger than the particles formed in a nebulizer.

When the physician orders aerosol inhalation, he also orders the drug to be administered, the quantity of the drug and the frequency of the treatment. The liter flow of oxygen that is necessary for aerosol therapy is usually 3 to 4 liters per minute. The exact flow is determined by the density of the spray. A treatment usually lasts 15 to 20 minutes; more exactly, it lasts until all the medicine has been inhaled.

Helium Inhalation. Helium in combination with oxygen (80:20) is sometimes required for dyspneic patients. Because helium is lighter than the nitrogen it replaces, it eases dyspneic breathing by lessening the work expenditure required of the patient.

Helium is supplied by mask, often a partial rebreathing mask. It may be administered at intervals or, if well tolerated by the patient, for prolonged periods.

Respirators

Respirators are mechanical aids to breathing which function by changing the pressure exerted upon the patient's chest, thereby forcing him to exhale (when pressure is increased) and to inhale (when pressure is decreased). Respirators are run by electricity, but most have hand pump arrangements for use should the electricity fail.

A variety of respirators are available commercially. The iron lung is one type. The patient lies within the iron lung with only his head exposed to the atmosphere. Portable respirators fit over the patient's chest and thus permit him greater freedom of movement.

Other respirators are used to prevent or treat respiratory disorders. Most provide intermittent positive pressure breathing assistance. They may be used for deep-breathing exercises, to increase tidal volume of inspired air, or to administer aerosol medications. An inhalation therapist usually assists patients with IPPB treatments, but sometimes this is a nursing function.

Postural Drainage

Postural drainage is done to facilitate the drainage of secretions from the respiratory tract. The position of the patient for postural drainage depends on the areas of the lung to be drained. For drainage from the lower lobes, the patient assumes a position in which his chest is lower than his hips so that gravity will assist the movement of the mucus. Several special postural drainage beds are now available. If a special bed is not available, one way of assuming this position is for the patient to lie in a prone position across the bed with the waist at the edge of the bed. The upper part of the body is supported by the arms, which rest on a chair at the side of the bed. A receptacle for sputum is put on the chair in front of the patient.

Another position assumed by hospital patients who require postural drainage is a prone position over the knee break of the bed. The patient lies facing the bottom of the bed so that his waist is at the knee break and his head and chest incline downward.

Postural drainage is carried out to drain sputum from the lungs and to obtain a specimen of sputum. It is ordered by the physician, usually for 10 to 15 minutes, three to four times daily, for therapeutic purposes.

Percussion of the chest helps to dislodge mucus and is frequently done prior to the treatment. For more detailed instructions on techniques used in postural drainage, the nurse is referred to Secor's monograph on *Patient Care in Respiratory Problems* (pp. 147–152).

GUIDE TO ASSESSING NURSING NEEDS

1. Does the patient complain of difficulty in breathing? How long has he had this condition?
2. Is he anxious about his ability to breathe? What can the nurse do to alleviate his anxiety?
3. What are his respirations like in rate, depth, regularity and sound? Is he using accessory muscles of respiration in breathing?
4. Does he show signs of cyanosis?
5. Does his condition require immediate medical or nursing intervention? What measures should the nurse institute first?
6. Has the specific causal factor for the dyspnea been identified? Which of the five processes involved in respiration have been impaired in function?
7. Is the patient's airway clear? Does he need suctioning or other measures to clear the airway?
8. Is the patient receiving an adequate supply of oxygen? Has oxygen therapy been ordered? If so, by what method of administration?
9. What position is best for this patient to promote maximal ventilatory efficiency?
10. Is the patient distressed by coughing?
11. Is he bringing up sputum?
12. Is the patient showing signs of restlessness? Of mental confusion?
13. Have diagnostic tests and examinations been ordered for this patient? What are the patient's learning needs relative to these? What are the nurses's responsibilities?
14. Has the patient or his family other learning needs (for example, needs relative to the patient's activities, measures to prevent dyspnea, or the use of equipment for his treatment)?

GUIDE TO
EVALUATING THE
EFFECTIVENESS OF
NURSING ACTION

1. Is the patient breathing more easily?
2. Has his anxiety been relieved?
3. Is his airway patent?
4. Has his ventilatory efficiency been improved?
5. Have distressing symptoms such as coughing been relieved?
6. Has cyanosis been lessened?
7. Is the patient able to bring up sputum sufficient to clear the bronchial tree?
8. Are his activities commensurate with his level of tolerance?
9. Has he (or his family) gained the knowledge and skills necessary to prevent further attacks of dyspnea or to continue his treatment at home?

STUDY
VOCABULARY

Acapnia	Hemoptysis	Singultus
Asphyxia	Humidity	Sputum
Cyanosis	Hyperpnea	Syncope
Dyspnea	Hypoxemia	Transudation
Eupnea	Hypoxia	Vertigo
Expectorate	Orthopnea	

STUDY
SITUATION

Mr. R. S. Rowlands is a 38 year old patient who has been in the hospital for three weeks. His medical diagnosis is acute bronchial asthma. When he was admitted his breathing was dyspneic, he appeared cyanotic and his respiratory rate varied from 28 to 34 respirations per minute.

Mr. Rowlands did not want his bed to be flat; he demanded five pillows from the nurse and spent most of his time bent forward in bed. He was thin and appeared anxious. The physician ordered an oxygen mask for Mr. Rowlands, who liked to use the oxygen and to turn it on and off himself.

1. What factors should be taken into consideration in explaining to this patient how to use the oxygen equipment?
2. By what means can the patient's need for oxygen be ascertained?
3. For what reason might the patient demand five pillows, and why would he like to handle the oxygen himself?
4. What nursing measures might ease this patient's breathing?
5. How can the effectiveness of these measures be evaluated?
6. What objectives could help to guide the nursing care of this patient?
7. What observations should you make about this patient?
8. What are his nursing needs? How would you meet these needs?

BIBLIOGRAPHY

Ahlstrom, Pearl: Raising Sputum Specimens. *The American Journal of Nursing,* 65:109–110, March, 1965.
Ayres, S. M., and Stanley Giannelli: *Care of the Critically Ill.* New York, Appleton-Century-Crofts, 1967.

Beland, Irene L.: *Clinical Nursing: Pathophysiological and Psychosocial Approaches*. New York, The Macmillan Company, 1965.

Black, V. C.: Helping the Patient to Ventilate. *Nursing Research, 17*:31–33, October, 1969.

Griffith, Elizabeth W.: Nursing Process: A Patient with Respiratory Dysfunction. *Nursing Clinics of North America,* 6:1:145–154, March, 1971.

Guyton, Arthur C.: *Textbook of Medical Physiology*. Fourth edition. Philadelphia, W. B. Saunders Company, 1971.

Kurihara, Marie: Assessment and Maintenance of Adequate Respiration. *Nursing Clinics of North America,* 3:1:65–67, March, 1968.

MacBryde, Cyril M. and Robert S. Blacklow (eds.): *Signs and Symptoms: Applied Pathologic Physiology and Clinical Interpretation*. Fifth edition. Philadelphia, J. B. Lippincott Company, 1970.

Nordmark, Madelyn T., and Anne W. Rohweder: *Scientific Foundations of Nursing*. Second edition. Philadelphia, J. B. Lippincott Company, 1967.

Secor, Jane: *Patient Care in Respiratory Problems*. Saunders Monographs in Clinical Nursing, Vol. 1. Philadelphia, W. B. Saunders Company, 1969.

Sutton, Audrey L.: *Bedside Nursing Techniques in Medicine and Surgery*. Second edition. Philadelphia, W. B. Saunders Company, 1969.

Waligara, Sister Barbara Marie: The Effect of Nasal and Oral Breathing upon Naso-Pharyngeal Oxygen Concentrations. *Nursing Research, 19*:75, January-February, 1970.

26 THE CARE OF PATIENTS WHO HAVE ANOREXIA, NAUSEA OR VOMITING

The nurse should be able to:

Define the terms *anorexia, nausea* and *vomiting*

Use appropriate terminology in recording and reporting observations about patients with these symptoms

Describe the anatomical structures and physiological mechanisms involved in these symptoms

Explain the etiology of these conditions

Describe signs and symptoms that commonly accompany anorexia, nausea and vomiting

Assess the nursing needs of patients with these symptoms

Establish goals for nursing action

Determine priorities for care

Describe appropriate nursing action including measures to prevent these symptoms, to assist in maintaining hydration and nutritional status, and to provide the patient with comfort and support

Establish criteria for evaluating the effectiveness of nursing action

THE CARE OF PATIENTS 26
WHO HAVE ANOREXIA,
NAUSEA OR VOMITING

INTRODUCTION

Anorexia, nausea and vomiting refer to varying degrees of distress of the upper gastrointestinal tract. *Anorexia* means loss of appetite, or lack of the desire for food, and it involves the subjective perception of a distaste for food. The individual often expresses this by saying "I don't feel like eating." This may be the first indication of a disorder of the gastrointestinal tract. Anorexia may precede nausea. In *nausea*, there is not only a distaste for food but the mere thought of food becomes repelling and, in addition, the individual usually complains of an uncomfortable sensation in the region of the stomach. This uncomfortable sensation is frequently described as "feeling sick," a lay term often used for nausea. In most cases, nausea precedes vomiting. *Vomiting* is the forceful ejection of the stomach's contents.

Anorexia, nausea and vomiting are common manifestations of disease. They can indicate disturbances of the gastrointestinal tract itself or of almost any system of the body. They can also reflect the body's reaction to stress. Situations which the individual perceives as stressful, whether these are pleasant or unpleasant, can, and often do, produce these symptoms. Cultural values can also affect a person's reaction to food. Eating habits, personal likes and dislikes, and the social significance of food in different cultures, can all be related to these symptoms (see Chapter 14).

THE PHYSIOLOGY OF ANOREXIA, NAUSEA AND VOMITING

The symptoms of anorexia, nausea and vomiting are considered by many to be sequential stages of the same physical phenomenon, although any one of the three may occur by itself in the absence of the other two.

Anorexia has been defined as a loss of appetite. Appetite is the pleasant sensation of a desire for food. Although appetite and hunger frequently occur together, they are not the same, hunger being an uncomfortable sensation which indicates a physiological need for nourishment, whereas appetite is a learned response. As such, appetite is closely related to cultural and social values. To a large extent, one's appetite is conditioned by previous pleasant experiences with food. A number of different stimuli will arouse the appetite. These include olfactory stimuli, such as the pleasant odor of something cooking; visual stimuli, such as an attractively served meal; auditory stimuli, including the clatter of pots and pans in the kitchen as dinner is being prepared; or gustatory stimuli. One may taste a sample of food, for example, find it agreeable, and the appetite is whetted for more.

Appetite, or the feeling of a desire for food, is accompanied by certain visceral changes. These include increased gastric tone and accelerated hydrochloric acid secretion in the stomach. The individual frequently experiences an increase in salivation also as the mouth "waters" for food.

When a person loses his appetite, or suffers from anorexia, it has been noted that specific visceral changes occur. There is usually a hypofunctioning of the stomach; gastric tone is lessened, and the secretion of hydrochloric acid is decreased. It has also been observed that the stomach of the anorectic patient is pale in comparison with those of people with normal appetites.

These same physiological findings have been observed in individuals suffering from nausea, except that, in the case of the nauseated person, they are more pronounced. In nausea, there is a relaxation of the walls of the stomach, and gastric secretions and muscular contractions cease. Because of this relaxation, the stomach usually sits lower in the abdominal cavity than it does normally. At the same time as the muscles of the stomach are in a relaxed state, the muscular wall of the intestine shows increased contractility, and contents from the duodenum may be regurgitated back into the stomach.

Most people locate the sensation of nausea as being in the epigastric region. The uncomfortable feeling in this area is usually accompanied by other symptoms of a distressing nature. Frequently there is increased perspiration and greatly increased salivation. Beads of perspiration may be evident on the person's forehead or upper lip, and he may state that his mouth is full of saliva. The individual's blood pressure usually drops and his pulse and respirations are rapid. Tachycardia may be followed by bradycardia. Some people feel faint, some complain of vertigo (dizziness) and headache. *Retching*, that is, an unproductive attempt at vomiting, may occur several times before vomiting actually takes place.

The act of vomiting involves a sequence of events which culminates in the forceful ejection of the stomach's contents. Initially there is a relaxation of the upper portion of the stomach, including the cardiac sphincter. This is followed by strong contractile waves in the lower portion of the stomach, which effectively close off the pyloric sphincter and prevent the stomach contents from passing into the duodenum. Subsequently, the diaphragm and the abdominal muscles contract. The strong contractions of these muscles during the act of vomiting account for the feeling of "soreness" which many people experience as an after effect of vomiting. With the simultaneous contraction of the diaphragm and the abdominal muscles, intraabdominal pressure is greatly increased and the stomach is literally squeezed between the two sets of muscles. The contents in the relaxed upper portion of the stomach are then forced upward through the esophagus and out through the mouth. Normally, the glottis is closed and respirations cease during the act of vomiting in order to prevent the vomitus from being aspirated (entering the lungs).

THE ETIOLOGY OF ANOREXIA, NAUSEA AND VOMITING

The primary center controlling vomiting is located in the medulla oblongata. It is felt that stimulation of this center may give rise to anorexia, nausea or vomiting, depending on the degree or intensity of the stimulus. Thus, a person who does not feel like eating may become nauseated at the sight of food and may vomit if he tries to eat it. However, vomiting is not always preceded by nausea, and it is felt, therefore, that only certain areas in the vomiting center are directly involved with nausea. The vomiting center may be stimulated by a number of factors. These include chemical stimuli, impulses from the cerebral cortex and impulses arising from receptors in the viscera.

Chemical Stimuli

A number of different chemical agents may give rise to anorexia, nausea and vomiting. Among these are many common drugs such as digitalis (frequently used in the treatment of people with heart conditions); a number of the narcotics, as, for example, morphine; and many drugs used as anesthetics. When giving a patient any medication, in fact, it is important to note whether nausea and vomiting are listed as possible side effects of the drug, and, if so, to watch for these symptoms in the patient. The drug apomorphine, because of its specific action on the vomiting center, is often administered when it is considered desirable to rid the stomach of its contents—if, for example, the individual has ingested a poisonous substance. Other toxic substances such as bacterial toxins which are circulating in the blood stream may also stimulate the vomiting center. It is believed that circulating toxic chemical agents activate a chemoreceptor trigger zone which is located in the fourth ventricle. When this zone is excited, it transmits impulses to the primary vomiting center where the symptoms of anorexia, nausea and vomiting are initiated.

It is felt that this chemoreceptor trigger zone also plays a part in the motion-sickness which bothers many travelers. A disturbance in motion, such as one experiences with the rolling motion of a ship at sea or with any rapid change in direction of the body, stimulates receptors in the labyrinth of the ear. These receptors send out impulses which are carried by the vestibular nerve to the cerebellum, and thence to the chemoreceptor zone in the fourth ventricle. Impulses from this zone are then transmitted to the vomiting center in the medulla.[1]

Impulses from the Cerebral Cortex

It was mentioned in the introduction to this chapter that stressful situations may give rise to anorexia, nausea or vomiting. The situation need not necessarily be unpleasant. An individual may be "too excited to eat" and, in countless poems and romantic novels, the person in love is described as someone with no appetite (among other symptoms). However, it is in connection with unpleasantly stressful situations that the symptoms of anorexia, nausea and vomiting are most often noted. Worry over a pending examination, pain, anxiety and fear may all give rise to these symptoms. Similarly, other psychic factors such as the sight of something particularly abhorrent, unpleasant odors or even extremely loud noise can also take away one's appetite, make one feel nauseated, or cause vomiting. It is felt that these psychic stimuli originating in the cerebral cortex activate the vomiting center directly, rather than being transmitted through the chemoreceptor trigger zone.

Impulses Arising from the Viscera

The parts of the body containing receptors which initiate vomiting are the stomach, duodenum, uterus, kidneys, heart, pharynx and semicircular canals of the ear. The gag reflex is a familiar example of a reaction to stimulation of the receptors in the pharynx. The stimuli which give rise to anorexia, nausea and vomiting are irritation of the receptors, as, for example, the tickling of the back of the throat to induce vomiting; the eating of irritating food; stretching of the organ, as occurs as when a child stretches his stomach by overeating and promptly vomits; or pressure on the receptors. Irritation of the gastrointestinal tract by infectious, chemical or mechanical agents, and distention of or trauma to other viscera are felt to affect the vomiting center directly, rather than being relayed through the chemoreceptor zone.

SYMPTOMS ACCOMPANYING ANOREXIA, NAUSEA AND VOMITING

Anorexia and nausea are subjective symptoms; hence their identification is highly dependent on the individual's

---

[1]Arthur C. Guyton: *Textbook of Medical Physiology.* Fourth edition. Philadelphia, W. B. Saunders Company, 1971, p. 780.

ability to communicate his discomfort. "I'm not hungry" or "I don't feel like eating" are ways of expressing a reluctance to eat. The person who says "I feel sick" or "I feel sick to my stomach" is usually putting into words his feeling of nausea. The nurse can supplement the patient's observations by noting his reactions to food. Does he seem to anticipate and enjoy his meals? Does he simply toy with food while he actually eats very little? Or, does he push the food away at mealtimes without touching it? Such behavior can indicate that a person is anorectic and perhaps nauseated. Sometimes concomitant with a lack of interest in food are listlessness and apathy.

As noted in the section on physiology, the person with nausea may show outward signs of his distress. The nurse should observe the individual for such signs as pallor, excessive perspiration, and increased salivation. Usually a person who is nauseated becomes pale and obviously uncomfortable. Beads of perspiration may show on the upper lip, or excessive perspiration be noted on other parts of the body. The nurse may note, if she takes the person's pulse, a marked acceleration in pulse rate.

Vomiting is usually preceded by nausea. Prior to vomiting a person frequently becomes very pale and perspires profusely. He may complain of neurological symptoms such as vertigo and tingling sensations in his fingers and toes. He may also describe pain in the epigastric region.

In projectile vomiting the impulse to vomit is very sudden, occurring with little or no warning (that is, with no symptoms of nausea beforehand). Moreover, the ejection of the stomach's contents is more forceful than in ordinary vomiting. This type of vomiting is often seen in patients with head injuries when there is increased intracranial pressure.

A concomitant of gastrointestinal disturbances is deterioration of the patient's nutritional status. Food and fluids, specifically the chloride ions, are lost as a result of vomiting the gastric juices. Prolonged deficiency in nourishment and fluids results in dehydration and malnutrition, which, in turn, can cause constipation. The patient can be expected to be constipated because of the fluid withdrawn from the feces in an effort by the body to compensate for the lowered fluid intake or fluid loss. There will probably also be a decrease in the amount of urine excreted, the urine being concentrated as a result.

A person who suffers from anorexia or nausea over a period of time loses weight and, in addition to showing signs of dehydration and malnutrition, will become weak and listless owing to inadequate intake of nutrients. The individual who has experienced prolonged vomiting will show more pronounced effects due not only to the lack of intake but also to the loss of food and fluids through vomiting. This individual may show a marked weight loss and rapidly progressive signs of weakness and prostration as well as signs of fluid and electrolyte imbalance (see Chapter 29). Prolonged vomiting in children is more serious than in adults because of the relatively greater loss of fluids and electrolytes proportionate to their body weight.

ASSESSING THE NURSING NEEDS OF PATIENTS WITH ANOREXIA, NAUSEA AND VOMITING

In determining the nursing needs of the individual suffering from anorexia, nausea or vomiting, the nurse may gather information from both the patient and his family. Pertinent information includes the nature of the patient's discomfort, the length of time the person has had these symptoms, the severity of the symptoms, and their relationship to eating habits, personal life-style and emotional stress. Specific causal factors should be identified, if possible; that is, has the patient eaten something that disagreed with him? Is he taking any medication which may have gastrointestinal side effects? Is he under emotional stress? The family can often explain many of the patient's cultural or religious beliefs that may affect his appetite and eating habits. Thus, the orthodox Jewish patient may not want to eat dairy products and meat at the same meal. The Chinese person may prefer rice and tea with his meals, and may leave the standard hospital food untouched.

The individual should also be observed for the signs and symptoms which accompany anorexia, nausea and vomiting as these have just been detailed. Vomiting should be evaluated in terms of both the nature of the vomiting and the characteristics of the vomitus (material vomited). In relation to vomiting, the nurse should determine its type, that is, whether it is projectile or regurgitated (ordinary vomiting): whether it is preceded by feelings of nausea; its frequency; and its occurrence in relation to intake of food, the administration of drugs, and the individual's emotional state. Characteristics of the vomitus which should be noted are: amount; color; consistency (that is, watery, liquid, or solid); the presence of undigested food, blood or other foreign substances; and odor.[2]

Specific diagnostic tests may be ordered by the physician. It is quite usual for a specimen of the vomitus to be sent to the laboratory for examination. Frequently it is examined for blood. Microscopic examination reveals occult blood, that is, blood which is present in the specimen but hidden to the naked eye. The nurse's responsibility includes seeing that a correctly labeled specimen is sent to the laboratory in the designated container.

Blood chemistry tests can also be significant. The patient who is vomiting is losing hydrochloric acid (HCl) and therefore H^+ ions. He is in danger then of developing alkalosis. An examination of the blood gases may be ordered to determine the acid-base balance (see Chapter 29). A decrease in blood chlor-

ides (hypochloremia) is also likely to occur as Cl^- ions are lost along with the H^+ ions. Prolonged vomiting may cause severe sodium depletion as well.

PRINCIPLES BASIC TO THE CARE OF PATIENTS WITH ANOREXIA, NAUSEA OR VOMITING

A healthy body requires a balanced diet, which includes the intake of sufficient nutrients as well as approximately 2500 cc. of fluid in every 24 hour period.

Factors in the individual's external environment and within his internal environment (that is, within the body itself) can cause anorexia, nausea and vomiting.

Anorexia, nausea and vomiting can often be modified by nursing intervention.

Normally, 150 cc. of fluid are lost directly from the gastrointestinal tract in a 24 hour period. This loss can be greatly increased by vomiting or suctioning, which also causes a loss of electrolytes.

OBJECTIVES OF NURSING INTERVENTION

Nursing action in the care of patients with anorexia, nausea or vomiting is directed towards three basic goals: the prevention of these symptoms, whenever possible; the maintenance of hydration and nutritional status; and the maintenance of the patient's comfort and hygiene.

DETERMINING PRIORITIES FOR NURSING ACTION

In determining priorities for nursing intervention, the immediate situation must be assessed and appropriate action instituted. The patient who is vomiting, for example, needs prompt attention, directed primarily at relieving the symptom, providing him with comfort and support and preventing complications.

[2]Madelyn T. Nordmark and Anne W. Rohweder: *Scientific Foundations of Nursing.* Second edition. Philadelphia, J. B. Lippincott Company, 1967, p. 79.

The nurse can assist the vomiting patient by holding a curved basin (emesis basin) under his chin to catch the vomitus, and supporting his head and shoulders. Most people find it easier to vomit when they are in a sitting position with the head bent over the basin. If the patient is lying down, his head should be turned to one side and his body placed in a side-lying position if possible. Again, the head should be supported. The patient who is in a dorsal recumbent position can choke and aspirate vomitus unless his head is raised and supported so that the vomitus can drain out of the mouth. In postoperative vomiting, the patient will find it less painful if the nurse supports his incision with her hands while he vomits.

The nurse should stay with the patient while he is vomiting. Vomiting is an unpleasant experience. Not only is it physically distressing but there is a loss of control and dignity which most people find embarrassing. The nurse can do much to reassure the patient by a calm acceptance of the situation and sympathetic yet efficient ministrations. For the patient's own feelings of dignity, and because most people find it distressing to watch someone vomiting, the patient should be screened from the view of others. Curtains can be quickly drawn around the patient's bed, or the door of his room closed to ensure privacy.

While the patient is vomiting, the nurse should provide him with tissues and help him to wipe his mouth. After he has stopped vomiting, mouth care and a hand and face wash will help him to feel more comfortable and relaxed. Any linen that has been soiled should be changed. The room should be aired and the patient allowed to rest.

With most patients who are anorectic or nauseated, the immediate problem is usually to prevent the aggravation of the symptoms. The nauseated individual usually feels better lying down in a cool and quiet room with adequate ventilation. If this is not possible, the person should be encouraged to sit quietly and take a few deep breaths.

This helps to relax the diaphragm. Measures to take the person's mind off his gastrointestinal problems may also help.

GENERAL PREVENTIVE MEASURES

The prevention of anorexia, nausea and vomiting involves a consideration of both the patient and his environment. The nursing care measures that are effective in the prevention of these disorders are often specific to the causes which have been discussed. The nurse can often assist the patient to identify situations and stimuli which induce the symptoms, and she can then modify or eliminate these from the patient's environment. Frequently the patient is aware of events or subjective experiences, such as pain, which elicit nausea and vomiting.

An environment that is clean and pleasant is helpful in the stimulation of appetite and the prevention of nausea and vomiting. If the patient eats while he is in bed, the nurse can provide him with a clean table that is free of equipment. The emesis basin should be kept out of sight. If the patient feels more secure with it nearby, it can be kept within easy reach.

Unpleasant odors, sights and sounds are noxious stimuli which may contribute to anorexia, nausea or vomiting. To dissipate unpleasant odors, a well ventilated room is important, and the use of deodorants may be necessary at times. Vomitus is always removed immediately and treatment trays are covered and placed as inconspicuously as possible. Bedpans and urinals are kept covered and out of sight; for esthetic and hygienic reasons they are not placed on the patient's bedside table. Unpleasant sounds are avoided whenever possible.

It is important to allow for personal hygiene prior to meals. Most people like to wash their hands and freshen up before they eat. Sick people, in this regard, are no different from those who are well, and personal cleanliness is perhaps more important in the case of the person who has anorexia, or a tendency to become nauseated. Personal hygiene should include the use of the washroom, or the bedpan, and an opportunity for the patient to wash his hands (and face) and clean his teeth or rinse his mouth if he so desires.

Other measures which stimulate a person's appetite and prevent nausea are those which provide physical comfort. These include the prevention or elimination of pain; appropriate positioning; exercise or inactivity, whichever an individual needs, just prior to a meal; good oral hygiene; reduction of fever; a comfortable temperature and adequate ventilation within the room; and refraining from unpleasant nursing measures just prior to eating. Emotional discomfort can also affect a person's appetite. Worry, fear and excitement can inhibit the desire for food and also delay the passage of food through the gastrointestinal tract. This latter point is important to remember with preoperative patients since it may be a contributing factor in postoperative nausea and vomiting.[3] Explanations and psychological support help the patient to deal with anxieties and cope with life situations.

In discussing measures which prevent anorexia, nausea and vomiting, the use of tonics to improve the appetite and of antiemetic drugs to control nausea and vomiting must be included. Most physicians have their own preferences about tonics to improve the appetite. These are usually ordered 20 to 30 minutes before meals or may be given once or twice daily. Antiemetic drugs have a specific action on the vomiting center, and they may be given 20 minutes to half an hour before mealtime or otherwise as ordered. Many people who are susceptible to motion-sickness travel much more comfortably if they take an antiemetic medicine shortly before embarking on a plane trip or other journey. It is well to re-

member that these drugs usually produce some drowsiness as a side effect.

Many people find the isolation of the sickroom lonely. They are much more likely to anticipate their meals with pleasure when these are partaken of in pleasant company. Some hospitals have dining rooms where patients can eat together in a situation analogous to dining at home. For the patient at home or confined to bed in hospital, someone to chat with at mealtime often makes for a pleasant interlude that encourages the patient to eat.

MAINTENANCE OF HYDRATION AND NUTRITIONAL STATUS

Helping the patient to maintain a satisfactory hydration and nutritional status is an important nursing function. Encouraging the individual to take fluids regularly helps him to attain adequate fluid intake. If he has difficulty in retaining fluids, giving him small amounts of fluid at frequent intervals is preferable to giving a large volume all at once. Patients who have been vomiting are usually permitted clear fluids only until vomiting subsides. Ginger ale and clear tea are frequently tolerated much better than other fluids when the stomach is upset. When other fluids are introduced into the patient's diet, those that are high in carbohydrate and protein are preferable because of the body's need for energy and tissue-building nutrients.

People who are anorectic or nauseated may become more so when confronted with large servings of food. Small portions, attractively served, are usually more appealing. It is often necessary to cater to the individual's particular food preferences to encourage him to eat. Patients should also be assisted with their meals if they are unable to manage alone. Today when hospital meals are frequently served by someone other than a nurse, it is perhaps more important than ever for the nurse to visit each patient at mealtime and offer whatever assistance is needed.

[3]Howard S. Downs: The Control of Vomiting. *The American Journal of Nursing*, 66:1:81, January, 1966.

All too often meals are left untouched or little is consumed because the patient could not cut his meat, butter his bread, or open one of the numerous cartons and containers that are used nowadays in meal service.

For patients who are unable to tolerate food and fluids by mouth or are taking an insufficient quantity, parenteral fluids may be prescribed. In some cases the patient is fed through a tube which is inserted into the stomach. This latter method of feeding is called a *gastric gavage*.

Many patients with gastrointestinal problems require gastric suction. This is a method of removing the gastric contents by means of suction apparatus. Patients on gastric suction are usually maintained with intravenous feedings to provide them with fluids and nourishment.

In some instances, it may be necessary to cleanse the stomach before further food and fluids can be taken, particularly if the individual has ingested some noxious substance. The procedure for washing out the stomach is called *gastric lavage*. This procedure is also frequently carried out prior to gastric surgery.

The description of a technique for carrying out each of these nursing measures is detailed later in this chapter.

Regarding the maintenance of fluid and electrolyte balance, the accurate recording and reporting of fluid intake and output is essential. Both parenteral and oral intake must be accurately assessed. The patient can often help to record the amount of fluid he drinks. If the patient is receiving gastric tube feedings, the amount given must be recorded accurately. On the output side, the amount of emesis should be measured or estimated when measurement is not feasible. In addition, drainage and suction returns should be included in the total output.

When the patient is receiving supplementary fluids such as intravenous or interstitial therapy, the nurse is also responsible for the care specific to this therapy (see Chapter 29).

COMFORT AND HYGIENE MEASURES

Most of the comfort and hygiene needs of patients with anorexia, nausea and vomiting have been discussed in previous sections of this chapter. Cleanliness of both the patient and his environment is an important factor in the prevention of these symptoms. The nurse· can contribute to the patient's comfort by seeing that his clothing and his bed linen are kept clean and fresh. Adequate bathing is essential, and oral hygiene of particular importance. Rinsing of the mouth, especially after vomiting, helps to remove any traces of vomitus and to give the patient a more comfortable feeling. If the patient is unable to tolerate food or fluids, good mouth care is essential to the prevention of complications (see Chapter 13 and also Chapter 23).

SPECIFIC TECHNIQUES

Gastrointestinal Intubation

Gastrointestinal intubation has been used for many years; as early as 1905, Lyons carried out duodenal drainage.[4] The primary reasons for the insertion of a tube into the stomach or the intestine are:

1. To establish a means of draining the stomach or intestine by suction. This is often done when a patient has an obstruction of the gastrointestinal tract or has undergone surgery of the tract.

2. For diagnostic purposes. For example, to identify malignant cells or microorganisms such as the tubercle bacillus in the gastric washings.

3. To aspirate the stomach contents. For example, after the ingestion of poisonous materials.

4. To establish a route for feeding the patient who is unable to take nourishment by mouth.

---

[4]W. Grobin: Gastrointestinal Intubation. *The Canadian Nurse*, 55:107, February, 1959.

Kinds of Tubes. There are many kinds of tubes used for gastrointestinal intubation. The Miller-Abbott tube and the Cantor tube are commonly used for decompression of the intestine. The *Miller-Abbott tube* has a double lumen and a weighted tip with a balloon attached. The tube is inserted by a physician into the stomach and passed through the pylorus into the intestine. Once it is positioned in the intestine, the balloon is blown up with air, and the tube is subsequently propelled onward by the peristaltic waves of the intestine. An adaptation of this tube is the addition of a bag containing 4 cc. of mercury, which weights the tube and facilitates its passage into the small intestine. The modified tube is called the *Harris tube.*

The *Cantor tube* also has a bag of mercury at its tip. It is a single lumen tube with a number of holes on the sides which allow suction to be applied along the intestinal tract.

The *Levin tube* is commonly used for gastric intubation. The tip of the tube is solid but there are several holes on the side. It is normally passed through the nose of the patient into his stomach. The insertion of a Levin tube is usually the physician's responsibility; however, when there is no gastric disease and the patient is conscious, the nurse often inserts the Levin tube.

The Insertion of a Levin Tube. Before the insertion of a Levin tube, the procedure is explained to the patient. Not only do most patients want to know how they can help, but explanations frequently allay fear. The passage of a tube is painless, but it sometimes stimulates the gag reflex as it passes over the nasopharyngeal area. If the patient breathes deeply at the first sign of gagging, he is less likely to become nauseated and vomit.

In the preparation of the equipment, the rubber Levin tube is placed in a bowl of chipped ice. This makes the tube more rigid (because cold causes molecules to come together) and thus more easily directed on insertion. It also lubricates the tube. Usually a plastic Levin tube is sufficiently rigid for insertion, but it must also be lubricated with water.

In addition to the ice and the Levin tube, a protective covering, a kidney basin, tissues and a syringe are required. The syringe is used to withdraw the stomach's contents after the Levin tube has been inserted. This also determines the tube's position inside the patient.

If it is possible, the patient assumes Fowler's position. In this position the passage of the tube is facilitated by the pull of gravity; it also makes it easier for the patient to spit out vomitus if this becomes necessary during the insertion of the tube.

The kidney basin and tissues are required because the patient may vomit. As noted previously, stimulation of the glossopharyngeal nerve endings in the posterior pharynx transmits impulses to the vomiting center in the medulla of the brain.

As a guide to the distance to which the tube is to be inserted, the nurse measures the distance from the patient's nose to an earlobe and then to the umbilicus. This distance is roughly equal to the distance from the lips to the stomach. The nurse then marks this distance on the tube with a piece of adhesive tape.

As a lubricant for the Levin tube, water has two advantages: (1) it moistens the tube and thus permits smoother passage of the tube over the mucous membranes and (2) if the tube enters the lungs, the water is not likely to become a focus of irritation. Some agencies suggest that a water-soluble lubricant be used; such lubricants are less dangerous to the lungs than oil base lubricants.

The Levin tube is never forced upon encountering an obstruction. Not only is force unpleasant to the patient, but the mucous membrane that lines the gastrointestinal tract is easily damaged and provides a likely site for infection.

While the nurse is inserting the Levin tube the patient swallows. Swallowing helps to pass the tube down the esophagus into the patient's stomach by setting up peristaltic waves. If the patient finds it difficult to swallow, the nurse can give him ice chips to suck, provided that this is not contraindicated by his physical condition.

The stomach is never empty; it always contains at least a little gastric juice, which is secreted by the glands in the walls of the stomach. Therefore the position of the tube can be ascertained by aspirating with the syringe. The obtainment of gastric contents verifies that the tube is positioned in the patient's stomach. If gastric juice cannot be obtained, the following tests should be performed:

Place the free end of the tube in a container of water. Continuous bubbling usually indicates that the tube is in the patient's lungs.

Hold the end of the tube to the ear. A crackling sound usually indicates that the tube is in the patient's lungs.

Ask the patient to hum. If the tube is in the patient's lungs he will not be able to do this.

If the patient becomes dyspneic during the insertion of a tube, it should be removed immediately. Cyanosis and dyspnea often indicate that the tube has entered the trachea. Once it has been ascertained that the Levin tube is in the patient's stomach, the tube is secured to the patient's face with a small piece of adhesive tape.

The Irrigation of a Levin Tube. The purpose of the irrigation of a Levin tube is to wash the lumen of the tube in order to maintain a clear passage. Usually this is not a sterile procedure unless the patient has just had stomach surgery. The order to irrigate the Levin tube is issued by the physician. Irrigations are ordered for regular intervals, or they are done only when the tube becomes blocked. In either case it is important to watch the patient closely and note whether the tube becomes occluded. If the patient is on gastric suction, the most obvious sign of blockage is a lack of gastric returns from the tube. In addition, the patient is likely to feel uncomfortable and his abdomen will be distended.

After the nurse has provided the explanation that the patient requires and has reassured him that this is a painless measure, she assembles the necessary equipment. She requires a syringe, usually a 20 cc. or 30 cc. syringe, or an Asepto syringe; the irrigating solution specifically designated by the physician, often water or normal saline, and a receptacle for the returned irrigation fluid.

Between 15 and 30 cc. of fluid is injected into the tube before the plunger is gently drawn back to withdraw the fluid. Because the mucous membrane lining of the stomach is easily damaged, the fluid is injected and withdrawn very gently. This measure is repeated until the tube is cleared. If fresh blood appears as a result of the irrigating, the measure is terminated and the information is reported to the physician. During the irrigation the nurse observes the color and consistency of the returning fluid. This is recorded on the patient's chart.

Gastric Suction

The purpose of gastric suction is to remove the contents of the patient's stomach. It is indicated as a measure to prevent or relieve distention and vomiting, to remove blood postoperatively and to remove the stomach contents of patients who have gastrointestinal obstructions. It may also be used as a measure to cleanse the stomach prior to gastric surgery.

Generally speaking, there are two types of gastric suction: continuous and intermittent. Continuous suction is applied continuously; intermittent suction is turned on and off as the patient requires or, usually, on the physician's order.

There are four basic ways of supplying suction. First, there is the electric suction machine, which is a portable machine that can be brought to the patient. It is run by electricity and the amount of suction can usually be regulated. The second method of supplying suction is by means of suction apparatus built into the wall. Many modern hospitals have suction outlets at the head of the patient's bed. The pressure of these systems can also be regulated by the nursing personnel.

The third method of supplying suction is by the use of the principle of displacement of water. Systems based on this method do not require electricity and are simple to construct. There are both two- and three-bottle systems. Simply explained, the water falls by gravity from bottle B to bottle A (see the accompanying illustration). This creates a vacuum in bottle B. If bottle B is connected directly to the patient's gastric tube, the vacuum is transmitted to his stomach, with the result that the stomach's contents flow to bottle B, that is, from a high pressure area to a low pressure area. If, on the other hand, bottle B is connected to bottle C, and bottle C is connected to the patient's gastric tube, then the stomach contents will be received in bottle C.

A fourth means of supplying suction is by the Gomco Thermotic pump, which is electrically operated but motorless. This pump provides intermittent suction through the alternate contraction and expansion of air.

When a patient requires gastric suction, he is likely to find the gastric tube irritating to his throat, and he is not likely to be able to take fluids by mouth. Therefore he requires special care for his mouth and nose in order that they do not become dry, cracked and subsequently infected. To ease the irritation by the tube on the patient's throat, the physician may order anesthetic lozenges.

Since gastric suction returns are an important part of the patient's fluid output, the nurse measures the amount of drainage accurately, and she notes the clarity, color and consistency of the drainage. These observations are

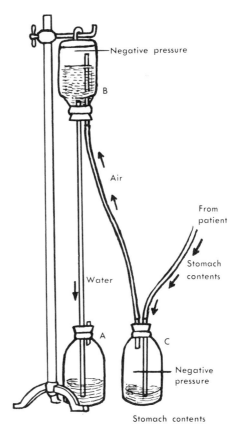

The water displacement method of producing suction.

charted on the patient's record. Any untoward changes in the patient's suction returns, such as bright red returns, or in the patient's condition, such as an accelerated pulse, are reported to the physician.

Gastric Lavage

Gastric lavage is the washing out of the stomach. It is done prior to some types of gastric surgery and as a means of removing noxious substances which have been ingested. The latter is often an emergency procedure, carried out in the emergency department of the hospitals or in the doctor's office.

For a gastric lavage a special tube is frequently used. It has a larger lumen than the Levin tube, and it may have a funnel at one end to facilitate the administration of the fluid for washing the patient's stomach. Because the lavage tube has a larger lumen than the Levin tube, it is usually inserted through the patient's mouth into his stomach by the physician. When a Levin tube is used, it can be inserted through the patient's nose or through his mouth.

The equipment required for a gastric lavage consists of the lavage tube and funnel, the solution ordered by the physician, a pail to receive stomach contents, ice in which to place the tube (see Gastrointestinal Intubation), a kidney basin for vomitus and a protective covering for the patient.

The physician usually administers 500 cc. of solution into the patient's stomach, and then he inverts the funnel to allow the stomach's contents to empty into the pail. To create a siphon, the tube is pinched while some of the fluid is still in it, and then it is lowered and inverted below the level of the patient's body and held inside the pail. Gravity drains the fluid from the tubing, and the vacuum thus established in the tubing draws the liquid from the patient's stomach. The washing is repeated until the physician considers that the stomach is satisfactorily cleansed.

During the lavage the nurse notes the reaction of the patient, the amount and kind of solution used and the amount, color and consistency of the returns. These observations are charted in the patient's record. Following gastric lavage, the patient usually needs a mouthwash.

Gastric Gavage

A gastric gavage is a feeding given to a patient through a tube which is inserted either through his nose or mouth into his stomach. It is done when the patient is unable to take food orally. The feeding can be given in two ways: at intervals ordered by the physician, for example, every four hours, or as a continuous drip over the 24 hour period. The latter method is usually indicated when the patient has diarrhea, gastric irritability or a reflex bowel disturbance.

The food used for a gavage feeding is usually given as a thick liquid. A typical tube feeding might include powdered milk, cream, cereal, strained meats and vegetables, orange juice, corn oil, sugar, iodized salt, vitamin compounds and water.[5] The feeding may be made up using different amounts of various nutrients in order to meet the patient's dietary needs.

It is the physician's responsibility to order the type of nourishment that the patient requires. In some health agencies a regular house diet is mixed in a blending machine so that it can be fed by gavage tube.

Often the patient who is to receive a gavage feeding has a Levin tube already inserted. If this is not the case, the physician usually inserts the tube (see Gastrointestinal Intubation). The nurse explains to the patient that feeding through the tube is painless and will provide him with adequate water and nourishment.

The nurse heats the feeding to 37° C. (98° F.). This temperature can be tested by putting a drop of feeding on the inner

---

[5]*Diet Manual.* Third edition. Saskatoon, Saskatchewan, University Hospital, 1970, p. 367.

aspect of the wrist. If it feels just warm to her, it will be approximately the correct temperature. Food that is at body temperature is most easily tolerated. Sometimes the physician requests that the stomach be aspirated prior to a new feeding to determine if the food is being passed into the intestinal tract. Before commencing the feeding the nurse injects a small amount of water into the tube to make sure that the lumen is clear. A disposable feeding bag may be used or the feeding may be injected by syringe. If a disposable bag is used it may be hung on an intravenous standard, and the rate of flow adjusted as desired. If the syringe method is used, care is taken to allow as little air as possible to be injected into the patient's stomach. The feeding should always be given slowly. Usually the gavage feeding flows through the tubing by gravitational force; however, if it does not do this readily, slight pressure can be applied on the plunger of the syringe. After the completion of the feeding, a small amount of water is again inserted into the tubing in order to clear the lumen of the tube of the gavage feeding. Some patients learn to administer their own gavage feedings.

The nurse records the amount of the gavage feeding that the patient has taken as well as the amount of water that was administered. Should the patient start to gag or vomit during the gavage feeding, the feeding is terminated and the situation is reported to the physician and recorded in the patient's record.

If the patient is to have a continuous gavage, a Baron food pump or a burette (glass or plastic container) and tubing may be used. The burette is hung to the side of the patient at a level just above him. The nurse adjusts the rate of flow of the gavage feeding as the physician has ordered. She also maintains a level of gavage fluid in the burette. The patient is observed at frequent intervals for any untoward signs resulting from the feeding.

GUIDE TO ASSESSING NURSING NEEDS

1. What is the nature of the patient's discomfort? Is he anorectic, nauseated or has he been vomiting?
2. How long has he had this discomfort? Is it related to a specific cause such as particular foods, medications or stressful situations?
3. Does the patient have other distressing symptoms such as headache or pain?
4. If the patient is vomiting, what is the nature of the vomitus, its amount? How often does he vomit?
5. How much food and fluid is the patient taking?
6. Does he show signs of poor nutritional status? Of dehydration?
7. Have specific laboratory tests been ordered? If so, what are the nurse's responsibilities relative to these? What learning needs does the patient have in regard to them?
8. Have specific diagnostic or therapeutic measures been prescribed? If so, what is the nurse's responsibility relative to these? What are the patient's learning needs?
9. Are there factors in the environment which contribute to the patient's discomfort? Can these be modified?
10. What nursing measures can contribute to the patient's comfort and hygiene?

GUIDE TO EVALUATING THE EFFECTIVENESS OF NURSING ACTION

1. Is the patient comfortable?
2. Is he obtaining adequate food and fluids for his nutritional needs?
3. Do laboratory tests reflect adequate hydration? For example, does the level of blood chlorides and blood pH indicate electrolyte balance and does the specific gravity of the urine indicate hydration?
4. Have the distressing symptoms been alleviated? That is, has vomiting stopped? Is nausea less troublesome? Is the patient beginning to have an appetite again?

STUDY VOCABULARY

Anorexia	Hunger	Projectile
Appetite	Hypochloremia	Wretching
Cachectic	Hypoglycemia	Vertigo
Emesis	Nausea	Vomitus

STUDY SITUATION

Mrs. W. Stanley had her appendix removed three days ago. Since she returned from the operating room, she has been nauseated continually and vomits after every meal. Mrs. Stanley says she has severe pain in her operative area, and she is reluctant to eat and to get out of bed. The doctor has ordered that she get up and walk to the bathroom at least three times a day and that she eat a normal diet, with adequate fluids in between meals.

1. What are the possible reasons for this patient's nausea and vomiting?
2. What nursing care measures might alleviate her symptoms?
3. What specific observations should the nurse make about the patient?
4. When the patient says she does not want to get out of bed, what should the nurse do?
5. How could the nurse possibly increase Mrs. Stanley's appetite?
6. What dangers and complications can be concomitant with vomiting?
7. By what criteria can the nurse evaluate the effectiveness of her nursing care?
8. What is an adequate intake of fluid for this patient, and how could you best gain her cooperation in taking this amount?

BIBLIOGRAPHY

Diet Manual. Third edition. Saskatoon, Saskatchewan, University Hospital, 1970.

Downs, Howard S.: The Control of Vomiting. *The American Journal of Nursing,* 66:1:76–82, January, 1966.

Grobin, W.: Gastrointestinal Intubation. *The Canadian Nurse,* 55:106–108, February, 1959.

Guyton, Arthur C.: *Textbook of Medical Physiology.* Fourth edition. Philadelphia, W. B. Saunders Company, 1971.

MacBryde, Cyril M., and Robert S. Blacklow (eds.): *Signs and Symptoms: Applied Pathologic Physiology and Clinical Interpretation.* Fifth edition. Philadelphia, J. B. Lippincott Company, 1970.

Monagle, J. E.: Nutrition and Health—A Critical Evaluation. *Canadian Journal of Public Health*, 56:488, November, 1965.

Nordmark, Madelyn T., and Anne W. Rohweder: *Scientific Foundations of Nursing*, Second edition. Philadelphia, J. B. Lippincott Company, 1967.

Olson, Edith V., et al.: The Hazards of Immobility. *The American Journal of Nursing*, 67:4:780–797, April, 1967.

Sodeman, William A., and William A. Sodeman, Jr.: *Pathologic Physiology, Mechanisms of Disease*. Fourth edition. Philadelphia, W. B. Saunders Company, 1967.

Sutton, Audrey L.: *Bedside Nursing Techniques in Medicine and Surgery*. Second edition. Philadelphia, W. B. Saunders Company, 1969.

27 THE CARE OF PATIENTS WHO HAVE URINARY PROBLEMS

The nurse should be able to:

Describe the anatomical structures and physiological mechanisms involved in the excretion of urine

Explain factors which can cause disturbances of urinary functioning

List signs and symptoms which are frequently observed in patients with urinary problems

Describe methods to assess the nursing needs of patients with urinary problems

List principles from the biophysical and social sciences relevant to the care of patients with urinary problems

Cite principal objectives in the care of these patients

Identify situations requiring priority action in the nursing care of patients with urinary problems

Describe the nurse's role in assisting with measures that reduce the workload on the kidneys

Describe nursing measures to minimize the effects of kidney impairment on the body

Describe nursing measures to facilitate the elimination of urine from the bladder

Describe measures to assist the patient in the reestablishment of a normal voiding pattern

Describe specific nursing techniques frequently used in the care of patients with urinary problems

INTRODUCTION

People who have urinary problems are usually considerably distressed; their symptoms are often uncomfortable, sometimes inconvenient and occasionally embarrassing. A person may find it necessary to void more often than normally, sometimes with acute urgency. He may have difficulty in voiding, or he may even experience pain on voiding. Some patients find it necessary to get up at night in order to urinate (nocturia).

Most people have difficulty in discussing urinary problems, possibly because of the intimate anatomical connection between the urinary and reproductive systems and early toilet training experiences. Even though the patient who has urinary disturbances is acutely uncomfortable, he is often reluctant to talk about the cause of his discomfort to a nurse. The topic of elimination of waste products by the urinary system is usually considered by patients to be a subject discussed only with a physician. Thus symptoms of urinary problems may be a source of social embarrassment and go unattended for some time. If the nurse can discuss these symptoms without showing signs of embarrassment herself, that is, by discussing them as forthrightly as any other type of symptom, this can help to put the patient at ease.

THE PHYSIOLOGY OF THE URINARY TRACT

Urinary problems can involve any part of the urinary tract: the kidneys, the ureters, the bladder or the urethra. The kidneys are complex organs whose chief functions are the elimination of waste products of body metabolism and the control of the concentration of the various constituents of body fluid, including the blood. These functions are accomplished through an efficient filtering system which removes the excess water, acid and other wastes from the blood as it passes through the kidney. The blood retains the essential elements needed by the body through selective reabsorption. Blood comes to the kidney through the renal artery and is filtered in the glomeruli of the nephrons. The filtrate contains water, the waste products of metabolism, electrolytes and glucose. These products pass along the nephron's tubules, where some solutes and water are reabsorbed. The tubules also secrete substances such as drugs into the urine.

The body can continue to function effectively even though a considerable amount of kidney tisssue has been damaged, indeed, even though one kidney is not functioning at all. The factors which adversely affect the efficiency of kidney functioning include infections of the kidney, disturbances in blood circulation to the kidney, hormone disturbances and growths within the kidney itself. As a result of impaired kidney function there can be retention of metabolic wastes and a disturbance in the water and electrolyte balance of the body.

Interference with the function of the ureters can also cause urinary disturbances. The ureters are long, narrow muscular tubes which serve to transport urine from the kidneys to its storehouse, the bladder. Strictures of the ureter and blockage of the ureter by stones are common pathological conditions. When a kidney is displaced from its normal position, this can cause a kink in the ureter which obstructs the passage of urine. A tumor in the abdomen can also cause a stricture in the ureter. Finally,

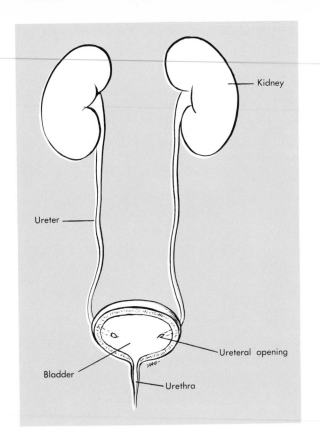

The urinary system.

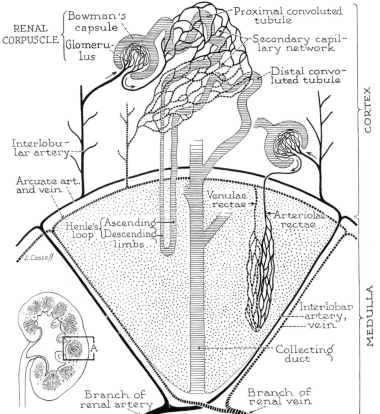

A nephron. (From B. G. King and M. J. Showers: Human Anatomy and Physiology. Sixth edition. Philadelphia, W. B. Saunders Company, 1969.)

380

ureters are susceptible to infections descending from the pelvis of a kidney or ascending from the bladder.

The chief function of the bladder is to retain urine until it can be excreted. The average adult bladder holds from 300 to 500 cc of urine; however, the bladder has been known to hold from 3000 to 4000 cc. of urine. The bladder is a hollow muscular organ whose efficient functioning is dependent upon the maintenance of muscle tone in the bladder wall and upon the integrity of the nervous system innervating the bladder. Stimulation of the bladder is transmitted by the sympathetic nervous system through the hypogastric nerves and by the parasympathetic nervous system through the pelvic nerves. The act of voiding is essentially parasympathetic in origin, involving the contraction of the detrusor muscle (bladder wall muscle) and relaxation of the internal sphincter of the bladder. The stimulus initiating this act is a stretch reflex stimulus that is evoked by an increase in pressure within the bladder as it fills with urine.

Micturition (voiding) is essentially a cord reflex, although it is subject to control by the higher centers of the brain. The acts of initiating and stopping micturition are normally under voluntary control via a second external sphincter muscle. Anxiety mediated through the parasysmpathetic nerves can stimulate voiding, at times with loss of control. Injury to the spinal cord can interfere with the transmission of nerve impulses to and from the bladder and thus cause loss of control over voiding. It is possible, however, for some patients with such injuries to establish an automatic bladder by utilizing the micturition reflex.

Women, particularly, are prone to bladder infections because of the shortness of the female urethra. Stasis or urine in the bladder, because of retention, is another predisposing factor in infections and also in the formation of bladder stones.

The chief function of the urethra is to provide a passageway through which urine can be voided from the bladder.

The urethra is a short, hollow muscular tube approximately $1\frac{1}{2}$ to 2 inches long in the female and 7 to 9 inches in the male. The urethra is susceptible to infection and strictures in the same way as are the ureters. In older men hypertrophy (increase in size) of the prostate gland, which surrounds the urethra, is common. The prostate gland is also a common site for malignancies. Thus anything that interferes with the patency of the lumen of the urethra can interfere with the act of voiding.

The entire urinary tract is lined with mucous membrane; therefore, infection initiated in any part of the urinary tract can very quickly involve the entire urinary system.

Normal urine has a pH of 4.8 to 8.0. It is slightly acidic. It contains creatinine, uric acid, urea and a few white blood cells. Normal urine does not contain bacteria, red blood cells, sugar, albumin, acetone, casts, pus or calculi. Calculi are stones which form in the urinary tract.

In appearance, urine is clear and straw or light amber in color. The darker the color the more concentrated it is. The specific gravity is usually 1.003 to 1.030. Urine normally has a faintly aromatic odor.

THE ETIOLOGY OF URINARY PROBLEMS

Infection is one of the most common causes of urinary disturbances. Because the entire urinary system is lined with a continuous mucous membrane, an infection that initiates in one part of the system can travel rapidly to all parts of the tract. Bacteria commonly found in the large intestine, colibacillus for example, are common causes of urinary tract infection. The proximity of the outlets of the gastrointestinal and the urinary tracts contributes to this transfer.

Disturbances in the circulatory system also can have an effect upon kidney function. Heart disease and diseases of the venous and arterial systems often interfere with the circulation of blood to the kidneys. Normally, 170 liters of blood are filtered through the adult kidneys in one day. From this filtration process approximately 1½ to 2 liters of urine are formed and excreted. Any disease that interferes with the circulation of blood through the kidney can result in the impairment of kidney functioning.

Obstructions may occur in almost any part of the urinary tract. Most commonly they are seen in the pelvis of the kidney, in the ureter and, in the male, in the prostatic section of the urethra. Blockage of the urinary tract, whether it is because of a malignancy or stones, hinders the excretion of urine.

Hormone disturbances, such as disturbances in the functioning of the adrenal or pituitary glands can also have an adverse effect upon the kidneys. The antidiuretic hormone, aldosterone and possibly norepinephrine, affect the reabsorption of fluid within the kidney tubules.

A *generalized trauma* to the body or a systemic infection can also affect the kidneys. For example, in severe dehydration there is a depletion in the amount of fluid within the body which can severely disturb kidney function, even to the point of failure.

Any *generalized muscular disturbance* can also affect urinary tract function. Specific dysfunctions of the muscles of the bladder, the ureters or the urethra can cause urinary symptoms such as retention of urine or poor urinary control.

Neurologic and psychogenic factors can interfere with normal kidney and bladder function. Drugs which depress the central nervous system, for example, can cause a loss of voluntary control over micturition. Hence, patients under heavy sedation and those undergoing general anesthesia may void by reflex action when the bladder is full. Damage to the spinal cord or to the pathways that transmit impulses from the spinal cord to the brain may also result in the loss of voluntary control over voiding. Emotion may also cause urinary dysfunction. Anxiety, for example, can be mediated through the parasympathetic nervous system and result in urinary frequency.

SIGNS AND SYMPTOMS OF URINARY PROBLEMS

The signs and symptoms of urinary dysfunction can appear as localized disturbances in the passage of urine or as generalized symptoms resulting from a disturbance in the elimination of waste products from the body.

Localized Symptoms

Of the localized symptoms the following are frequently seen:

Urinary incontinence, or involuntary voiding, is a common urinary problem. Sometimes there is a complete inability to control the flow of urine and as a result a constant dribbling. This is not only demoralizing and embarrassing, but the urine can be a source of irritation to the skin in the anogenital area. Urinary incontinence sometimes occurs temporarily after an operation. It can also occur as a result of diseases of the nerves and muscles of the bladder. Nursing measures are chiefly concerned with helping the patient to reestablish control over voiding and with preventing secondary complications such as decubitus ulcers which may occur as a result of skin irritation.

Urinary retention is another common urinary problem. In retention the urine is formed in the kidneys, but the patient is unable to excrete it from his bladder. As a consequence his bladder becomes distended and he feels increasingly uncomfortable. Some patients have *retention with overflow;* they void small amounts of urine frequently but continue to have distended bladders. Urinary retention predisposes a patient to bladder infection (cystitis).

Urinary retention can be identified by checking the patient's voiding pattern. If the patient voids 30 to 50 cc. of urine every 1 to 2 hours he is probably retaining urine. In addition, a distended bladder can often be palpated. With the patient in the dorsal recumbent position, palpation just superior to the symphysis pubis reveals a firm distention.

Percussion with the fingers causes the dull sound indicative of a full bladder.

Dysuria means difficulty in voiding or pain on voiding. It can be a result of a blockage within the urinary tract or an infection of the bladder or urethra. Sometimes a patient describes a burning sensation upon voiding.

Oliguria is the passage of a lessened amount of urine. This condition can be caused by dehydration or an impairment of the circulation of blood to the kidney. A lowered efficiency of the kidney or a blockage within the urinary tract can also result in oliguria.

Polyuria is the passage of an increased amount of urine. It can be caused by failure of the tubules to reabsorb water or by a disturbance in the hormone balance of the body. The latter can result in an increased elimination of fluids from the body, that is, above the normal level expected. The average adult loses approximately 1500 cc. of water through the kidneys in a 24 hour period.

Renal anuria (suppression of urine) is a condition in which there is an absence of urinary excretion from the kidneys. If this condition is prolonged, toxic substances build up within the body and the patient eventually dies. The formation of less than 25 cc. of urine an hour is considered to be inadequate for an adult. Normal urine formation in the kidney is 60 to 120 cc. per hour.

In both renal anuria and urinary retention the patient is unable to void; however, in urinary retention the urine is retained in the bladder, whereas in renal anuria the urine never reaches the bladder. Normally when the bladder contains between 300 to 500 cc. of urine, an awareness of the need to void occurs.

Foreign substances in the urine may be found upon examination in the laboratory. Blood in the urine may appear as a smoky brown discoloration *(hematuria)*. A cloudy, whitish urine usually indicates the presence of pus *(pyuria)*, and albumin in the urine *(albuminuria)* also causes a cloudy appearance. The presence of protein in the urine *(proteinuria)* is usually due to either tissue disintegration or an increase in glomerular permeability. *Casts*, on the other hand, are coagulated protein from the lumen of the kidney tubules. Sugar in the urine *(glycosuria)* is seen when the body is unable to utilize all the sugar that is ingested.

Generalized Symptoms

In addition to the localized signs and symptoms, generalized symptoms are also indicative of impairment in the function of the kidneys.

When there is a severe reduction in the ability of the kidneys to function, the patient usually develops *uremia*. This condition may occur as a result of an acute renal shutdown, due to trauma or infection for example, or because of a chronic kidney disorder. The impairment in renal functioning has several effects on the body. Water is retained and there is a resultant edema of body tissues. The acid-base balance is disturbed, and the patient may develop acidosis due to failure of the kidneys to remove the acidic waste products of metabolism. Potassium excretion is impaired, with a resulting high concentration of potassium in body fluids, and there is usually also retention of the nonprotein nitrogenous waste products of metabolism as well, particularly of urea, whence the condition derived its name.

Edema is due to the retention of water and possibly sodium in the body. It is usually first observed in the soft tissues around the eyes and then in the dependent areas of the body, for example, the ankles and the feet. In patients who remain in bed, edema can also be noted in the dependent sacral area. Generalized edema can follow edema of these dependent areas. In situations in which there is extensive renal damage, the edema can be pitting, that is when pressure is placed upon the skin a small depression remains after the pressure has been released.

Another generalized symptom which can indicate kidney dysfunction is a *pallor with a powdery appearance of the skin.* This is due to an attempt by the body to utilize other avenues for the elimination of wastes, with a resultant deposit of salts upon the skin. Patients who have acute renal failure often exhibit this *urea frost.*

Lassitude, headache, and other cerebral symptoms can also result from the accumulation of waste products within the body. The sensorium (sensory areas of the brain), however, is usually unaffected.

When the kidneys are inhibited in the elimination of excess acid from the body, the lungs attempt to compensate for this. As a result there are *respiratory changes* involving the character and the rate of the respirations. The respirations become deeper, the rate of the respirations increases and sometimes the patient's breath has the odor of urine.

Another important change that can often be seen is the *retention of potassium ions.* As a result, not only can severe weakness and eventually voluntary muscle paralysis be observed, but there are disturbances in the myocardium (heart muscle) which are manifested by an irregular pulse as well. There are also significant *changes in blood chemistry.* The concentration of urea in the blood (BUN) may increase from a normal of 15–25 mg. per 100 ml. to as much as 200 mg. per 100 ml. in severe cases of uremia. Similarly, the blood creatinine may rise from a normal of 1.2 mg. per 100 ml. to 13 mg. per 100 ml. The extent of the increase in blood levels of these substances provides an indication of the severity of the kidney impairment. The blood urea nitrogen and the blood creatinine are increased in the blood plasma.

ASSESSING THE NURSING NEEDS OF PATIENTS WITH URINARY PROBLEMS

In identifying the nursing needs of patients with urinary problems, the nurse can usually obtain a good deal of pertinent information from the patient. He may describe sensations of pain related to voiding, for example, or he may have noted disturbances in the normal pattern of voiding. The patient may be distressed by frequency or urgency in the need to void, or conversely, he may find micturition difficult. Patients are usually aware, too, of changes in the amount of urine. When there is either suppression of urine formation in the kidneys, or retention of urine in the bladder, the amount of urine voided may be small. On the other hand, in some types of disease conditions, there may be copious amounts of urine formed and excreted. Some patients find that their sleep is disturbed because of the need to urinate. This may happen when kidney function is impaired and there is a loss of the normal ability of the kidneys to vary the concentration of urine. The patient may also be the first to notice abnormalities such as the presence of blood or pus in the urine. Often patients are reluctant to discuss urinary problems and they may need encouragement to express their needs. It is important to minimize the patient's feelings of embarrassment by ensuring privacy and a quiet place for discussion.

The nurse can supplement the information she obtains from the patient with her own observations. The characteristics of urine which should be noted are its color, odor, consistency and amount, and the presence of abnormal constituents. Normal urine is clear and straw-colored. It has the consistency of water and is usually slightly aromatic in odor. If the urine is lighter than normal in color, this may be due to either an abnormally high intake of fluids or a diminution of the concentrating power of the kidneys. A dark, brownish color usually indicates a more concentrated urine. Urine may also be almost orange in color in some conditions because of the presence of bile salts. Urine sometimes has a sweetish odor, often described as "fruity," which is characteristic of the presence of acetone. Blood in the urine may be observed as bright red, or the urine may be smoky in color. Another abnormal constituent which may be noted by visual observation is pus, which usually indicates an infection in the urinary tract.

In addition to observing the character and amount of the patient's urine, the nurse should be alert to the signs and symptoms of urinary dysfunction as these have been described in the previous section of this chapter. One of the primary responsibilities in the nursing care of patients with urinary problems is the observation and recording of pertinent facts. The early detection of edema, of changes in the pigmentation of the skin, or of signs of central nervous system or neuromuscular dysfunction can contribute significantly to the physician's plan of care for the patient.

An important part of the nurse's responsibility is often the exact measurement of the patient's fluid intake and output. These fluids are usually measured in cubic centimeters and recorded on a fluid balance sheet on the patient's chart. Occasionally it is also necessary to record the amount of fluid ingested as part of the patient's food and the amount lost in perspiration and feces, but these are rare situations. Normally fluid output includes all liquid drainage (for example, gastric suction, vomitus, bleeding, or diarrhea) and urine excretion.

Numerous diagnostic laboratory tests are performed on urine to evaluate kidney function. Some tests indicate the rate of glomerular filtration, tubular reabsorption and excretion by the kidneys.

A routine *urinalysis* is probably the most common urine examination. It includes microscopic examination and tests of pH, specific gravity, albumin and sugar.

Urine Test	*Normal Results*
pH	4.8 to 8.0
Specific gravity	1.003 to 1.030
Albumin	Negative
Sugar	Negative
Microscopic examination	(Female) few red blood cells; few casts
	Straw to light amber

Blood in urine may be obvious or hidden. Laboratory tests can detect intact red blood cells and dissolved hemoglobin (hemoglobinuria).

Nurses are frequently called upon in the clinical areas to perform some of the more routine laboratory tests on urine. Thus, a nurse may be requested to carry out a test for specific gravity or to test the patient's urine for the presence of sugar or acetone.

Tests of renal function include the phenolsulfonphthalein test, the Fishberg concentration test, concentration and dilution tests and the urea clearance test. Generally speaking, most of these tests have special requirements as to the food and fluid intake of the patient, the hours when urine specimens are to be collected and, perhaps, definite times when blood specimens are to be collected. It is important that the patient understand his needs relative to these tests and how he can help with them.

Urine cultures are done to determine the presence of a urinary infection. Normally a catheter specimen is required for culture, unless the physician feels a clean voided specimen will suffice. Urine is normally sterile.

When a midstream specimen from the male patient is needed, the patient cleanses the urinary meatus with an antiseptic solution. He voids some urine, which is discarded, and then collects the midstream urine in a sterile container. The latter part of stream is also discarded.

Obtaining a midstream specimen from a female patient is more difficult. The labia and vestibule are first cleansed with an antiseptic solution. Then, after a cotton plug is placed in the entrance of the vagina, the patient voids. The first and latter parts of the stream are caught in a discard container. The midstream specimen is caught in a sterile container. Most female patients find it easier to obtain this specimen when the toilet is used for discarded urine.

Some tests of urine are concerned with physiological processes other than those of the urinary tract. The Aschheim-Zondek test, the Friedman test and the frog test are tests for pregnancy. The Bence-Jones protein test is carried out as an aid in the diagnosis of bone tumors; the 5-Hydroxyindoleacetic acid test reveals the presence of a carcinoid tumor. The level of 17-ketosteroid excretion is a measure of adrenal function, and the d-xylose tolerance test indicates the ability of the gastrointestinal tract to absorb nutrients.

Some blood tests are also indicative of kidney function. The nonprotein nitrogen test (N.P.N.) measures the ability of the kidney to remove urea, creatine, etc., from the blood. The blood urea nitrogen (B.U.N.) test is a more sensitive test of kidney function. For each of these tests, 5 cc. of venous blood is collected.

There are many examinations of the urinary tract. A cystoscopy is the examination of a patient's bladder with a lighted instrument which is inserted up the urethra. The intravenous pyelogram and retrograde pyelogram outline the pelves, calices, ureters and urinary bladder by means of a contrast media which is visible on an x-ray.

PRINCIPLES RELEVANT TO THE CARE OF PATIENTS WITH URINARY PROBLEMS

Most of the nitrogenous wastes of cellular metabolism are eliminated by the kidneys.

The kidneys play an important role in maintaining the fluid and electrolyte balance of body tissues and fluids.

The average adult loses approximately 1500 cc. of fluid from the kidneys in a 24 hour period.

The awareness of the need to void normally occurs when the bladder contains from 300 to 500 cc. of urine.

Mucous membrane lines the urinary tract.

Previous learning influences an individual's attitudes and behavior relative to elimination.

The excretion of urine is normally an independent function in the adult.

OBJECTIVES OF NURSING CARE

The goals of nursing care of the patient with urinary problems depend to a large extent on the nature of the problem. If there is impairment of kidney functioning, nursing measures are directed toward assisting to reduce the workload of the kidneys until such time as they are able to resume normal activity, and assisting to minimize the effects of impaired kidney functioning on the body. In this, the nurse is guided by the physician's plan of therapy for the patient.

If the problem is one of interference with the elimination of urine, rather than impaired kidney functioning, nursing measures are directed toward facilitating the elimination of urine from the bladder and assisting in the reestablishment of a normal voiding pattern.

In all types of urinary problems, an important aim of nursing care is to provide emotional and physical comfort measures which the patient finds supportive.

DETERMINING PRIORITIES FOR NURSING ACTION

When a patient has an impairment in kidney functioning, the body's ability to eliminate the nitrogenous waste products of protein metabolism is decreased. The accumulation of these waste products within the body constitutes a serious threat to the patient's life. One of the most important aspects of nursing care for patients with renal disorders is the constant monitoring of fluid intake and output. If there is a decrease in fluid loss below the levels considered safe, this fact should be reported promptly so that appropriate therapy can be instituted. In assessing the safety levels for the patient, the nurse is guided by the physician's estimate for this particular patient, but it is helpful for her to remember that the normal urine output in an adult is approximately 1500 cc. per day. An output of less than 25 cc. per hour (600 cc. in a 24 hour period) is considered inadequate for a normal adult.

If the patient's problem is one that causes interference with the excretion of urine from the bladder, it is important that he be watched for signs of urine retention. Although some adult bladders have been known to hold up to 3000 to 4000 cc. of fluid, not all bladders will contain this quantity and there is a danger of rupture when the bladder content is considerably below this point. The early detection of urinary retention is therefore vitally important. (The identification of urinary retention is discussed in the section on signs and symptoms of urinary problems earlier in the chapter.) It should be reported promptly so that appropriate medical or nursing intervention can be started. Frequently, it is left up to the nurse to initiate action; that is, the physician may leave an order for catheterization of the patient every eight hours as needed (p.r.n.). When catheterization is needed, it should be done promptly. A patient should never be left with a distended bladder.

ASSISTING WITH MEASURES TO REDUCE THE WORKLOAD ON THE KIDNEYS

The principal functions of the kidneys are to control the concentration of the various constituents of body fluid and to eliminate the waste products of metabolism, chiefly the nitrogenous wastes of cellular metabolism. When kidney function is impaired, various measures may be instituted to relieve them of some of their workload. Often, the patient is put to bed to minimize activity and, hence, lessen cellular metabolism. Unless the patient is losing large amounts of protein in the urine (which occurs in some conditions), he is usually given a low-protein diet, again, to minimize the amount of nitrogenous wastes from protein metabolism which need to be eliminated. There may also be restrictions placed on the sodium and potassium in his diet,

since sodium contributes to fluid retention, and the accumulation of potassium, which a damaged kidney cannot excrete (or has a lessened ability to excrete), may cause serious neuromuscular disturbances. The patient's fluid intake may be limited to prevent or lessen edema. It is important for the nurse to see that instructions regarding both food and fluid intake for the patient are followed exactly. Patients with renal disorders often suffer from anorexia and may need encouragement to eat their meals. The patient should be made aware of the importance of adhering to the diet and fluid intake that has been ordered for him, since this is part of his therapy. Many patients can help to keep track of their fluid intake; by encouraging them to participate in their care in this way, the nurse can often gain their cooperation.

Sometimes, in order to put the kidneys at rest and give them a chance to recover when there has been extensive tissue damage, or to maintain patients whose kidneys are no longer functioning, an artificial kidney is used. In the artificial kidney, blood is continually removed from an artery and allowed to circulate through a channel with a thin membrane through which a *dialyzing fluid* removes the impurities from it before it is returned to the patient through a vein. This process is called *renal dialysis*. There are several different types of machine for renal dialysis now available on the market, including a unit for home use. Some patients require renal dialysis for a short period of time, to tide them over an acute episode, but many people without functioning kidneys have been maintained over a period of years with an artificial kidney. Frequently, these patients come into an outpatient department or a clinic for dialysis every few days. In addition to renal dialysis, other methods of removing impurities from body fluids are occasionally used, such as peritoneal or gastrointestinal dialysis. In these techniques, large amounts of dialyzing fluid are injected into the peritoneal cavity or inserted into the gastrointestinal tract and later removed. Dialysis occurs in these cases through the mucous membrane. For additional detail on the use of the renal dialysis machine, the nurse is referred to Audrey Sutton's *Bedside Nursing Techniques in Medicine and Surgery*, Chapter 15, pp. 278–281.

The experience of undergoing renal dialysis can be very frightening for the patient. Often the individual is very ill, and the large and complicated machinery that is used can provoke much anxiety. Usually there are a number of people involved in operating the machine, in taking samples for laboratory analysis and in supervising technical details, and this too can be alarming to the patient. A simple explanation of the procedure frequently helps the patient to understand what is happening to him. The nurse should always be mindful of the patient's needs for encouragement and supportive care. The presence of someone who is interested in him as an individual as well as in the technical aspects of his care can be very reassuring.

MEASURES TO MINIMIZE THE EFFECTS OF RENAL IMPAIRMENT ON THE BODY

When there is impairment of kidney function, the individual's fluid and electrolyte balance is disturbed. There is usually a retention of fluid in the tissues, and the patient's fluid intake is frequently restricted to minimize this tendency. When edema is present, the nurse should remember that edematous tissue is more prone to break down than normal tissue is, and therefore nursing measures to maintain the integrity of the skin are especially important. Patients who are confined to bed require particular attention to prevent the development of pressure areas. Fluids tend to collect in dependent parts of the body, such as the sacral area in bed patients, and also the lower limbs. These areas should be carefully watched for signs of impending tissue breakdown, and measures should be taken to prevent this. (See Chapter 11 for a

discussion of measures to prevent the formation of decubitus ulcers.)

Meticulous skin care is important in the care of patients with renal impairment, not only as a factor in maintaining skin integrity, but also to cleanse the skin of perspiration. When the body is hampered in the elimination of waste products through the kidneys, increased amounts of nitrogenous wastes are excreted through sensible and insensible perspiration. This may cause a crystal-like product to gather on the skin, which can create an unpleasant odor. As a result, bathing is particularly important for the patient's cleanliness and comfort.

To compensate for the lessened ability of the kidneys to excrete excess acid, an increased amount of carbonic acid is eliminated through the respiratory tract. Measures to facilitate breathing are therefore important. When the patient is in bed, his position should be such that maximum expansion of the chest is possible. The room should be well-ventilated, and an adequate supply of oxygen ensured. (See Chapter 25 for a discussion of measures to facilitate respiration.)

The accumulation of nitrogenous wastes due to the kidneys' lessened ability to excrete these may cause disturbances in neuromuscular functioning. Headache and lethargy are not uncommon, and in severe cases of renal impairment, the patient may become disoriented and subsequently comatose. In these cases, the safety needs of the patient must be especially kept in mind. Although the sensorium usually remains clear even in patients with considerable kidney damage, it is always wise to watch for signs of mental confusion, particularly in older patients. Measures such as crib sides to protect the confused patient from injuring himself and the application of mitts to prevent him from pulling at catheters or other tubing are frequently needed. (See Chapter 15 for a discussion of the safety needs of confused patients.)

Weakness of the muscles may result from the retention of potassium ions, and the patient usually fatigues easily.

Because the heart is a muscular organ, it is usually affected by potassium retention. Readings of the apical heart beat are frequently ordered to assist in monitoring cardiac function in patients with renal disorders.

MEASURES TO FACILITATE THE ELIMINATION OF URINE FROM THE BLADDER

To maintain adequate urinary elimination is important to physiological functioning. For the patient who has difficulty in voiding, there are certain nursing measures which can be provided to assist him. In addition to urinary catheterization, which is carried out as ordered by the physician, there are also measures to stimulate the act of micturition. Some ways in which this is done are:

1. Helping the patient to assume a natural position for voiding.

2. Providing a commode or, preferably, assisting the patient to the bathroom if this is possible (male patients frequently find it easier to void when they are standing rather than sitting or lying down)

3. Running water within the patient's hearing

4. Providing water in which he can dangle his fingers

5. Providing privacy and setting aside a time for voiding

6. Providing a warm bedpan or urinal

7. Applying a warm hot water bottle to the patient's lower abdomen

8. Pouring warm water over the perineum

9. Relieving pain

10. Applying ice

It has long been accepted that warmth applied to the bladder and perineal areas will help to relax the muscles used in voiding and therefore facilitate this process. There is also reason to believe, however, that the application of ice may also accomplish the same purpose.

Unless the physician has expressly ordered the insertion of a urinary catheter, the foregoing measures are tried before catheterization is considered. Catheterization is the insertion of a sterile tube into the bladder to drain off urine. The techniques of catheterization and the various types of catheters used are described in the section on specific nursing care measures later in this chapter.

The excretion of urine is normally an independent function for an adult. Consequently, the necessity for help in voiding can represent a return to a dependency state similar to that of a child. For some people this is difficult to accept and may produce anxiety. Patients who cannot void or those who void without control are frequently embarrassed as well as anxious. The nurse can offer support by providing explanations of the cause of the patient's problem within the context designated by the physician. The patient should be taught to respond to the urge for voiding promptly, rather than to wait. It is important, in this regard, for the nurse to answer the patient's call signal promptly also so that the patient is not kept waiting for a urinal or a bedpan. At no time should the nurse show impatience or a lack of understanding of the patient's distress.

MEASURES TO ASSIST IN THE REESTABLISHMENT OF A NORMAL VOIDING PATTERN

Some patients with urinary problems have difficulty in voiding; others may suffer from urinary incontinence. For those patients whose ability to control voiding has been lessened, the nurse can often assist them to train their bladders to function at regular and predictable times. For the nurse to be able to assist the patient in this, she should know his normal pattern of voiding. What are the times when he voids and when is he usually dry?

The patient is encouraged to assume as natural a position as possible for voiding and to void at regular times, preferably at his normal voiding periods. There is considerable debate whether the effort involved in getting on and off the bedpan exceeds that involved in getting out of bed and using a commode. Many women patients find it easier to void when they use a bedside commode, and male patients find it easier if they stand at the side of the bed to use a urinal. If permissible, these measures often help the patient in regaining a normal pattern of voiding.

The patient can be assisted to void by the various means just described. In addition to those already mentioned, digital pressure at the side of the urinary meatus or a circular movement over the bladder can often stimulate urination. If the patient has had a catheter in place over a period of time, he will need to have it clamped for intervals of two to three hours in order to increase the muscle tone before bladder training is initiated. The patient can expect accidents during a bladder training regime; nevertheless, many people do develop a regular voiding pattern.

It has already been mentioned that the patient should be encouraged to void as soon as he feels the urge to do so. The importance of having nursing personnel answer the patient's call signal promptly cannot be overemphasized. The patient should not be kept waiting or allowed to become incontinent because his request for a bedpan or a urinal went unheeded.

If an accident does occur, the patient's bedding should be changed at once. This has the psychological advantage of encouraging the patient to keep his bed dry, if it is not allowed to stay wet. Changing wet linen also helps to prevent skin irritation and the development of unpleasant odors.

In a bladder retraining program, it is essential that the patient have an adequate intake of fluids to stimulate the secretion of sufficient urine to distend the bladder enough so that the micturition reflex is initiated at regular times. Normally, the urge to void is felt when the bladder contains 300 to 500 cc. of urine. The provision of fluids at regular intervals helps to ensure an adequate intake; under normal circumstances, a minimum of 1500 cc. should be maintained and preferably more if the patient can tolerate a larger amount.

Patients on a bladder retraining regime have much need for both physical and emotional support. They usually require physical assistance from nursing personnel when they need to use a bedpan, commode or toilet. The dependence on others and the lack of control over such a basic function as voiding can be very distressing to the patient. Since both the patient and his family will probably need help, the nurse must understand the meaning that urinary problems have for them. Sympathy, tolerance and patience are all required of the nurse in helping patients with urinary problems.

SPECIFIC NURSING TECHNIQUES

Urinary Catheterization of the Female Patient

A urinary catheterization is the introduction of a narrow tube, called a urinary catheter, through the urethra into the bladder in order to remove urine. It is ordered by the physician, although it is usually carried out by a female nurse for the female patient and by a male nurse, an orderly or the physician for the male patient. This does not mean, however, that a female nurse might not find it necessary to catheterize a male patient on occasion.

The purpose of urinary catheterization may be to obtain a sterile urine specimen for laboratory examination or to empty a patient's bladder preoperatively so that the danger of incising the bladder is lessened. A urinary catheterization is also ordered postoperatively for a patient who is unable to void. Normally the act of voiding is a spinal cord reflex subject to voluntary control by the cerebrum. After surgery, however, some patients have difficulty in voiding. This is particularly true when anxiety is mediated through the hypothalamus and the sympathetic nervous system to the nerves which supply the bladder muscles.

Another reason for a urinary catheterization is to insert a retention or indwelling catheter in order to prevent uncontrollable voiding or voiding upon an operative area. Elderly patients and patients who have had cerebral vascular accidents sometimes have difficulty controlling their voiding. A patient who has surgery on her perineum will probably have an indwelling catheter inserted postoperatively in order to prevent the urine from irritating the operative area.

Equipment. A catheter is a hollow tube made of rubber, plastic, glass, metal or silk. Plastic catheters are becoming increasingly popular. Catheters are graded in size according to the French scale; No. 14 and No. 16 catheters are commonly used for the catheterization of the adult female patient. The larger the number, the larger is the lumen of the catheter. It is, of course, safest to use the correct size of catheter, but should the nurse be unsure about which size to use, she should use a smaller size in order not to harm the mucous membrane of the urethra or to cause the patient discomfort. The larger the lumen of the catheter, the more quickly will urine flow from the bladder, but usually this is not of great importance unless the patient's bladder is greatly distended. In any case, a clamp can be used to regulate the flow of urine according to the physician's order.

There are many kinds of catheters available. Retention or indwelling catheters are inserted into the patient's bladder and are kept in place by an inflated balloon or a rubber ring which is larger than the bladder orifice. These catheters may have a single lumen, as in the mushroom catheter, a double lumen or even a triple lumen, as in the Foley-Alcock catheter. The latter type of catheter is used for continuous irrigations, in which the fluid flows continuously up one lumen to the bladder and down a second lumen into a receptacle. The third lumen is connected to the inflated balloon which keeps the catheter in place. A straight catheter is usually used when the purpose of the catheterization is to remove urine rather than to have the patient retain the catheter.

The equipment for a urinary catheterization should be sterile. Because of the continuous mucous membrane lining throughout the urinary tract and because the warm mucous membrane is a likely place for the propagation of bacteria, an aseptic technique is carried out throughout the entire catheterization procedure. Disposable, prepackaged catheterization sets are available. If these are not used, then the set that is used is checked to see that it is sterile (see Chapter 16).

A catheterization set contains, at a minimum, the catheter, a receptacle for the urine and materials for cleansing the labia and urinary meatus of the patient. Some agencies suggest that the nurse use sterile rubber gloves during the catheterization procedure, whereas others suggest that sterile forceps may be used for the insertion of the catheter. In either case it is important that the catheter remain sterile during its insertion up the urethra into the patient's bladder.

The nurse needs to have a good light in order to visualize the urinary meatus and prevent contamination. Either an extension lamp or an extendible lamp can be used to illuminate the perineal area.

Since urinary catheterization can be an embarrassing measure, it is important that the nurse protect the patient from unnecessary exposure. The positions that are most often used for the catheterization are the dorsal recumbent or lithotomy positions, although some authorities are now advocating that a side-lying position be used, with the patient's knees flexed and the upper leg higher than the lower. Once the patient assumes the position that is to be used, she is covered with drapes in such a way that her legs and body are adequately covered. Then only the perineal area is exposed. In her explanation to the patient, the nurse assures her that the catheterization is usually painless but that the patient may experience a feeling of wanting to urinate because the catheter irritates the ureth-

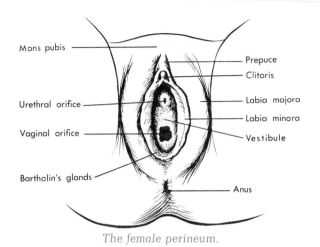

The female perineum.

ra. Discomfort is minimized if the patient is relaxed.

Preparation of the Patient. In explaining a urinary catheterization, the nurse must be guided by the needs of the patient. Some patients want a detailed explanation; others simply want assurance that it is a painless measure. From inexperience many patients want to know whether it will hurt, how long it will take and where the tube goes. The nurse should rarely assume a knowledge of anatomy on the patient's part; indeed, she may be surprised at some of the beliefs people have. That sterile technique is maintained is important to the patient's safety, but the patient probably has little awareness of this.

If the patient needs a retention catheter, she probably requires reassurance that she will be able to move about freely in bed and, very often, will still be able to get out of bed. The length of time a retention catheter remains in place depends upon the reason for its insertion; this matter is left to the physician's judgment. Points which can prove helpful to the patient with a retention catheter are:

1. Usually the patient should drink a large amount of fluid, approximately 3000 cc. per day.

2. The patient may move freely in bed.

3. The patient should not lie on the catheter tubing.

4. It is normal to have a feeling of wanting to void for a while while the catheter is in place.

After the patient has been properly draped, a sterile towel is placed between the patient's legs to make it easier to maintain sterile technique. The receptacle for the urine is then placed on the towel near the urinary meatus. It is advantageous if this receptacle is lower than the patient's bladder so that the urine will flow easily from the bladder to the receptacle by the force of gravity. All the equipment is placed conveniently.

CLEANSING THE PERINEAL AREA. Trauma to the mucous membrane of the urinary tract and the admission of bacteria to the urinary tract can result in a local or a generalized infection. Therefore, the patient's perineal area is cleansed thoroughly. There are many different ways suggested to do this; soap and water and a variety of antiseptics are used. Regardless of the method used, the patient's labia must be as clean as possible, and the urinary meatus as free from bacteria as possible.

The following are guides to cleansing the perineal area:

1. If the area is obviously soiled wash with soap and water and then dry. All soap is carefully removed, because it can inactivate some disinfectants.

2. Use a mild, nonirritating disinfectant such as aqueous Zephiran in a 1:1000 solution.

3. Use each swab just once, cleansing from the cleanest area (near the symphysis pubis) toward the most contaminated area (near the rectum).

4. Cleanse the outer labia, the inner labia and then the vestibule of the perineum. A minimum of five sponges is needed.

5. Once the vestibule has been cleansed, the labia must not touch it until the catheter has been inserted. It is necessary to keep the labia separated with the fingers for adequate visualization and to prevent unwanted contamination of the catheter.

Insertion of the Catheter. The catheter used in a urinary catheterization should be smooth so that it will not damage the mucous membrane of the urethra. In order to facilitate the passage of the catheter up the urethra, a water soluble lubricant is used. The lubricant is applied to the catheter prior to its insertion into the urethra.

With sterile forceps, sterile gloves or sterile gauze, the urinary catheter is picked up approximately 4 inches from the tip and inserted gently into the urethra. The catheter should be inserted 1½ to 2½ inches into the urethra, that is, the distance from the urinary meatus to the bladder. If any resistance is met during the passage of the catheter, it is withdrawn and the situation is reported to the physician.

The other end of the catheter lies in the sterile receptacle between the patient's legs and is held in place until the patient's bladder is empty or until the urine specimen has been obtained. If the patient has a large amount of retained urine, the distended bladder should be emptied gradually. Not all fluid should be drained off at once or there is danger of decompressing the bladder too quickly. The sudden release from pressure may result in injury to the organ itself or may cause a generalized reaction within the body, characterized by chills, an elevated temperature and, occasionally, shock. These complications can be avoided by clamping off the catheter at intervals to allow time for the bladder to adjust to the changes in pressure caused by withdrawing the urine from it. Once the urine has been obtained, the catheter is pinched and withdrawn slowly. The patient is assisted with drying the perineal area and assuming a comfortable position before the equipment is removed.

A description of the urine is recorded. This includes the amount, the color, the clarity and any unusual characteristics. If the urine has an unusual odor, if the nurse encountered any difficulty during the urinary catheterization or if the patient experienced any unusual discomfort, these observations are also charted.

Urinary Catheterization of the Male Patient

Usually this measure is carried out by the physician, orderly, or male nurse; however, on occasion a female nurse may have to catheterize a male patient. This can be particularly embarrassing to the patient, but he will be helped by an understanding, competent manner on the part of the nurse. The equipment that is necessary is similar to that used for a female urinary catheterization. The

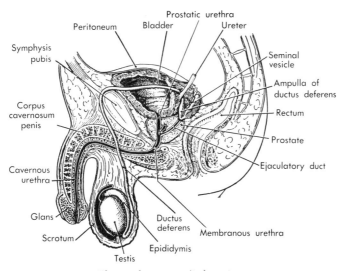

The male urogenital system.

use of sterile rubber gloves is advised to facilitate the maintenance of sterile technique.

The downward curvature of the prepubic urethra of the male can be straightened by lifting the penis and, with slight traction, holding it perpendicular to the patient's body. The patient lies in the dorsal recumbent position, his knees flexed and his legs slightly rotated externally to expose the penis. The draping and placing of the equipment are similar to that used for a female catheterization.

After the catheter and the urethral orifice are lubricated, the penis is extended vertically as described and then the catheter is inserted. It is inserted approximately 20 cm., that is, into the patient's bladder. When, in the course of the insertion, the catheter meets the resistance of Guérin's fold or the pouch of the fossa navicularis, the resistance can be bypassed by twisting the catheter. If the catheter encounters resistance at the vesical sphincters, it should not be forced, but held firmly until the sphincters relax. Once the catheter is in place the procedure is similar to that for a female catheterization.

Insertion of a Retention Catheter

If a patient requires an indwelling catheter, a syringe, sterile water for the inflation of the balloon of the catheter, connecting tubing and a receptacle for the draining urine are needed, in addition to the equipment used in a simple catheterization. After the indwelling catheter is inserted into the patient's bladder, the balloon is filled with the amount of sterile water that it is designed to hold. After the water has been injected, slight tension is placed upon the catheter to make sure that it is in place and that it will not come out of the patient's bladder easily. If the balloon is in the patient's urethra, the nurse will encounter considerable difficulty in filling the balloon and the patient will complain of discomfort. In such cases, the catheter is inserted a little farther into the bladder and the fluid is again injected into the balloon.

Once the indwelling catheter is safely in the patient's bladder, it is attached to the connecting tubing, the other end of which is in a receptacle, which is often attached to the patient's bed. Sterile technique is maintained while connecting the tubing.

The receptacle for the urine is situated at a level lower than the patient so that the urine flows readily by force of gravity. The tubing should not loop below the receptacle, because a kink may be formed which occludes the lumen. Also, the urine then has to flow against gravity. The tubing is pinned to the bed in such a manner that the lumen of the tubing is patent. This can be accomplished by pinching a piece of sheet on either side of the tubing and pinning the sides over the tubing. The tubing that lies on the top of the bed should be kept flat to facilitate drainage. Sometimes the catheter tubing is taped to the patient's thigh to avoid pulling on the catheter as the patient moves about in bed. The nurse should make sure that the patient's leg is never resting on the tubing, since this will occlude the lumen. Also, the lowest point of the tubing should always be above the level of urine in the drainage bottle, or, again, the urine is forced to run uphill, against the force of gravity.

For the patient with an indwelling catheter, the physician may order continuous or intermittent drainage. If he orders continuous drainage, then the catheter is attached to the tubing, and the urine is allowed to drain freely into the receptacle that is provided. If intermittent drainage is ordered, then the tubing is clamped at designated intervals.

Urine receptacles are available commercially which attach to the upper leg and can be used to receive urine from a catheter while the patient is walking around. These leg bags are usually disposed of when they accumulate urine and are replaced by clean, sterile bags.

When the patient requires continuous or intermittent drainage, many agencies now use disposable closed drainage sets. When these are used, the urine bag is simply emptied when full, or at regular intervals, and the tubing is left untouched until the entire set is either removed or changed. If closed drainage sets are not used, it is necessary to change the tubing and urine receptacle regularly to prevent the accumulation of salt deposits and the development of unpleasant odors. The urine receptacle is often changed daily and the tubing every few days.

When tubing is changed or the catheter is disconnected from the tubing for a period of time, for example, when the patient is to be up and walking around, or when a bladder irrigation is to be done, it is vitally important that the sterility of both the catheter and tubing be maintained. Small disposable urinary adaptor protectors are now available. These provide a sterile cover for both tubing and catheter when these are disconnected.

Urinary catheters are usually changed at the physician's order. They are never changed without good reason because of the danger of infection to the patient. If there is any obstruction to urine flow which is not cleared by an irrigation, the catheter should be replaced. Other signs that a catheter may need to be changed are:

1. Insufficient urine in the drainage bottle in comparison with the fluid intake of the patient. Generally, over a 24 hour period the normal urine output is approximately 1500 cc. urine with a similar intake of fluid.

2. Abdominal distention just above the symphysis pubis which on palpation indicates a full bladder (see discussion of urinary retention, p. 382).

Urinary Bladder Irrigation

The procedure of bladder irrigation is not used as commonly today as in times past. It is now felt by many physicians that the danger of introducing infection into the bladder during the course of the irrigation is sufficiently hazardous to offset many of the benefits. When a bladder irrigation is ordered, the importance of maintaining sterile technique during the procedure cannot be overstressed.

A physician might order urinary bladder irrigations for a patient who has an indwelling catheter. The purpose of the irrigations is to cleanse the bladder or to apply an antiseptic solution to the lining of the bladder.

This nursing measure is a sterile procedure similar to urinary catheterization. The equipment required includes a container for the irrigation solution, a receptacle for the returned irrigation solution and a syringe with a tip that fits into the urinary catheter. The solutions that are used for irrigations vary considerably; sterile water, sterile normal saline and many antiseptic solutions are used. The irrigating fluid is usually administered at room temperature unless the physician orders otherwise.

Sterile equipment is used for the bladder irrigation, and sterile technique is maintained throughout this nursing measure. The end of the catheter and the end of the tubing are kept sterile while the bladder is irrigated. Frequently they are put in a sterile container placed close to the patient's leg.

After the tubing has been disconnected from the catheter, a small amount of sterile solution is introduced into the bladder. This is done by using either a funnel or an Asepto syringe. The amount of solution that is recommended for insertion varies in different agencies, many suggesting that no more than 50 to 100 cc. be introduced at any one time. The solution is always administered gently in order not to damage the mucous membrane lining. The fluid should be allowed to run in slowly and the syringe or funnel should be kept low to prevent undue pressure being exerted on the walls of the bladder. The catheter is pinched off before the syringe (or funnel) is completely empty to prevent the introduction of air into the bladder. The fluid is then withdrawn by permitting it to drain from the catheter into a basin. This procedure, the administration of fluid and its return, is repeated until all of the solution ordered has been used or until the return flow is clear.

In recording this nursing measure

the nurse notes and records the strength and kind of solution used in the bladder irrigation and the character of the return flow. Was the return flow cloudy or colored? These observations are charted in the patient's record.

Urinary Bladder Instillation

Some patients require a urinary bladder instillation. Usually this procedure involves the administration of an antiseptic solution or a medication directly into the bladder. It is generally carried out for patients who have indwelling catheters. For this nursing measure the equipment required consists of a sterile syringe and the medication that is ordered by the physician. After the nurse has disconnected the catheter from the tubing, she inserts the medication directly into the catheter and then clamps the catheter, usually for an hour, so that the solution is retained in the patient's bladder.

GUIDE TO ASSESSING NURSING NEEDS

1. Is the patient voiding an amount of urine that is normal in relation to his intake and concomitant with good health?
2. Does he have difficulty in voiding?
3. Does he have difficulty in discussing his urinary problems?
4. Does he show signs and symptoms of renal impairment?
5. Does he show signs of urinary retention?
6. Is he incontinent?
7. Do the laboratory reports show increased levels of non-protein nitrogen in the blood? Abnormalities in the urine?
8. Does the patient need help with his diet and fluid intake?
9. Does the patient need an explanation of laboratory tests and nursing care measures?
10. Does the patient or his family need skills or knowledge in order to prevent a recurrence of his condition or to improve the patient's health?

GUIDE TO EVALUATING THE EFFECTIVENESS OF NURSING ACTION

1. Is the patient taking the required amount of fluids to maintain adequate fluid balance?
2. Are the laboratory test result showing improvement?
3. Is the patient's skin in good condition?
4. Is he getting sufficient rest?
5. Is he taking an adequate diet?
6. Is he comfortable — free from pain, restlessness and anxiety?

STUDY VOCABULARY

Albuminuria	Glycosuria	Polyuria
Anuria	Hematuria	Proteinuria
Calculi	Hemoglobinuria	Pyuria
Casts	Incontinence	Retention
Cystoscopy	Micturition	Suppression
Dysuria	Nocturia	Uremia
Edema	Oliguria	

STUDY SITUATION

Mrs. Smith needs an indwelling catheter prior to her surgery tomorrow. Mrs. Smith is an intelligent person; she understands the purpose of her surgery but she has never had a urinary catheterization. The catheter is to be inserted the next morning.

That afternoon Mrs. Smith's husband comes to the nursing unit desk greatly disturbed. His wife has told him that she has to have a tube inserted and he does not understand why. In talking with Mr. Smith, the nurse learns that his mother had had a tube inserted and she died two days later.

1. What are Mr. Smith's needs relative to his wife's care?
2. What factors should the nurse include in her explanation?
3. What should the nurse include in her explanation to Mrs. Smith? Why?
4. What principles guide the nurse regarding a urinary catheterization?
5. Why is a urinary catheterization a distressing measure?
6. What nursing care measures would be essential for Mrs. Smith as a result of the indwelling catheter?
7. How can the nurse evaluate the effectiveness of her nursing care after the catheterization?

BIBLIOGRAPHY

Bergstrom, N. S.: Ice Application to Induce Voiding. *The American Journal of Nursing,* 69:283, February, 1969.

Bland, John H.: *Clinical Metabolism of Body Water and Electrolytes.* Philadelphia, W. B. Saunders Company, 1963.

Cummings, J. W.: Home Dialysis—Feelings, Facts, Fantasies: The Pressures and How Patients Respond. *The American Journal of Nursing,* 70:70–76, January, 1970.

Delehanty, L., et al.: Achieving Bladder Control. *The American Journal of Nursing,* 70:312, February, 1970.

Garb, Solomon: *Laboratory Tests in Common Use.* Fourth edition. New York, Springer Publishing Company, 1966.

Guyton, Arthur C.: *Textbook of Medical Physiology.* Fourth edition. Philadelphia, W. B. Saunders Company, 1971.

MacKinnon, Harold A.: Urinary Drainage: The Problem of Asepsis. *The American Journal of Nursing,* 65:8:112 August, 1965.

Nordmark, Madelyn T., and Anne W. Rohweder: *Scientific Foundations of Nursing.* Second edition. St. Louis, The C. V. Mosby Company, 1967.

Sawyer, Janet R.: *Nursing Care of Patients with Urologic Diseases.* St. Louis, The C. V. Mosby Company, 1963.

Saxon, Jean: Techniques for Bowel and Bladder Training. *The American Journal of Nursing,* 62:69–71, September, 1962.

Symposium on Patient Care in Kidney and Urinary Tract Disease. *Nursing Clinics of North America,* 4:393, September, 1969.

Sodeman, William A., and William A. Sodeman, Jr. (eds.): *Pathologic Physiology: Mechanisms of Disease.* Fourth edition. Philadelphia, W. B. Saunders Company, 1967.

Sutton, Audrey L.: *Bedside Nursing Techniques in Medicine and Surgery.* Second edition. Philadelphia, W. B. Saunders Company, 1969.

Thornton, George F., and Vincent T. Andriole: Bacteriuria During Indwelling Catheter Drainage. *Journal of the American Medical Association, 214:* 339–342, October 12, 1970.

28 THE CARE OF PATIENTS WHO HAVE PAIN

The nurse should be able to:

Describe the physiological mechanisms for receiving, trans-
  mitting and interpreting pain sensations
Explain present thinking regarding the cause of pain by vari-
  ous types of stimuli
List major types of pain
Differentiate between pain perception and pain reaction
List factors which affect pain perception
Describe physiological manifestations of the pain reaction
List factors influencing an individual's behavioral response
  to pain
Assess the nursing needs of patients who have pain
List principles relevant to the care of patients in pain
Establish goals for nursing action
Determine priorities for care
Describe appropriate nursing action, including measures to
  eliminate or minimize painful stimuli, measures to allevi-
  ate pain and measures to assist patients to handle pain
Establish criteria for evaluating the effectiveness of nursing
  action

INTRODUCTION

Of all of the signs and symptoms of illness, pain is perhaps the most common and the most important. Pain is a sensation that is caused by the action of stimuli of a harmful nature. People who have pain experience varying degrees of distress, from a mild feeling of discomfort to an acute feeling of agony that obliterates all other sensations.

Although distressing, pain is in most instances a protective mechanism that warns the individual that body tissues are being damaged or are about to be damaged. The point at which pain is first felt is called the *pain perception threshold.* In controlled laboratory experiments, it has been found that this threshold is remarkably similar in most individuals under normal circumstances; that is, people subjected to an increasing amount of a painful stimulus, such as an increasing degree of heat applied to an area of the body, report feeling pain at almost exactly the same point of intensity of the stimulus. Yet, this threshold may be altered by a person's physical condition or by his emotional state at the time the pain is experienced.

Then, too, each person's reaction to pain is highly individualistic. Some people accept pain with stoical indifference; others react to similar pain with weeping or other outward displays of suffering. Also, the same individual may react to pain differently under different circumstances. The way in which an individual reacts to pain at any given time appears to be influenced by a number of factors: physical, emotional and cultural.

The reasons for the anomalies in both the perception of pain and the reaction of people to it has intrigued physiologists, psychologists and sociologists for many years. Although pain is such a common symptom of illness, there are still large gaps in our knowledge concerning the mechanisms for receiving, transmitting, interpreting and reacting to pain sensations. Recent research in the fields of neurophysiology, experimental psychology, sociology and nursing has increased our understanding of the phenomenon of pain and contributed to our ability to help people in pain. However, there are still many unanswered questions for which different theories have been proposed.

THE PHYSIOLOGY OF PAIN

It is generally agreed that pain begins with the stimulation of sensory nerve endings located on the body's surface or in the deeper structures. Although it has been traditionally assumed that there were specific receptors for pain, as for touch and temperature, there seems to be evidence that pain is not a pure sensation. Rather, it may be caused by intense stimulation of all types of sensory receptors. Thus, a hot water bottle may feel comfortably warm in one instance but in another, if the temperature of the water it contains is too high, the heat may be painful. Similarly, stroking or patting of the skin with a light pressure may be soothing, whereas rough massage can hurt.

The sensory nerve endings appear to be differentially sensitive to painful stimuli; that is, some are more sensitive to pain than others. Also, some areas of the body are richly supplied with free sensory nerve endings which are sensitive to painful stimuli while other areas are not. The skin has an abundant supply, as have some of the internal organs such as the arterial walls, the joints and the periosteum. Other organs have fewer receptors which are sensitive to pain; the brain and the alveoli of the lungs have none.

Once a pain impulse is initiated by the stimulation of a sensory receptor, the impulse is transmitted rapidly via first-level neurons to the lateral portion of filaments in the spinothalamic tracts of the spinal cord and thence to the thalamus. In the thalamus, there is a crude sorting-out and evaluation of the pain impulses, which are then transmitted via third-level neurons to higher centers in the brain. Between the thalamus and the sensory areas of the cerebral cortex where pain is perceived, it is believed that there is a further sorting-out and evaluation of the sensory impressions. Not all impressions reach the cortex; a person can only focus his attention on a limited number of stimuli at any one time. It is believed that the reticular system of the brain performs the function of evaluating the sensory impressions received in the thalamus and forwarding on to the cortex those of sufficient importance to merit attention.[1] Once the impression reaches the cortex, the person becomes aware of the pain. Action is then set in motion to counteract the noxious stimulus which has caused the pain.

In some instances, the stimulus is of sufficient intensity for a response to be initiated at the cord level. For example, the slightest touch of a hot stove causes a reflex reaction, and the individual withdraws his hand immediately.

Sometimes pain is perceived in one area of the body although the stimulus for its origin was in another area. Pain that is initiated in a deep visceral organ,

for example, may be perceived by the individual on a surface area, or sometimes pain appears to be transferred from one surface area to another. This is called *referred pain.* The pain of myocardial infarction (a blockage in one of the blood vessels supplying the heart muscle) typically gives rise to feelings of pain in the left shoulder and down the left arm of the afflicted individual, in addition to the pain felt in the region of the heart.

The physiological mechanism of referred pain is more complicated than the mechanism just described for the perception of pain. In referred pain, the fibers carrying pain impulses from the viscera are believed to synapse (join together) with other neurons in the spinal cord. If the pain stimulus from the visceral organs is sufficiently intense, the sensation tends to spread over into some areas that normally receive stimuli only from the skin. Thus the individual has the sensation of pain coming from the skin rather than, or as well as, from the viscera.

THE SPINAL-GATING HYPOTHESIS

An interesting theory about pain which is receiving a considerable amount of attention at the present time is called the *spinal-gating hypothesis.* The proponents of this theory contend that the mechanism of pain is not so simple as the explanation just given would indicate. They suggest that in addition to the pain excitory impulses which are traveling upward through the spinal cord, there are also pain inhibiting impulses traveling downward. These inhibiting impulses, it is believed, are carried by larger (in diameter) specialized fibers which run parallel to the small afferent fibers conducting pain excitory impulses. It is felt that when the large fibers are stimulated, they counteract the effect of the small fibers. The net effect of the pain excitory and pain inhibiting impulses is evaluated and forwarded to higher

---

[1]Albert F. Hanken: Pain and Systems Analysis. *Nursing Research,* 15:2:140, Spring 1966.

centers of the brain. Thus, under certain circumstances pain impulses would be permitted to pass through the "spinal gate" and up to the perceptory levels in the brain, while under other circumstances their passage would be blocked. At the present time this theory has been neither proved nor disproved.

THE ETIOLOGY OF PAIN

Generally speaking, any stimulus that causes tissue damage, or is perceived by the individual as potentially causing injury to body tissues, causes pain. Thus, pain may result from a number of different kinds of damaging stimuli, including irritating chemical substances, mechanical trauma, thermal extremes or ischemia (lack of blood flow to a part), as well as from psychogenic factors.

Chemical Irritants

Direct stimulation of free sensory nerve endings by irritating chemical substances will cause pain. A common example of this is the pain that occurs when one spills a drop of acid on the skin. Also, it is now believed that whenever tissues are damaged, certain chemical substances are liberated by the injured cells. Some of these substances trigger the inflammatory response (see Chapter 22). Others, it is felt, excite pain receptors in the damaged area. These substances are believed to include *histamine* and peptides of the *bradykinin* group. They are sometimes referred to simply as *kinins*.[2] Thus, in the case of the acid burn, there is usually an initial sharp, stinging pain, caused by the chemical irritation of the nerve endings by the acid, followed by a longer-lasting pain that is due to the action of substances released by cells that have been damaged by the acid.

---

[2]Cyril M. MacBryde and Robert S. Blacklow (eds.): *Signs and Symptoms: Applied Pathologic Physiology and Clinical Interpretation.* Fifth edition. Philadelphia, J. B. Lippincott Company, 1970, p. 47.

Ischemia

Other chemical irritants that are believed to cause pain are the acidic waste products of cellular metabolism. When these substances accumulate as, for example, in areas of the body where blood supply to a part is not sufficient to carry them away, pain is believed to result from the irritating effect of these substances on free nerve endings. This helps to explain the pain in ischemic areas where blood supply has been cut off or impaired and metabolic waste products accumulate. Another factor in the pain of ischemia is the death of tissue cells in the area, resulting from the loss of blood supply. The decaying cells also liberate irritating chemical substances, as already discussed, and this would contribute to the pain.

Mechanical Trauma

Pain may be incurred by physical force or other mechanical means. When an individual is driving a nail into the wall, for example, the hammer may accidentally hit the thumb instead of the nailhead. The resulting bruise and painful thumb are familiar to most of us. The pain is felt to be caused in this instance by pressure on the nerve endings initially, with chemical irritation from the kinins released by damaged cells as a factor in the continued pain of the bruised tissues.

Pain may also result from *stretching or contraction* of body tissues, or from prolonged pressure on the tissues. Distention of a hollow organ such as the stomach is a common example of stretching of the tissues. If a person eats a very big meal as, for example, at Thanksgiving or Christmas, he may develop considerable discomfort in the region of his stomach. It is believed that stretching of the tissues causes pain because of two possible factors: stretching of the nerve endings in the sensory receptors and the occlusion of small blood vessels in the stretched tissue, which results in localized ischemia.

When *tissues are contracted* as, for

example, in a muscle spasm, there is constriction of small blood vessels in the area with, again, localized ischemia resulting. There may also be stretching of the nerve endings. In addition, in prolonged muscular contraction, cellular metabolism is greatly increased, with a resultant buildup in metabolic waste products which the constricted blood vessels cannot carry away. As already stated, these metabolic waste products are believed to be chemically irritating to sensory nerve endings and therefore to cause pain.

Continued pressure on any body structure causes tissue damage and concomitant pain. The pain is felt to be due to pressure on the nerve endings and also to localized ischemia resulting from the occlusion of small blood vessels in the tissues being pressed. Even the prolonged pressure of sitting too long in the classroom may cause pain unless one changes position or stretches occasionally. Normally a person alters his position every few minutes. This is a conditioned response to the perception of pain sensations which are felt whenever pressure is exerted on any one area for too long. People who have impaired pain perception, for example, unconscious or paralyzed patients, may not feel these pain sensations. The individual does not therefore of his own accord alter his position, and pressure areas can easily develop. For this reason, it is particularly important that the patient is turned frequently and that other measures are taken to prevent prolonged pressure on any part of the body (see Chapter 11).

Thermal Causes of Pain

Extremes of heat and cold cause pain. They also damage body tissues. Everyone is familiar with the burn which is caused by excessive heat, and with the pain that results from even a small burn on the tip of the finger. Here, the initial burning pain probably results from the intensity of the thermal stimulus. The lingering after-pain is felt to be due to the destruction of tissue and the re-

lease of irritating chemical substances from the injured cells. Because burns are one of the most frequent causes of accidental injury to patients, the nurse must be ever alert to protect patients from the danger of solutions that are too hot, heating pads that are set at too high a temperature and the like (see Chapter 20). Again, these precautions are especially important when the patient's pain perception is impaired.

Extreme cold, particularly if there is freezing of body tissues, as in frostbite, also causes tissue damage and accompanying pain. Cold constricts the blood vessels in the affected tissue and may completely cut off the blood supply. The pain in a frostbitten nose or fingers is most severe when the blood flow is returning and the constricted vessels are being dilated.

Psychogenic Pain

Pain may be experienced by an individual in the absence of any physiological basis for it. This occurs in a *conversion reaction*, for example, in which emotional disorders are experienced by the patient as bodily symptoms rather than as mental ones. Pain may also arise from the physiological accompaniments of psychogenic disorders, as in the tension headache caused by contraction of the muscles in the back of the neck and vasodilatation of blood vessels in the head.

CLASSIFICATION OF PAIN

Pain can be classified as superficial, deep or visceral. *Superficial pain* is usually described as having either a burning or a pricking quality. It arises from stimulation of receptors in the skin or the mucous membranes of the body. As a rule, an individual is able to localize surface pain fairly accurately because of the large number of free sensory nerve endings on the surface of the body.

Deep pain arises from the deeper structures of the body such as the muscles, tendons, joints and fasciae. It is usually described as dull, aching, cramping, gnawing or boring. Muscles and tendons are particularly sensitive to pain and may give rise to pain of considerable intensity.

Visceral pain may be perceived as originating in the organ itself, or pain may be felt at a site far removed from the affected viscera through the mechanism of referred pain. It is usually more difficult to localize visceral pain because there are fewer sensory nerve endings in the viscera than on the skin or mucous membranes. The nature of the pain experienced is sometimes highly specific to the particular organ involved and the pathological process that is taking place. In myocardial infarction, for example, the pain is often described as constricting, viselike or compressing. Pain in hollow muscular organs frequently gives rise to sensations of griping, cramping or twisting. In the case of a peptic ulcer, the patient often describes pain as having a gnawing, burning or sometimes knifelike quality. An accurate description of the nature of the pain as reported by the patient often helps the physician to diagnose the cause of the patient's condition. The nurse should be careful, however, not to put her own interpretation on the patient's description nor to suggest words for the patient to use. It is far better to record and report the patient's pain as he describes it in his own words.

The nurse may also hear the term, *central pain*, used. This type of pain arises from injury to sensory nerves, the neural pathways or the areas in the brain which are concerned with pain perception. It is often very difficult for the patient to describe this type of pain since it is usually unlike anything he has experienced before. Some people have, however, described it as gnawing, burning or crushing.[3]

There are also cases of *phantom pain* such as the pain that a patient feels in his toes after the limb has been amputated. This is felt to be due to the per-

sistence of the pain sensation or a "pain memory" after the cause for it is removed.

PAIN PERCEPTION AND PAIN REACTION

There are always two aspects to pain: pain perception and pain reaction. The pain perception threshold, although remarkably the same in most individuals under normal circumstances, may be altered by certain physical and emotional factors. Pain reaction, or the way in which a person reacts to pain, varies considerably from one individual to another and within the same individual under different circumstances. The two aspects of pain can be dissociated. For example, in certain conditions a physician may not be able to do anything about a person's perception of pain, but he may be able to treat the reaction to pain.

Pain Perception

The ability to perceive pain is dependent upon the integrity of the nerve fibers which receive, transmit and interpret pain impulses. Thus, injury to sensory nerves, the sensory tracts in the spinal cord, the thalamus, or sensory areas in the cerebral cortex will interfere with pain perception. A patient who has had a spinal cord injury, for example, and is paralyzed from the waist down does not feel pain in the lower half of his body. This patient must then be protected from harmful stimuli to which a person with normal pain perception would respond by taking suitable action to prevent injury to body tissues. For example, paraplegic patients must be taught to alter their position frequently when they are sitting in a wheelchair, or they soon develop decubitus ulcers. The nurse must also take special precautions to protect paralyzed or unconscious patients from the pressure of tight bed coverings which may cause foot drop, among other distressing effects.

---

[3]Ibid., p. 57.

Sometimes pain perception seems to be facilitated. In some disease conditions affecting the central nervous system, for example, in a neuritis in which the nervous tissue is inflamed, the individual often becomes hypersensitive to painful stimuli. Also, with the prolonged application of painful stimuli, the neural pathways appear to become worn and the pain perception centers hypersensitive. Thus, a person who suffers from continuous pain becomes more, rather than less, sensitive to it.

Areas of the body adjacent to injured areas are usually more sensitive to pain than normal tissue is. The skin adjacent to a wound area, for example, is usually very tender. It is felt that in these cases there is a spillover of pain impulses into neighboring pathways, much the same as in the case of referred pain. There is also the factor of engorgement of the tissues in the wounded area due to the inflammatory process, and this may cause pressure on sensory nerve endings in the surrounding tissue.

Tissues that are already damaged react to additional painful stimuli, even of minimal intensity, much more readily than does normal intact tissue. The sensitivity of the sunburned skin is usually cited as an example of this phenomenon, which might be considered as a case of stimulus overload.

On the other hand, intense pain in one part of the body may raise the pain threshold in other areas. A person who is suffering considerable pain from a broken leg, for example, may not be aware of pain from an abrasion on his elbow. This is probably due to selective perception, the stimulus of greater priority (or intensity) taking precedence in attention over the less intense, or less significant, stimulus.

The pain perception threshold is also altered by an individual's level of consciousness. The unconscious person, for example, the patient under a general anesthetic, does not feel pain. The ability to perceive pain, as tested by a person's reaction to a pinprick or to supraorbital pressure, is frequently used to determine a patient's level of consciousness. Both pain perception and pain reaction may be altered by the emotional state of the individual and by the amount of attention that is focused on the pain. These points are discussed later.

Pain Reaction

There are both physiological and behavioral manifestations in the reaction to pain. The *physiological manifestations* are those of the "alarm reaction" of the body to the threat of danger from any harmful stimulus (see Chapter 3). Among the signs and symptoms that the nurse can observe are pallor, elevated blood pressure, and increased tension of the skeletal muscles. Gastrointestinal functioning may also be impaired. The person in pain usually does not want to eat, and nausea and vomiting are not uncommon accompaniments of pain. Restlessness and irritability are frequently seen. The patient who is in pain cannot rest and he cannot sleep.

With severe pain of any sort, the body's defenses may collapse. In such an event, the nurse may observe signs of weakness and prostration in the patient. His blood pressure may drop and his pulse become weak and slow. There may be increased pallor, and the patient is often described as being "white as a ghost." Collapse and loss of consciousness may ensue.

The *behavioral responses to pain* differ much more widely from one individual to another than do the physiological manifestations. Everyone has observed the individual who "never flinches" even though the pain he experiences is intense. Such behavior is usually much admired in our Western society. On the other hand, some people react to pain with loud groans, weeping, screaming, thrashing about or violent attempts to remove themselves from the source of pain.

A person's reaction to pain is influenced by a number of factors. The individual's physical condition, his emotional state and the way in which he has been conditioned to respond to pain will all affect his reaction to pain in a particular situation.

If a person is tired, or weakened physically, his resistance and control over his reactions are lessened. He may then react to a minimal stimulus with an exaggerated response that is out of all proportion to the intensity of the stimulus. When one is tired, even a small cut on the finger may seem too much to endure, and tears or profanity may be evoked. Thus, the harassed mother who is attempting to cook dinner and, at the same time, look after small children may suffer a slight burn at the stove and promptly burst into tears.

Conversely, in extreme exhaustion, the individual's attention span is markedly reduced and he may not be able to concentrate his attention on any one stimulus for a sufficient length of time to react to it. Thus, the severely sunburned sailor who has been adrift in an open boat may not complain of pain at all, or, if he does, his mind soon wanders from it to other things.

The emotional state of the individual also modifies his reaction to pain. Anxiety and fear aggravate it. This is understandable since anxiety, fear and pain all provoke the same physiological "alarm reaction" in the body in response to stimuli that threaten the individual's safety. Certainly, if anxiety is relieved, the patient's reaction to pain is considerably lessened. If there is a strong emotional response to stimuli other than the pain-producing one, however, this emotional state may block out the awareness of pain. A football player injured during a game may not notice that he has been hurt until the game is over. In this case, excitement and the desire to win may be so intense as to demand the individual's full attention so that the sensory impressions of pain from the injury become of lesser priority and he does not perceive them. A similar explanation could account for the numerous reports of soldiers wounded in battle who state that they did not feel pain even though they had injuries of considerable extent. The overriding fear during the battle and the

necessity for self-preservation at all costs may take precedence over impressions from any other sensory stimulation so that pain is not perceived. Pleasurable emotions tend to nullify pain perception so that the person who is in a happy or contented mood does not usually seem to feel pain to the same extent as the worried patient.

Then, too, an individual's emotional makeup, his cultural and social background and his early home and school training have a great deal to do with his behavior in response to painful stimuli. There has been much study by sociologists, for example, of the differing reactions of various cultural groups to pain.[4] The North American Indian is often cited as an example of a member of a cultural group in which stoical indifference to pain is a highly valued characteristic. Among people of Latin origin, on the other hand, an open display of suffering is usually permitted as the socially approved response to pain.

In our Western society, very strong values are placed on bravery, endurance and the ability to bear pain with silent fortitude. Children in our culture are taught very early that they are expected not to cry when they are hurt. "Be brave," "Don't be a sissy," and "Only babies cry," are the frequent admonishments of mothers to young children. Even children from differing ethnic groups, in which the open display of suffering is permitted, soon learn from their teachers and from their peer groups in school and on the playground that they must react to pain in the accepted North American manner or be scorned by their fellows.

The nurse who has been raised in this framework of "only babies cry" may find herself reacting negatively to the patient who does not handle his pain in the "approved" manner. If she realizes that her reaction is normal and a reflection of her social values, which are different from those of the patient, she is in a better position to analyze and accept her own feelings. These feelings

[4]Mark Zborowski: *People in Pain.* San Francisco, Jossey-Bass Inc., 1969.

then need not interfere with her acceptance and support of the patient.

ASSESSING THE NURSING NEEDS OF PATIENTS WHO HAVE PAIN

Pain is probably the most personal and the most distressing of all the symptoms of disease. Only the individual who is experiencing the pain really knows what it is like. The primary source of information about the pain he is having then is always the patient. Other sources the nurse can use include her own observations of the patient and those of other members of the health team.

Information Obtained from the Patient

In gathering information about the patient's pain, the nurse should ascertain, whenever possible, the following aspects of the pain experience:
1. The quality of the pain
2. The location of the pain
3. The intensity of the pain
4. The time it occurs and its duration
5. Any factors which appear to precipitate the pain
6. Any measures which relieve it or measures which the patient has tried to relieve it

Quality. Patients use many descriptive terms when talking about pain. A number of the terms commonly used have been mentioned earlier in the chapter in the section on classification of pain. Frequently patients describe pain in terms of something that is familiar to them. Thus, pain may be likened to the cutting action of a knife, if it is a sharp, piercing pain; or to "hammers pounding inside the head" in certain types of headache. In recording and reporting pain, the nurse should use the exact words the patient has used in order to convey an accurate description of the pain as the patient perceives it.

Location. The patient is usually able to localize superficial pain fairly accurately and also pain arising from bones, muscles, joints and blood vessels. Visceral pain is more difficult to localize. Often, the patient complains of pain generally in the epigastric region, or in the lower part of the abdomen, in the chest, or the lower back when a visceral organ is affected. Often, too, the pain from viscera is referred to a surface area. An exact description of the location of the pain is of considerable assistance to the physician in diagnosing the patient's condition, and to the nurse in planning her care.

Intensity. The degree of pain felt by the patient is also important in assessing his nursing needs and the need for medical or nursing intervention. Certain tissues are more sensitive to pain than others; for example, muscle tissue appears to be highly responsive to painful stimuli, and the pain from bruised or ischemic muscles may be excruciating. Hence, it is necessary to use great care in moving patients who have disorders involving the musculoskeletal system.

When the intensity of the patient's pain changes abruptly, it is usually an indication that the nature of his condition has altered. For example, when an inflamed appendix ruptures, or a peptic ulcer perforates, the patient usually experiences very sharp and severe pain which persists and is quite different both in quality and intensity from the pain felt previously.

Time and Duration. An accurate description of the patient's pain should include when it occurs, how long it lasts, and whether it is an intermittent pain that recurs or a steady pain that continues. Pain is often most severe at night, when a person is alone. A possible explanation for this is that, in the absence of other people or activities to distract him, the individual's full attention is then focused on his discomfort. The duration of the pain is very important. An example of this may be found in obstetrics, in which the length of the interval between pains and the time each pain lasts are significant in assessing the patient's progress in labor, the muscular contractions of the uterus becoming stronger and closer together as delivery becomes imminent.

Precipitating Factors. Pain is often related to the patient's activities. In some cardiac conditions, pain may be brought on by exertion, and in planning the patient's care, it is important to know how much activity the patient can tolerate. Sometimes it is necessary to space nursing measures to allow the patient to rest between activities. For example, it may be wise in some cases to leave the patient's bath until an hour or so after breakfast in order to give him time to rest after the exertion of eating a meal. With patients who have musculoskeletal problems, pain is frequently associated with movement of the affected structure. Again, it is important to know exactly what movement precipitates pain, both for medical assessment of the patient's condition and for planning care to minimize the patient's discomfort. Pain in the gastrointestinal tract may be precipitated by eating certain foods. Or pain may be related to an intolerance of factors in the environment. Noise may bring on a headache, for example. Very often the patient is able to identify the specific factor or factors which cause pain, and these should be recorded and reported, again using the patient's own words in preference to an interpretation of what he says.

Measures Which Relieve Pain. Frequently, the patient has tried a number of measures to relieve his pain before he seeks medical help. The nurse should ascertain the measures he has tried and the effectiveness of these is relieving his pain. For example, does rest relieve the pain that is brought on by exertion? Does holding the limb in a certain way prevent pain on movement? This type of information is of value both to the physician in his assessment of the patient's condition and the development of a plan of therapy, and to the nurse in her determination of nursing measures which will help to alleviate pain.

Information Obtained Through Observation

The nurse can supplement the information she obtains from the patient with her observations of his reaction to the pain. She should be alert to the physiological manifestations of pain as these have just been described. Very often the patient's facial expression and posture will indicate that he is having pain. The patient in pain often has a typical facial grimace: his brows are knotted, his facial muscles are tense and drawn and his mouth is often drawn downward. In addition, he may assume a characteristic position to minimize the

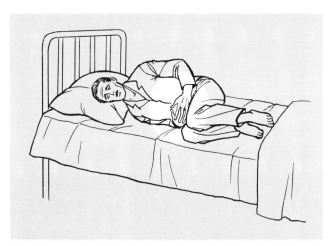

A person who is experiencing pain may assume a position indicative of the site of the pain.

pain. With abdominal pain, the patient may draw up his knees and curl into a ball; for a sore arm he may hold the affected part. In severe pain patients sometimes lie rigidly because any movement intensifies the discomfort. Some patients, because of their training to bear pain in stoical silence, do not like to complain of pain. As a result, the nurse may find it difficult to identify even the existence of pain. Pallor, muscular tension (as in the drawn facial muscles or a clenching of the fists), posture, inactivity and profuse perspiration may be the only outward evidences of pain in these people.

The nurse may, however, often note other behavior in patients who are having pain. Restlessness and increased sensitivity to stimuli in the environment, such as noise and bright lights, are frequently indicative of pain. The patient in pain often shows evidence of increased emotional tension as well; he may react with irritability and bad humor to people or things that disturb him. Pain usually prevents people from sleeping or resting comfortably, and, because pain is usually worse at night, insomnia may be a problem. Nursing measures to ensure that the patient is relieved of pain are important in order to enable him to rest.

Information from Other Sources

Frequently pain is the principal symptom which prompts people to seek medical help. The physician then has usually investigated the nature of the patient's pain, and the nurse can often obtain much information from the physician himself or from the notes he has made on the patient's record. Of particular importance are notations made regarding factors which precipitate pain, since the nurse may be able to institute measures to eliminate or minimize these factors.

The observations made by all members of the nursing team who are caring for the patient contribute to the total picture of the patient's pain. These observations should be accurately reported and recorded so that all staff members are aware of measures that prevent, minimize or alleviate the patient's pain, as well as factors that aggravate it.

In addition, other members of the health team, such as the physical therapist, can often contribute information about the patient's pain. The physical therapist usually assists in assessing the patient's mobility and functional ability and can provide guidance to nursing personnel on activities which the patient can tolerate without pain. The patient's family too can be helpful in regard to the nature of the patient's pain, factors that precipitate it and measures which help to alleviate it. Some people are reluctant to admit that they have pain, or may try to minimize its severity when talking to medical personnel, usually again because of their cultural background; yet they have often confided the extent of their suffering to their wife or husband. Or, the wife may be aware of such evidences of her husband's discomfort as his inability to sleep or his restlessness and increased irritability.

PRINCIPLES RELEVANT TO THE CARE OF PATIENTS IN PAIN

Pain has a protective function in warning a person of present or potential damage to body tissues.

Pain may be caused by a number of different kinds of stimuli.

Tissues of the body differ in their sensitivity to painful stimuli.

Severe pain can cause collapse of the body's adaptive mechanisms.

The ability to perceive pain is dependent upon the integrity of the neural structures which receive, transmit and interpret pain impulses.

Pain perception may be altered by certain physical and emotional factors.

A person's reaction to pain is highly individualized and depends on a number of factors — physical, emotional and cultural.

OBJECTIVES FOR NURSING INTERVENTION

Nursing action for the patient who is having pain is directed primarily toward three goals:
1. Eliminating or minimizing the stimuli that are causing pain
2. Alleviating pain
3. Assisting the patient to handle pain

DETERMINING PRIORITIES FOR NURSING ACTION

The relief of pain is always a matter of priority for nursing action. However, there are some circumstances in which it is more urgent than others, when the prompt treatment of pain is essential to save a person's life or to prevent damage to body structures. Severe pain can cause a collapse of the body's adaptive mechanisms. Hence, the presence of severe pain in a patient requires immediate intervention. The nurses's judgment of the patient's condition is extremely important. If she observes signs of weakness and prostration such as markedly increased pallor, a lowered blood pressure and weakened pulse in a patient who is having pain, the physician should be notified immediately so that his guidance can be obtained on the measures to be taken. He may wish the administration of analgesics discontinued and other measures such as intravenous infusion with supportive drug therapy instituted. Or he may feel that the patient's condition warrants immediate surgical intervention.

The action of pain-relieving drugs is more effective if these are administered before the pain reaches a peak. Early intervention at the beginning of pain, then, can often prevent a serious attack. This is important in such conditions as myocardial infarction, or biliary or renal colic (stones in the bile duct or the ureter of the kidney), in which the pain can mount to agonizing proportions. The patient's request for pain relief should be answered without delay.[5]

Another situation in which the prompt relief of pain is imperative is in the care of the surgical patient. The restlessness that accompanies increasing pain can sometimes cause damage to newly sutured tissues. The patient should therefore be kept comfortable at all times during the immediate postoperative period. Analgesics for the relief of pain are usually prescribed every three to four hours as needed (p.r.n.) for the first 48 hours following surgery. The nurse's judicious administration of these medications can make the patient's recovery from surgery much easier.

The relief of pain is not always, of course, a matter of administering a medication. Many times nursing measures such as changing the patient's position, straightening his bed, or helping him to overcome his anxiety are equally effective in alleviating pain. In exercising judgment as to the appropriate measures to be taken, the nurse utilizes her knowledge about the patient's medical condition and also her knowledge of each individual patient and his reaction to pain.

MEASURES TO ELIMINATE OR MINIMIZE PAINFUL STIMULI

Whenever possible, it is always better to prevent pain than to treat it. One cannot always do this, of course. Many times pain is the chief reason a person has sought medical help. Investigation of the cause of pain and elimination of its source frequently constitute a major part of the patient's total care. The nurse can often help to control the extent of his suffering, however, through eliminating or minimizing known causes of pain and discomfort.

Pain is usually a warning signal that body tissues are being damaged or are about to be damaged. When exertion brings on pain, the patient's activities may need to be curtailed to prevent

[5]Virginia Jarratt: The Keeper of the Keys. *The American Journal of Nursing*, 65:7:68–70, July, 1965.

further injury to body cells. The patient with a heart condition, for example, must learn to moderate his activities to prevent further damage to the heart and concomitant pain. The activities of the surgical patient, to use another example, are usually restricted until the wounded tissues have healed sufficiently that normal movement will not disturb the healing process.

It is not possible to curtail all movement that is painful, though, nor is it always wise. The dangers of immobility in people who are sick have been well documented and referred to many times throughout this text. The postoperative patient, for example, must move about and must breathe deeply and cough to prevent respiratory complications, even though these activities cause him some pain. The nurse's actions are then directed toward minimizing the patient's discomfort. Supporting the patient's incision can lessen pain when he coughs or breathes deeply. The nurse may use her hands to support the incision, or sometimes a pillow held firmly against the operative area will accomplish the

same purpose. A binder may be needed to provide support to the operative area when the patient is up and walking around.

Whenever it is necessary to lift or turn a patient for whom movement is painful, the utmost gentleness should be used. The nurse should always make certain that she has sufficient help in moving the patient so that he is not subjected to unnecessary pain or discomfort. Supporting a painful limb while turning the patient can help to minimize his discomfort. In addition, devices such as a "turning sheet" which is placed under the patient can sometimes be used to advantage to prevent excessive handling of painful limbs.

All the comfort measures which have been discussed in earlier chapters are important in eliminating sources of pain for the patient. For example, helping a patient to change his position relieves muscle strain and also prevents pressure on any particular part of the body for too long a period of time. Positioning to maintain good body alignment aids in preventing painful muscu-

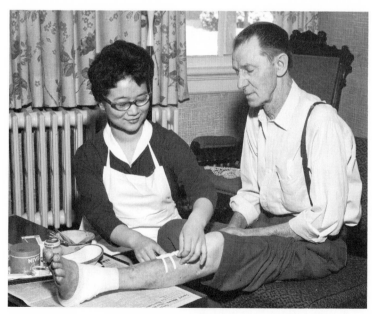

Changing a patient's dressing helps to eliminate irritating stimuli that can cause pain.

lar contractures. A soothing back rub will often help to relax a patient and ease muscular tension. Also, helping the patient to stay dry and comfortable and relieving any sources of irritation can aid in eliminating stimuli that can cause pain.

The nurse should remember too that helping the patient to meet his basic physiological needs can eliminate many existing or potential sources of pain. For example, food can prevent or relieve the uncomfortable muscular contractions of an empty stomach. Seeing that the patient is taking sufficient fluids helps to prevent the distressing effects of dehydration (see Chapter 29). The pain caused by a distended bladder and the discomfort of constipation are both preventable by nursing action and may be relieved by specific nursing techniques (see Chapters 24 and 27). Ensuring that the patient gets sufficient rest and sleep is an important consideration also, since fatigue lowers a person's resistance and control, thereby increasing his reaction to painful stimuli.

MEASURES TO ALLEVIATE PAIN

In determining the most appropriate action to alleviate pain, the nurse must take into consideration both the physical pain the patient is experiencing and the emotional distress that accompanies it. It is often difficult to assess how much of the pain is caused by psychological factors and how much is due to physical pain. Measures that focus on relieving the emotional component can often dispel pain in themselves, or can enhance the effectiveness of physical measures.

Psychological Measures

In some instances, dramatic results have been obtained in pain relief with the use of purely psychological measures. Hypnosis, for example, has been a successful form of treatment for some patients, and sometimes "placebos"

(which contain no drugs) are as effective as the administration of analgesics. In both hypnosis and placebo administration, *suggestion* is the key factor in relieving the patient's pain.

Distraction is helpful sometimes in lessening an individual's awareness of painful stimuli. Pain is accentuated when attention is focused on it. The individual who is engaged in activities such as reading, watching an interesting television program or talking with other people has a number of sensory impressions competing for his attention, and his awareness of pain sensations may thus be lessened. It should be remembered that, if a patient does not have diversional activities, he becomes much preoccupied with his own self. Mild discomforts which might otherwise not be noted assume major importance. In planning situations or activities that are diversional, though, the nurse must assess them carefully to ensure that they are neither irritating to the patient nor fatiguing. Visitors are sometimes helpful in distracting patients from their discomfort. However, the nurse should be aware of the individual patient's preference in this regard; some prefer not to have visitors because they find them tiring or irritating.

Changing a person's attitude toward a potentially painful experience can alter his reaction to pain. The success of "natural childbirth" methods in obstetrics illustrates this point. These methods are based largely on the preparation of the expectant mother to anticipate childbirth as a joyful event rather than as a cause of pain and suffering. It should be noted that this approach does much to eliminate the fear of childbirth.

The extent to which anxiety and fear are contributing factors in pain is difficult to determine. Both anxiety and fear intensify the reaction to pain so that, if these can be successfully reduced, the individual is often relieved of much of his distress. Measures to assist in relieving anxiety were discussed in Chapter 9, and it is suggested that, at this point, the student may find it helpful to review that chapter.

A number of studies in recent years have demonstrated that the nurse's interaction with the patient is a significant factor in the relief of pain. Such actions as talking with the patient, using comfort measures, or positive suggestion coupled with a comfort measure, have all been used with success in various situations. To be effective, however, these actions must be based on a feeling of trust and confidence that has been established between the patient and the nurse. The student may find it helpful in this regard to read the reports of some of the studies which have been done on nursing approaches to the patient in pain. A number of these reports are listed in the bibliography at the end of this chapter.

Physical Measures

Psychological measures will not, of course, relieve all pain. In some cases, the physiological cause of pain can be ameliorated by using physical agents. The pain-relieving actions of *heat* and *cold*, for example, are well known (see Chapter 20). In general, heat tends to relieve pain through increasing circulation in the part of the body to which it is applied. Hence, heat is often effective in the relief of muscular aches and pains, since the increased circulation helps to carry away metabolic waste products which are felt to be a factor in causing muscular pain. A warm bath, for example, often helps to relieve aching muscles after a person has engaged in strenuous exercise. Cold has the opposite effect of heat, that is, it decreases peripheral circulation. In doing so, it helps to reduce swelling and therefore pressure on sensory nerve endings. An ice collar is frequently used to relieve pain following operations on the throat when the tissues are swollen and painful. Cold is also used sometimes as a local anesthetic agent. The intense cold in this case serves to deaden sensory nerve endings, thus preventing the transmission of pain impulses.

Therapeutic baths are also used to relieve pain. Sometimes the bath is a means of applying heat or cold to the body. Sometimes it is a vehicle for other agents as, for example, in the colloid baths that are frequently used for people with irritating skin conditions (see Chapter 20).

Massage has had a long history of use in the treatment of pain of muscular origin. The effect of massage is similar to that of heat in that it increases circulation to a part, thereby accelerating removal of the waste products of cellular metabolism.

Then, too, there are the numerous *pharmacological agents* that are used for pain relief. These tend to fall into two groups: those that are "specifics" for certain conditions and those which have a general analgesic effect. Among the specifics are the muscle relaxants, such as meprobamate, which is used in conditions such as spastic paralysis, and phenylbutazone, which is a central nervous system depressant frequently prescribed for patients with arthritic conditions.

The principal drugs used as general analgesics include the narcotics, such as morphine, codeine and their derivatives; synthetic compounds such as Demerol and Darvon; and the analgesic-antipyretic group of drugs, of which aspirin is by far the most widely used. Considerable controversy still exists over the physiological reason for the effectiveness of these drugs in pain relief. The narcotics, we know, have a depressant action on the central nervous system. Some experts believe that these drugs act on the cortico-thalamic pathways and the perceptive areas of the brain to cause a reduction in pain sensations. Others feel that the action of morphine and the other narcotics is principally that of mood alteration, so that the person remains aware of the pain, but his reaction to it is diminished. Morphine, its derivatives, and some of the stronger synthetic compounds such as Demerol, are used in cases of severe pain; codeine for pain of lesser intensity. Tranquilizing drugs, such as Phenergan and chlorpromazine, are sometimes given at the same time as a narcotic. Their action appears to enhance the pain-relieving properties of the narcotic so that a smaller dosage of the analgesic may be used.

With regard to the analgesic-antipyretic group of drugs, most experts seem to agree that these agents in some way block the transmission of pain impulses, probably in the thalamic pathways, thus decreasing the perception of pain. Aspirin and other drugs of this group are used extensively for the relief of minor aches and pains.[6]

The nurse's responsibility in the administration of analgesics is a crucial one. Sometimes prescriptions are written for analgesics to be given every four hours, or at other specified times (as, for example, is frequently the case with patients who have arthritic and rheumatoid disorders). In most instances, however, the orders are written as *p.r.n.*, and the nurse must use her judgment as to the time of administration and the interval between medications. Many times the nurse is faced too with the decision of which of two or three analgesic orders to use for a patient. He may, for example, have morphine sulphate, Darvon and aspirin all prescribed for pain relief. If the patient is having pain, the nurse must then decide on the medication to be used in this particular situation or whether, in fact, the patient may be made comfortable by measures other than drugs. In making this decision, the nurse is guided by her knowledge of the disease process the patient has, her understanding of the factors causing his pain and her knowledge of the individual patient. A patient who is suffering from incurable cancer and is in the terminal stages of illness may require a strong narcotic to effectively relieve his pain. For the person who has a simple headache, aspirin may be sufficient to bring relief. Sometimes, changing the patient's position is all that is needed to make him more comfortable.

MEASURES TO ASSIST THE PATIENT TO HANDLE PAIN

One of the nurse's most important functions is the provision of psychological support for the patient in pain. Discussing the meaning pain holds for the patient is one way of doing this. Sometimes the nurse will find that it is not really pain which is bothering the patient but something else. He may be concerned with the results of his surgery, for instance, and view anything that he thinks is unusual as indicative that he has an incurable condition. Possibly the patient may be worried about his ability to tolerate pain, particularly if he has been raised with the Western ethic of stoicism.

Knowing what to expect in the way of pain often enables a person to prepare himself to cope with the situation; it also removes much of the fear of the unknown so that anxiety is lessened. Many diagnostic and therapeutic procedures which patients have to undergo are uncomfortable or even painful. If it is known that a patient is scheduled for an examination or treatment that is potentially painful, it is usually better to explain to the patient exactly what is going to be done, the nature of the pain he may experience and what he can do to assist. If the individual understands also why the procedure is necessary, he is usually much better able to cooperate. Explanations of this sort can often help to change the individual's attitude toward the painful experience, since pain that is viewed as an aid in getting better is usually more tolerable than pain inflicted for reasons a person does not understand.

Even with children, telling them that a procedure is going to hurt a little, and what the hurt will be like, is much preferable to telling them that it is not going to hurt and then proceeding to inflict pain. The latter course of action can destroy a child's trust in medical

---

[6]For a more extensive coverage of analgesics, the nurse is referred to *The Drug, The Nurse, The Patient* by Mary W. Falconer, Mabelclaire R. Norman, H. Robert Patterson, and Edward A. Gustafson. Fourth edition. Philadelphia, W. B. Saunders Company, 1971, pp. 121–131.

personnel. A factual explanation of exactly what is going to happen to them can usually eliminate much fear for both adults and children.

Reassuring the patient that pain will not be beyond his level of tolerance is sometimes advisable. "If it hurts too much, we will give you something to relieve the pain" is an example of words that can sometimes be used. Touch, for instance, placing a hand on the patient's arm, is often helpful when a patient is undergoing a painful procedure. The nurse should be careful in the use of touch, however. Some patients dislike it, particularly if they are striving to maintain their independence. Many, however, are grateful for a hand to hold when pain seems too much to bear alone.

Enabling the patient to retain a measure of control over the situation can also be helpful in minimizing the reaction to pain. "Tell me when it hurts and we will stop for a minute" is one way of doing this. Involving the patient in some part of the activity, such as holding a piece of the equipment, can help to make him feel a participating member of the health team rather than an object of its actions. Again, distraction can sometimes be used. If the patient is concentrating on taking deep breaths, for example, his attention will not be entirely focused on his pain.

After a painful experience is over, the nurse should make certain that the patient is settled comfortably. Evidence of the painful procedure, such as the dressing tray, should be removed as soon as possible. Some nurses have found that staying with the patient and allowing him to talk over the experience helps him to put it into perspective.[7]

Helping the patient who suffers pain over a long period of time, for instance, the patient with a chronic disease condition, is frequently a challenge to nursing personnel. The nurse can often help to minimize his pain, if not always to completely alleviate it, by some of the measures discussed in previous sections. The nurse can also make certain that in her care of the patient she does not aggravate his pain. She can, for example, use gentleness when handling painful limbs and remove potential sources of pain and discomfort. It has been suggested too that helping the patient to find a meaning for his suffering can be of assistance to the patient in handling chronic pain.[8] In this regard, many patients have found their spiritual counsellor of considerable help and some have benefited from psychiatric counselling.

EVALUATING THE EFFECTIVENESS OF NURSING ACTION

Because pain is a very personal experience, the nurse must rely to a large extent on the patient for an assessment of the effectiveness of pain relieving measures. The patient can, for example, tell the nurse if the pain is gone or is lessened in intensity and whether he feels more comfortable. The nurse can also supplement the patient's observations with her own. She may note that muscular tension has eased and the patient appears more relaxed. His restlessness and irritability may be observably lessened. Or, the alleviation of pain may be inferred because the patient is sleeping quietly or resting comfortably. Sometimes, the effect of pain relief may be that the patient is able to enjoy activities, such as meals or visitors, that he did not enjoy when he was in pain. Checking to see if pain-relieving measures were effective is important. If they were not effective, the nurse must then reassess the situation and try an alternative course of action.

[7]For further suggestions on helping patients to handle pain, the student is referred to the article, Nursing Intervention for Bodily Pain, by Margo McCaffery and Fay Moss in *The American Journal of Nursing*, 67:6:1224–1227, June, 1967.

[8]The Loneliness of Suffering. *The Canadian Nurse*, 61:4:299, May, 1965.

GUIDE TO ASSESSING NURSING NEEDS

1. What words does the patient use to describe his pain?
2. Where does the patient feel pain? Can he describe its exact location?
3. How severe is the pain? Does its intensity vary?
4. When does the pain occur? How long does it last? Is it intermittent or steady?
5. Has the cause of the patient's pain been identified?
6. Is the patient aware of any factors which precipitate the pain? Which aggravate it or relieve it?
7. Are there observable signs of pain, for example, evidence of muscular tension, protective posture, pallor, diaphoresis?
8. Are there signs that would lead you to suspect that the patient's pain has been sufficiently intense to cause a collapse of the body's adaptive mechanisms, such as a lowered blood pressure or weakened pulse?
9. Is the patient restless, irritable? Does he have difficulty in getting to sleep?
10. Are the patient's basic physiological needs being met?
11. Are there factors which might cause the patient to be anxious or fearful?
12. How much exertion can the patient tolerate without pain? Are there certain movements or activities which are painful?
13. Does he have to undergo any procedures which may be painful?
14. What measures have been prescribed for relief of the patient's pain?

GUIDE TO EVALUATING THE EFFECTIVENESS OF NURSING ACTION

1. Does the patient state that he is more comfortable? Has the pain gone or lessened in intensity?
2. Does the patient appear more comfortable, that is, is he more relaxed, less restless and irritable?
3. Has the patient been able to get to sleep without difficulty? Or to rest quietly?
4. Is he able to enjoy his usual activities?

STUDY VOCABULARY

Analgesic	Pain perception
Bradykinin	Pain perception threshold
Central pain	Pain reaction
Conversion reaction	Phantom pain
Deep pain	Referred pain
Histamine	Superficial pain
Ischemia	Visceral pain

STUDY SITUATION

Mrs. Jean Roberts is admitted to the hospital after an automobile accident in which she has possibly fractured her ribs. Mrs. Roberts' husband was also injured at the same time, and he is admitted to a nearby nursing unit. He has a fractured pelvis. Mrs. Roberts is 33 years old, has three small children at home and is in a great deal of pain upon admission. Her physician does not wish to bind her chest at this time. His orders include:

Demerol 100 mg. I.M. q.4.h. p.r.n.
Seconal gr. 1½ q.h.s.
Up and about as desired
Food and fluids as desired
Chest x-rays as soon as possible

1. What observations would indicate to the nurse that the patient has pain?
2. What should the nurse include in her recording of this patient's pain? Give an example of the recording.
3. What are the nursing care objectives for this patient?
4. What factors would enter into this patient's perception of and reaction to pain?
5. Describe the physiology of this patient's pain.
6. Outline nursing objectives for this patient.
7. What specific nursing care measures might help alleviate pain?
8. By what criteria can the nurse evaluate the success of the nursing care?

BIBLIOGRAPHY

Baer, Eva, Lois Jean Davitz and Renee Liab: Inferences of Physical Pain and Psychological Distress. *Nursing Research,* 19:5:338–401, September-October, 1970.

Beecher, H. K.: Anxiety and Pain. *Journal of the American Medical Association,* 209:7:1080, August 18, 1969.

Billars, Karen S.: You Have Pain? I Think This Will Help. *The American Journal of Nursing,* 70:10:2143–2145, October, 1970.

Chambers, Wildan G., and Geraldine G. Price: Influence of Nurse Upon Effects of Analgesics Administered. *Nursing Research,* 16:3:228–233, Summer, 1967.

Ewing, Gerald. Pain. *The Canadian Nurse,* 61:6:443–445, June, 1965.

Falconer, Mary W., Mabelclaire R. Norman, H. Robert Patterson and Edward A. Gustafson: *The Drug, The Nurse, The Patient.* Fourth edition. Philadelphia, W. B. Saunders Company, 1970.

Francis, Gloria M., and Barbara Munjas: *Promotion of Psychological Comfort.* Dubuque, Iowa, William C. Brown Company, Publishers, 1968.

Graffam, Shirley Ruth: Nurse Response to the Patient in Distress — Development of an Instrument. *Nursing Research,* 19:4:331–336, July-August, 1970.

Guyton, Arthur C.: *Textbook of Medical Physiology.* Fourth edition. Philadelphia, W. B. Saunders Company, 1971.

Hanken, Albert F.: Pain and Systems Analysis. *Nursing Research,* 15:2:139–143, Spring, 1966.

Jarratt, Virginia.: The Keeper of the Keys. *The American Journal of Nursing,* 65:7:68–70, July, 1965.

MacBryde, Cyril M., and Robert S. Blacklow (eds.): *Signs and Symptoms: Applied Pathologic Physiology and Clinical Interpretation.* Fifth edition. Philadelphia, J. B. Lippincott Company, 1970.

McBride, Mary Angela B.: Nursing Approach, Pain and Relief: An Exploratory Experiment. *Nursing Research,* 16:4:337–341, Fall, 1967.

McCaffery, Margo, and Fay Moss: Nursing Intervention for Bodily Pain. *The American Journal of Nursing,* 67:6:1224–1227, June, 1967.

Moss, Fay T., and Burton Meyer: The Effects of Nursing Interaction Upon Pain Relief in Patients. *Nursing Research,* 15:4:303–306, Fall, 1966.

Nordmark, Madelyn T., and Anne W. Rohweder: *Scientific Foundations of Nursing.* Second edition. Philadelphia, J. B. Lippincott Company, 1967.

Pain. *Medical World News*, December 11, 1970, pp. 26–32.

Pepin, Sister Irene, and Del Howe: Nursing the Patient in Pain. *The Canadian Nurse, 61*:6:446–448, June, 1965.

The Loneliness of Suffering. *The Canadian Nurse, 61*:4:299, May, 1965.

Walike, B. C., and Burton Meyer: Relations Between Placebo Reactivity and Selected Personality Factors. *Nursing Research, 15*:303–306, Fall, 1966.

Zborowski, Mark: *People in Pain,* San Francisco, Jossey-Bass Inc., 1969.

29 THE CARE OF PATIENTS WHO HAVE FLUID AND ELECTROLYTE PROBLEMS

The nurse should be able to:

Describe the distribution of fluid and the major electrolytes
    in the body
Identify the normal methods of fluid and electrolyte intake
    and output to and from the body
Explain the principal factors regulating fluid and electrolyte
    balance in the body
Identify the principal mechanisms which maintain the body's
    acid-base balance
List common causes of fluid and electrolyte imbalance
Assess the nursing needs of patients with fluid and electro-
    lyte problems
List signs and symptoms of common problems of fluid and
    electrolyte imbalance
Recognize significant laboratory findings which may be in-
    dicative of fluid and electrolyte imbalance
List principles relevant to fluid and electrolyte balance
Establish goals for nursing action
Determine priorities for care
Describe appropriate nursing action including measures to
    assist patients to maintain fluid and electrolyte balance
    and to assist in the restoration of a balance if a disturbance
    has occurred
Establish criteria for evaluating the effectiveness of nursing
    action

INTRODUCTION

Water has been called the indispensable nutrient.[1] Approximately 50 to 70 per cent of the total body weight of an adult is made up of water and its dissolved constituents; 70 to 80 per cent of the total body weight of the newborn is similarly in a fluid state. The fluid system plays an essential role in the body. Its principal functions are (1) the transportation of oxygen and nutrients to the cells and the removal of waste products from them and (2) the maintenance of a stable physical and chemical environment within the body.

Important in the latter function are the electrolytes. The student will recall from her chemistry courses that electrolytes are compounds which in water solution separate into particles, each capable of carrying an electrical charge. A cation is a positively charged particle; an anion is a negatively charged one. The chief cations in body fluids are sodium, potassium, calcium and magnesium, while chloride, phosphate, bicarbonate and sulfate are the principal anions. The electrolytes in body fluids are important in the chemical reactions that occur within cells. They also help to regulate the permeability of cell membranes, thus controlling the diffusion of various materials across the membrane. They are vital to the maintenance of the body's acid-base balance and are also essential in the transmission of electrical energy within the body. Without the calcium ion, for example, muscle contraction could not occur.

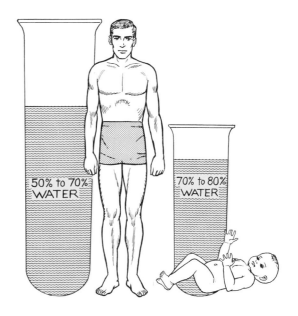

50% to 70% WATER

70% to 80% WATER

Under normal circumstances, the body maintains a very precise fluid and electrolyte balance. Both the volume and the constituents of body fluids vary but little from day to day, and usually return to a state of equilibrium within a very few days following any minor disturbance.

Serious fluid and electrolyte imbalance may occur, however, as a result of a number of pathological conditions. The nature of the imbalance may be one of excess or insufficiency. An individual may, for example, retain an excess amount of fluid in the tissues and become edematous. On the other hand, he may lose an inordinate amount of fluids, through persistent vomiting, for example, and become dehydrated. Whenever fluids are lost or retained in excessive amounts, there is an accompanying loss or retention of electrolytes so that both fluid and electrolyte balance are disturbed.

Disturbances in fluid and electrolyte

[1]James R. Robinson: Water, the Indispensable Nutrient. *Nutrition Today*, pp. 16–25, Spring, 1970.

balance cause serious repercussions within the body. Both the transportation and regulatory functions of the fluid system are likely to be affected. The cells may not get sufficient nourishment, for instance, or there may be an accumulation of waste products due to inefficiency of the mechanism for their removal. The body's acid-base balance may be upset and temperature regulation impaired (see Chapter 23). There may also be interference with the transfer of materials across the cell membrane so that a shift occurs in the distribution of fluids and electrolytes. Activities within the body which depend on the transmission of electrical energy, such as muscle contraction and the relay of nervous impulses, may also show impairment of function.

Whenever there is a disturbance in fluid and electrolyte balance, the body attempts to compensate for the lack or the excess, whichever the case may be, by bringing into play various adaptive mechanisms. A very common example of this occurs in the person who perspires heavily on a hot day and then finds that he is thirsty for extra fluids to replace those he has lost through sweating. The body has a number of adaptive mechanisms in addition to thirst; these are discussed later in this chapter.

If the imbalance is too great, however, or persists over a prolonged period of time, the body's adaptive mechanisms may not be able to cope. In this event, the body's defenses collapse and prostration ensues. This may happen, for example, when there is a continuous loss of fluids with no replacement, or a very sudden large loss, as in a massive hemorrhage.

THE PHYSIOLOGY OF FLUID AND ELECTROLYTE BALANCE

To understand the physiology of fluid and electrolytes in the body, the following areas should be included:

1. The distribution of fluid and electrolytes within the body
2. The methods of intake and output of fluids to and from the body

3. The factors that affect fluid and electrolyte balance within the body
4. The maintenance of the acid-base balance of the body

THE DISTRIBUTION OF FLUID AND ELECTROLYTES. Fluid within the body is generally considered to be distributed in what may be termed two basic compartments. First it is within the cells of the body. This fluid, termed *intracellular fluid*, accounts for approximately 40 to 50 per cent of the total body weight. Secondly there is fluid outside the cells of the body; this is *extracellular fluid*. There are two basic kinds of extracellular fluid: *intravascular fluid*, which accounts for 5 per cent of the total body weight, and *interstitial fluid*, which accounts for 15 per cent of the total body weight. The interstitial (intercellular) fluid is the fluid in the spaces between the cells. Intravascular fluid is the fluid inside the blood and lymph vessels.

There is a constant shift of fluid from one compartment to another as it performs its function of transporting nutrients and oxygen to the cells and removing wastes and manufactured products from the cells. The amount of fluid in the circulating blood and the total amount of fluid within the cells must be maintained at a fairly constant volume in health. In cases of dehydration the body fluid is drawn from within the cells and routed into the blood vessels. This explains why a patient who is unable to retain fluids owing to prolonged vomiting soon loses the elasticity of his subcutaneous tissue, his skin becoming loose and flabby.

The principal electrolytes contained in extracellular and intracellular fluid are shown in Table 1. It can readily be seen that the electrolyte composition of the two types of fluid is quite different. In intracellular fluid, as, for example, in muscle and blood cells, potassium is the most important cation. Sodium and magnesium are present in lesser concentrations, and calcium is absent. In extracellular fluid, such as blood serum and interstitial fluid, on the other hand, sodium is the chief cation. Potassium, magnesium and calcium are present in lesser amounts.

TABLE 1.   THE ELECTROLYTE CONTENT OF BODY FLUIDS*

Constituent	Extracellular Fluid Concentration (mEq./L.)	Intracellular Fluid Concentration (mEq./L.)
Na$^+$	137	10
K$^+$	5	141
Ca^{++}	5	0
Mg^{++}	3	62
Cl$^-$	103	4
HCO$_3^-$	28	10
PO$_4^{---}$	4	75
SO$_4^{--}$	1	2

*Data from Arthur C. Guyton: *Function of the Human Body.* Third edition. W. B. Saunders Company, 1969, p. 45.

Among the anions, chloride and the carbonates are more plentiful in the extracellular fluids, while the phosphates predominate in the intracellular fluid. Sulfates are present in lesser amounts in both intracellular and extracellular fluids.

The electrolyte composition of the two types of extracellular fluid, that is, the interstitial fluid and the intravascular fluid, is essentially the same in so far as principal anions and cations are concerned. The fluid within the blood vessels does however contain a much greater concentration of protein than is found in the interstitial fluid. Normal serum values of various electrolytes are shown on pages 426 and 427, in the discussion of signs and symptoms of imbalance.

Methods of Fluid Intake and Output

A person derives fluid and electrolytes from three main sources: the fluid that is ingested as fluid, the fluid content of the various foods that are eaten and the water that is formed as a byproduct of the body's oxidation of foods and body substances. The total daily intake of water under normal circumstances is approximately 2000 to 3000 cc.

Water is lost from the body through the skin by perspiration, through the lungs in expirations and from the kidneys in the urine. In addition, a small amount of fluid is excreted in the feces.

The total daily loss of water from the body in normal circumstances is approximately 2000 to 3000 cc., depending largely upon the amount of fluid intake. It is lost as follows:

In urine: daily 1000 to 1500 cc.
In feces: daily 100 to 200 cc.
From the skin: daily 600 to 700 cc.
From the lungs: daily 400 to 500 cc.[2]

The balance between the fluid ingested and the fluid excreted is maintained within a very narrow range. The intake usually equals the output over a three day period even though it may not always be equal over a single 24 hour period.

Factors Affecting Fluid and Electrolyte Balance

The main forces at work in holding water within the various compartments of the fluid system of the body are generated by proteins and electrolytes. In the intravascular compartment (blood vessels) the force is generated largely by the serum albumin, in the intercellular fluid by the sodium ion and within the cells by protoplasm. Water passes freely through the capillary walls and membranes, but the protein molecules and the sodium ions do not move as freely. These substances exert an osmotic pressure which tends to hold water in the respective compartments. Osmotic pressure is that pressure exerted by particles which tends to draw a solvent toward it. A patient who has lost a great deal of serum albumin through malnutrition tends to become edematous, since fluid is drawn from the blood plasma into the intercellular spaces. This happens because the main force holding the water in the blood vessels has been lost.

By far the most important regulatory mechanism operating to maintain the body's fluid balance is the kidneys.

[2]Mary W. Falconer, Mabelclaire R. Norman, H. Robert Patterson and Edward A. Gustafson: *The Drug, The Nurse, The Patient.* Fourth edition. Philadelphia, W. B. Saunders Company, 1970, p. 277.

When the intake of fluid is insufficient or when there is an excessive loss of fluid from the body, the amount of urine that is excreted is decreased. Conversely, when an excess amount of fluid is ingested, urine output increases. This is accomplished through the selective reabsorption of water in the tubules of the kidney.

The kidney also exerts the main control over the sodium and potassium balance of the body through the selective reabsorption of these ions in the tubules. When sodium and potassium need to be retained, increasing amounts are reabsorbed. Excess sodium and potassium are excreted in the urine. If there is an acute shortage of sodium in the body, the excretion of this ion through the urine may be cut to almost zero. In the case of potassium, however, there appears to be an obligatory excretion of a certain amount in the urine.[3] Thus, there is always some potassium in the daily urine output even though the body reserves may be dangerously low. This factor is taken into account by the physician when he is planning replacement therapy.

The control of fluid and electrolyte balance by the kidneys is influenced by two sets of hormones. The *antidiuretic hormone* (ADH), which is produced primarily in the anterior hypothalamus and stored in the pituitary gland, is a major factor in controlling water reabsorption. When the body takes in an insufficient quantity, or there is water deprivation from other sources, the secretion of ADH is stimulated. This in turn causes increased reabsorption of water in the kidney tubules and a lessened volume of urinary output. *Aldosterone*, one of several steroid hormones produced in the adrenal cortex, exerts a major influence in promoting the retention of sodium and the excretion of potassium. Aldosterone secretion appears to be stimulated by such factors as a lessened sodium intake, an

excess of potassium, muscular activity, trauma and emotional tension.[4]

The gastrointestinal tract also helps to regulate fluid and electrolyte balance. The manner in which this is done is similar to the action of the kidneys, that is, through the selective reabsorption of water and solutes, the reabsorption taking place principally in the small intestine. Although the volume of digestive juices secreted into the gastrointestinal tract each day is considerable (approximately 8200 cc.), all but about 100 to 200 cc. of fluid are reabsorbed. Under normal circumstances, only a small amount of the body's daily fluid loss is from the gastrointestinal tract in the feces, and the loss of electrolytes by this route is normally negligible. Both fluid and electrolytes may be lost in considerable quantity, however, in such conditions as vomiting and diarrhea.

Thirst is another of the regulatory mechanisms operating to maintain fluid balance. Thirst is the desire for more fluids. It usually indicates a basic physiological need for water, although it may sometimes occur as a result of dryness of the mucous membranes of the mouth and throat from other causes such as mouth-breathing. In cases in which thirst is due to a simple dryness of the oropharynx rather than a basic lack of water in the body, it may be relieved by measures to keep the mucous membranes moist. Good oral hygiene can usually relieve this dryness.

"True thirst," due to a basic lack of water, usually occurs when body cells are dehydrated, extracellular volume is lessened (as in a hemorrhage), or certain centers in the hypothalamus are stimulated.[5] It is felt that the thirst mechanism is closely related to the control of water balance by the antidiuretic hormone. When the body is suffering from a lack of water, the thirst mechanism operates to increase the intake of water, while ADH restricts the loss of water through urinary output.

The lungs are also important in the regulation of fluid and electrolyte bal-

[3]Cyril M. MacBryde and Robert S. Blacklow (eds.): *Signs and Symptoms: Applied Pathologic Physiology and Clinical Interpretation.* Fifth edition. Philadelphia, J. B. Lippincott Company, 1970, p. 787.

[4]Ibid., p. 774.
[5]Ibid., p. 757.

ance. Ordinarily, the amount of water lost from respiration is quite small. Whenever respirations are increased in rate and depth, however, the amount of water loss via this route is also increased and may become a significant factor to consider. This may occur with strenuous muscular exercise, for example, in fevers or any condition in which respirations are considerably increased, or when the air that is breathed is very dry. This last point is important to remember in the administration of inhalation therapy. Oxygen, or other substances given by inhalation, should always be humidified in order to counterbalance the loss of water through expiration. The loss of electrolytes through respiration is normally minimal, although the lungs can play an important role in maintaining the acid-base balance of the body, as discussed later.

Water and the Maintenance of Acid-Base Balance

Intimately connected with the water balance of the body is the maintenance of the acid-base balance. Normally the blood and other body fluids are maintained in a slightly basic state (pH 7.35 to 7.45). The principal agent in the control of the acid-base balance of the plasma is the kidneys, which vary the acidity of the urine in response to the body's need to throw off excess acid or base. The lungs also influence the acid-base balance of the body through their control of carbonic acid. The lungs aid in elimination through the conversion of carbonate to carbonic acid. When large amounts of fluid are lost from the body, there can be disturbance of the acid-base balance. When large amounts of base are lost, acidosis develops; when large amounts of acid are lost, alkalosis develops.

THE ETIOLOGY OF FLUID AND ELECTROLYTE IMBALANCE

There are many conditions in which an imbalance of body fluids and electrolytes may occur. It is perhaps helpful here to group the causes of imbalance under five general headings.

Insufficient Intake

The sources of water and electrolytes for the body are the food and fluids ingested. Any disturbance in the source of nourishment is reflected in the body. Sometimes people who are anorectic and nauseated also show a disturbed fluid and electrolyte balance, particularly when these symptoms are prolonged.

Disturbances of the Gastrointestinal Tract

A very large volume of fluid in the form of digestive juices is secreted into the gastrointestinal tract each day. Almost all of this fluid is reabsorbed during the process of digestion. Interference with the normal processes of secretion and reabsorption can result in serious fluid and electrolyte imbalance. The nature of the imbalance depends to a large extent on the portion of the gastrointestinal tract affected. In order to appreciate the significance of this point, it is helpful to keep in mind both the volume and the electrolyte composition of the various digestive juices. The approximate volumes of the principal digestive juices are as follows:

Saliva	1500 cc. per day
Gastric secretion	2500 cc. per day
Intestinal secretion	3000 cc. per day
Pancreatic secretion	700 cc. per day
Bile	500 cc. per day

Total 8200 cc. per day[6]

The major components that are involved in electrolyte and acid-base balance are found in the gastric and in-

---

[6]Joseph I. Routh, Darrell P. Eyman and Donald J. Burton: Essentials of General, Organic and Biochemistry. Philadelphia, W. B. Saunders Company, 1969, p. 673.

testinal secretions. Gastric juice contains large quantities of hydrochloric acid and a significant amount of sodium. Gastric mucus contains a high proportion of sodium and chloride and a relatively small amount of carbonate. Thus, when fluids are lost from the stomach through vomiting, there may be a significant loss of acid as well. Prolonged vomiting may cause severe sodium depletion and loss of the chloride ion also. Gastric suction removes hydrochloric acid and fluids; gastric washings can severely deplete the store of chloride ions, particularly if these washings are done with water rather than normal saline. All gastric tube irrigations as well as gastric washings should therefore be done with isotonic saline to prevent the depletion of these electrolytes.

Pancreatic juice, bile and the intestinal secretions are predominantly base and contain relatively large amounts of carbonate, as well as sodium and chloride. In addition, a large proportion of the total volume of potassium excreted from the body daily is via the gastrointestinal tract in the feces. Thus, diarrhea results in the loss of fluids, generally, and in the loss of sodium and chloride ions as well as of the base secreted in the intestine. Severe diarrhea depletes the body's potassium also.

Disturbances of Kidney Function

Because the kidney is so intimately concerned with the regulation of fluid and electrolyte balance, any impairment in renal function may disturb this balance. Damage to the kidney itself may interfere with its ability to reabsorb water and electrolytes in the tubules. An imbalance in the antidiuretic hormone (caused by pituitary gland dysfunction, for example) affects kidney functioning, particularly the reabsorption of water. Similarly, an imbalance in aldosterone (which may result from steroid therapy, for example) affects sodium retention and potassium excretion by the kidneys. The kidneys are also affected by disturbances in cardiovascular function. An insufficient flow

of blood through the kidneys due to a poorly functioning heart, for example, hampers the efficiency of the kidneys in that there may not be enough blood circulating through the kidneys to produce an adequate amount of glomerular filtrate. Retention of fluid in body tissues may then occur. This is evidenced by edema, which is a frequent accompaniment of many cardiac conditions.

Excessive Perspiration or Evaporation

One of the largest variables in the amount of water lost from the body daily is the volume of perspiration. This may range from zero to several liters per day, depending on the amount of physical activity of the individual, the temperature of the environment, the presence of fever or the like. When there is excessive perspiration, two protective mechanisms are brought into play: thirst, which increases the amount of fluid intake, and adjustment of the water output by the kidneys.[7]

When fluids are lost through sweating, there is a loss of sodium chloride as well. Hence, people who live in hot climates, and those who must work in temperatures above normal, are frequently advised to take salt tablets to replace that lost through perspiration. As a person becomes acclimatized to higher environmental temperatures, however, the body usually adjusts by lessening the salt content of sweat so that the loss of sodium and chloride ions by this route is minimized.

Hemorrhage, Burns and Body Trauma

In hemorrhage, not only fluid, but a percentage of all the blood elements are lost. The total circulatory volume is decreased and, in a large hemorrhage, the body's adaptive mechanisms may collapse and shock may ensue.

---

[7]MacBryde and Blacklow, op. cit., p. 770.

In burns, as well as in some trauma to the body (including surgical trauma), fluids and electrolytes are lost from the general circulation as these tend to accumulate in the interstitial spaces. Fluids are removed from the plasma, sodium is depleted throughout the body generally, and potassium is released in excessive amounts from the damaged cells. Proteins are also depleted. Therefore, there is a need to replace not only fluids but also sodium, potassium and proteins in order to restore a balance.

ASSESSING THE NURSING NEEDS OF PATIENTS WITH FLUID AND ELECTROLYTE PROBLEMS

In order to assess the needs of the patient with fluid and electrolyte problems, the nurse should be aware of factors in the patient's history which could cause an imbalance. She should be alert to signs and symptoms in the patient which could be indicative of fluid and electrolyte imbalance and she should be able to identify significant laboratory findings. In addition, the nurse should know the physician's plan of therapy for the patient and understand the rationale on which this plan is based.

Information Obtained from the Patient

Significant factors in the patient's history which alert the nurse to the possibility of fluid and electrolyte imbalance include recent changes in the individual's usual patterns of intake and output or the presence of any one of the health problems already mentioned. When taking the nursing history, the nurse should obtain information about the patient's normal habits of food and fluid intake and output. How many glasses of water does he usually drink per day, for example? How many cups of tea or coffee? What types of fluids does he like? What foods does he usually eat? This type of information not only provides base-line data with which

to compare but also helps the nurse to plan the patient's care to prevent fluid and electrolyte imbalances from developing or to assist in correcting those which have occurred.

In addition to obtaining information about usual habits, the nurse should ascertain if there have been any recent alterations in the individual's pattern of intake and output. Has the patient been suffering from anorexia, for example, and not taking the usual amount of food and fluid? Has he noticed that he is not voiding as much as usual or, conversely, has been voiding more than usual? Is he taking any medications which could affect fluid and electrolyte balance, as for example, steroids?

The patient's medical history provides the nurse with much valuable information about existing or potential fluid and electrolyte problems. The person who has had a history of nausea and vomiting over several days, for example, is likely to show disturbances resulting from the loss of fluids generally, the loss of acid from gastric secretions and possibly a depletion of the sodium ions as well. The patient who is admitted for surgery may develop fluid and electrolyte imbalance postoperatively and will need careful observation on the part of the nurse to detect signs and symptoms of impending imbalance. The history notes made by the physician on the patient's record can alert the nurse to the presence of any of the health problems discussed in the section on etiology as possible causes of fluid and electrolyte imbalance.

Information Obtained by Observation

Although fluid and electrolyte disturbances are usually the result of other disorders in the body, they may in themselves give rise to specific signs and symptoms which are indicative of the nature of the imbalance. The signs and symptoms of common problems caused by an insufficiency or an excess of fluid and the major electrolytes in the body are shown in Table 2.

TABLE 2.   INDICATIONS OF COMMON PROBLEMS OF FLUID
AND ELECTROLYTE BALANCE*

Component	Insufficiency	Normal	Excess

Fluid Volume
Common symptoms
	Dehydration
	  dry skin and mucous
	    membranes
	  wrinkling of tongue
	  thirst
	  scanty urine
	  weight loss
	  low blood pressure
	  weak pulse
			Generalized edema
			  puffiness of skin
			
			lessened urine output
			weight gain
			high blood pressure
			bounding pulse
			dyspnea, with moist
			  breathing

Significant laboratory findings	Increased hemoglobin and hematocrit	14–18 Gm./100 ml. (men) 12–18 Gm./100 ml. (women) 45%	

Primary Base Bicarbonate
Common symptoms
	Metabolic acidosis
	  shortness of breath
	  rapid deep respirations
	
	  weakness
	  mental confusion
	  stupor
	  coma
	  sweet, fruity odor to
	    breath
			Metabolic alkalosis
			
			  slow shallow respira-
			    tions
			  hypertonic muscles
			  irregular pulse
			  convulsions

Significant laboratory
findings
	Urine pH below 6.0
	Plasma pH below 7.35
	Plasma bicarbonates
	  below 25 mEq./L.
		5.0–7.0
		7.35–7.45
		
		25–29 mEq./L.
			Urine pH above 7.0
			Plasma pH above 7.45
			Plasma bicarbonates
			  above 29 mEq./L.

Primary Carbonic Acid
Common symptoms
	Respiratory alkalosis
	  rapid deep breathing
	
	  tetany
	  unconsciousness
			Respiratory acidosis
			  respiratory embarrass-
			    ment with cyanosis
			  weakness
			  disorientation

Significant laboratory findings	As in metabolic alkalosis		As in metabolic acidosis

Protein
Common symptoms
	Protein deficit
	  anorexia
	  pallor
	  fatigue
	  mental and emotional
	    depression
	  weight loss
	  loss of muscle tone
			no adverse effects

Significant laboratory
findings
	Hemoglobin depressed
	
	Red blood cell count
	  depressed
	Plasma albumin
	  below 4 mEq./L.
		14–18 Gm./100 ml. (men)
		12–16 Gm./100 ml. (women)
		
		4,500,000–5,000,000/cu. mm.
		
		16 mEq./L.	

*Sources of information:
  Falconer, Mary W., Mabelclaire R. Norman, H. Robert Patterson and Edward A. Gustafson: *The Drug, the Nurse, the Patient.* Fourth edition. Philadelphia, W. B. Saunders Company, 1970, pp. 276–284.
  MacBryde, Cyril M., and Robert S. Blacklow (eds.): *Signs and Symptoms: Applied Pathologic Physiology and Clinical Interpretation.* Fifth edition. Philadelphia, J. B. Lippincott Company, 1970.

TABLE 2. INDICATIONS OF COMMON PROBLEMS OF FLUID
AND ELECTROLYTE BALANCE (Continued)

Component	Insufficiency	Normal	Excess
Sodium			
Common symptoms	Hyponatremia apprehension abdominal cramps low blood pressure scanty urine cold clammy skin convulsions rapid thready pulse		Hypernatremia excitement scanty urine hot dry skin sometimes convul- sions elevated temperature
Significant laboratory findings	Plasma sodium below 137 mEq./L. Specific gravity of urine below 1.010	142 mEq./L. 1.010–1.030	Plasma sodium above 147 mEq./L. Specific gravity of urine above 1.030
Potassium			
Common symptoms	Hypokalemia anorexia abdominal distention soft muscles weak pulse disorientation		Hyperkalemia intestinal colic diarrhea weakness slow pulse irritability
Significant laboratory findings	Plasma potassium below 4 mEq./L. Specific changes in electrocardiogram	5 mEq./L.	Plasma potassium above 5.6 mEq./L. Characteristic changes in electrocardiogram in severe cases
Calcium			
Common symptoms	Calcium deficit muscle cramps tetany progressing to convulsions tingling in extremities		Calcium excess relaxed muscles flank pain deep thigh pain
Significant laboratory findings	Plasma calcium below 4.5 mEq./L. Changes in electro- cardiogram	5 mEq./L.	Plasma calcium above 5.8 mEq./L. Changes in electro- cardiogram
Magnesium			
Common symptoms	Magnesium deficit disorientation confusion hallucinations high blood pressure slow pulse hyperactive deep re- flexes tremors		Magnesium excess depression of central nervous system loss of deep tendon reflexes
Significant laboratory findings	Plasma magnesium below 1.4 mEq./L.	3 mEq./L.	Plasma magnesium above 4 mEq./L. (moderate excess) above 10 mEq./L. (severe excess)

Of particular importance to the nurse is an awareness of the early signs of dehydration in a patient. His tongue is often dry and furry. He may complain of thirst, his skin tissues usually appear to be loose and flabby (loss of tissue turgor), and the mucous membranes appear dry. The patient frequently complains of fatigue also. The nurse will note that the patient's urine is scanty in amount and darker in color than normal urine. If the dehydration progresses, evidence of a greater degree of imbalance may be noted. Fluid is first drawn from the interstitial spaces and then from within the cells in order to maintain an adequate blood volume. However, as dehydration advances, the blood volume may be lessened also, and the patient's pulse may then become weak and his blood pressure low. He may experience a feeling of faintness, and sometimes signs of mental confusion are evident. With moderately advanced dehydration, the individual's temperature is usually elevated and there is a marked weight loss as well. In the most extreme cases of dehydration the patient may go into shock which progresses to a comatose state. There is usually evidence of kidney failure at this stage (see Chapter 27).

Also important to the nurse is the early recognition of retention of fluid in the body tissues. Edema may be localized or it may be general. Generalized edema can usually be observed first in the soft tissues around the eyes and in dependent areas of the body. If the individual is up and walking around, the edema may be noted first in the feet and ankles. With bed patients, the nurse may notice edema particularly around the sacral area. The patient's skin appears puffy and soft to the touch. The edematous patient usually shows a gain in weight which is due to the extra fluid he is retaining. When there is marked edema, the blood volume becomes increased, with a resultant rise in blood pressure. The lungs may be affected since the lungs are a low pressure area in the circulatory system and extra fluids tend to accumulate there. Thus, the patient may show symptoms of dyspnea with moist and noisy breathing. When there is a retention of fluids, there is usually a lessened volume of urine output.

Information Obtained from Diagnostic Tests

Diagnostic tests for patients who have fluid and electrolyte problems usually involve the laboratory examination of specimens of blood and urine. Electrolyte levels in the blood serum can be determined after the collection of approximately 5 cc. of venous blood. Potassium, sodium, calcium, and magnesium concentrations are frequently measured. The normal values for these ions in blood serum are shown in Table 2, together with values indicative of marked excess or insufficiency.

A blood gas analysis is often carried out to assess the acid-base balance. For this, 5 cc. of arterial blood is withdrawn. Measurement of the pH, PCO_2 and standard PCO_3 is usually ordered. pH indicates the overall acid-base balance of the body (normal 7.35–7.45). PCO_2 is the pressure of carbon dioxide dissolved in the plasma and indicates carbonic acid retention (normal 35–40 mm. Hg). Standard PCO_3 measures the amount of bicarbonate buffer (normal 25–29 mEq./liter). Often a PO_2 reading is requested; it measures the oxygen tension, normally 95–100 mm. Hg.

Diagnostic tests of the urine are done to measure the fluid and electrolyte balance. Tests for acetone and diacetic acid may indicate a disturbance in the metabolism that results in a type of acidosis. Urine is examined to test for the excretion of chlorides and sometimes potassium. The specific gravity of urine indicates the concentration of dissolved materials such as waste products and can reflect the degree of hydration of the patient. Other urine and kidney tests are more likely to assess kidney functioning, which may or may not be a contributing factor to fluid and electrolyte imbalance.

PRINCIPLES RELEVANT TO FLUID AND ELECTROLYTE BALANCE

The average adult requires 2500 cc. of water in a 24 hour period.

Normally, fluid intake is balanced against fluid loss.

When fluids are lost or retained in excessive amounts, there is an accompanying loss of electrolytes.

The signs and symptoms accompanying electrolyte imbalance vary according to the excess or deficiency of the specific electrolyte.

The specific electrolytes lost from the body in any fluid loss depend on the route of the loss.

OBJECTIVES OF NURSING INTERVENTION

The basic objectives of care for the patient with fluid and electrolyte problems are to assist the patient to maintain a homeostatic balance insofar as this is possible or to restore a balance that has been disturbed.

DETERMINING PRIORITIES FOR NURSING ACTION

Disturbances of fluid and electrolyte balance can have serious effects on body functioning. The nurse must be particularly observant in noting early signs and symptoms of imbalance. These should be reported promptly to the physician so that appropriate therapy can be instituted to correct the situation before it becomes too advanced.

Children in particular show signs of dehydration with accompanying electrolyte imbalance very rapidly in acute illnesses. A child who has been vomiting and has had diarrhea at home for even a few days may be brought into hospital in a state of acute dehydration. He will need immediate medical and nursing intervention.

It should be noted that in the case of a sudden hemorrhage, there is no time for the development of early symptoms and the patient may show signs of circulatory collapse very suddenly. Again, prompt intervention is essential to save the person's life.

The consequences of marked imbalance of fluid and the major electrolytes in the body have been documented throughout the chapter. It should be stressed therefore that all measures to maintain or restore fluid and electrolyte balance should receive priority from the nurse.

MEASURES TO MAINTAIN FLUID AND ELECTROLYTE BALANCE

Ensuring Adequate Food and Fluid Intake

Of primary importance in the nursing care of the patient with fluid and electrolyte problems is the maintenance of a therapeutic fluid intake. In many instances the physician orders the exact amount of oral fluid for a patient. Sometimes, however, it is a nursing function to judge the oral fluid needs of the patient; for example, the nurse determines that the patient with a fever or an infection requires large amounts of fluid (at least 3000 cc. per day).

Generally speaking, if the patient is dehydrated, or has lost an excessive amount of fluids, he should be encouraged to take extra. Additional fluid intake may be contraindicated in some cases, however. If the patient is nauseated or vomiting, for example, it is not reasonable to expect that he can tolerate oral fluids. Patients with kidney or heart conditions may require restriction of their fluid intake. The nurse should be aware of the physician's objectives in medical therapy and never push or force fluids beyond the limit prescribed

People normally get electrolytes from the food and fluids they ingest. Therefore, to maintain good electrolyte balance, adequate nutrition is essential. When the patient is deficient in certain electrolytes or extra are needed in the body these may be administered by medication. For example, calcium tablets are frequently ordered for pregnant women because of the heavy demands for additional calcium to promote growth of the fetus.

In addition, it is not unusual for restricted electrolyte intake to be pre-scribed; for example, the physician might order a salt-free diet for a patient. The usual purpose here is to restrict the oral intake of sodium (Na^+). It is frequently the nurse's responsibility to help the patient to understand the necessity for the restriction and to help him plan meals with this in mind. Most people are able to assume the responsi-bility for restricting their diets. Never-theless, in hospitals it is not unknown for a helpful roommate to lend his salt shaker to a person on a restricted salt diet.

Monitoring Fluid Intake and Output

With patients who have existing or potential fluid and electrolyte problems, it is essential to monitor fluid intake and output accurately. Normal fluid intake of the adult during a 24 hour period is about 2500 cc. When the physician wishes to know the fluid intake of a particular patient, accurate measures are made of all the fluid he is given. This includes fluid given orally, intra-venously, interstitially and rectally. Most hospitals provide chart forms for recording fluid balance.

Body fluids are normally excreted through the kidneys, the intestine, the lungs and the skin. In recording the amount of fluid output, the nurse meas-ures the amount of the patient's urine accurately. In addition, she measures any drainage, such as bile drainage and suction returns. In some instances, significant amounts of fluid lost in the feces, from wounds or by perspiration are also recorded.

It is difficult to obtain an exact record of fluid intake and output in all cases. Most hospitals have charts or written material which show the estimated fluid content of the drinking glasses, cups, soup bowls and other utensils usually used in the agency. However, it re-quires the cooperation of all personnel to maintain an accurate record of the patient's total fluid intake. The patient can often help to keep his own record,

particularly if he understands the need for doing this.

An accurate recording of output is usually more difficult. For example, the amount of fluid loss from perspiration may be considerable in the patient with a fever, yet measuring this is not easy. The nurse should, however, record the fact that the patient is perspiring pro-fusely and draw this to the attention of the physician. Often the amount of fluid lost from wounds can only be esti-mated. Sometimes, the number of dress-ing pads that are soaked through is helpful in assessing the extent of wound drainage.

When drainage tubing is irrigated, or such procedures as gastric washings or bladder irrigation are done, the amount of fluid inserted must always be in-cluded in the calculations of fluid intake and output.

Keeping an accurate record of urine output can also present some problems. When patients have bathroom privi-leges, it is necessary to place a meas-ured container in the bathroom and to enlist the patient's cooperation in col-lecting urine and, if feasible, measuring the amount voided. Patients who are incontinent of urine and feces present additional problems in the assessment of fluid losses. The nurse must watch these patients carefully for fluid reten-tion or excessive fluid loss.

The urine output of the average adult is 1500 cc. in a 24 hour period. When urine output is less than 25 cc. or more than 500 cc. per hour, it generally is abnormal. Abnormalities of either ex-cess or inadequate urine output should be drawn to the attention of the pa-tient's physician so that appropriate therapy can be instituted.

Observing for Signs and Symptoms of Imbalance

In assisting in the maintenance of fluid and electrolyte balance, the nurse must be alert to early indications of imbalance. Observations of the degree of hydration of the patient are noted and recorded. The nurse should watch par-

2-8738   RIVERSIDE HOSPITAL OF OTTAWA

FLUID BALANCE WORK SHEET

TOTAL 24 hr Intake _4090 cc_ Date _Sept 1/71_

NORTH   JANE   SP 1249
223 TREE RD   OTT   234-7566-600
NORTH   RICHARD   HUS
SAME
1.9.71 1PM   F 30 M SURG   RC
420   1

Time	Type	Amount	Time	Type	Amount	Time	Type	Amount
11:30 - 7:30			**7:15 - 3:45**			**3:15 - 11:45**		
12 mn.	I/v 5% D/w	200 cc	8 am	Juice	100	5 pm	I/v 5% D/w	200 cc
	I/v 5% D/s 1000cc put up.	—		Coffee	130		absorbed & discontinued	
				H₂O	150			
			8³⁰ am	I/v D/s 5%	150 cc	5³⁰	Soup	170
12¹⁵ am	H₂O	100 cc		I/v D/w 1000cc put up.			Tea	130
			10 am	Milk	100 cc		Milk	200
7 am	i/v D/s	850 cc	12 noon	Soup	170	8³⁰	Tea	130
7¹⁵ am	Tea	130 cc		Tea	130		Gingerale	200
			3³⁰ pm	H₂O	50			
				I/v D/w 5%	800			
Total		1280 cc	Total		1780 cc	Total		1030 cc
Oral		230	Oral		830	Oral		830
I.V.		1050	I.V.		950	I.V.		200
T.B.A.		150 cc	T.B.A.		200 cc	T.B.A.		/

Total 24 Hr Output

Time	Type	Amount	Time	Type	Amount	Time	Type	Amount
12 mn	Urine	300	9 am	Urine	200	6 pm	Urine	300
			12 noon	Urine	600			
7 am	Urine	700				10 pm	Urine	600
			3 pm	Urine	500			
Total	1000 cc		Total	1300 cc		Total	900 cc	
Urine	1000		Urine	1300		Urine	900	
Other	/		Other	/		Other	/	

Large Glass = 200 cc   Soup Bowl = 170 cc
Small Glass = 100 cc   Cup = 130 cc

A sample fluid balance work sheet. (Courtesy of the Riverside Hospital of Ottawa.)

ticularly for early signs of dehydration or fluid retention, as these were outlined in the section on assessment of nursing needs.

When observing for indications of electrolyte imbalance, the nurse should have an understanding of the patient's medical condition and the potential problems that may occur. If she is aware, for example, that the patient has a condition involving dysfunction of the adrenal cortex or impairment of renal function, she should observe him carefully for signs of sodium and potassium imbalance. Potassium in the blood plasma is maintained at a fairly constant volume even when there is a significant loss of the ion from the cells. Thus the body may be seriously depleted of potassium before significant changes can be noted in the blood plasma level, which is the only tabulated measurement. Therefore, the nurse should be alert to the early signs and symptoms of potassium deficiency such as muscular weakness, irregularities of the pulse or nervous irritability.

When the nurse is aware of potential problems, her observations are more directed and purposeful. She knows what to look for and her observations can be of inestimable assistance to the physician in diagnosing the patient's condition and planning therapy.

ASSISTING IN THE RESTORATION OF FLUID AND ELECTROLYTE BALANCE

General Considerations

Whenever a disturbance in fluid or electrolyte balance occurs, steps must be taken to restore homeostasis. Since the principal sources of fluid and electrolytes are the food and fluids a person takes in, adjustments in diet or fluid intake or both may be sufficient to rectify a mild imbalance. In the case of deficiencies of specific electrolytes, supplements may be given in the form of medications. Often, however, fluid loss is too extensive and the accompanying loss of electrolytes too great to be corrected by oral intake alone, or this method of replacement may be contraindicated. Fluids and electrolytes may then be administered by other routes, by intravenous infusion, by blood transfusion, or by interstitial or rectal infusion. The decisions of route to be used and the type of solution to be administered are made by the physician. His decisions are based on his knowledge of the patient's condition and the particular factors causing the imbalance. The patient's intake and output record is of considerable assistance to the physician in assessing the extent of fluid loss and in calculating the balance between intake and output. The nurse's observations of the patient's state of hydration, of his nutritional status and of signs and symptoms of impending fluid and electrolyte imbalance also contribute significantly to the physician's assessment of the need for replacement or corrective therapy.

The care of the patient with fluid and electrolyte problems includes good supportive nursing measures as well as assistance with curative measures. Hygiene is of particular importance for patients with these problems. The patient's physical comfort is largely dependent upon his feeling of cleanliness and freshness. Profuse diaphoresis may necessitate frequent changes and baths; dry, scaly skin and mucous membranes are lubricated with emollient creams. One of the dangers of cracked lips and dry mouth is the increased risk of secondary infections.

The overhydrated patient, in particular, should turn in bed regularly to promote circulation and adequate nourishment of all tissues. The presence of edema or even the weight of the patient can restrict circulation to particular areas, thus predisposing the area to tissue death and the formation of decubitus ulcers.

SPECIFIC MEASURES

Intravenous Infusion

The infusion of fluids directly into a vein is often indicated when a patient is unable to take fluids orally. Infusion permits the patient to obtain many fluids, electrolytes and nutrients that are necessary to life. In addition, it has the advantage of rapid absorption, which is particularly important in the administration of some medications.

Many kinds of intravenous fluid are available for infusion. It is the physician's decision as to which kind of fluid the patient needs. For example, a patient may require 5 per cent dextrose in water, normal saline or 10 per cent dextrose in normal saline. Usually intravenous fluid is provided in 250, 500 or 1000 cc. containers.

In some states of the United States, only the physician is permitted to start an intravenous infusion; in others it is a responsibility of the graduate nurse. Often hospitals have policies regarding the kinds of infusions which nurses can initiate. Sometimes the physician orders the addition of drugs such as norepinephrine, vitamin C, potassium chloride, Neo-Synephrine or nitrogen mustard to an intravenous solution. It is the responsibility of the nurse to know which she is permitted to add and which drugs the physician must administer.

The choice of site for an intravenous infusion is dependent upon a number of factors. The condition of the patient's veins as well as his comfort must be considered. Often the cephalic and basilic veins in the inner aspect of the elbow and the saphenous vein at the ankle are used. These *cephalic* and *basilic* sites may require extension of the patient's arm, which can be uncomfortable after a prolonged period. If, however, these veins are entered along the shaft of radius and ulna (bones of the forearm), the bones provide a natural splint and make extension of the elbow unnecessary.

Prior to starting an intravenous infusion, the tubing is attached to the intravenous flask. Sterile precautions are taken throughout this procedure in order to protect the patient from infection. In addition to the flask and the intravenous tubing, the nurse requires a tourniquet, an antiseptic swab, a sterile syringe, a standard to hold the flask and a receptacle for the discarded fluid.

After the tubing has been attached to the intravenous flask, the flask is hung upon the standard and the fluid is then run through the tubing before the tubing is clamped. By running the fluid through the tubing, air is removed so that it will not be introduced into the patient's vein. Air injected into a vein can result in an air embolus. An embolus is a clot or plug in a blood vessel which has been transported from another place by the blood and which can result in the blocking of blood flow.

A tourniquet is applied to the patient's arm above the intravenous site. At the same time, the patient clenches and unclenches his fist. These measures distend the veins in his arm to make them more accessible for venipuncture. The injection site is cleansed with antiseptic and then a sterile needle (No. 18, 19, 20 or 21) is attached to the syringe and inserted at a 45 degree angle, bevel up, into the vein. Some resistance to the needle is encountered at the skin, but the subcutaneous tissues and veins offer very little resistance. The patient perceives pain when the needle goes through the skin but little discomfort thereafter. The plunger of the syringe is drawn back to ascertain the position of the needle in the vein by obtaining blood. Then the syringe is disconnected, and the tubing is attached to the needle. The rate of flow is then established. Depending upon the patient's condition, the rate of flow may be from 40 to 100 drops per minute. The usual rate is 80 drops per minute. The rate of flow for an intravenous infusion is ordered by the physician.

The tubing and the needle are then attached to the arm by adhesive tape. The patient can be provided with an arm board to immobilize his arm if this is necessary. Whenever the site of the needle insertion is near a joint, as, for example, the elbow or the wrist, it is wise to use an armboard to prevent the needle from being dislodged with the patient's movement. It is very difficult to maintain immobility of a part without support such as a board provides. To

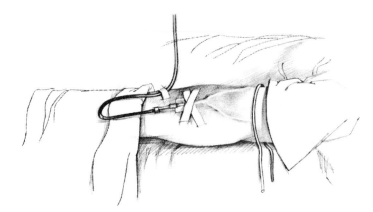

The site of an intravenous infusion.

be effective the armboard should reach from above the elbow joint to the end of the fingertips. The board should always be padded for the patient's comfort and safety.

If intravenous fluids are to be administered over a prolonged period of time, polyethylene tubing (Intra-cath) may be used instead of a needle for an infusion; the tubing fits through the needle, which is removed after the tubing has been inserted into the vein. Tubing is more flexible than a needle, but it must be checked to make certain that it does not become dislodged and move down the patient's vein, particularly when it is being removed.

Often with children, and sometimes with adult patients whose surface veins are inaccessible or unsuitable for infusion, it is necessary to make a small incision in order to locate an appropriate site for the needle insertion. In these cases, a "cut-down" will be used by the physician. This technique is not carried out by nursing personnel although the nurse should have the equipment ready and assist the physician as needed.

It may be necessary to vary the height of the intravenous flask according to the pressure with which one wishes the fluid to enter the vein. The higher the flask, the stronger is the gravitational pull on the fluid, and the greater the pressure it exerts. Usually 3 feet above bed level is an adequate height for most intravenous infusions.

Frequently it is the nurse's responsibility to adjust the rate of flow of the intravenous solution. Various methods of deriving the number of cubic centimeters per minute are used, the objective being to divide the total amount of solution equally over the time period prescribed for the infusion. For example, if 250 cc. of fluid are to be given over a two hour period, the rate of flow should be approximately 30 cc. per minute to allow all of the fluid to run through in two hours.

During an intravenous infusion, the patient is observed for any untoward effects. Specifically, the nurse should note the site of the intravenous for swelling, redness or pain. These reactions can indicate that the needle has slipped out of the patient's vein with the result that the fluid is flowing into the surrounding tissues. Patients are also observed for signs of overhydration or cardiac overload. Tachycardia, hypertension or dyspnea can indicate cardiac overload and consequently are reported to the physician immediately.

The nurse records on the patient's chart the amount and the kind of intravenous fluid being administered, as well as the name of the person who initiated the procedure. The site of the intravenous puncture and the rate of flow are also recorded. In this way another site can be chosen for the next infusion. Generally the sites are chosen by starting from the distal and working toward the proximal areas so that previous infusion sites will not impede the flow of solution in the veins.

Several problems may be encountered in the administration of intravenous fluids. If the fluid stops running or flows spasmodically, the needle may have become dislodged, or the bevel of the needle (or the end of the plastic tubing) may be resting against the wall of the patient's vein. Slight alteration of the position of the needle or tubing can often correct this. If the intravenous

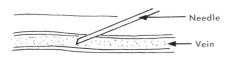

solution flows into the interstitial spaces, the infusion must be restarted with another sterile needle. The nurse can tell if the infusion has gone into the interstitial spaces by the edema which forms around the injection site when fluid infiltrates the subcutaneous tissues. Another problem is the appearance of air bubbles in the tubing. When this happens the tubing can be disconnected at the needle and the fluid allowed to run through the tubing until the bubbles are expelled.

Discontinuing an Intravenous Infusion. To discontinue an intravenous infusion, an antiseptic swab for cleansing the open area is needed. The intravenous tubing is clamped, and then the adhesive tape on the patient's arm is loosened. The needle is removed quickly from the patient's vein, the antiseptic swab is placed over the puncture wound and digital pressure is applied until the bleeding stops. If plastic tubing has been used instead of a needle, it is withdrawn carefully and checked to make sure that none of the tube remains in the patient's vein. Since the length of the tube that was inserted is often recorded in the patient's chart, the length of the removed tube can be checked against this record.

Whenever bleeding persists from the intravenous site, pressure is prolonged by means of a small dressing in order to prevent bleeding into the tissues and resultant ecchymosis (escape of blood into the surrounding tissue). Subsequently, the kind and amount of fluid that was infused is recorded, as is the time that the intravenous infusion was terminated.

Blood Transfusion

Prior to a blood transfusion, the patient's blood is typed. There are many blood groupings beyond the basic A, AB, B and O types. The Rh factor is determined along with the blood group. Usually 5 cc. of blood is taken for typing.

Blood transfusions are usually started by a physician or a specially qualified nurse. Initiating a transfusion is similar to starting an intravenous infusion. A careful check is always made to be certain that the patient is getting the right blood. Usually this means that two nurses check the number on the blood bottle against the number on the duplicate request form on the patient's record, and the name on the requisition against the name of the patient's record and identification band. In some hospitals it is also necessary to check the patient's hospital identity number on the blood bottle, the blood requisition, the chart and the identification band.

A No. 18 needle is usually used for a blood transfusion, and the rate of flow of the blood is normally 40 drops per minute. Special note is made of the patient's reaction and condition; at any sign of urticaria, chills, backache or respiratory or circulatory distress, the transfusion is terminated and the physician notified. Because most reactions to a blood transfusion occur within a short time after it has been started, the nurse should stay with the patient for the first 15 minutes.

Recording the initiation of a blood transfusion should include the time it was started, the amount of blood, the number on the bottle of blood and the name of the person who initiated the transfusion. Termination of the blood transfusion is similar to the termination of the intravenous infusion.

On occasion a patient requires a phlebotomy, that is, an opening into a vein in order to remove blood. This measure is carried out by the physician, usually to decrease blood volume, for example, to relieve dyspnea caused by congestion of blood in the lungs. For this procedure, empty bottles to receive the blood are required, in addition to the equipment that is needed to enter a vein.

Interstitial Infusion

Interstitial infusion, hypodermoclysis and subcutaneous infusion are synonymous terms referring to the administration of large amounts of fluid into subcutaneous tissue. This measure is generally indicated when a patient is unable to take fluids orally, rectally or intravenously. Its purpose is to supply the patient with fluids, electrolytes and occasionally nourishment. Hyaluronidase is often added to the fluid to hasten its absorption. This enzyme breaks down the hyaluronic acid of the connective tissue.

Whether the initiation of an interstitial infusion is the responsibility of the nurse or the physician is dependent upon the policy of the specific agency. The usual sites for the administration of an interstitial infusion are just below the scapula, the abdominal wall above the crest of the ilium, the lower aspect of the breast and the anterior aspect of the thigh.

The equipment that is used is similar to that used in intravenous infusions. A No. 19, 20, 21 or 22 needle is used. If the physician wishes to increase the rate of administration of the fluid, two sites can be used simultaneously. After the equipment has been set up (see Intravenous Infusion), the needle is inserted into the skin at a 20 degree angle. It is then taped in place and the flow of the fluid is adjusted in accordance with the physician's order. The usual rate of flow for an interstitial infusion is 60 to 120 drops per minute. The rate is dependent upon the ability of the individual to absorb the fluid. Thin people usually absorb fluid more easily than obese people, because they have fewer fat cells.

The nurse assists the patient to assume a comfortable position, since this treatment is often lengthy. Observations are indicated to detect untoward symptoms, particularly those related to circulatory collapse, for example, an accelerated, weak pulse. The patient should also be watched for signs of respiratory difficulty that could indicate overhydration, such as dyspnea or moist and noisy breathing. Sometimes the infusion is poorly absorbed and the nurse may notice that tissues at the site of injection are becoming edematous. If untoward symptoms develop, the infusion should be stopped and the physician notified promptly. Because of the site of interstitial infusions, adequate draping is necessary for the patient's comfort.

At the termination of an infusion the needle is removed and a small antiseptic dressing is taped over the wound with slight pressure to prevent leakage of the fluid. The nurse records the time of initiation and termination of the infusion, as well as the type of fluid, the amount of fluid absorbed, the addition of any medications, the rate of flow and the patient's reaction to the treatment. Again it is wise to record the site of the infusion so that the injection sites can be changed for subsequent infusions.

Rectal Infusion

Rectal infusion, proctoclysis and Murphy drip are all terms which refer to the instillation of fluid via the rectum. This treatment is indicated when the patient is unable to take fluids orally and intravenous and interstitial infusions are contraindicated. A hypotonic solution is slowly instilled into the rectum, from which it is absorbed. Because the solution is hypotonic it is drawn across the mucous membrane lining by osmosis.

GUIDES TO ASSESSING NURSING NEEDS

1. What is the patient's usual pattern of fluid intake and output?
2. Have there been any recent changes in this pattern? Has the patient been anorectic, for example, and not taking the usual amount of food and fluid? Has he noticed that he has a lessened amount of urine output? An increased amount?
3. Has he noticed any loss or gain in weight recently?
4. Does he have a health problem which could cause fluid and electrolyte imbalance? For example, has he been nauseated or vomiting, has he had diarrhea? Does he have a kidney problem? A cardiac condition? Has he lost large amounts of fluid from any cause?
5. Is he taking any medication which could affect fluid and electrolyte balance?
6. Does he show signs or symptoms of dehydration? Of fluid retention?
7. Are there signs or symptoms which would lead you to suspect an excess or insufficiency of specific electrolytes in this patient?
8. Do laboratory tests such as blood gases, electrolyte and urine tests show findings indicative of fluid or electrolyte imbalance?
9. Has measurement of intake and output been ordered for this patient? If so, are the totals of intake and output normal for a 24 hour period?
10. Are there restrictions on the patient's fluid or electrolyte intake? Does he need help to plan a diet to meet these restrictions?
11. Is the patient receiving medications to supplement or replace electrolytes?
12. Have parenteral fluids been prescribed? If so, why have they been ordered? What are the nurse's responsibilities in their administration? Are there special precautions to be observed with any of these?

GUIDES TO EVALUATING THE EFFECTIVENESS OF NURSING ACTION

1. Is the patient taking adequate nourishment to meet his fluid and electrolyte needs?
2. In his urine output compatible with his fluid intake?
3. If there are restrictions on the patient's fluid or electrolyte intake, are these being observed?
4. If parenteral fluids have been prescribed, have they been given at the correct time? Have sterile precautions been observed in their administration? Is the infusion flowing at the proper rate?
5. Have the patient's hygiene needs been met?
6. Is his skin in good condition?

STUDY VOCABULARY

Anion	Ecchymosis	Embolus
Cation	Electrolyte	Hypercalcemia

Hyperkalemia   Hypodermoclysis   Hyponatremia
Hypernatremia   Hypokalemia   Tissue turgor
Hypocalcemia

**STUDY
SITUATION**

Mr. R. Miller is admitted to a medical nursing unit of a large city hospital late one evening. His diagnosis was tentatively given as dehydration and emaciation. The physician ordered an examination of a specimen of his blood to determine sodium and potassium concentrations and arterial blood gases. He also ordered an intravenous infusion of 1000 cc. of 5 per cent dextrose in normal saline to be started at midnight and to be run at 80 drops per minute. Mr. Miller is 83 years old. He is very thin and says he has not eaten well in many months. He appears frightened; this is his first admission to a hospital.

The results of Mr. Miller's blood tests are as follows: sodium, 82 mEq./L.; potassium, 7.2 mEq./L.; plasma bicarbonates, 22 mEq./L.

1. What are dehydration and emaciation?
2. What symptoms might you expect Mr. Miller to exhibit? Why?
3. Compare the results of his laboratory tests with normal values?
4. How long can you expect this patient's intravenous infusion to run?
5. What factor should be taken into consideration in explaining the intravenous infusion to this patient?
6. What observations should you make regarding his intravenous infusion?
7. What are the objectives of the nursing care for Mr. Miller?
8. Outline a nursing care plan for this patient and include the reasons.
9. How can you evaluate the nursing care for this patient?

BIBLIOGRAPHY

Abbey, June C.: Nursing Observations of Fluid Imbalance. *Nursing Clinics of North America*, 3:1:77–86, March, 1968.
Falconer, Mary W., Mabelclaire R. Norman, H. Robert Patterson and Edward A. Gustafson: *The Drug, The Nurse, The Patient.* Fourth edition. Philadelphia. W. B. Saunders Company, 1970.
Fenton, Mary: What to Do About Thirst. *American Journal of Nursing*, 69:5: 1014–1017, May, 1969.
Guyton, Arthur C.: *Function of the Human Body.* Third edition. Philadelphia, W. B. Saunders Company, 1969.
Heath, Joleen K.: A Conceptual Basis for Assessing Body Water Status. *Nursing Clinics of North America*, 6:1:189–198, March, 1971.
MacBryde, Cyril M., and Robert S. Blacklow (eds.): *Signs and Symptoms: Applied Pathologic Physiology and Clinical Interpretation.* Fifth edition. Philadelphia, J. B. Lippincott Company, 1970.
Metheny, N. M., and W. D. Snively, Jr.: *Nurses' Handbook of Fluid Balance.* Philadelphia, J. B. Lippincott Company, 1967.
Nordmark, Madelyn T., and Anne W. Rohweder: *Scientific Foundations of Nursing.* Second edition. Philadelphia, J. B. Lippincott Company, 1967.

Reed, Gretchen, and Vincent F. Sheppard: *Fluid and Electrolyte Balance: A Programmed Text*. Philadelphia, W. B. Saunders Company, 1971.

Robinson, James R.: Water, the Indispensable Nutrient. *Nutrition Today*, pp. 16–25, Spring, 1970.

Routh, Joseph I., Darrell P. Eyman, and Donald J. Burton: *Essentials of General, Organic and Biochemistry*. Philadelphia, W. B. Saunders Company, 1969.

30 THE CARE OF TERMINALLY ILL PATIENTS

THE CARE OF TERMINALLY 30
ILL PATIENTS

INTRODUCTION

Inextricably involved in nursing is the preservation of life, the alleviation of suffering and the restoration of health. Our society exalts health, life and youth. Death is a subject which generally is avoided; even when it is imminent, it is frequently denied. Yet death is a not infrequent occurrence on hospital wards or among the sick in the community. Nurses and physicians, by the very nature of their work, encounter the presence of death more often than most people do in the normal course of their lives.

The frequency of the encounter does not, however, make it easier. The care of the terminally ill patient and the conforting and consoling of the patient's family, whether death is sudden or follows a lengthy illness, presents one of the most difficult situations in nursing practice. It is particularly distressing for the young student who has possibly never been face to face with the realities of death before in her life. Her own natural feelings of grief over the loss of the patient are something she has to work through in much the same way as the patient and his family do. It is helpful, then, if she understands the nature of the process of grieving so that she is better able to handle her own reactions and to help the patient and his family to meet their needs.

THE STAGES OF DYING

In her book, *On Death and Dying*, Dr. Elisabeth Kubler-Ross suggests that

there are five stages that most people go through when they learn that they are going to die. These are: denial, anger, bargaining, depression and acceptance.[1]

The first stage is one of nonacceptance. This is not happening to them! Surely, there must be some mistake. Often the patient seeks reassurance from the nurse and questions her regarding what the doctor has said. While the decision of what to tell the patient belongs to the physician, and the nurse accepts his guidance in this area, she should know what the patient and his family have been told so that she can provide support. Throughout the denial stage, the nurse must accept the fact that the patient is not yet ready to acknowledge the seriousness of his illness. Some patients maintain this denial up to the point of impending death, and continue to talk optimistically of future plans and of what they are going to do when they get better. Nursing personnel often mistakenly admire this type of behavior, considering that the patient is being "very brave," although in fact, it is usually more difficult for this patient when the time comes when he can no longer deny that death is near. Many patients, however, are aware of their prognosis, even though they have never been told in words, and yet they may pretend not to know. Often, they maintain a façade of cheerfulness for the benefit of their families, whom they sense are uncomfortable

---

[1]Elisabeth Kubler-Ross: *On Death and Dying.* New York, The Macmillan Company, 1969.

talking about death, or because they feel that they are expected to behave in this manner by the hospital staff. For these patients, it is frequently a relief to drop the façade in the presence of someone whom they feel understands what they are going through. It should be pointed out, however, that most patients appear to prefer to hold onto some hope – that a new cure may be found or a miracle happen – even though they do not rationally expect one.

Once the person has passed the stage of denial, he usually goes through an understandable period of anger and hostility. Why should this be happening to him? What did he do to deserve this punishment? At this point, the patient often lashes out at those nearest to him, the physicians, the nurses, the hospital, his family. He may be highly critical of the care he is receiving. If the nurse is aware that there is nothing personal in his attack, that he is in reality angry at God and whatever fates there be rather than at those who are caring for him, it is easier for her to have patience and tolerance with his behavior. The patient's family will usually go through this stage of anger and hostility also, and may take out their feelings on the staff. It is helpful to remember that this too is a normal reaction and one which the nurse should not counter with defensiveness or hostility on her part.

The third stage of dying is often one of bargaining. From early childhood, one is taught that good behavior is rewarded and bad actions are punished. Therefore, promising to be very good may bring about a reversal of the decision that death is due. The nurse may hear the patient say that he would do anything – repent his sins, make up for previous errors – if he can just live a little longer or, perhaps, have a day free of pain. The nurse is probably personally familiar with the bargaining process; she has perhaps stated to herself or prayed that if she could just pass this exam she would faithfully study every night in the future. The nurse cannot change the patient's prognosis, of course, but the relief of pain is usually something which she can do some-

thing about. The patient should be kept as comfortable as possible. The effectiveness of analgesic drugs is generally considered to be better if these are given regularly every three to four hours rather than waiting for the patient to request them when pain becomes unbearable.[2] Some analgesics have the unfortunate side effect of clouding the consciousness. Consequently the patient may ask that they be withheld near the time of death so that he can think and talk clearly. The nurse is guided by the physician's orders, but in most instances, the physician and the nurse follow the patient's wishes in this respect.

When the patient realizes that his bargaining efforts are of no avail, he usually enters into a depressed phase. This again is a normal reaction, as the individual contemplates all that he has held dear in life and mourns its loss. During this stage the patient may be very concerned about how his family is going to manage when he is gone, and he may be anxious to "put his affairs in order." Sometimes it is difficult for him to discuss these matters with members of his family, who frequently react very emotionally to any talk of death. In this case, a third party such as the chaplain, a social worker or a close friend of the patient may be the best person to deal with these practical concerns. During this stage of depression, the patient may not want to talk a great deal. He may wish to see only those nearest and dearest to him. Because of his withdrawal, however, the nurse should not take it for granted that he wishes to be left all alone. The presence of someone who sympathetically cares for him is reassuring. Many hospitals permit a member of the family to stay with a patient who is seriously ill, or family members to visit as often as they wish. A terminally ill patient is often placed in a single room so that the patient and his family may have

---

[2]Eleanor E. Drummond: Communication and Comfort for the Dying Patient. *Nursing Clinics of North America,* 5:1:55–63, March, 1970.

privacy. Yet often, this contributes to the patient's sense of isolation. By stopping in to see the patient at frequent intervals, if he has no family members with him, or spending time with him as her schedule permits, the nurse can help to overcome the patient's feelings of isolation.

The final stage of the dying process comes when the patient has accepted that he is going to die soon and he is prepared for it. By this time, the patient is usually tired but at peace. At this stage, it is the patient's family who usually require the most support. Patient's families react to death and dying in a variety of ways. They too go through the same stages as the patient does, but not always at the same time. When relatives are with a terminally ill person, they are often at a loss as to what to say and how to act. It is not uncommon to see even imminent death denied by a family. The nurse can often help the family by such actions as ensuring them privacy, permitting them access to the patient, and showing them small kindnesses in ministering to their comfort as well as to the patient's.

It is important to the family that they feel the patient is receiving the best care possible. Helping the patient to die in a dignified and peaceful manner is perhaps one of the most valuable contributions the nurse can make to the comfort of both the patient and the members of his family.

At times, it is up to the nurse to tell the family that a patient has died. It is best told to the family group in privacy. The nurse should anticipate that they will be upset and will look to her for supportive understanding. Many agencies have a small prayer room or a chapel where the nurse may take grieving families so that they can be alone for a while. With all cultural groups, there are certain rituals that are performed at the time of death, and these help the family to work through their grief. The nurse should be aware of these rituals and make provisions to ensure that they can be carried out. Often, family members will want to go in and pay their last respects to the dead person, and this should be permitted. Some ethnic groups expect that the members of the immediate family will be very vocal in their outpouring of grief. With others, a more stoical behavior is expected. Regardless of the cultural background, however, the death of an immediate family member is one situation in which crying is considered not only permissible but helpful in the grieving process.

THE SPIRITUAL NEEDS OF THE TERMINALLY ILL PATIENT

Terminally ill patients have many needs: emotional, spiritual and physical. Perhaps the need which can best guide the nurse is the need of a patient to die gracefully. In describing a way to acquire a positive approach to death, Saunders advises us "to look continually at the patients, not at their need but at their courage, not at their dependence but at their dignity."[3]

In gaining the strength and courage to face death with dignity many people find their religious beliefs of inestimable assistance. Often patients and their families seek support from representatives of their religious faith. Even patients who profess not to believe in a Superior Being may find the visits of a chaplain comforting. The nurse is frequently the person who first identifies the spiritual needs of the patient and she may be called upon to act as a liaison between the patient and the chaplain. Many hospitals maintain a list of clergymen of the different faiths who may be called if the patient does not have his own spiritual counsellor, or the hospital may have its own chaplain. Nurses too may feel the need to talk over their feelings about death and the dying patient with someone and often find the chaplain a helpful person in this regard.

---

[3]Cicely Saunders: The Last Stages of Life. *The American Journal of Nursing*, 65:70, March, 1965.

THE PHYSICAL NEEDS OF THE TERMINALLY ILL PATIENT

The physical needs of the dying person are similar to the needs of any seriously ill patient. Unless death occurs suddenly, there is usually a progressive failure of the body's systems and senses as the individual becomes weaker. The following changes take place:

1. Loss of muscle tone
2. Progressive cessation of peristalsis
3. Slowing of blood circulation
4. Labored respirations
5. Loss of the senses

Loss of muscle tone is usually manifested in the patient's inability to control defecation and urination. The sphincter muscles of the rectum and bladder relax, and as a result there is involuntary micturition and defecation. A retention catheter may be required, and absorbent pads can be used to help the patient keep dry and comfortable. Since patients are often embarrassed about their inability to control these functions, it is important that the nurse be discrete and understanding in her care. Deodorants are frequently used to keep the air in the patient's room fresh and free from unpleasant odors.

Involuntary micturition and defecation predispose the patient to decubitus ulcers. By helping the patient to keep dry and clean and to change his position regularly, the nurse can usually prevent these complications.

Because of the progressive loss of muscle tone the dying patient finds it increasingly difficult to maintain his position in bed without support. If the patient is conscious, Fowler's position is usually indicated in order to increase the depth of ventilation of the lungs. If he is unconscious, a semiprone position promotes the drainage of mucus from his mouth. Family members may become anxious when they see the patient positioned in this manner, and it is wise to explain to them the reasons for it. Regardless of the position that the nurse judges to be most beneficial, the patient will need supportive measures, such as pillows, to maintain it (see Chapter 13). If possible, the various parts of the body should be kept out of dependent positions to prevent the pooling of blood.

The inability to swallow (dysphagia) is also characteristic of the loss of muscle tone in the dying patient. Mucus tends to accumulate in the patient's throat, and as a result the air passing through it causes a typical gurgling sound, "the death rattle." Throat suctioning usually helps to keep his airway patent.

There is a *progressive diminution in peristalsis* of the gastrointestinal tract of the dying patient. His desire for food is usually minimal, but he may want frequent sips of water. His mouth may be dry, owing to dehydration and perhaps to a slight fever which sometimes precedes death. Good oral hygiene is essential. Because of the reduced peristalsis, flatus accumulates in the stomach and intestines, often distending the patient's abdomen and causing nausea. More than a few sips of water at a time can, as a consequence, cause vomiting. Dying patients are often given nourishment and fluids parenterally but rarely are sips of fluid contraindicated.

As *blood circulation slows*, the patient's extremities appear cyanosed or mottled and feel cold and clammy to the touch, although he probably perceives warmth and his temperature is above normal. When circulation is considerably decreased, the effectiveness of the administration of analgesics, intramuscularly or hypodermically, is decreased. As a consequence the patient may require analgesics in an intravenous solution.

Respiratory embarrassment is alleviated by throat suctioning, by positioning (such as Fowler's position) and by the administration of oxygen. Aside from its effect on the patient, respiratory difficulty is one of the most distressing signs that his family has to witness.

There are also *alterations in the senses* of the dying patient. His vision frequently becomes blurred, and as a result the patient prefers a lighted room, rather than the darkened room that so often comes to mind. His eyes may need special attention also. Frequently secretions tend to gather, and these should be removed with absorbent cotton dipped in normal saline to prevent crusting. Sometimes, however, the eyes become dry and it may be necessary to instill some sterile ophthalmic ointment onto the lower conjunctivae to keep them lubricated.

Hearing is considered to be the last sense to leave the body; hence the patient who cannot respond verbally often understands what people are saying. When people talk to a dying person, they should take care to speak distinctly in a normal voice. Whispering is to be avoided, because it may disturb the patient to realize that people are talking and yet he is unable to understand what they are saying.

Varying degrees of consciousness precede death: Drowsiness is a state of sleepiness, stupor is a state of unconsciousness from which one can be aroused and coma is an unconscious state from which one cannot be aroused. The patient may remain conscious and rational until the moment of death, or he may become unconscious or confused several days or even weeks prior to death.

For the comfort of the dying patient and his family, the patient's room is kept clear and tidy. Frequently the dying patient is given a private room on the nursing unit of the hospital so that he and his family may have privacy.

Some patients experience pain while they are critically ill. Generally in such cases the physician orders an analgesic to prevent discomfort.

SIGNS OF IMMINENT DEATH

Certain signs are indicative of the imminence of death. The patient's reflexes gradually disappear and he is unable to move. His respirations become increasingly difficult; Cheyne-Stokes respirations may occur. Typically his face assumes a pinched expression, and often a faint cyanotic pattern becomes discernible in the skin of his face. The patient's skin feels cold and clammy and his pulse accelerates and becomes weaker. With increasing anoxia, the pupils become dilated and fixed. Low blood pressure, an elevated temperature and a rapid respiration rate are often seen.

SIGNS OF DEATH

Death is considered to have occurred when the patient's respirations and heart have ceased to function for several minutes. Usually breathing stops first; the heart stops beating a few minutes later.

In this day of cardiac massage and mouth-to-mouth resuscitation, it is not unusual for a patient "to die" only to revive and walk out of the hospital.

Nursing personnel should note for the medical record the exact time that respirations cease and the heart stops beating. A physician pronounces the patient dead.

For the purpose of human transplants, it has become necessary to have a more precise definition than the cessation of respiration and heart beat as the absolute signs of death. The absence of brain wave activity as measured by the electroencephalogram is usually used to confirm that death has occurred.

CARE AFTER DEATH

In caring for the body of the patient after death, whatever procedures are carried out are performed with dignity and respect. In some religious faiths, only family members are permitted to care for the body of the deceased. Generally, however, this is a nursing responsibility. Although each agency usually has its own specific procedures, there are some general guidelines for the care of the body after death which are fairly universal.

The body is generally placed in a supine position in bed with one pillow under the head. The head is slightly elevated to prevent postmortem hypostasis of blood, which could discolor the face. The body is positioned immediately after death and before rigor mortis sets in.

Rigor mortis, a stiffening of the body after death, is a result of a chemical action within the muscles in which glycogen is coagulated and lactic acid is produced. It generally occurs shortly after death, progressing from the jaw, down the trunk to the extremities. Once rigor mortis has set in, the body remains rigid for one to six days.

When relatives wish to see the body, the nurse first tidies the room and removes extraneous equipment. The body should appear clean, comfortable and peaceful. A slightly shaded room affords a comforting effect.

In some hospitals it is the policy to insert dentures immediately after death; other institutions send the dentures with the body to the morgue, where they are inserted later by the mortician. In most institutions, rings are removed; if a ring cannot be removed it is taped in place and a notation is made on the patient's chart and on the form which goes with the body to the morgue.

The preparation of the body by the nurse involves the application of pads to the perineal area or the insertion of packing into the rectum and vagina. Rarely is it necessary to bathe the body; this procedure is carried out by the mortician. It is, however, necessary to cleanse the body of any blood or drainage which may have accumulated after death.

At most hospitals bodies are labeled twice: one label is attached to the ankles, the other to the shroud in which the body is wrapped. If the ankles and wrists are to be tied together, they should be well padded in order to prevent bruising. In some areas it is the practice to treat the body as if the patient were still living, and no shroud is used. When the preparation of the body is complete it is taken to the hospital morgue. If the hospital does not have a morgue, the mortician should be notified to come for the body.

The patient's valuables and clothes should, whenever possible, be sent home with the relatives. If there is no one present who can assume responsibility for these, valuables should be placed in the hospital safe and the clothes labeled and stored until such time as the family collects them.

The family of the deceased may be asked by the physician to sign a permission for an autopsy (postmortem examination). Under some circumstances an autopsy is required by law. For example, when a patient dies within 24 hours of admission to a hospital or when he dies as a result of injury or accident, some states require an autopsy. It is usually not the nurse's responsibility to secure permission for an autopsy. She may, however, be called upon to explain to the family the reasons for the autopsy.

The death certificate is signed by the physician and then sent to the local health department. If the deceased has had a communicable disease, special regulations are observed regarding the care and disposition of the body.

GUIDE TO ASSESSING NURSING NEEDS

1. Is the patient aware of his prognosis?
2. What have the patient and his family been told about his prognosis?
3. Does the patient have any special requests?
4. Does the patient wish to have a chaplain visit him?
5. Is the patient in pain?
6. Is he lonely?
7. What needs do the family have which the nurse can help to meet?

STUDY VOCABULARY	Autopsy	Drowsiness	Rigor mortis
	Coma	Dysphagia	Stupor

STUDY SITUATION

Mr. John Edwards is in a hospital with a malignancy which the doctors consider terminal. He is 93 years old and has three sons and seven grandchildren. Mr. Edwards has been in a stuporous state and upon waking he complains of pain.

1. What are some of the nursing needs of this patient?
2. What is stupor?
3. What needs of the family could be met by the nurse?
4. Which other members of the health team might be able to assist Mr. Edwards and his family?
5. How can you evaluate Mr. Edwards' nursing care?

BIBLIOGRAPHY

Beland, Irene L.: *Clinical Nursing: Pathophysiological and Psychosocial Approaches.* New York, The Macmillan Company, 1965.

Davidson, Ramona P.: Let's Talk About Death—To Give Care in Terminal Illness. *The American Journal of Nursing,* 66:74–75, January, 1966.

Drummond, Eleanor E.: Communication and Comfort for the Dying Patient. *Nursing Clinics of North America,* 5:1:55–63, March, 1970.

Engel, George L.: Grief and Grieving. *The American Journal of Nursing,* 64:93–98, September, 1964.

Foltá, Jeanette R.: The Perception of Death. *Nursing Research,* 14:232–235, Summer, 1965.

Fox, Jean E.: Reflections on Cancer Nursing. *The American Journal of Nursing,* 66:1317–1319, June, 1966.

Kneisl, Carol R.: Thoughtful Care for the Dying. *The American Journal of Nursing,* 68:550–553, March, 1968.

Kubler-Ross, Elisabeth: *On Death and Dying.* New York, The Macmillan Company, 1969.

Lewis, Wilma R.: A Time to Die. *Nursing Forum,* 4:7–27, 1965.

Mead, Margaret: The Right to Die. *Nursing Outlook,* 16:20, October, 1968.

Quint, Jeanne C.: Obstacles to Helping the Dying. *The American Journal of Nursing,* 66:1568–1571, July 1966.

Saunders, Cicely: The Last Stages of Life. *The American Journal of Nursing,* 65:70–75, March, 1965.

Shephard, Melba W.: This I Believe . . . About Questioning the Right to Die. *Nursing Outlook,* 16:22–25, October, 1968.

Skipper, James K., and Robert C. Leonard (eds.): *Social Interaction and Patient Care.* Philadelphia, J. B. Lippincott Company, 1965.

Spitzer, Stephan P., and Jeanette R. Folta: Death in a Hospital. *Nursing Forum,* 3:85–92, 1964.

Verwoerdt, Adrian, and Ruby Wilson: Communication with Fatally Ill Patients. *The American Journal of Nursing,* 67:2307–2309, November, 1967.

Wagner, Berniece M.: Teaching Students to Work with the Dying. *The American Journal of Nursing,* 64:128–129, November, 1964.

APPENDIX

Word or Phrase	Abbreviation	Meaning
ad		to, up to
ad libitum	ad lib.	at pleasure
ana	aa	of each
ante cibum	a.c.	before meals
aqua		water
bene		well
bis in die	b.i.d.	twice daily
cum	$\overline{c}$	with
divide	div.	divide
dosis	dos.	a dose
fac		make
fiat, fiant	ft.	let there be made
gutta	gtt.	a drop
hora	h.	an hour
hora somni	h.s.	just before going to sleep
mane et nocte	m. et n.	morning and night
misce	M.	mix
non repetatur	n.r.	not to be repeated
numero	no.	number
omne die	o.d.	every day
omne mane	o.m.	every morning
omne nocte	o.n.	every night
pilula	pil.	pill
pone		place
post cibum	p.c.	after meals

---

*Harold N. Wright: *Prescription Writing and Medical Jurisprudence.* Sixth edition. Minneapolis, Burgess Publishing Company, 1962, pp. 11–12.

449

Word or Phrase	Abbreviation	Meaning
pro re nata	p.r.n.	as occasion requires
pulvis	pulv.	powder
quantum sufficiat	q.s.	a sufficient quantity
quaque die	q.d.	every day
quaque hora	q.h.	every hour
quaque nocte	q.n.	every night
quaque 3 hora	q.3.h.	every three hours
quater in die	q.i.d.	four times a day
semel in die	s.i.d.	once a day
signa	sig.	sign, write
si opus sit	s.o.s.	if necessary
statim	stat.	immediately
tabella	tab.	tablet
talis, tales		such
ter in die	t.i.d.	three times a day

PREFIXES AND SUFFIXES IN MEDICAL TERMINOLOGY

Prefix	Meaning
adeno-	gland
arthro-	joint
chole-	bile
chondro-	cartilage
colpo-	vagina
cranio-	skull
entero-	intestine
gastro-	stomach
hystero-	uterus
laparo-	loin
litho-	stone
masto-	breast
myo-	muscle
nephro-	kidney
neuro-	nerve
osteo-	bone
phleb-	vein
pneumo-	air
pyelo-	pelvis, basin
salpingo-	tube
teno-	tendon
thoraco-	chest
trachel-	neck

Suffix

-ectomy	a cutting out or excision
-oscopy	examination by means of a lighted instrument
-ostomy	formation of a fistula or opening
-otomy	a cutting or an incision
-pexy	fixation
-plasty	molding
-rhaphy	a suturing of

GLOSSARY

abduction. movement away from the central axis of the body.

abrasion. an area of the body rubbed bare of skin or mucous membrane.

abscess. a localized collection of pus in a cavity formed by the disintegration of tissue.

acapnia. a condition of decreased carbon dioxide in the blood.

acetone. a colorless liquid with a pleasant ethereal odor. It is found in small quantities in normal urine and is used as a solvent for fats, resins, rubber and plastics.

acidosis. a condition in which there is an excessive proportion of acid in the blood and a reduced reserve of alkali (bicarbonate).

acne. an inflammatory disease of the sebaceous glands.

acromion process. the outward extension of the spine of the scapula, forming the point of the shoulder.

acute. having a short and relatively severe course.

adaptation mechanism. the reaction of the body to disturbances in its equilibrium.

addiction. the state of being given to some habit, as a drug habit.

adduction. movement toward the central axis of the body.

adhesion. a fibrous band or structure by which parts may abnormally adhere.

adipose. of a fatty nature.

adrenal gland. endocrine gland located atop the kidney.

adrenocortical hormone. a hormone secreted by the cortex of the adrenal gland.

agitate. to excite the mind or feelings; to move with irregular, rapid or violent action.

alarm reaction. mobilization of the body's defense forces in response to physiological or psychological stress.

albuminuria. the presence of protein in the urine, in the form of white blood cells.

aldosterone. a hormone secreted by the cortex of the adrenal glands; a mineralocorticoid.

alkalosis. a condition in which there is an excess of alkali such as bicarbonate in the blood

alveolus (i). an air sac of the lungs formed by the terminal dilatations of a bronchiole.

ambulate. to move about; to walk from place to place.

ameba. a minute one-celled animal organism of the phylum Protozoa.

amino acid. the structural unit of protein.

anabolism. the synthesis of compounds by the cells.

anaerobe. a microorganism that grows in the absence or near absence of oxygen.

analgesic. relieving pain; a pain-relieving agent.

anemia. a condition in which the blood is deficient in hemoglobin or red blood cells.

aneroid. containing no liquid.

anesthesia. loss of feeling or sensation.

anion. a negatively charged ion.

anogenital. pertaining to the area around the anus and genitalia.

anorexia. loss of appetite.

anoxemia. a decrease in the amount of oxygen in the blood below physiological levels.

anoxia. a decrease in the amount of oxygen in the tissues below physiological levels.

antecubital. situated in front of the cubitus or forearm.

anthelmintic. destructive to worms.

antibiotic. a chemical substance produced by microorganisms which has the capacity to destroy or inhibit the growth of other microorganisms.

antibody. a substance formed in the body in response to an antigen.

antidiuretic hormone. a hormone produced by the posterior pituitary gland which inhibits the secretion of urine.

antigen. a substance which stimulates the production of antibodies within the body.

antipyretic. an agent which reduces fever.

antisepsis. the prevention of sepsis by inhibiting the growth of microorganisms.

anuria. the absence of urinary excretion from the body.

anus. the distal orifice of the alimentary canal.

anxiety. an emotional response to danger of unknown origin.

aortic receptor. a nerve ending in the aortic arch which is sensitive to changes in blood pressure.

apathy. lack of feeling or emotion.

apical beat. the beat of the heart as it is felt over the apex.

apnea. a period of cessation of breathing.

apomorphine. an alkaloid which is a powerful emetic and relaxant.

appendicitis. inflammation of the vermiform appendix.

appetite. desire for food.

arachnoidal granulations. the capillary-like projections of the arachnoid membrane.

arachnoid membrane. a membrane between the pia mater and dura mater surrounding the brain and spinal cord.

areolar connective tissue. loose connective tissue widely distributed in the body.

Aschheim-Zondek test. a pregnancy test in which urine from a female is injected into mice.

ascites. abnormal accumulation of fluid in the peritoneal cavity.

asepsis. freedom from infection, that is, from pathogenic organisms.

asphyxia. suffocation; a condition in which there is anoxia and an increase in carbon dioxide tension in the blood and tissues.

aspiration. the act of breathing or drawing in; the removal of fluids or gases from a cavity by suction.

asthma. a condition marked by periodic attacks of dyspnea, with wheezing and a sense of constriction.

astringent. an agent which causes contraction and arrests discharges.

asymmetric. not symmetrical; lack of correspondence in paired organs.

atelectasis. incomplete expansion of the lungs at birth or collapse of the adult lung.

atrioventricular valve. the valve between the atrium and the ventricle of the heart.

atrophy. a wasting away or diminution in the size of a cell, tissue, organ or other part.

auscultation.   observation by listening for body sounds.

autonomic.   self-functioning; independent.

autonomy.   the condition of being functionally independent.

bactericidal.   capable of destroying bacteria.

bacteriostatic.   capable of inhibiting the growth or multiplication of bacteria.

bacterium(a).   any microorganism of the order Eubacteriales.

barrier technique.   medical aseptic practices to control the spread of pathogenic bacteria and contribute to their destruction.

basal metabolism.   the rate of energy expenditure of the body at rest.

basic need.   a need that is necessary for survival, as the need for air.

basilic vein.   superficial vein of the arm.

Bence-Jones protein test.   examination of urine to detect bone tumors.

binder.   a type of bandage.

biopsy.   the removal and examination of tissue or other material from the living body.

Biot's respirations.   irregular respirations as to speed and depth; pauses may be associated with a sigh.

bleb.   a skin vesicle filled with fluid.

blister.   a collection of fluid in the epidermis causing an elevation of the outer layer (stratum corneum).

boil.   furuncle; a painful nodule in the skin caused by bacteria and often having a central core.

bolus.   a mass of food ready to be swallowed or a mass passing along the intestines.

bradycardia.   a very slow heart beat, reflected in a pulse of under 60 beats per minute.

bradykinin.   chemical substance released by damaged cells which excites pain receptors.

bradypnea.   an abnormal decrease in the respiratory rate.

bronchoscopy.   inspection of the bronchi with a lighted instrument (bronchoscope).

bronchus(i).   one of the two main branches of the trachea; also the divisions of the main bronchi within the lungs.

burette.   a graduated glass.

cachexia.   a general physical wasting, often associated with chronic disease.

calculus(i).   a stone formed in various parts of the body such as the gallbladder or kidney.

calorie.   a unit of heat. One small calorie is the amount of heat required to raise the temperature of 1 gm. of water 1° C. A large calorie is the amount of heat required to raise the temperature of 1 kg. of water 1° C.

calyx(ices).   a cup-shaped organ or cavity; in the kidney, one of the recesses in the pelvis.

cannula.   a tube for insertion into the body, often made of a hard substance, and the lumen of which contains a trochar during the insertion.

canthus.   the angle formed at either end of the eye by the upper and lower eyelids.

cardiac sphincter.   the band of circular fibers situated at the opening of the esophagus into the stomach.

carminative.   a medicine which relieves flatulence.

carotid receptors. nerve endings located in the carotid sinuses and carotid bodies which are sensitive to changes in blood pressure, excess blood CO_2 and blood pH.

carrier. an individual who harbors disease organisms in his body and yet does not manifest symptoms but who can pass on the infection.

cast. coagulated protein in the urine, passed from the lumen of the kidney tubules.

catabolism. a destructive process within the cells in which complex substances are converted into simpler substances.

cathartic. a medicine which hastens bowel evacuation.

catheter. a tube used to withdraw fluid from body cavities, as from the urinary bladder.

cation. a positively charged ion.

central pain. pain arising from injury to sensory nerves, neural pathways or areas in the brain concerned with pain perception.

cephalic vein. a superficial vein on the thumb side of the arm.

cerebral cortex. the outer layer (gray matter) of the largest part of the brain (cerebrum).

cerebrospinal fluid. the fluid which surrounds the brain and spinal cord.

cerumen. wax found in the ears.

cervix. a necklike structure; the lower narrow portion of the uterus.

Cheyne-Stokes respirations. respirations with rhythmical variations in intensity occurring in cycles, often with periods of apnea.

chill. involuntary contractions of the voluntary muscles, with shivering and shaking.

chordotomy. surgical division of the anterolateral tracts of the spinal cord.

choroid plexus. a network of capillaries found in the ventricles of the brain which produce the cerebrospinal fluid.

cicatrization. a healing process which leaves a scar.

cilium(a). a minute hairlike process attached to the free surface of a cell, as in the nose.

cinefluorography. the production of a motion picture record of a sequence of fluoroscopic images.

circumcision. removal of all or part of the foreskin of the penis.

circumduction. circular movement, as of a limb or an eye.

cisterna. a closed space serving as a reservoir.

cisterna magna. an extension of the subarachnoid space below and behind the corpus callosum.

cisternal puncture. the insertion of a needle into the cisterna magna.

clavicle. the collar bone. It articulates with the sternum and the scapula.

clean. denoting the absence of disease-producing microorganisms.

cognition. the process by which we become aware through thought or perception, including reasoning and understanding.

cohesion. a force which unites particles.

collagen. an albuminoid supportive protein found in connective tissue.

coma. a state of unconsciousness from which an individual cannot be aroused.

commode. a portable toilet-like structure.

communicable disease. a disease capable of being transmitted from one person to another.

compress. a pad or cloth that is folded and applied to press upon a body part.

concave. rounded inward or hollowed.

concurrent disinfection. on-going measures to control the spread of infection during the time the patient is considered infectious.

conditioned. learned through repetition of a stimulus, as in Pavlov's experiment.

conduction. the transfer of sound waves, heat, nerve impulses or electricity.

congestion. an abnormal accumulation of blood in a part.

consciousness. the normal state of awareness.

constant fever. an elevated temperature which remains at essentially the same level.

constipation. abnormal delay in the passage of feces.

contact. a person who is known to have been sufficiently near an infected person to be exposed to the transfer of infectious organisms.

contaminate. to soil or make unclean.

context. the environment; the portions of a discourse that precede or follow a word or words.

contracture. a shortening or distortion of muscle tissue.

convection. transmission of heat in liquids or gases.

conversion reaction. a condition in which emotional disorders are experienced as physical symptoms.

conversive. pertaining to a change in the state of energy, as from electricity to heat.

corneal reflex. closing of the eyelids as a result of irritation of the cornea.

counterirritant. an agent applied to the skin to produce a reaction which relieves irritation.

covert. hidden; covered.

creatinin. nitrogenous waste excreted in the urine.

crisis. the rapid fall of a fever.

cultural shock. stress caused by exposure to customs and social values at variance with one's own.

culture. those aspects of society which include knowledge, beliefs, art, morals, laws and customs.

curative aspects. pertaining to diagnostic therapeutic and rehabilitative measures in health care.

custom. a practice that is common to many or to a place or class or that is habitual to an individual.

cyanosis. a bluish tinge in the skin or mucous membrane.

cyst. a sac, usually containing a liquid or semisolid material.

cystitis. inflammation of the urinary bladder.

cystoscopy. examination of the urinary bladder with a lighted instrument.

debilitated. enfeebled; lacking strength.

deceleration. the state of moving at decreasing speed.

decubitus ulcer. a bedsore.

deep pain. pain arising from deeper structures of the body, such as muscles, tendons, joints.

defecation. the evacuation of feces.

dehydration. removal of water from the body or tissues.

delirious. suffering from mental confusion, incoherence and physical restlessness.

dependency. having to rely on others for the satisfaction of basic needs.

detergent. an agent which purifies or cleanses.

detrusor muscle. the three layers of smooth muscle of the urinary bladder.

diacetic acid.   acetoacetic acid; an acid excreted in the urine.

diagnosis.   the determination of the nature of a disease.

diaphoresis.   profuse perspiration.

diarrhea.   undue frequency of the passage of feces, with the discharge of loose stools.

diastolic blood pressure.   the pressure in the arteries when the ventricles of the heart are relaxed.

diathermy.   the generation of heat in the tissues by the application of high frequency electric currents.

dietitian.   a person educated in the use of diet in health and disease.

differentiation.   distinguishing of one thing or disease from another on the basis of differences.

digital.   pertaining to the fingers.

disassociate.   to separate; to detach from association.

discipline.   a field of study.

disinfection.   the destruction of disease-producing microorganisms.

disorientation.   a state of mental confusion; a lack of awareness of time, place or person.

distal.   farther from a point of reference or point of attachment.

diuretic.   a substance which increases the secretion of urine in the kidneys.

doctor's order sheet.   a written record of the orders given by the physician for the patient's treatment.

dorsal.   pertaining to the back; posterior.

dorsal recumbent.   supine; lying on one's back.

drowsiness.   readiness to fall asleep.

drug.   a chemical compound used for diagnosis or therapy or as a preventive measure.

duodenum.   the first part of the small intestine.

dysphagia.   difficulty in swallowing.

dyspnea.   difficult breathing.

dysuria.   difficulty in voiding or pain on voiding.

ecchymosis.   extravasation of blood into the tissues.

edema.   the presence of excessive amounts of fluid in the intercellular spaces.

efferent.   carrying outward from the center.

electrocardiogram.   a graphic tracing of the electrical current produced by the contraction of the heart muscle.

electroencephalogram.   a record of the electrical impulses produced by the brain.

electrolyte.   a compound which in an aqueous solution is able to conduct an electrical current.

emaciation.   abnormal leanness; a state of wasting away.

embolus.   a clot in a blood vessel which has been transported from another vessel.

emesis.   vomiting.

emollient.   softening or soothing.

emphysema.   a condition in which the pulmonary alveoli are distended or rupture as a result of air pressure.

emulsion.   a liquid which is distributed throughout another liquid in small globules.

endemic.   present at all times among a particular people or within a particular country.

endogenous.   developing from within.

endogenous spread.   the transfer of microorganisms from one area of a person's body to another.

endothelium.   the layer of squamous cells which lines the blood vessels.

enema.   a liqud to be injected into the rectum.

enteric.   pertaining to the intestines.

enteroclysis.   the injection of a nutrient or medicine into the bowel.

environment.   the sum total of the external surroundings and influences.

epidemic.   attacking many people in a region at the same time; widely diffused and rapidly spreading.

epididymitis.   inflammation of the epididymis, the oblong body containing a duct attached to the testicle.

epinephrine.   a hormone produced by the medulla of the adrenal gland or prepared synthetically; a vasopressor.

epistaxis.   nosebleed.

equilibrium.   a static or dynamic state of balance between opposing forces or actions.

erythema.   redness of the skin due to congestion of the capillaries.

esophagus.   the canal extending from the pharynx to the stomach.

etiology.   the study of the causes of disease.

eupnea.   normal, regular or effortless breathing.

eversion.   a turning outward.

excoriation.   the loss of superficial layers of skin.

excreta.   waste materials excreted by the body.

exogenous.   developing from outside.

expectorate.   to bring mucus up from the lungs or trachea.

expiration.   the act of expelling air from the lungs (breathing out).

expressive activities.   those activities of the nurse which contribute to the comfort and well-being of the patient.

extension.   the act of straightening a limb.

extracellular.   situated outside the cells.

extravasation.   the escape of blood from a vessel into the tissues.

exudate.   a substance produced on or in a tissue by disease or a vital process.

fastigium (stadium).   the high point of a fever.

fear.   an emotional response to a known and identifiable danger.

feces.   excreta discharged from the intestines.

femur.   the leg bone extending from the pelvis to the knee.

fibrin.   a protein substance which forms an essential part of a blood clot.

fibroplasia.   the formation of fibrous tissue.

Fishberg concentration test.   a special urine test to determine specific gravity.

fissure.   a deep cleft or groove.

fistula.   an abnormal passage leading from an abscess or hollow organ to the body surface or from one hollow organ to another.

flatulence.   distention of the stomach or the intestines with air or gases.

flatus.   gas in the intestines or stomach.

flexion.   the act of bending.

fluoroscopy.   examination of structures of the body such as the stomach by means of roentgen rays and a fluorescent screen.

fomite.   a substance other than food which can harbor microorganisms.

fossa navicularis. a widened area of the lumen of the male urethra just superior to the meatus; a depression on the internal pterygoid process of the sphenoid bone.

frequency. in reference to voiding, abnormally short intervals between times of voding.

friction. the force which opposes motion.

Friedman test. a test for pregnancy which involves the injection of urine into rabbits.

frontal plane. the plane that divides the body into dorsal and ventral sections.

fulcrum. the fixed point of a lever.

functional pathology. referring to diseases which have no apparent physical basis.

gastrocolic reflex. mass peristalsis of the colon stimulated from the stomach.

gastroenteritis. inflammation of the stomach and intestines.

gastroscopy. the examination of the stomach with a lighted instrument.

gavage. feeding through a stomach tube.

genitalia. the reproductive organs; generally, the external reproductive organs.

geriatric. pertaining to old age.

glomerulus. a tuft of capillaries such as that of the nephron of the kidney.

glossopharyngeal nerve. the ninth cranial nerve; the nerve serving the tongue and pharynx.

glottis. the vocal apparatus of the larynx.

glycerol. glycerin; a byproduct of the breakdown of fats.

glycogen. a polysaccharide stored in cells after the breakdown of carbohydrate.

glycosuria. the presence of glucose in the urine.

granulation tissue. tissue formed in wounds.

gravity. the force which pulls all objects toward the center of the earth.

Guérin's fold. a fold of mucous membrane occasionally seen in the fossa navicularis of the urethra.

gynecology. the branch of medicine which deals with diseases of the female reproductive tract.

halitosis. foul odor of the breath.

health team. all those who participate in providing health care services.

hectic (septic) fever. an intermittent fever with wide variations in temperature elevation but in which the temperature falls to normal during each 24 hour period.

hematemesis. the vomiting of blood.

hematuria. the discharge of blood in the urine.

hemoglobin. the red pigment of the red blood cell which carries oxygen.

hemoglobinuria. hemoglobin in the urine.

hemoptysis. the spitting up of blood or of blood-tinged sputum.

hemorrhage. bleeding; the escape of a large amount of blood from the blood vessels.

hemorrhoid. enlarged, often-infected, veins and sinuses at or near the anus.

hemothorax. a collection of blood in the thoracic cavity.

herbalist. a nonmedical practitioner of the healing arts who makes use of herbs (plants) to treat disease.

Hering-Breuer reflex. the reflex which limits respiratory inspirations and expirations.

hierarchy. an arrangement in a graded series.

homeostasis. a tendency to uniformity or stability in body states; dynamic equilibrium.

host. an animal or plant which harbors or nourishes another organism.

humidity. the degree of moisture in the air.

hunger. an uncomfortable feeling which indicates a need for nourishment.

hyaluronidase. an enzyme which initiates the hydrolysis of the cement material (hyaluronic acid) of the tissues.

hydration. the act of combining with water; the state of having adequate body fluids.

hydraulic. pertaining to the action of liquids.

hydrostatic. pertaining to fluids in a state of equilibrium.

hydrostatic pressure. the pressure of liquids.

hyperalgesia. excessive sensitiveness to pain.

hypercalcemia. an excessive amount of calcium in the blood.

hyperemia. excessive blood in any part of the body.

hypertension. an abnormally high blood pressure.

hyperglycemia. an increased concentration of glucose in the blood.

hyperkalemia. an excessive amount of potassium in the blood.

hypernatremia. an excessive amount of sodium in the blood.

hyperplasia. an abnormal increase in the number of cells in a tissue or organ.

hyperpnea. an abnormal increase in the rate and depth of respirations.

hyperthermia. an abnormally high body temperature; fever.

hypertonicity. a state characterized by excessive tone or activity.

hypertrophy. an abnormal increase in the size of an organ or tissue as a result of an increase in the size of the cells.

hypervolemia. an abnormal increase in blood volume.

hypocalcemia. a decrease in the amount of serum calcium.

hypochloremia. a reduced concentration of chlorides in the blood.

hypodermoclysis. the introduction of fluids into the subcutaneous tissues.

hypogastric nerve. the nerve trunk of the autonomic nervous system which serves the abdominal viscera.

hypoglycemia. a reduction in the amount of glucose in the blood.

hypokalemia. a reduction in the amount of potassium in the blood.

hyponatremia. a decrease in the amount of sodium in the blood.

hypotension. an abnormally low blood pressure.

hypothalamus. part of the diencephalon of the brain, from which fibers of the autonomic nervous system extend to the thalamus, neurohypophysis, etc.

hypothermia. an abnormally low body temperature.

hypoxemia. a reduction in the oxygen content of the blood.

hypoxia. a reduction in the oxygen content of the tissues.

immunity. the condition of being protected against a particular disease.

impaction. the condition of being firmly lodged or wedged.

incontinence. inability to restrain a natural discharge, as urine or feces.

infection. the invasion of the body by disease-producing microorganisms and the body's reaction to their presence.

infestation. invasion of the body by arthropods, including insects, mites and ticks.

inflammation. a condition of the tissues in reaction to injury.

infusion. the therapeutic introduction of a fluid into a vein or part of the body.

inguinal hernia. the protrusion of an organ or tissue through an abnormal opening into the inguinal canal.

inhalation therapist. a technician who is skilled in the performance of diagnostic procedures and therapeutic measures dealing with the respiratory tract.

insertion (of a muscle). the place of attachment of a muscle to the bone that it moves.

inspection. observation by use of the sense of sight.

inspiration. the act of taking air into the lungs.

instillation. the dropping of a liquid into a cavity such as the ear.

instrumental tasks. nursing activities which provide the patient with technical assistance required to regain his health.

insulator. a material or substance which prevents or inhibits conduction, as of heat.

intercostal. located between the ribs.

intermittent (quotidian) fever. fever which falls to normal at sometime during a 24 hour period.

intern. a graduate of a basic professional program (medicine, nursing, etc.) who is receiving a planned program of clinical experience, usually in order to complete requirements for licensure.

interstitial. located between the cells of tissue.

intracellular. located within the cells.

intradermal. located within the dermis.

intramuscular. located within the muscle tissue.

intraosseous. located within the bone.

intravascular. located within a vessel.

intravenous. located within a vein.

intravertebral. intraspinal.

intrathecal. located within the spinal canal.

intubation. the insertion of a tube.

inversion. a turning inward.

inward rotation. a turning of a bone upon its axis toward the midline.

irradiation. exposure to x-rays or radioactive matter such as radium.

irrational. confused as to time, place or person; not possessing normal judgment.

irritant. an agent applied to the skin to produce a reaction.

ischemia. localized anemia due to an obstruction to the inflow of blood.

isolation. the separation of one person, material or object from others.

isometric exercise. exercise in which muscle tension is increased but the muscles are not shortened and the body parts are not moved.

isotonic. pertaining to equal tone or pressure; pertaining to solutions having equal osmotic pressure.

isotonic exercise. exercise in which the muscle is shortened and body parts are moved.

jaundice. a condition in which yellowish pigment is deposited in the skin, tissues and body fluid.

ketone.   a compound containing the carbonyl group.

17-ketosteroid.   a type of hormone classed as an androgen and excreted in the urine. It is partially produced in the adrenal cortex and partially derived from testosterone.

kilogram.   a unit of weight equal to 1000 grams or approximately 2.2 pounds.

kinesiology.   the science of motion.

Kussmaul's breathing.   air hunger; dyspnea occurring periodically without cyanosis.

languor.   listlessness; lassitude.

lassitude.   weariness; fatigue; languor.

lateral.   relating to the side; situated away from the midline.

lavage.   therapeutic washing out of an organ such as the stomach.

lethargy.   abnormal drowsiness; state of being lazy or indifferent.

leukocyte.   white blood cell.

lever.   a rigid bar which revolves around a fixed point.

ligament.   a band of connective tissue that connects bones or supports organs.

lumbar puncture.   the introduction of a needle into the subarachnoid space in the lumbar section of the spinal cord for diagnostic or therapeutic purposes.

lumen.   the cavity of a tubular organ.

lymph nodes.   an accumulation of densely packed lymphatic tissue.

lymphatic.   pertaining to or containing lymph.

lysis.   the gradual fall of an elevated temperature.

malaise.   a vague sense of debility or lack of health.

malignancy.   a tendency to progress in virulence.

malnutrition.   a disorder of nutrition.

manometer.   an instrument for measuring the pressure of liquids or gases.

massage.   systematic stroking and kneading of the tissues.

meatus.   an opening.

medial.   pertaining to the middle; situated toward the midline.

medical asepsis.   practices which are carried out in order to keep microorganisms within a given area.

medical diagnosis.   the physician's opinion as to the nature of a patient's illness.

medicament.   an agent used in therapy; medicine; drug.

medicine.   any drug or remedy.

medulla oblongata.   the part of the rhombencephalon which attaches to the spinal cord and contains a number of the vital centers.

meniscus.   a crescent-shaped structure; the surface of a liquid column.

menstrual.   pertaining to the monthly flow of blood from the female genital tract.

metabolism.   the sum of all physical and chemical processes by which living substance is produced and maintained.

microorganism.   an organism which can be seen only by means of a microscope.

microwave.   an electromagnetic wave of high frequency and short wave length.

micturition.   voiding.

minim.   a unit of volume equal to 1/60 part of a fluid dram.

mold.   a type of fungus.

morbid.   pertaining to disease.

morbidity.   the relative incidence of disease.
mortality.   the quality of being subject to death.
mortality rate.   the death rate.
Mosaic Law.   writings attributed to Moses.
mucoid.   a moist viscid protein substance.
myelography.   the x-ray examination of the spinal cord by using a contrast medium.
myocardium.   heart muscle.

narcotic.   a drug which relieves pain or induces sleep or stupor.
nasopharynx.   the upper part of the pharynx continuous with the nasal passage.
naturopath.   a nonmedical practitioner of the healing arts who makes use of physical forces such as heat and massage to cure disease.
nausea.   stomach distress accompanied by an urge to vomit.
necrosis.   localized death of tissue.
need.   something an individual perceives as being useful or necessary.
neoplasm.   any new and abnormal growth.
Neo-Synephrine.   phenylephrine hydrochloride, an adrenergic drug which produces vasoconstriction.
nephron.   functional unit of the kidney.
neuron.   functional unit of the nervous system.
nitrogen mustard.   an agent used therapeutically to inhibit the growth of abnormal new cells, as white blood cells in leukemia. It is very irritating to tissues.
nocturia.   excessive urination at night.
norepinephrine.   a hormone produced by the adrenal medulla.
norm.   a fixed or ideal standard.
nurse's aide.   a member of the nursing team who assists professional and practical nurses either directly in the care of patients or through maintenance of a clean and comfortable physical environment.
nursing action.   those measures which nurses carry out to help patients in the achievement of health goals.
nursing care plan.   a plan of care for a patient.
nursing diagnosis.   an assessment of those needs of patients which a nurse can help to meet through nursing action.
nursing history.   a written record of information about a patient obtained by the nurse through interview and observation.
nursing orderly.   a member of the nursing team who assists in the personal care of male patients and who may perform simple nursing tasks.
nursing process.   the series of steps the nurse takes in planning and giving nursing care.
nutrient.   nourishing; a substance affording nourishment.
nutritionist.   a member of the health team whose special area of expertise is nutrition, usually employed in other than institutional agencies to teach and counsel people about nutrition and provide consultive services for other health workers.

obese.   corpulent; excessively fat.
objective symptom.   evidence of a disease process or dysfunction of the body which can be observed and described by other people.

obstetrics.   that branch of medical science which deals with birth and its antecedents and sequelae.

occult.   hidden.

occupational therapist.   a member of the health team who assists patients to develop new skills or to regain skills lessened or lost through illness.

oliguria.   secretion of a diminished amount of urine.

ophthalmoscope.   an instrument used to examine the interior of the eye.

organic.   of, relating to or containing living organisms.

organic pathology.   pertaining to disease processes which can be identified physically, as, for example, tumors or communicable diseases.

oriented.   aware of time, place and person.

orifice.   entrance or outlet of any body cavity.

origin (of muscle).   the fixed end or attachment of a muscle.

oropharynx.   that division of the pharynx between the soft palate and the epiglottis.

orthopnea.   the inability to breathe except when in a sitting position.

osmosis.   passage of a solvent through a membrane from a lesser to a greater concentration of two solutions.

otoscope.   an instrument used to inspect the ear.

outward rotation.   a circular motion directed away from the midline.

ovulation.   the discharge of an ovum from the ovary.

pain.   unpleasant sensation resulting from the stimulation of specialized nerve endings.

pain perception threshold.   the level of stimulation at which pain is first experienced.

palliative.   affording relief but not cure.

palpation.   examination by using one's fingers (sense of touch).

pandemic.   widespread epidemic disease.

Papanicolaou smear.   a cytologic test in which cells are taken from the cervix for examination, chiefly to detect malignancy.

papillary reflex.   tactile response of the skin.

paracentesis.   the removal of fluid from the peritoneal cavity.

paralysis.   loss or impairment of motor or sensory function due to neural or muscular disease.

parasite.   a plant or animal which lives upon or within another living organism.

parasympathetic nervous system.   the craniosacral part of the autonomic nervous system.

parenteral.   occurring outside the alimentary tract.

Parkinson's disease.   a chronic condition marked by muscular rigidity and tremor.

parotid glands.   salivary glands situated near the ear.

parotitis.   inflammation of the parotid glands; mumps.

patent.   open; unobstructed.

pathogen.   a disease-producing microorganism or material.

pathogenic.   capable of producing disease.

pathology.   the branch of medicine which deals with the nature of disease.

patient.   a person with a health problem.

patient's record.   a written record of a person's medical history, examinations, tests, diagnosis, prognosis, therapy and response to therapy while he is a patient.

peer.   one of equal standing.

pelvis (of kidney).   funnel-shaped cavity of the kidney.

penance.   repentance for sin.

percussion.   examination by tapping the body.

perineum.   the area between the anus and the posterior part of the genitalia; entire anogenital area.

periosteum.   fibrous membrane surrounding bone.

peripheral.   outward or toward the surface.

peristalsis.   wormlike movement by which the alimentary tract propels its contents along.

peritoneal cavity.   the potential space between the layers of the peritoneum.

peritoneum.   the serous membrane lining the abdominal cavity.

peritonitis.   inflammation of the peritoneum.

petechia.   a pinpoint of blood in the skin or mucous membrane.

Petri dish.   a shallow glass receptacle for growing bacterial cultures.

phantom pain.   pain believed to be caused by a pain "memory," after the cause of the pain has been removed, as pain in amputated limbs.

phenosulfophthalein.   a chemical used to test the function of the kidneys.

phlebotomy.   an opening into a vein made in order to remove blood.

physical therapist.   a member of the health team who assists in assessment of patients' functional ability and carries out therapeutic and rehabilitative measures dealing particularly with the musculoskeletal system.

physiology.   the science which deals with the function of living organisms and their parts.

plantar flexion.   a reflex in which an irritation of the sole of the foot contracts the toes; extension of the foot away from the body.

plasma.   the fluid portion of blood.

pleura.   the serous membrane lining the thoracic cavity.

pleural cavity.   the potential space between the plurae.

pneumothorax.   the accumulation of gas or air in the pleural cavity.

poliomyelitis.   a virus disease which when serious can involve the central nervous system, with resultant paralysis.

polydipsia.   excessive thirst.

polyethylene.   a lightweight plastic resistant to chemicals and moisture and having insulating properties.

polypnea.   an abnormal increase in the respiratory rate.

polyuria.   secretion of an increased amount of urine.

popliteal space.   posterior surface of the knee.

posterior fornix (of the vagina).   a vaultlike space at the back of the vagina.

posture.   the relationship of the various parts of the body at rest or in any phase of motion.

precordium.   the region over the heart or stomach.

preoptic center.   the nerve center anterior to the optic center.

prepubic urethra.   the part of the male urethra inferior to the pubis.

preventive.   directed at; averting the occurrence of.

proctoclysis.   Murphy drip; the slow injection of a large amount of liquid into the rectum.

proctoscopy.   examination of the rectum and the anus by means of a lighted instrument.

progesterone.   a hormone produced by the corpus luteum of the ovary.

prognosis.   medical opinion as to the outcome of a disease process.

proliferation.   growth by rapid reproduction.

prophylactic.   preventive.

prostate.   a gland which surrounds the male urethra just below the bladder.

prostration.   extreme exhaustion.

proteinuria.   the presence of protein in the urine.

protoplasm.   the living substance of cells.

proximal.   closer to the point of reference or to the point of attachment.

pruritus.   intense itching.

psychiatry.   the branch of medicine which deals with disorders that are mental, emotional or behavioral.

psychology.   the science of mind and mental processes.

psychosomatic.   concerning the mind and the body.

pulse deficit.   the difference between the apical rate and the pulse rate.

pulse pressure.   the difference between the systolic and diastolic blood pressures.

pupil.   the opening in the center of the iris of the eye.

purulent.   containing pus.

pus.   the thick liquid product of inflammation, composed of leukocytes, liquid, tissue debris and microorganisms.

pyemia.   a general septicemia in which there is pus in the blood.

pyloric sphincter.   the thickened layer of circular fibers which surrounds the opening between the stomach and the duodenum.

pyrexia.   fever.

pyrogen.   a fever-producing substance.

pyuria.   pus in the urine.

Queckenstedt's sign.   when the veins on either side of the neck are compressed, the pressure of the cerebrospinal fluid rises in a normal person.

radiation.   treatment with x-rays, radium or other radioactive matter.

radiopaque.   not permitting the passage of roentgen rays.

rapport.   a relationship marked by accord or affinity.

reciprocal.   given in return; mutual.

rectum.   the distal portion of the large intestine.

referred pain.   pain perceived in one area of the body when the stimulus for its origin is in another area.

regimen.   a regulated pattern of activity.

rehabilitation.   the restoration of the ill or injured to function at their full capacity.

relapsing fever.   a fever in which there is one or more days of normalcy between febrile periods.

remittent fever.   a fever with marked variations but in which the temperature does not reach normal.

renal.   relating to the kidney.

resident.   a qualified medical practitioner who is resident in a hospital, usually while preparing for practice in a medical specialty.

residual volume.   the amount of air remaining in the lungs after a forceful expiration.

resuscitation.   restoration to life or consciousness.

retention (of urine).   a condition in which urine is accumulated in the bladder and not excreted.

rickettsiae. minute rod-shaped microorganisms of the family Rickettsiaceae.

rigor mortis. the stiffening of a dead body.

roentgen. the unit of measurement of x-radiation.

role. the pattern of behavior that is expected of an individual in a particular group or situation.

rubefacient. reddening of the skin; an agent that reddens the skin.

ruga(e). a ridge, wrinkle or fold.

sacrament. a formal religious act.

sagittal plane. the plane which divides the body into right and left sections.

sanguineous. pertaining to blood.

saphenous veins. superficial veins of the legs.

sclerosis. an induration or hardening.

scored. marked with significant notches, lines or grooves.

secretion. a product of a gland.

secularism. indifference to religion.

sedative. tending to calm or tranquilize; a sedative agent.

semantics. the study of meaning in language.

semicircular canal. an organ within the temporal bone which functions to give the sense of equilibrium.

semilunar valves. pulmonary and aortic valves of the heart.

senility. the feebleness of body and mind incident to old age.

sensitivity. responsiveness to various stimuli; frequently used to refer to the responsiveness of bacteria to specific antibiotic agents.

septic. due to or produced by putrefaction.

septic fever. hectic fever.

serum. the clear portion of an animal liquid; the liquid part of blood as distinct from the solid particles.

shock. a condition of acute peripheral circulatory failure.

sigmoidoscopy. examination of the sigmoid colon with a lighted instrument.

sign. an objective symptom which can be detected through special examination.

singultus. hiccup.

smear. a specimen for microscopic study prepared by spreading the specimen across a glass slide.

social worker. a member of the health team who assists in evaluating the psychosocial situation of patients and helps them with their social problems.

sociology. the science of the social institutions and relationships.

sordes. a collection of bacteria, food particles and epithelial tissue in the mouth.

spasm. involuntary contraction of a muscle or a group of muscles.

speculum. an instrument for opening to view a cavity or canal.

sphincter. a ringlike muscle which closes a natural orifice.

sphygmomanometer. an instrument used to measure blood pressure in the arteries.

spinothalamic tract. the neural pathway along the spinal cord to the thalamus.

spore. the reproductive element of a microorganism which is surrounded by a thick wall.

sprain. the wrenching of a joint resulting in injury to its attachments.

sputum. matter ejected from the respiratory tract, often from the lungs.

stammering. hesitant speech.

stasis. stagnation of fluid such as blood.

stenosis. a narrowing or constriction.

sterile. free from microorganisms.

sterilization. the destruction by heat or chemicals of all forms of bacteria, spores, fungi and viruses.

sternum. the breastbone.

stertorous. noisy breathing.

stethoscope. an instrument used to transmit sounds, as the heart beat.

stomatitis. inflammation of the oral mucosa.

stopcock. a valve for stopping or regulating the flow of fluids or gases.

strain. the overstretching or overexertion of muscles; a group of organisms within a species or variety.

stressor. any factor which disturbs the body's equilibrium.

stricture. an abnormal narrowing of a passage or canal.

stroke volume output. the amount of blood ejected by the heart with each beat.

stupor. partial or nearly complete unconsciousness.

stuttering. spasmodic repetition of the same syllable when speaking.

subarachnoid space. the space beneath the arachnoid tissue.

subjective symptom. evidence of disease or bodily dysfunction which can be perceived only by the patient.

sublingual. situated under the tongue.

subscapular. situated below the scapula.

sulfanilamide. a drug used in infections.

superficial pain. pain arising from stimulation of receptors in the skin or mucous membranes.

supine. lying on the back.

suppression. the sudden stoppage of a secretion, excretion or normal discharge.

suppuration. the formation of pus.

supraoptic. pertaining to the area above the eye.

supraorbital. situated above the orbit of the eye.

surgery. that branch of medicine that treats diseases by operative procedures.

surgical asepsis. practices carried out to keep an area free of microorganisms.

suture. a surgical stitch.

sympathetic nervous system. the thoracolumbar branch of the autonomic nervous system.

symptom. evidence of a disease process or a disturbed body function.

synapse. juncture of nerve cells; to form a synapse.

syncope. a faint.

syndrome. a group of symptoms which commonly occur together.

synthesis. the process of putting together parts of a whole.

systolic blood pressure. the pressure of the blood in the arteries at the time of ventricular contraction.

tachycardia. an accelerated heart beat, with a pulse rate of over 100 per minute.

tachypnea. abnormal increase in the respiratory rate.

tenacious. adhesive.

tenesmus. ineffectual and painful straining at stool or urination.

terminal disinfection. measures taken to destroy pathogenic bacteria in an area that has been vacated by a patient with an infection.

tetany.   tonic spasm of the muscles.

thalamus.   part of the diencephalon of the brain; one of its functions is the relay of sensory impulses.

therapeutic environment.   an environment which helps a patient grow, learn and return to health.

therapy.   treatment that is remedial.

thoracentesis.   the insertion of a cannula into the pleural cavity.

thrombus.   a clot within a blood vessel which remains at the point of its formation.

thyroxin.   a hormone produced by the thyroid gland.

tidal volume.   the amount of air normally inhaled and exhaled.

tissue turgor.   the condition of normal tissue fullness and resilience.

tolerance.   the ability to endure without ill effect.

tonsillectomy.   surgical removal of the palatine tonsils.

tonus.   the slight continuous contraction of muscle.

topical.   pertaining to local external application.

tourniquet.   an instrument to compress blood vessels in order to control circulation.

toxin.   any poisonous substance of microbic, vegetable or animal origin.

trachea.   the windpipe; the tube extending from the larynx to the bronchi.

tracheotomy.   a surgical incision into the trachea.

traction.   the act of drawing, as in applying a force along the axis of a bone.

transition.   a period of change.

transudation.   the passage of serum or other fluid through a membrane.

transverse plane.   the plane which divides the body into superior and inferior sections.

trauma.   injury.

trocar.   a sharp-pointed instrument often used with a cannula.

troche.   lozenge.

tumor.   an abnormal mass of tissue that arises from cells of preexistent tissue and possesses no physiologic function.

ulcer.   a break in the skin or mucous membrane with loss of surface tissue.

ultrasound.   those sound waves which have a frequency above that heard by the human ear.

ultraviolet.   pertaining to rays whose wavelengths lie between those of the violet rays and the roentgen rays.

umbilicus.   the site of attachment of the umbilical cord in the fetus.

urban.   relating to or characteristic of a city.

urea.   the final nitrogenous product of the decomposition of protein. It is formed in the liver and carried by the blood to the kidneys, where it is excreted.

uremia.   a condition in which the urinary constituents are found in the blood.

ureter.   the tube that carries the urine from the kidney to the bladder.

urethra.   the canal that conveys the urine from the bladder to the body's surface.

urobilin.   a brownish pigment normally found in feces.

urticaria.   a temporary condition of raised edematous patches of skin or mucous membrane which are itchy.

uterus.   the muscular organ of the female reproductive tract in which the fetus grows and is nourished.

vagina.   the canal in the female reproductive system extending from the cervix to the vulva.

variable.   a condition which is subject to change and which is assigned a set of values during an experiment.

vasoconstriction.   a narrowing of the lumen of the blood vessels, particularly the arterioles.

vasodilation.   an increase in the size of the lumen of the blood vessels, particularly the arterioles.

vector.   an organism which transmits a pathogen.

ventral.   anterior; situated toward the front when in anatomical position.

ventricle.   a cavity, such as those of the brain or heart.

ventriculography.   x-ray examination of the ventricles of the brain after the insertion of a radiolucent medium.

vermin.   external animal parasites such as lice.

vertigo.   dizziness.

vesicant.   an irritant that is used to produce a blister upon the skin.

vestibule.   a space of cavity at the entrance to a canal.

virulence.   the degree of pathogenicity of a microorganism.

virus.   a submicroscopic pathogen.

viscera.   plural of viscus.

visceral pain.   pain arising from the viscera.

viscosity.   the quality of being sticky.

viscus.   any large interior organ such as the stomach.

vital capacity.   the amount of air which can be expired after an inspiration.

volatile.   tending to evaporate rapidly.

vomitus.   emesis; matter ejected from the stomach via the mouth.

xiphoid process.   the inferior part of the sternum.

x-rays.   the visualization of parts of the body by roentgen rays.

yeast.   a minute fungus, particularly *Saccharomyces cerevisiae.*

INDEX